AF738755

THE CARDIOVASCULAR SYSTEM – PHYSIOLOGY, DIAGNOSTICS AND CLINICAL IMPLICATIONS

Edited by **David C. Gaze**

The Cardiovascular System – Physiology, Diagnostics and Clinical Implications
Edited by David C. Gaze

Published by InTech
Janeza Trdine 9, 51000 Rijeka, Croatia

Copyright © 2012 InTech
All chapters are distributed under the Creative Commons Attribution 3.0 license, which allows users to download, copy and build upon published articles even for commercial purposes, as long as the author and publisher are properly credited, which ensures maximum dissemination and a wider impact of our publications. After this work has been published by InTech, authors have the right to republish it, in whole or part, in any publication of which they are the author, and to make other personal use of the work. Any republication, referencing or personal use of the work must explicitly identify the original source.

As for readers, this license allows users to download, copy and build upon published chapters even for commercial purposes, as long as the author and publisher are properly credited, which ensures maximum dissemination and a wider impact of our publications.

Notice
Statements and opinions expressed in the chapters are these of the individual contributors and not necessarily those of the editors or publisher. No responsibility is accepted for the accuracy of information contained in the published chapters. The publisher assumes no responsibility for any damage or injury to persons or property arising out of the use of any materials, instructions, methods or ideas contained in the book.

Publishing Process Manager Iva Simcic

Technical Editor Teodora Smiljanic

Cover Designer InTech Design Team

Additional hard copies can be obtained from orders@intechopen.com

The Cardiovascular System – Physiology, Diagnostics and Clinical Implications,
Edited by David C. Gaze
p. cm.
ISBN 978-953-51-0534-3

We are IntechOpen,
the world's leading publisher of
Open Access books
Built by scientists, for scientists

4,000+
Open access books available

116,000+
International authors and editors

120M+
Downloads

151
Countries delivered to

Our authors are among the
Top 1%
most cited scientists

12.2%
Contributors from top 500 universities

WEB OF SCIENCE™

Selection of our books indexed in the Book Citation Index
in Web of Science™ Core Collection (BKCI)

Interested in publishing with us?
Contact book.department@intechopen.com

Numbers displayed above are based on latest data collected.
For more information visit www.intechopen.com

For EU product safety concerns:
IN TECH d.o.o., Prolaz Marije Krucifikse Kozulić 3, 51000 Rijeka, Croatia,
info@intechopen.com or visit our website at intechopen.com.

Meet the editor

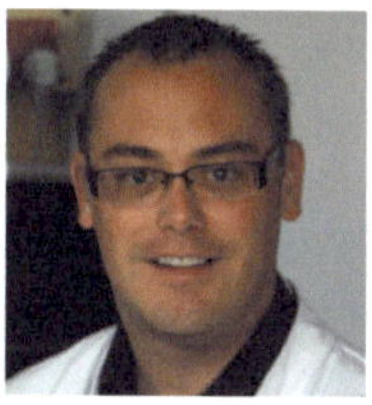

After undergraduate and postgraduate study in the North of England and London respectively, David Gaze works as a Research Biochemist in Clinical Blood Sciences at St George's Hospital and Medical School, London. His area of research interest is the development and clinical utility of cardiovascular biomarkers for assessment of patients with cardiovascular disease and cardiorenal disease. He has authored and co authored over 115 peer reviewed original papers, editorials and reviews, 145 conference proceedings and has authored two book chapters and a textbook on cardiac troponin. He has delivered over 25 invited international presentations. He received two NACB distinguished abstracts awards (2006/2008) and a diploma for oral presentation from the 17th IFCC–FESCC European Congress of Clinical Chemistry and Laboratory Medicine. He is a member of the American Association of Clinical Biochemistry; Member of the Association for Biochemistry; Associate member of the Royal Institute; Member of the Institute of Biomedical Sciences; Fellow of the Royal Society of Medicine and a member of the Pathological Society of Great Britain.

Contents

Preface

The cardiovascular system includes the heart located centrally in the thorax and the vessels of the body which carry blood. The cardiovascular (or circulatory) system supplies oxygen from inspired air, via the lungs to the tissues around the body. It is also responsible for the removal of the waste product, carbon dioxide via air expired from the lungs. The cardiovascular system also transports nutrients such as electrolytes, amino acids, enzymes, hormones which are integral to cellular respiration, metabolism and immunity.

This book is not meant to be an all encompassing text on cardiovascular physiology and pathology rather a selection of chapters from experts in the field who describe recent advances in basic and clinical sciences. As such, the text is divided into three main sections:

1. *Cardiovascular Physiology* – In this section, the control of the cardiovascular system is discussed in particular the heaemodynamic mechanisms controlling blood volume, flow and the regulation of systolic blood pressure. The next chapter investigates the molecular control of smooth muscle cell (SMC) differentiation marker genes by serum response factor (SRF) including the interaction of myocardin as a potent cofactor of SRF in SMC differentiation. The chapter also details the interaction of GATA-6, Klf4, LIM-only proteins CRP1 and 2 and PIAS-1 with SRF. The following chapter reports on trans fatty acids (TFA) and human health, detailing the biochemistry of trans fats as well as recommended daily intake. The chapter describes both animal and human studies of TFA. There are details on the analytical determination of TFA as well as their potential antioxidants. There is also a comprehensive overview of TFA and legislative control in food production and consumption. This is followed by a chapter on the control and coordination of vasomotor tone in the microcirculation; concentrating on the cellular membrane potential and potassium channels, the role of prostaglandins, nitric oxide and endothelium-derived hyperpolarizing factor as paracrine signalling in the wall of the vessel. There is also detail of the role of gap junctions in vascular smooth muscle and endothelium communication processes. The following chapter discusses the concept of hemodynamics, detailing the relationship between physical factors and the effect on blood flow through the vessel in laminar or turbulent flow patterns. The principles of

velocity, elasticity and compliance are described. Furthermore the clinical implications such as alteration to blood flow during atherosclerosis and arteriosclerosis are described. The penultimate chapter of this section describes the adenosinergic system in the mesenteric vessels which form the splanchnic circulation. The chapter details the role of adenosine from its production to tissue concentration controlled by nucleoside transporter membrane proteins, namely equilibrative and concentrative nucleoside transporters. The family member subtypes are of these transporter proteins are described thoroughly. The final chapter of section one concentrates on endothelial nitric oxide synthase (eNOS), nitric oxide (NO) and subsequent metabolic disturbances within the vascular system. An overview of vascular dysfunction is given along with the biochemistry of eNOS/NO. The endogenous eNOS and NO inhibitor asymmetric dimethylarginine and its role in the vascular system is also reviewed. The reader is also given the importance of lifestyle on the vascular system, concentrating on dietary habits and physical activity on the eNOS/NO system.

2. *Cardiovascular Diagnostics* – Section 2 is concerned with modalities used in the diagnosis and monitoring of parameters associated with the cardiovascular system. The first chapter entitled 'the diagnostic performance of cardiovascular system and evaluation of hemodynamic parameters based on heart cycle phase analysis describes the development and use of the electrocardiogram (ECG) and the rheogram. Furthermore the use of both the ECG and rheogram to assess cardiovascular function in normal and diseased states are described. The second chapter describes the biophysical phenomena of blood flow during indirect arterial pressure measurement. The role of the oscillogram in measuring systolic and diastolic arterial pressure is well described compared to the practice of auscultation of Korotkov sounds. The chapter also notes the peculiarities seen in some oscillogram readings. The third chapter describes the interrelation between changes of phase function of cardiac muscle concentration and the biochemical processes as an algorithm for identifying pathological processes within the cardiovascular system. In this chapter the authors outline their vision of the main biochemical processes determining the clinical meaning of the pathology diagnosed with the aid of the cardiac cycle analysis method. Selection of the therapeutic agents aimed at normalization of the diagnosed functional deviations taking into account the biochemical processes underlying these functions resulted in the recovery of the functions. The next chapter investigates computational intelligence techniques in cardiovascular diagnostics. Continual monitoring of cardiac function in the acute care setting can allow the detection of cardiac arrhythmias. Continuous wavelet transform and principal component analysis are described in detail. The application of these techniques within a multi-layer perceptron neural network is demonstrated. The final chapter of this section analyses the time course changes in the cardiovascular response to head-up tilt in fighter pilots. In this interesting chapter the authors describe the physiological adaptations that occur following frequent exposure to G-force acceleration. By

measuring mean arterial pressure, heart rate, stroke volume and total peripheral resistance, the authors compare the cardiovascular responses in fighter pilots compared to non-pilots.

3. ***Clinical Impact of Cardiovascular Physiology and Pathophysiology*** – The final section of this textbook relates physiology to pathophysiology, clinical presentation and implications of cardiovascular diseases. The first chapter of this section explores the relationship of cardiovascular health and exercise from both the European and North American perspectives, detailing the relationship between physical activity and life expectancy and discusses the pro-inflammatory state in relation to reduced physical activity and its relationship to cardiovascular disease. The second chapter reviews the global burden of cardiovascular disease and the associated risk factors, including lipid components, inflammatory markers, fibrinogen, smoking and dietary modification to reduce the incidence of cardiac disease. The next chapter details the associations between cardiac and cerebral vascular issues in patients with neurodegenerative diseases such as Alzheimer's disease. Risk factors such as hyperlipidemia, hypertension, diabetes and a history of smoking contribute to deterioration of cognitive function. A reduction of cerebral perfusion following ventricular dysfunction can also contribute to the advancement of cognitive decline. The 'French Paradox' of a low incidence of cardiovascular disease in people who consumed moderate red wine irrespective of the quantity of saturated fatty acids and describes the cardioprotective role of polyphenolic compounds is discussed in the next chapter. The fifth chapter in section 3 discusses the clinical implications of dermatological findings in patients who develop infective endocarditis, in particular the causative microorganisms, risk factors, the clinical signs and symptoms, and the clinical tools to aid diagnosis. The next chapter details the cardiovascular risk factors associated with the development of diabetes mellitus and the role of herbal drugs to control cardiac risk factors. The next chapter reviews the morphology and functional changes of the intestine in patients with heart failure identifying the systemic nature of heart failure. A comprehensive overview of the histological patterns observed and the pro inflammatory state of the gastrointestinal tract is presented. Chapter 20 describes the evaluation and treatment of hypotensive premature infants which is a common phenomenon in the first few weeks of life; describing the interplay between hypovolaemia, tissue hypoxia and myocardial dysfunction. The clinical presentation is described along with diagnostic modalities used to detect hypotensive cardiac problems, followed by the treatment regimens available to correct to the normotensive state. The next interesting chapter discusses the role of echocardiography in Sub-Saharan Africa. Access to echocardiography is common place in the developed world. In the remoteness of Africa, access to such diagnostic tests are rarely available due to cost, logistical access and the lack of trained sonographers. This chapter reviews the current usage of echocardiography to describe the epidemiology of cardiovascular disease in an otherwise neglected population. The final chapter to

this section and the whole book describes a study of cardiovascular functional parameters such as heart rate and blood pressure along with a psychophysiological assessment in females displaying defensive hostility demonstrating such women have higher heart rates and blood pressures if they were defensive compared to those with low hostility.

David C. Gaze
Dept of Chemical Pathology Clinical Blood Sciences,
St George's Healthcare NHS Trust, London
United Kingdom

Acknowledgements

I would like to acknowledge the tremendous efforts of the contributing authors to these chapters, especially when writing in English rather than their native tongue. I would also like to thank Ms Iva Simcic of InTECH publishers for keeping the production of this book active and to for steering me to complete the editorial review by the appropriate deadlines.

Section 1

Cardiovascular Physiology

1

Control of Cardiovascular System

Mikhail Rudenko, Olga Voronova, Vladimir Zernov,
Konstantin Mamberger, Dmitry Makedonsky,
Sergey Rudenko and Sergey Kolmakov
Russian New University,
Russia

1. Introduction

The main method of cognition of the performance of biological systems is their mathematical modeling. The essence of this method should reflect the principle of optimization in biology[9]. Any biosystem cannot function if its energy consumption is inadequately high.

The same is applicable to the blood circulatory system. Its main function is to transport blood throughout the body in order to maintain the proper gaseous exchange, deliver important substances to viscera and tissues in living body and remove decay products. It is impossible to study this function without due consideration of hemodynamic features. But how is the blood circulation provided? It is a question of principle, and so far no unambiguous answer has been given thereto.

The conventional interpretation of blood circulation is that blood flows through blood vessels under laminar flow conditions to which Poiseuille's law is applicable. But it is a matter of fact that this conventional interpretation concept is inadequate because it is not in compliance with the above principle of optimization in biology, according to which all processes in bio systems show their best performance, i.e., their highest efficiency. It is just the compliance with this principle that is the major criterion to be used for evaluation of adequacy of any theoretical models describing various systems in living body and their interactions both with each other and their external environment.

Significant progress in understanding of such phenomena is made after G. Poyedintsev and O.Voronova discovered the so called mode of elevated fluidity, i.e., the third flow conditions that show lesser losses of energy to overcome friction and that is noted for lesser friction losses and specific pattern of the flow[4].

It has been proved that the blood flow through the blood vessels is provided in "the third" flow mode that is the most efficient and therefore fully in compliance with the said principle of optimization.

The theory of the third mode is a foundation for the development of new mathematical models describing the performance of the blood circulation system. In addition, new methods of quantitative determination of a number of hemodynamic parameters and qualitative evaluation of some processes occurring in the system have been elaborated. The application of these methods in practice allows filling a lot of gaps in theoretical cardiology and creates at the same time a system of analysis of the functions of the cardiovascular system taking into account the relevant cause-effect relationship.

The detailed description of this theory is given in our book "Theoretical Principles of Heart Cycle Phase Analysis"[3]. Our intention is to outline herein the general principles of the performance of the cardiovascular system only.

2. Biophysical processes of formation of hemodynamic mechanism

2.1 Special features of hemodynamics and its regulation. Hemodynamic volumetric parameters

There two types of liquid flow conditions described in the classical fluid mechanics: the first type is the laminar flow, and the second one is the turbulent flow mode. In the 80th last century, a new theory of a specific liquid flow mode was developed by G.M. Poyedinstev and O.K. Voronova that was defined by them as the "elevated fluidity mode"[4]. Another name "the third flow mode" was given by the above discoverers to differ it from the two other modes well-known before. Being experts in solving technical problems of fluid mechanics, the authors succeeded in modeling the above elevated fluidity mode in a rigid pipe. For this purpose, hydraulic pulsators of specific design were used. It was established that the energy used to transport liquid in the third flow mode is several times less than it is the case under the laminar flow conditions[3]. Moreover, an efficiency of this process could be considerably increased when liquid is pumped under certain conditions through an elastic piping. The subsequent researches demonstrated that the physical processes producing the elevated fluidity mode and those in the blood circulation are identical. The mathematical tools used to describe "the third" flow mode was applied to describe the hemodynamic processes.

It was established by the authors that there are processes which are always observed in a rigid pipe at the initiation of a liquid flow from a quiescent state, as mentioned below. Whilst particles of liquid are starting their moving in the rigid pipe due to a difference in the static pressure, there a set of concentric waves of friction in the boundary layer is generating, the front of propagation of which is directed towards the pipe axis[3] (Fig. 1). Amplitudes of these waves depend on the diameter of the pipe, acoustic velocity in liquid and an initial difference in pressures at the pipe ends. The length of these traveling waves during this complex process continuously increases. The waves travel towards the axis of the pipe and degenerate. Finally, there a single wave remains only close to the pipe wall, the profile of which becomes parabolic that is typical for the laminar flow (s. Fig. 2 herein).

It should be noted that it is just within this short period of time, i.e., starting from the moment of the motion initiation from a quiescent state till the moment of formation of the laminar flow (s. positions E and F in Fig. 2 herein), when liquid flows in its optimum mode of elevated fluidity, considering it from the point of view of energy consumption (s. positions A, B, C, D in Fig 2 herein). The energy consumption under the laminar flow conditions to transport liquid in the pipe is significantly higher due to increase in the flow resistance.

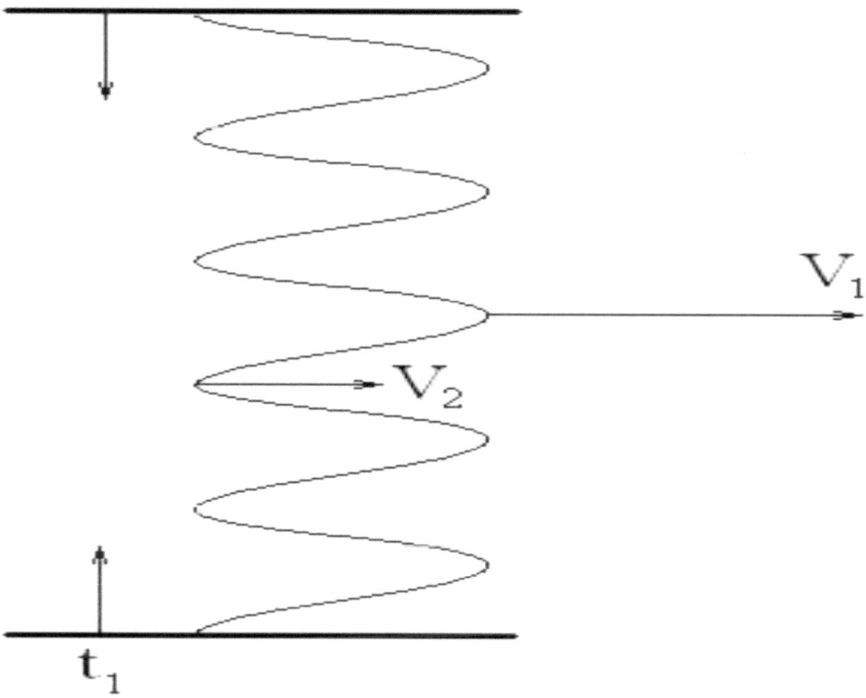

Fig. 1. Formation of concentric waves of friction at initiation of flow in a pipe (according to G.M. Poyedintsev and O.K.Voronova); t_1 - moment of pressure difference formation; V_1 - velocity of plasma in stagnated layers; V_2 – velocity of blood elements in accelerated layers

There is another phenomenon typical for the "third" flow mode. If liquid contains suspended particles similar to those in blood, during the development of the above mentioned wave process the particles are concentrated at the wave maxima, and the particle-free liquid is delivered to their minima, correspondingly[3]. When the liquid, patterned in such a way, flows along the pipe axis, the velocity of the concentric particle-loaded layers is twice what the liquid pattern-free layers reach. Vectors of velocity are parallel to the axis of the flow. And it is just a prerequisite to elevated fluidity of liquid with reduced friction between the liquid layers and the pipe wall. Figure 2 herein shows the locations of erythrocytes in the blood flow referring to each flow formation stage as mentioned above. At the beginning of the formation of the "third" flow mode, there ring-shaped alternating layers of the blood elements and plasma are available, while in the laminar mode all elements are accumulated in the center of the flow. In this case they are located very close to each other forming a thick mass. This process may result in an aggregation of erythrocytes and hemolysis. In order to avoid such pathological consequences, it is a must to manage the blood transportation in the "third" mode of flow, avoiding its transformation into a laminar one.

The theory gives a clue that it can be obtained when transporting liquid in a pulsating mode through an elastic pipe. According to this theory, the pipe clear width and the liquid flow velocity should be changed with every impulse under certain laws[3]. The laws of increasing in the pipe clear width and decreasing in the flow velocity with every impulse take the form as follows[4].

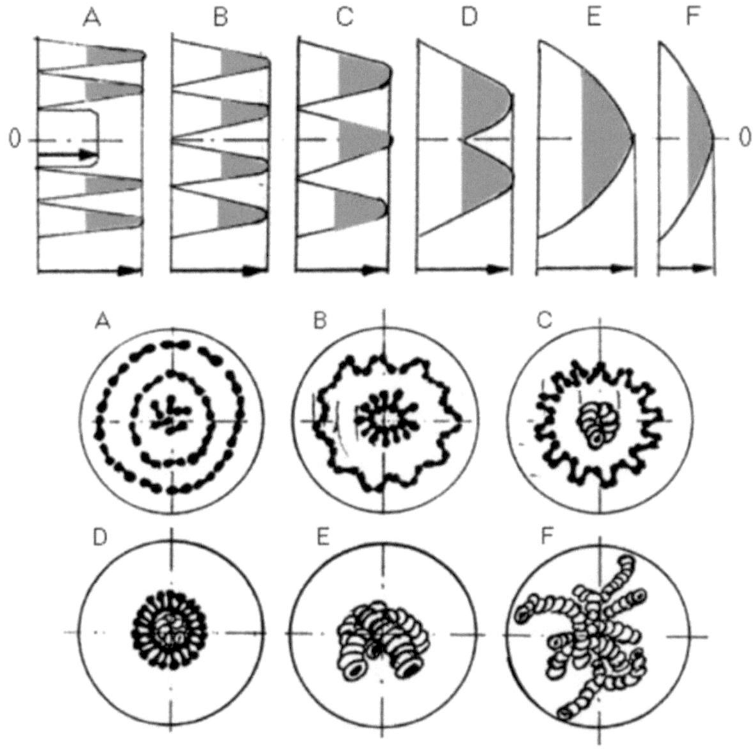

Fig. 2. Formation of two-phase pattern at the initiation of the flow from a quiescent state (according to G.M. Poyedintsev and O.K. Voronova), A-F – flow structure in corresponding sections

$$r_t = r_0 \left(\frac{t}{t_0} \right)^{1/5} \tag{1}$$

$$W_t = W_0 \left(\frac{t_0}{t} \right)^{2/5} \tag{2}$$

where r_t - current radius of the pipe increasing;

r_0 – initial radius (at $t = t_0$);

t - current time ($t \geq t_0$);

t_0 – time of acceleration of flow velocity up to maximum velocity in an impulse;

W_t - current value of liquid flow velocity;

W_0 - maximum value of velocity in an impulse (at $t = t_0$).

It is proved by the authors of this theory that the above conditions are met in the blood circulation system.

This is provided by changing in the clear width of blood vessels in every cardiac cycle and arterial pressure pulsating. The shape of the arterial pressure wave is given herein in Fig. 3 below.

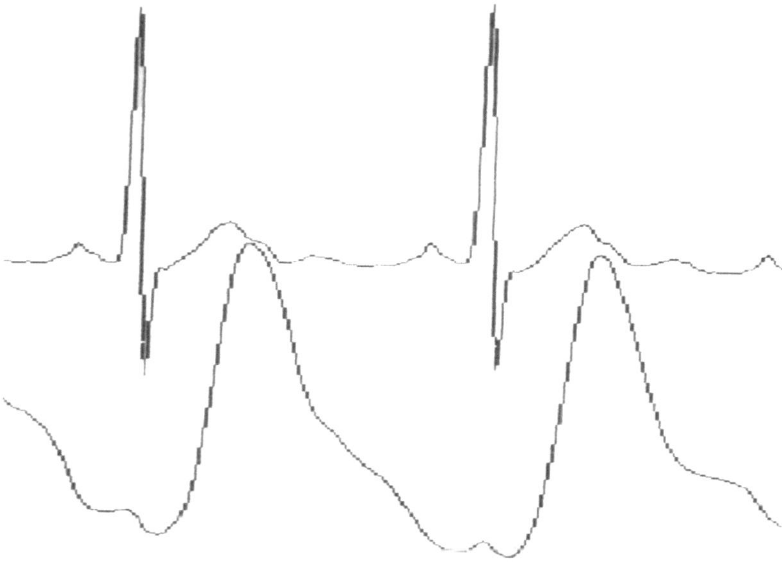

Fig. 3. Arterial pressure wave shape reography-recorded. ECG recorded simultaneously with Rheogram.

The foundation of hemodynamics is the phase mode of the heart performance. In one beat the heart changes its shape ten times that corresponds to the heart cycle phases[4].

The most efficient way is to evaluate the status of hemodynamics not only by values of integral parameters, i.e., stroke and minute volumes, but also phase-related volumes of blood entering or leaving the heart in the respective phase in a cardiac cycle.

So, the final formulae for calculation the volumes of blood in the phase of rapid and slow ejection, symbolized as PV3 and PV4, respectively, are as follows:

$$PV3=S\cdot(QR+RS)^2\cdot f_1(\alpha)\cdot[f_2(\alpha)+f_3(\alpha,\beta,\gamma,\delta)] \quad (ml); \qquad (3)$$

$$PV4=S\cdot(QR+RS)^2\cdot f_1(\alpha)\cdot f_4(\alpha,\beta,\gamma,\delta) \quad (ml), \qquad (4)$$

where S - cross-section of ascending aorta;
QR – phase duration according to ECG curve;
RS – phase duration according to ECG curve;

$$f_1(\alpha)=\frac{22072{,}5[(5\alpha-2)^3-27]}{(5\alpha-2)^5-243};$$

$$f_2(\alpha)=\frac{\alpha^5-1}{2};$$

$$f3(\alpha,\beta,\gamma,\delta)=\frac{1}{8}[\frac{10}{3}(4\alpha^2-\delta^2)(\beta^3-\alpha^3)+5\chi\delta(\beta^4-\alpha^4)-2\chi^2(\beta^5-\alpha^5)];$$

$$f_4(\alpha,\beta,\gamma,\delta)=\frac{1}{8}[5(\delta^2-\frac{8}{3}\alpha^2)(\beta^3-\alpha^3)+7{,}5\chi\delta(\beta^4-\alpha^4)+3\chi^2(\beta^5-\alpha^5)];$$

$$\alpha=(1+\frac{Em}{QR+RS})^{0,2};$$

$$\beta=(1+\frac{Em+Er}{QR+RS})^{0,2};$$

$$\chi=\frac{2(\alpha-1)}{\beta-\alpha};$$

$$\delta=\alpha(2+\chi).$$

Stroke volume SV is calculated by an equation as given below:

$$SV = PV3+ PV4=S\cdot(QR+RS)^2\cdot f_1(\alpha)\cdot[f_2(\alpha)+f_3(\alpha,\beta,\gamma,\delta)+f_4(\alpha,\beta,\gamma,\delta)] \quad (ml) \quad (5)$$

The minute stroke is computed as follows:

$$MV = SV\cdot HR \quad (l/min) \quad (6)$$

In similar way calculated are other phase-related volumes of blood as listed below:

PV1 - volume of blood entering the ventricle in premature diastole;
PV2 - volume of blood entering the ventricle in atrial systole;
PV5 - volume of blood pumped by ascending aorta as peristaltic pump.

So, the main parameters in hemodynamics are 7 volumes of blood entering or leaving the heart in different heart cycle phases. They are as follows: stroke volume SV, minute volume MV, two diastolic phase-related volumes PV1 and PV2, two systolic phase-related volumes PV3 and PV4, and PV5 as volume of blood pumped by the aorta.

The authors of this theory in their researches utilized relative phase volumes denoted by RV. Each relative phase volume is that expressed as a percentage of stroke volume SV. These relative parameters demonstrate contributions of each phase process to the formation of the stroke volume in general.

The above hemodynamic parameters should be used mainly in order to evaluate eventual deviations from their normal values, if any. The limits of normal values of hemodynamic parameters are not conditional, and they have their respective calculated values.

With respect to the normal values (the required parameters) in hemodynamics, they have been taken on the basis of the known data on ECG waves, intervals and segments for adults from the literature sources as given below:

1. The upper and lower limit of the QRS complex values:

$QRS_{max} = 0.1$ s. ; $QRS_{min} = 0.08$ s.

2. The upper and lower limit of the RS complex values:
   $RS_{max} = 0.05$ s. ; $RS_{min} = 0.035$ s.
3. The normal value of interval QT in every specific cardiac cycle is determined from the Bazett formula as follows:

$$QT = 0.37\ RR^{0.5}\text{, s (male);} \tag{7}$$

$$QT = 0.4\ RR^{0.5}\text{, s (female).} \tag{8}$$

4. Normal value $PQ_{cer.}$ is calculated from a formula as indicated below:

$$PQ_{cer.} = 1 / (10^{-6}\ 638{,}44\ HR^2 + 9{,}0787)\text{ s} \tag{9}$$

This equation has been produced according to the method of approximation of normal values $PQ_{cer.}$, as known from the sources, considering their dependence on heart rate (HR).

These values are used as initial values for calculations of an individual range of normal values of volumetric parameters in hemodynamics considering individual patient cases. In practice, for a better visualization of the data, it should be recommended to present them not only numerically but also graphically, as bar charts, as shown in Figure 4 herein. In the latter case, it is convenient to indicate the deviations from the normal value limits of the actually calculated values of hemodynamic parameters as percentage.

For example. On Figure 4 a), b), c) the result of hemodynamic parameters PV2 measuring - volume of blood entering the ventricle in atrial systole- is displayed as follows. Figure 4 a) in column "Blood volumes" shows the result of measuring 18,31 (ml). The second column "% of stroke volume" shows the deviation from the norm. It is 0% here. For quick associative perception of both these values and rapid highlighting of going beyond the bounds of norm parameter, there exists a dark green field with red light indicator to the right of this number in the column "indicators of measurement results". On the left and right sides of the dark green field we see the values of individual range of this hemodynamic parameter, calculated using equation 7, 8, 9. In this case, it is from 15.26 to 35,13 ml. Measured parameter of 18,31 ml is in the middle of the range, which corresponds to the 0% deviation from the norm. And the red light indicator that corresponds to this value is on the dark green background. Light green field - is a bound of "norm - pathology". Sides of this field correspond to excess or deficiency of more than 30% of norm. More than 30% excess requires special attention to the patient. As a rule, such patients needs hospital care. Figure 4 b) shows another patient's result, PV2 = 12,85 ml, and this result goes 15.84% beyond patient's individual norm 15,26 ... 35.13 ml. In this case red light indicates lack of blood volume, rather than redundancy. Lower (upper) than 30% value, but lower (upper) than normal value corridor, denotes further out-patient treatment for this patient. Fig. 4 c) shows a third patient with PV2 = 47,00 ml value, which goes 76.91% beyond his individual norm 10,72 ... 26.13 ml. Red light indicates the redundancy of blood volume. This patient should be examined by cardiac cycle phase analysis to identify the root causes of the disease. It's possible to identify these causes using ECG and RHEO for phase compensation mechanism of the cardio-vascular system determination.

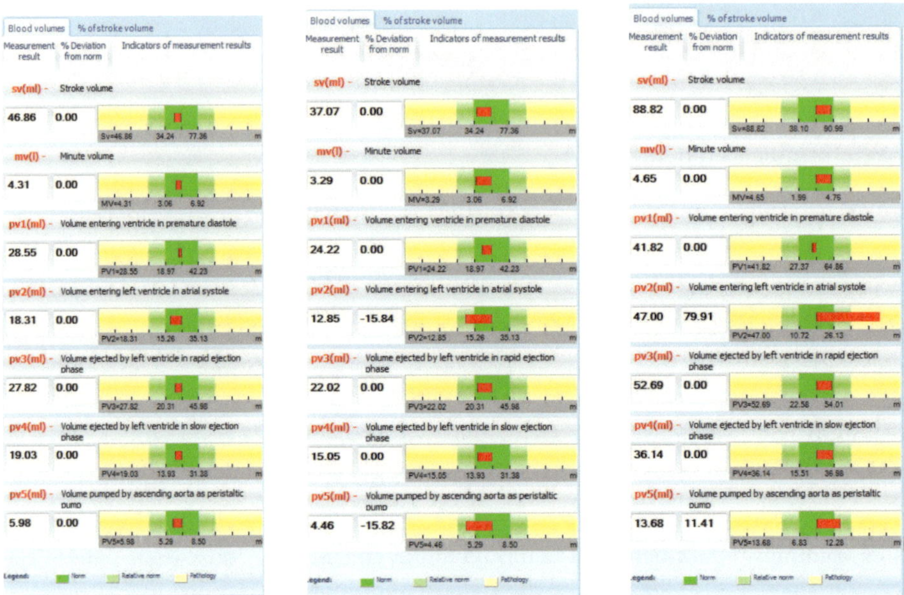
Blood volumes
% of stroke volume
Measurement result
% Deviation from norm
Indicators of measurement results
sv(ml) - Stroke volume
46.86 0.00
mv(l) - Minute volume
4.31 0.00
pv1(ml) - Volume entering ventricle in premature diastole
28.55 0.00
pv2(ml) - Volume entering left ventricle in atrial systole
18.31 0.00
pv3(ml) - Volume ejected by left ventricle in rapid ejection phase
27.82 0.00
pv4(ml) - Volume ejected by left ventricle in slow ejection phase
19.03 0.00
pv5(ml) - Volume pumped by ascending aorta as peristaltic pump
5.98 0.00
37.07 0.00
3.29 0.00
24.22 0.00
12.85 -15.84
22.02 0.00
15.05 0.00
4.46 -15.82
88.82 0.00
4.65 0.00
41.82 0.00
47.00 79.91
52.69 0.00
36.14 0.00
13.68 11.41

a) b) c)

Fig. 4. Displayed measured phase-related values and their qualitative representation as bar charts, with reference to normal values. This figure gives three different measuring cases

The values of phase-related blood volumes are influenced by the mechanism of compensation existing in the cardiovascular system[6]. This mechanism is responsible for the maintenance of the hemodynamic parameters within their respective norms. If any parameter goes far beyond its norm, it means that it is an indication of physiological problems of the respective phase process. In this case, the function in the next phase compensates for the changes in the functioning of the problematic phase[6]. It is the just the case with sportsmen whose cardiovascular system shows the proper performance.

Physical exercise may cause a deficiency in diastolic volumes of blood by more than 500 %.[4] Under the circumstances, the systolic phases undertake to compensate for the above deficiency. For this purpose, the mechanisms may be involved, the manifestations of which cannot be found even in a pathology case. Upon stress relieving, 1 minute later, all phase-related volumes are normalized again. This kind of the performance of the cardiovascular system hinders an identification of the cause of pathology at early stages for those who are not professional athletes.

As a rule, deviations due to pathology exceed the norm by more than 30 %. Patients, who receive their treatment at cardiology hospital, show sometimes deviations of 50 % and over. The only way to find the primary cause of any pathology, based on the manifestation of the compensation mechanism, can be a thorough analysis of the actual cause-relationship in every individual case.

The phase-related volumetric parameters in hemodynamics are the most informative characteristics of the performance of the cardiovascular system since they are capable of reflecting the coordinated operation of the heart and the associated blood vessels. Knowing their ratios and considering the actual anatomic and functional status of the heart and the blood vessels in every phase, we can produce very reliably a diagnosis of the actual status of the blood circulation system, reveal pathology and control the efficiency of therapy, if required.

The above mentioned evidence is really of fundamental importance. It should be taken into account when making diagnosis.

2.2 Mechanism of regulation of systolic pressure

The above mentioned main volumetric parameters should be complemented by another one: it is arterial pressure (AP). The cardiovascular system has its own mechanism to provide separate regulation of the systolic and diastolic pressures (AP)[8]. A narrowing in sectional areas of the blood vessels in total leads to a displacement of a certain volume of blood that is symbolized by ΔV. The displacement volume enters the ventricles in premature diastole phase T - P. During myocardium contraction phase R - S, the same volume is displaced via the closed aortic valve into the aorta. Actually, before the ejection of stroke volume SV into aorta, the total of displacement volume ΔV enters the aorta. Therefore, it is that the R - S phase, when ΔV can be ejected into the aorta, is preceded by that phase when the motion of the entire mass of blood is actuated, and this preceding phase is the Q - R interval, when the contraction of the septum occurs. It is just the phase when the blood flow becomes its directed vortex motion within the ventricle. Displacement volume ΔV contributes to moving against the total increased resistance of the blood vessels in the next phase which shows rapid blood ejection.

The blood circulation scheme is shown in Figure 5 herein. The anatomy of the heart is designed in such a way so that the displacement blood can penetrate without hindrance through the closed arteric valve into the aorta. It is determined not only by the configuration of the valves but also the mechanism of the contraction of the heart chambers that consists of three phases. Phase one among them is the contraction of the septum. Phase two provides for the contraction of the ventricle walls. Phase three is the phase of tension. The processes occurring therein are responsible for spinning the blood flows so that the penetration of the displacement blood through the closed valves into the aorta is assisted. Under normal conditions, when there is no displacement volume ΔV available, and, as a consequence, no penetration is required, upon completion of the phase of tension, stroke volume SV residing in the heart is supplied into the aorta. In this case, volume SV added to the volume of blood residing in the aorta creates the systolic pressure that produces a difference in pressures between the aorta and the periphery. Such mechanism required to overcome an increased blood flow resistance operates cyclically till the cause of blood vessel constriction disappears. The processes described above are typical for the mechanism of regulation of the diastolic arterial pressure. Various Rheogram curve shapes reflect this mechanism.

The anatomy design of the heart is determined by the phase mechanism of hemodynamics, i.e., the mechanism of the regulation of the diastolic pressure. This mechanism is responsible for elimination of general vasoconstriction difficulties in blood circulation. Causes of the said vasoconstriction cannot be diagnostically identified in this case.

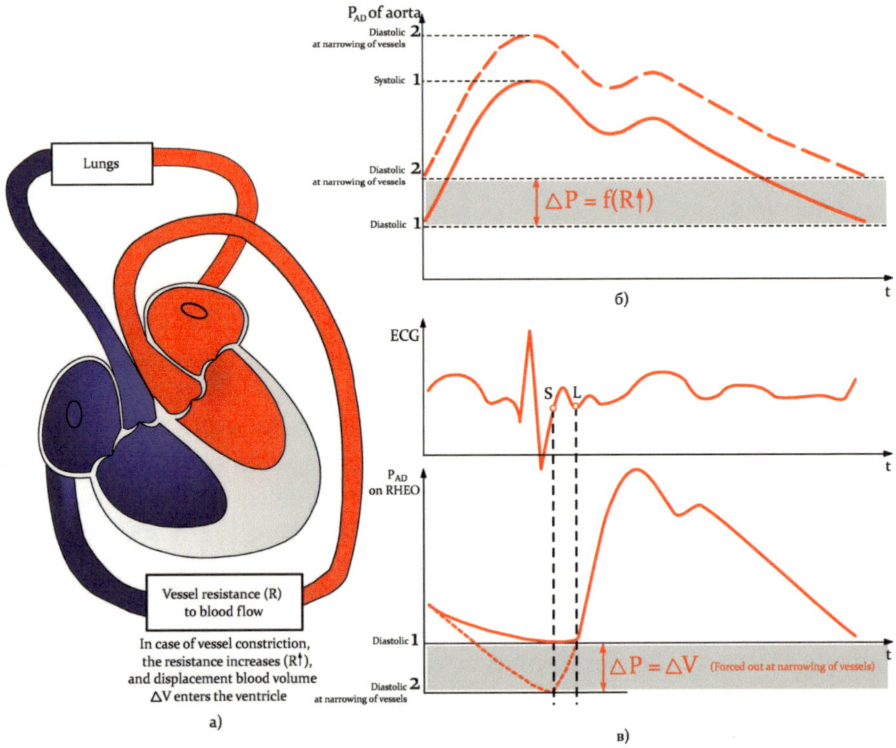

Fig. 5. a) Blood circulation scheme considering changes in blood vessel resistance. b) AP changes in aorta; c) Changes in AP identifiable on Rheo curve in phase of tension S-L, in proportion to displacement volume ΔV in blood vessel constriction

With synchronous recording of an ECG and a Rheo from the ascending aorta, provided that they are synchronized at wave point S on the ECG curve, the process of the regulation of diastolic pressure may manifest itself as an early AP rise on the respective Rheo curve in phases R - S and S - L.

2.3 Mechanism of regulation of systolic pressure

The mechanism of regulation of the systolic pressure differs significantly from that responsible for the regulation of the diastolic pressure. It has the function to provide a pre-requisite to the blood circulation in the blood vessels due to a difference in pressures between the aorta and veins and manage the transportation of an oxygen quantity as required by tissues and cells. For these purposes, several biophysical processes are engaged.

First and foremost, we should mention the process of myocardium contraction in tension phase S - L. The tension created in this phase presets the velocity of the blood flow during the blood ejection phase. Therefore, the initial velocity of the blood flow in the aorta depends on the degree of the myocardium tension.

The second important process is the phenomenon of an increase in the systolic pressure during the propagation of the AP wave throughout the arteries[1]. The systolic pressure in the aorta and that in the brachial artery may considerably differ from each other. On the normal conditions, the pressure increase is provided by the pumping function of the blood vessels and their increasing resistance.

An additional point to emphasize is that there is another biophysical phenomenon connected with hemodynamics. It is cavitation in blood that promotes blood volume expansion[2]. It may spread over very quickly within one heart cycle and is capable of considerably expanding the blood volume.

The cause of the systolic pressure buildup is a reduction in blood supply of some viscera. The pressure buildup is aimed at elimination of hindrances in blood supply in order to maintain the proper blood circulation. The blood supply mechanism of some viscera provides for protection from arterial overpressures. In the first place, the protection of the cerebral blood supply system should be mentioned. The cerebral blood vessels are anatomically connected with veins. During an increase in AP, the venous drainage is hindered, affecting the blood vessel constriction and limiting in such a way an excessive AP increase.

If for some reason a viscus is not sufficiently supplied with blood, it leads to a systolic AP growth. The venous drainage will be hindered. The first symptoms of this problem could be edema of legs. To solve this problem, required should be elimination of the cause of the improper blood supply to the affected viscus that should decrease the AP and, subsequently, normalize the venous drainage.

3. Phase structure of heart cycle according to ECG curve

Every heart cycle consists of 10 phases. Each phase undertakes its own functions[7].

The complete phase structure of an ECG is shown in Figure 6 herein.

Phase of atrial systole $P_H - P_K$;
Phase of closing of atrioventricular valve $P_K - Q$;
Phase of contraction of septum $Q - R$;
Phase of contraction of ventricle walls $R - S$;
Phase of tension of myocardium $S - L$;
Phase of rapid ejection $L - j$;
Phase of slow ejection $j - T_H$;
Phase of buildup of maximum systolic pressure in aorta $T_H - T_K$;
Phase of closing of aortic valve $T_K - U_H$;
Phase of premature diastole of ventricles $U_H - P_H$.

Each phase serves its purpose. But the phases may be grouped in a manner as follows:

Group of diastol4ic phases which are responsible for blood supply to the ventricles:

Phase of premature diastole of ventricles $U_H - P_H$;
Phase of atrial systole $P_H - P_K$;
Phase of closing of atrioventricular valve $P_K - Q$.

The phase of premature diastole contains a period of time equal to the duration of wave U which reflects an intensive filling of the coronary vessels with blood. It occurs in synchronism with filling of the ventricles.

The diastolic phases are described as hemodynamic values PV1 and PV2.

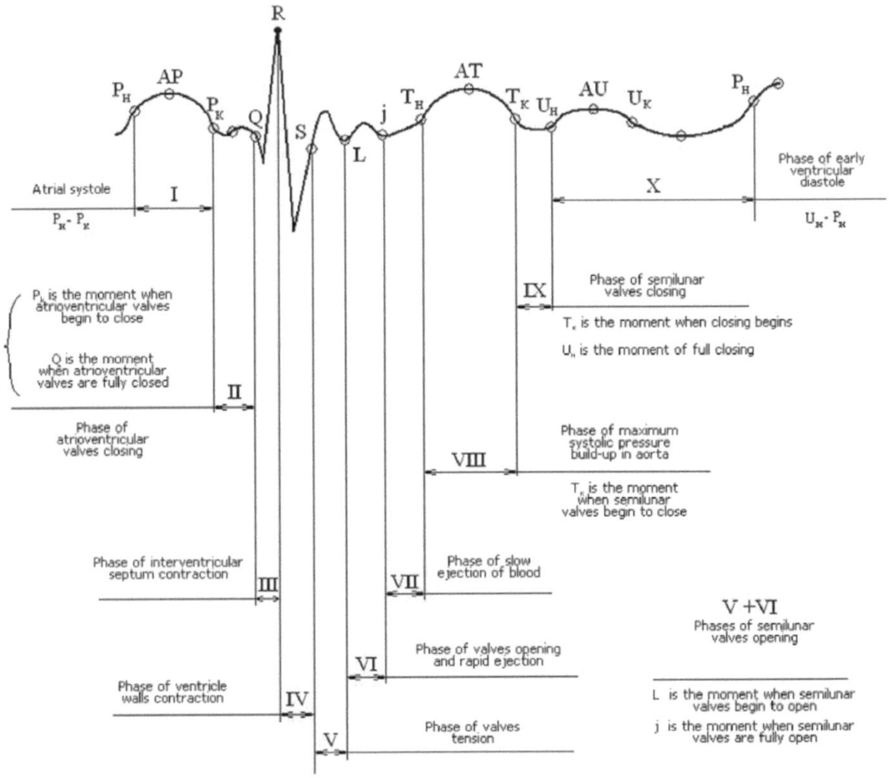

Fig. 6. Phase structure of ECG recorded from ascending aorta; Phase of atrial systole P_H - P_K; Phase of closing of atrioventricular valve P_K - Q; Phase of contraction of septum Q - R; Phase of contraction of ventricle walls R - S; Phase of tension of myocardium S - L; Phase of rapid ejection L - j; Phase of slow ejection j - T_H; Phase of buildup of maximum systolic pressure in aorta T_H - T_K; Phase of closing of aortic valve T_K - U_H; Phase of premature diastole of ventricles U_H - P_H

Group of systolic phases which provide for the conditions for the proper blood circulation. They can be divided into subgroups undertaking certain functions as given below:

Subgroup responsible for diastolic AP regulation:

Phase of contraction of septum Q - R;
Phase of contraction of ventricle walls R - S;
Phase of tension of myocardium S - L (partially).

Subgroup responsible for systolic AP regulation:

Phase of tension of myocardium S - L,
Phase of rapid ejection L - j.

Subgroup responsible for aorta pumping function control:

Phase of slow ejection j - T_H;
Phase of buildup of maximum systolic pressure in aorta T_H - T_K;

Phase of closing of aortic valve T_K - U_H;

The given systolic phases are characterized by hemodynamic values PV3, PV4 and SV.

Hemodynamic value MV is an indication of a blood flow rate.

Hemodynamic parameter PV5 shows what share of blood is pumped by the aorta operating as a peristaltic pump during the ejection of blood from the ventricles.

It should be noted that phase of slow ejection j - T_H is a time when the stroke volume of blood is distributed throughout the large blood vessel, i.e., the time of the aorta expansion. As our investigations demonstrate, in case of improper elasticity of the aorta this period of time is prolonged.

4. Phase structure of heart cycle on RHEO curve

An electrocardiogram reflects the most important hemodynamic processes. According to an ECG curve, it is possible to identify an intensity of the contraction of the muscles of the respective segment in the cardiovascular system by analyzing inflection points in the respective heart cycle phase and considering the respective phase amplitudes. However, it is required to understand how the flow of blood changes. For this purpose, rheography should be used. A rheogram shows changes in the arterial pressure. An ECG and a RHEO are produced by using signals of different nature. To record an ECG used is electric potential, and for RHEOgraphy employed are changes in amplitudes of high-frequency AC under the influence of changing blood volumes in blood circulation, which produce changes in the conductivity within the space between the recording electrodes.

There is no AP increase in myocardium tension phase S – L. The aortic valve opens at the moment denoted as L. The slope ratio of RHEO in phase of rapid ejection L – j is descriptive of the velocity of stroke volume travel, and, finally, decisive in governing the systolic AP.

5. Criteria for recording phases on ECG, Rheo and their derivatives

When considering an ECG as a complex signal, it should be pointed out that it consists of a number of single-period in-series sinusoidal signals connected. It is referred to a re-distribution of energy in bio systems in a not a stepwise, but sinusoidal way, showing half-periods as follows: energy increase, retardation, attenuation and development. Transition points of these processes should be at the same time the points of inflection of energy functions which are shown by the first derivative at their extrema. Similar processes occur in the cardiovascular system control. Figure 8 represents a schematic model of an ECG comprising the said in-series single-period sinusoidal waves.

Should an ECG curve be differentiated, 10 extrema on the derivative can be identified which correspond to the boundaries of the respective phases of the heart cycle. It should be mentioned that each phase shall be determined by the same criterion, i.e., by the respective local extremum on the derivative curve. Since a wavefront steepness varies, the respective amplitudes of the derivative extrema differ. The ECG phases are equivalent to those of energy variations responsible for the heart control. For illustration purposes, it is better to use graphic differentiation.

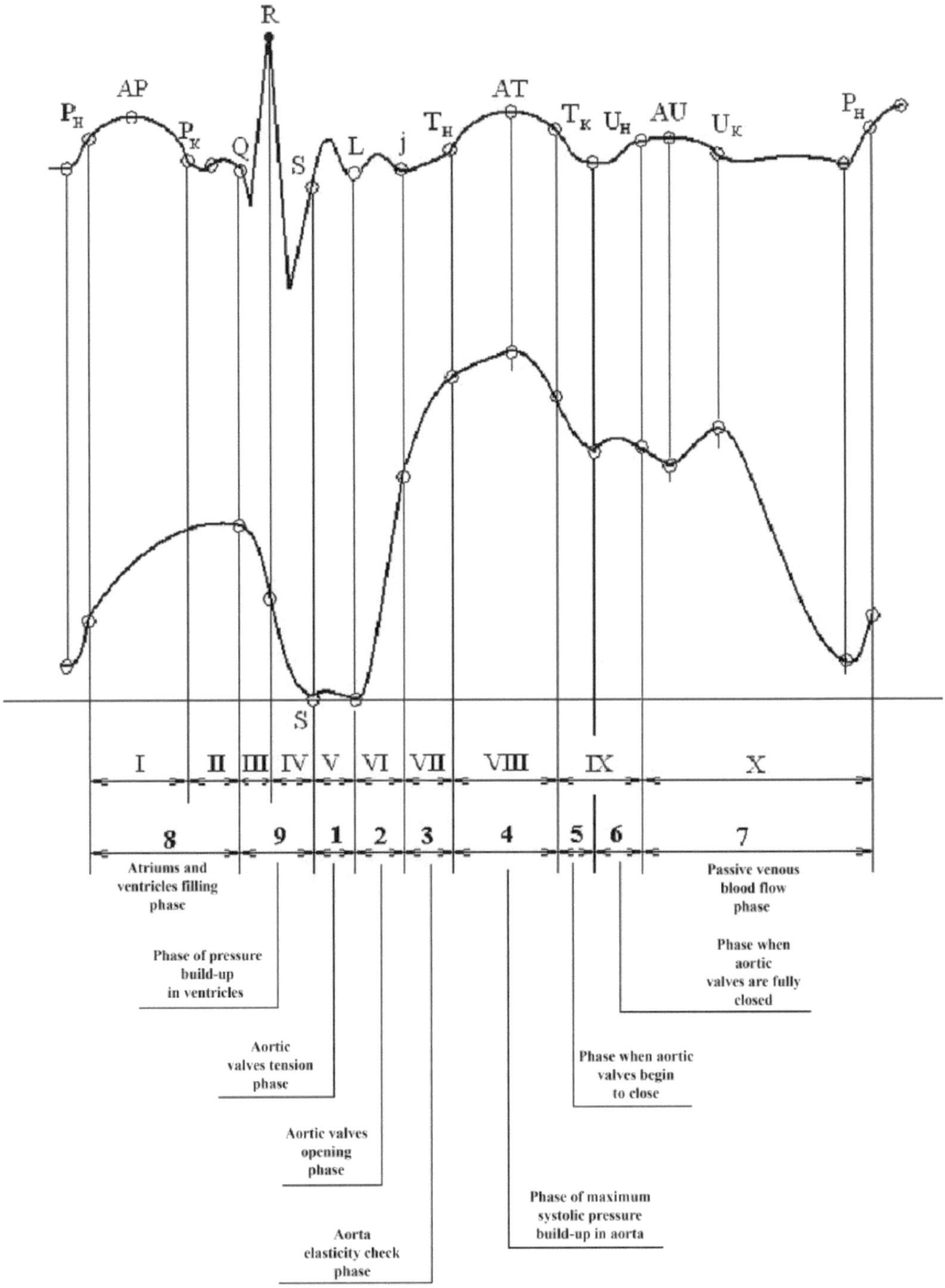

Fig. 7. Phase structure of RHEO recorded from ascending aorta

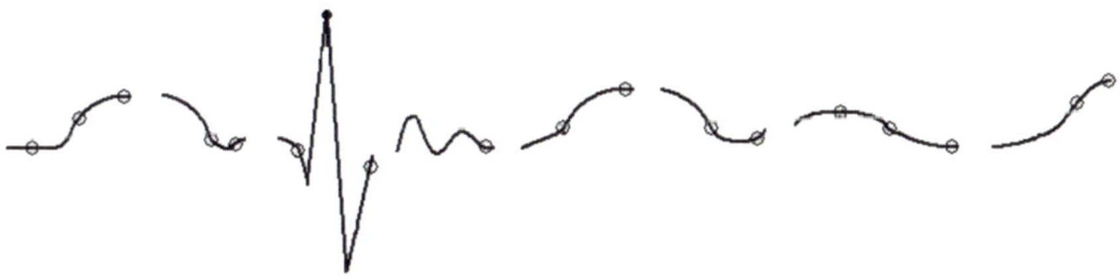

Fig. 8. Schematic model of ECG comprising in-series single-period sinusoidal variations

It is just the graphic differentiation that is capable of clearly illustrating all specific points of such complex signal like an ECG signal. Whereas it is practically impossible to detect visually on an ECG curve the inflection points, they can be easy identified on the derivative by local extrema without error. Figure 9 gives an ECG curve and its first derivative. It is evident that point P on the ECG curve corresponds to point P on the derivative that is found by the respective local extremum. In the same way point T should be identified. It is of great importance to localize point S. There are no other methods capable of identifying this point.

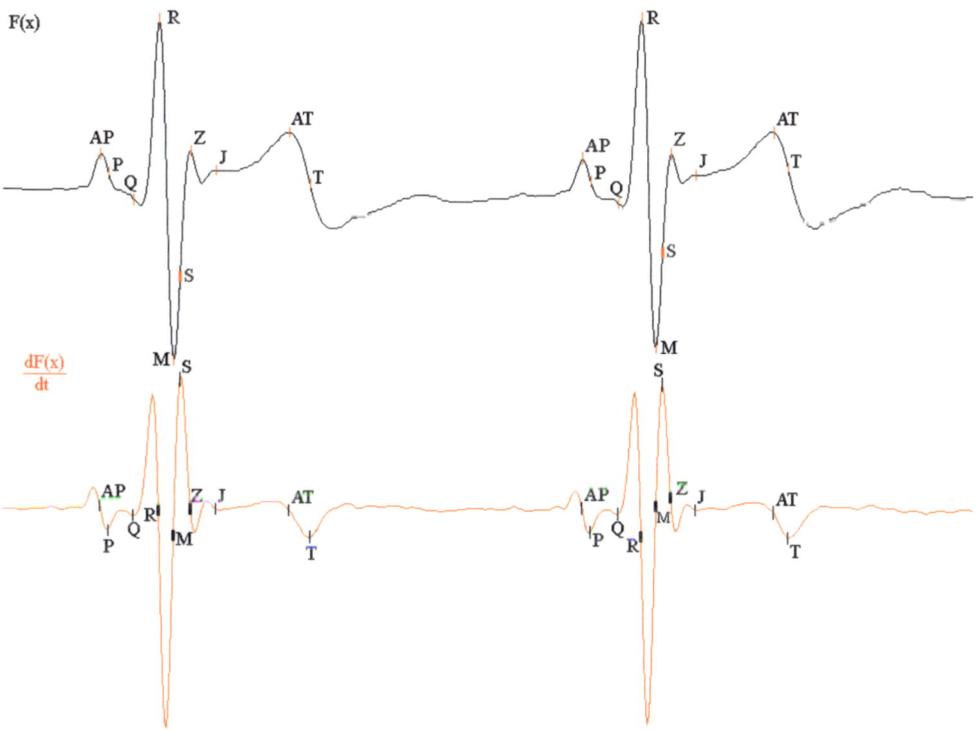

Fig. 9. Graphic differentiation of ECG curve. Shown are an ECG and its first derivative. Wave points on the ECG curve are its inflection points that correspond to the local extrema on the derivative

It is just the derivative that is capable of recognizing point S very clearly by the respective local positive extremum. The proposed procedure of identifying the above mentioned key points makes possible to develop a computer-assisted technology for measuring durations of every heart cycle phase.

For the same purpose, the second derivative may be used, too, but in this case there is no need to do it since the informative content of the heart cycle phase identifiable criteria with utilization of the first derivative is quite sufficient.

Some real ECG curves recorded from the aorta are given in Figure 10 herein. Wave points P, Q, S and T are marked on the curves which are reliably found according to the first derivative.

Figure 11 herein illustrates real ECG signals and the first derivative of this ECG. The ECG shape shown in this Figure is close to an ideal one. It is the matter of fact that in practice we deal with such ECG curves that significantly differ from the ideal ECG type represented herein. Therefore, it is the differentiation only that can very reliably identify the boundaries of every phase in every heart cycle.

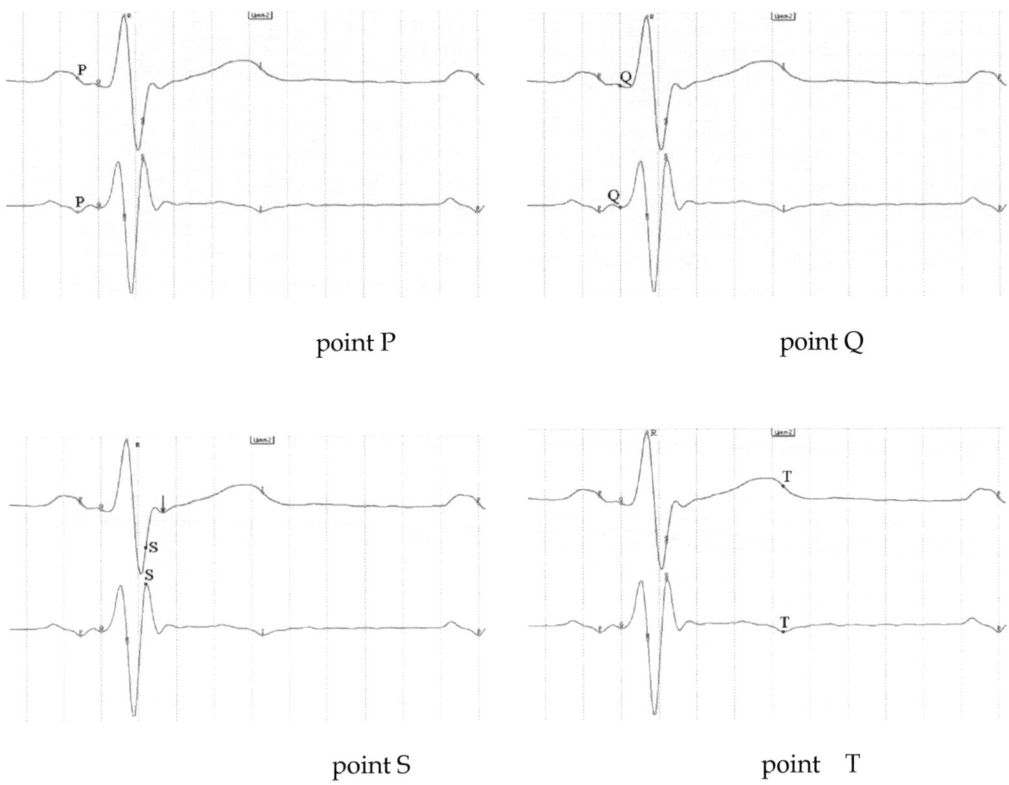

Fig. 10. Key points P, Q, S and T on ECG curve, characterizing the respective phases of the heart cycle and corresponding to the respective local extrema on the derivative

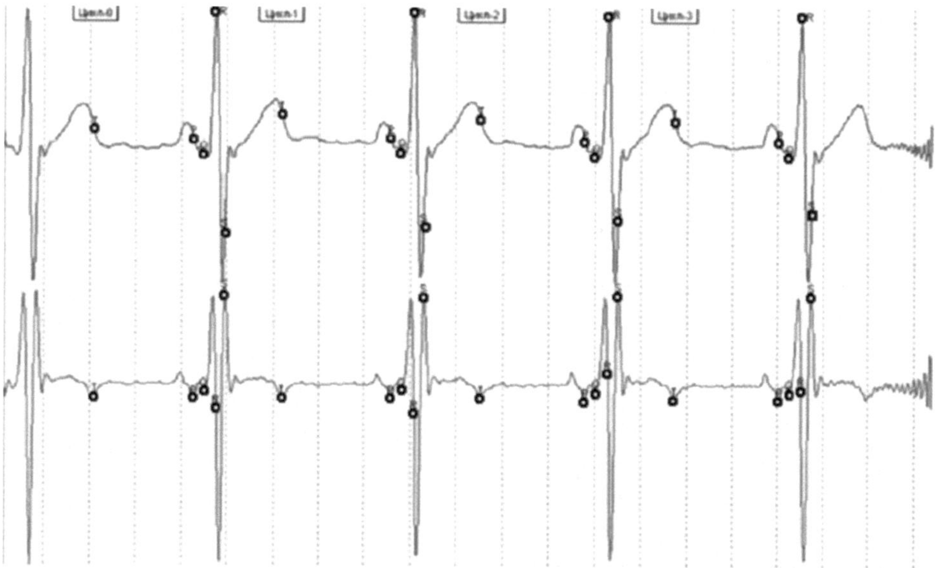

Fig. 11. Identification of phases on an ECG curve with use of the first derivative graph

6. Functions of cardiovascular system to be evaluated on the basis of heart cycle phase analysis

The complex of the functions of the cardiovascular system is a combination of the functions in every individual heart cycle phase. There is a certain logic design available explaining this. Every phase has its own significance but the basis of all phases is the mechanism of contraction or relaxation of muscles. Should metabolic disturbance in a muscle occur, its contraction or relaxation will be diminished. In this case, every next phase will undertake to compensate for this malfunction by enhancing its activity. The phase analysis gives us a clue to clearly identifying such imbalances.

In this connection, the following functions of the cardiovascular system should be mentioned:

№	Function	Regulated parameter
1	Contraction of septum	diastolic AP in the aorta
2	Contraction of myocardium;	diastolic AP in the aorta
3	Tension of myocardium muscles	systolic AP in the aorta
4	Elasticity of aorta	Maintain blood flow structure
5	condition of venous flow	
6	condition of pulmonary function	
7	whether pre-stroke conditions are available or not	
8	problems with coronary blood flow	

Table 1. Main functions and regulated parameters of cardiovascular system

Figure 12 given below demonstrates the relations between the heart cycle phases on an ECG & RHEO and the respective functions of the cardiovascular system. Although it seems that the hemodynamic mechanism as a whole and the performance of the cardiovascular system are very complicated, the heart cycle phase analysis allows establishing of cause-effect relationship of any pathology in every individual case within the shortest time. It is very important that it makes possible to detect the primary cause of a cardiac disease.

Figure 13 displays anatomic segments of the heart and their respective functions in every heart cycle phase.

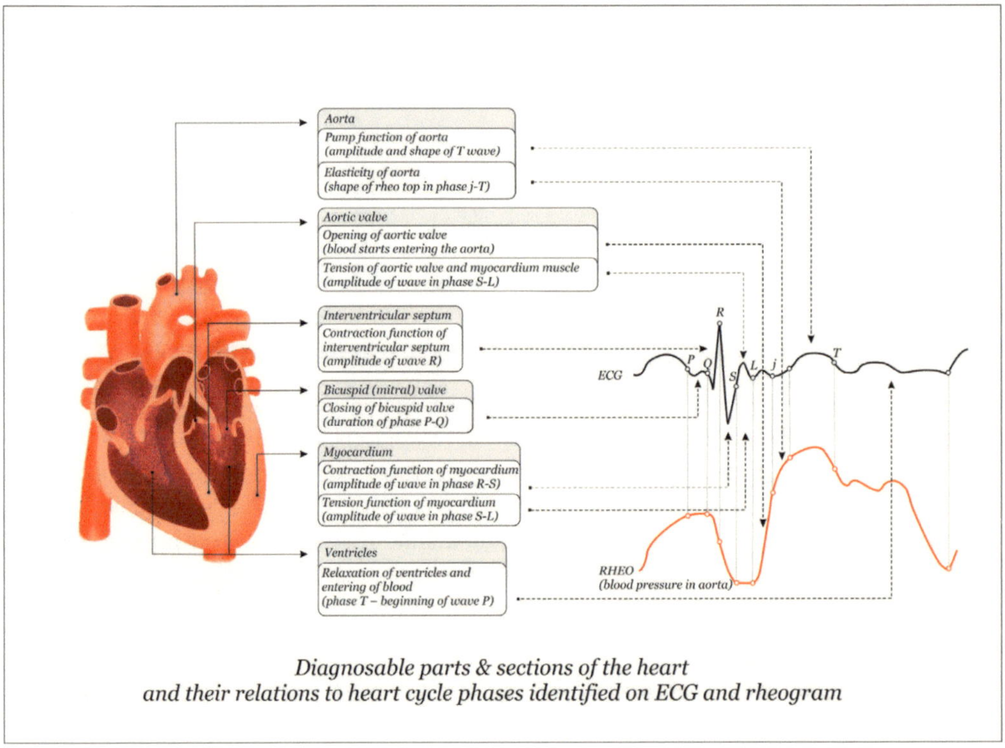

Fig. 12. Diagnosable heart segments with their functions and their relations to heart cycle phases on ECG and RHEO

7. Conclusion

Making progress in research of biophysical processes of the formation of the hemodynamic mechanism is possible only when theoretical models are tested for their compliance in practice, i.e., a model to be validated should show in practice its compliance with the requirements for all simulated functions. The results of many years' researches accumulated by our R & D team made it possible not only to develop an innovative, radically new theory of the heart cycle phase analysis but also provide metrology for such field of medical science as cardiology[4]. We have succeeded in solving the problem of indirect measuring technologies for hemodynamic parameters, including phase-related volumes, by the mathematical modeling.

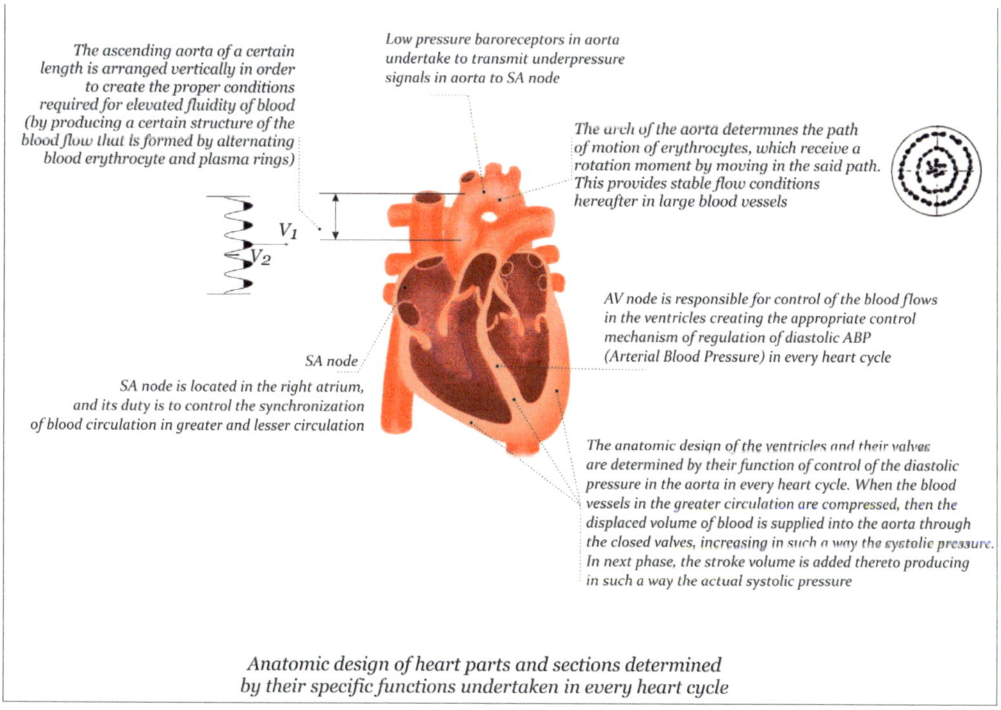

Fig. 13. Anatomical design of the heart predetermined by the required functions in every heart cycle

Our clinical studies offer a clearer view of how many difficult issues associated with biochemical reactions responsible for the stable maintenance of the hemodynamic and the entire performance of the cardiovascular system can be answered. This is a pre-requisite to developing and validating of new high-efficient therapy methods.

Hereby the authors would like to express their hope that within the nearest future we shall deal with a new research field, which is cardiometry. The basis of this science should create mathematical modeling and instrumentation technology.

8. Acknowledgements

The well-known recipe for success in any work is to create a team of like-minded researches working for the same cause. If the concept of their work is that the point of life is work, and if the work results encourage and motivate them, then success is assured. But our life is able to make its corrections. We regret to say that, one of the authors of our discovery, who originated the idea of the "third" mode of flow, died. We speak about Gustav M. Poyedintsev, a great mathematician and scientist. Our last book *Theoretical Principles of Heart Cycle Phase Analysis* published in 2007 was devoted to the memory of him and his work.

The other sad news has been received by us when we were working on this Chapter: Jaana Koponen-Kolmakova, another member of our R & D team, has departed this life. She was really an outstanding person! She was the General Manager of the Company CARDIOCODE-Finland. She remains in our memory for ever.

During our work we meet a lot of people who dedicate their life to science. We always enjoy communicating with them. This is a sort of people who deserve our special recognition and respect.

9. References

[1] Caro, C.; Padley, T.; Shroter, R. & Sid, W. (1981) *Blood Circulation Mechanics.* Mir. M. (fig.12.14).

[2] Goncharenko, A. & Goncharenko, S. (2005) Extrasensory Capabilities of Heart. Magazin "Technika Molodyozhi", No. 5, ISSN 0320 - 331 X Rosen, P. (1969) *The Principle of Optimization in Biology.* Mir.

[3] M. Rudenko, M.; Voronova, O. & Zernov. V. (2009). *Theoretical Principles of Heart Cycle Phase Analysis.* Fouqué Literaturverlag. ISBN 978-3-937909-57-8, Frankfurt a/M. München London - New York.

[4] Voronova, O. (1995). *Development of Models & Algorithms of Automated Transport Function of The Cardiovascular System.* Doctorate Thesis. Prepared by Mrs. O.K. Voronova, Ph.D., VGTU, Voronezh.

[5] Voronova, O. & Poyedintsev, G. Patent № 94031904 (RF). *Method of Determination of the Functional Status of the Left Sections of the Heart & their Associated Large Blood Vessels.*

[6] Rudenko, M.; Voronova, O. & Zernov. V. Innovation in cardiology. A new diagnostic standard establishing criteria of quantitative & qualitative evaluation of main parameters of the cardiac & cardiovascular system according to ECG and Rheo based on cardiac cycle phase analysis (for concurrent single-channel recording of cardiac signals from ascending aorta). (npre.2009.3667.1). *Nature Precedings.* Available from: http://precedings.nature.com/documents/3667/version/1/html

[7] Rudenko, M.; Voronova, O. & Zernov. V. (2009) Study of Hemodynamic Parameters Using Phase Analysis of the Cardiac Cycle. *Biomedical Engineering. Springer New York.* ISSN 0006-3398 (Print) 1573-8256 (Online). Volume 43, Number 4 / July, 2009. P. 151 -155.

[8] Rudenko, M.; Voronova, O. & Zernov. V. (2010) Innovation in theoretical cardiology. Phase mechanism of regulation of diastolic pressure. Arrhythmology Bulletin (Appendix B) – M. - P. 133.

[9] Rosen, P. (1969) *The Principle of Optimization in Biology.* Mir. M.

2

Molecular Control of Smooth Muscle Cell Differentiation Marker Genes by Serum Response Factor and Its Interacting Proteins

Tadashi Yoshida
Apheresis and Dialysis Center
School of Medicine, Keio University
Japan

1. Introduction

Vascular smooth muscle cells (SMCs) exhibit a wide range of different phenotypes at different stages of development (Owens, 1995; Owens et al., 2004; Yoshida & Owens, 2005). Even in mature animals, SMCs retain the capability to change their phenotype in response to multiple local environmental cues. The plasticity of SMCs enables them to play a critical role in physiological processes in the vasculature, as well as the pathogenesis of numerous vascular diseases including atherosclerosis, re-stenosis after percutaneous coronary intervention, aortic aneurysm, and hypertension. Thus, it is important to understand the precise mechanisms whereby SMCs exhibit different phenotypes under distinct conditions. Because one of the most remarkable differences among SMC subtypes is the difference in expression levels of SMC-specific/-selective genes, elucidation of the molecular mechanisms controlling SMC differentiation marker gene expression may shed light on this issue.

Most of SMC differentiation marker genes characterized to date, including *smooth muscle (SM) α-actin* (Mack & Owens, 1999), *SM-myosin heavy chain* (*SM-MHC*) (Madsen et al., 1998), *SM22α* (Li et al., 1996), and *h1-calponin* (Miano et al., 2000), have multiple highly conserved CC(A/T-rich)$_6$GG (CArG) elements in their promoter enhancer regions. Results of studies *in vivo* have shown that expression of these genes is dependent on the presence of CArG elements (Li et al., 1997; Mack & Owens, 1999; Manabe & Owens, 2001a). For example, expression of the *SM α-actin* gene requires a promoter-enhancer region from -2.6 kb to +2.8 kb to recapitulate the expression patterns of the endogenous gene, and mutation of any one of three conserved CArG elements within the regions abolishes the expression (Mack & Owens, 1999). Likewise, SMC-specific expression of the *SM-MHC* gene requires 4.2 kb of the 5′-flanking region, the entire first exon, and 11.5 kb of the first intronic sequence, and mutation of CArG elements in the 5′-flanking region abolishes the expression (Manabe & Owens, 2001a). These results indicate the critical roles of CArG elements in the regulation of SMC differentiation marker gene expression. Currently, it is reported that over 60 of SMC-specific/-selective genes possess CArG elements in the promoter-enhancer regions by in-silico analysis (Miano, 2003), although it is not fully determined how many CArG elements of them are functional.

The binding factor for CArG elements is the ubiquitously expressed transcription factor, serum response factor (SRF) (Norman et al., 1988). Knockout of the *SRF* gene in mice resulted in early embryonic lethality due to abnormal gastrulation and loss in key mesodermal markers (Arsenian et al., 1998), precluding the evaluation of requirement of SRF for SMC differentiation. Instead, conditional knockout of the *SRF* gene in the heart and SMCs exhibited the attenuation in cardiac trabeculation and the compact layer expansion, as well as decreases in SMC-specific/-selective genes including *SM α-actin* in aortic SMCs (Miano et al., 2004). Moreover, SRF has been shown to be required for differentiation of SMCs in an *in vitro* model of coronary SMC differentiation (Landerholm et al., 1999). Indeed, over-expression of dominant-negative forms of SRF inhibited the induction of SMC differentiation marker genes including *SM22α, h1-calponin,* and *SM α-actin* in proepicardial cells excised from quail embryos. As such, the preceding studies provide evidence indicating that the CArG-SRF complex plays an important role in the regulation of SMC differentiation marker gene expression. However, SRF was first cloned as a binding factor for the core sequences of serum response element (SRE) in the *c-fos* gene (Norman et al., 1988). Because the *c-fos* gene is known as one of the growth factor-inducible genes, major unresolved issues in the field are to identify the mechanisms whereby: (1) the CArG-SRF complex can simultaneously contribute to two disparate processes: induction of SMC differentiation marker gene expression versus activation of growth-regulated genes; and (2) the ubiquitously expressed SRF can contribute to SMC-specific/-selective expression of target genes.

To date, a number of factors have been reported to interact with SRF. Several recent studies suggest that these interactions are responsible for multiple actions of SRF. Therefore, this review article will summarize recent progress in our understanding of the transcriptional mechanisms involved in controlling expression of SMC differentiation marker genes by focusing on SRF and its interacting factors.

2. Myocardin is a potent co-factor of SRF for SMC differentiation marker gene expression

One of the major breakthroughs in the SMC field was the discovery of myocardin (Wang et al., 2001). Myocardin was cloned as a co-factor of SRF by a bioinformatics-based screen and found to be exclusively expressed in SMCs and cardiomyocytes (Chen et al., 2002; Du et al., 2003; Wang et al., 2001; Yoshida et al., 2003). It has two isoforms, and smooth muscle-enriched isoform consists of 856 amino acids (Creemers et al., 2006). Myocardin has several domains including three RPEL domains, a basic domain, a glutamine-rich domain, a SAP (Scaffold attachment factors A and B, Acinus, Protein inhibitor of activated STAT) domain, and a leucine zipper-like domain. It has been shown that leucine zipper-like domain is required for homodimerization of myocardin (Figure 1) (Wang et al., 2003), but the function of the other domains is not well understood. Transcriptional activation domain, TAD, is localized at the carboxy-terminal region, and deletion mutants that lack TAD behaved as dominant-negative forms (Wang et al., 2001; Yoshida et al., 2003). Over-expression of myocardin potently induces transcription of virtually all CArG-dependent SMC differentiation marker genes, including *SM α-actin, SM-MHC, SM22α, h1-calponin,* and *myosin light chain kinase* (*MLCK*) (Chen et al., 2002; Du et al., 2003; Wang et al., 2001; Wang et al., 2003; Yoshida et al., 2003). Mutation of CArG elements in the SMC promoters abolished the responsiveness to myocardin, suggesting that myocardin activates the transcription in a CArG-dependent manner. However, myocardin showed no DNA binding activity, but showed interaction with SRF. In addition, myocardin failed to activate the transcription of CArG-dependent genes in the absence of SRF (Du et al., 2003), demonstrating that myocardin is a co-activator of SRF. Over-expression of myocardin also induced the endogenous expression of SMC differentiation marker genes in cultured SMCs and non-SMCs, including 3T3 fibroblasts, L6 myoblasts, 3T3-L1 preadipocytes, COS cells, and undifferentiated embryonic stem cells (Chen et al., 2002; Du et al., 2003; Du et al., 2004; Wang et al., 2001; Wang et al., 2003; Yoshida et al., 2003; Yoshida et al., 2004b). However, forced expression of myocardin in non-SMCs was not sufficient to induce the full SMC differentiation program, because some SMC-enriched genes, which do not contain CArG elements in their promoter-enhancer region, were not induced (Yoshida et al., 2004b). Nevertheless, it was sufficient to establish a SMC-like contractile phenotype (Long et al., 2008). Either dominant-negative forms of myocardin or siRNA-induced suppression of myocardin decreased the transcription of SMC differentiation marker genes in cultured SMCs (Du et al., 2003; Wang et al., 2003; Yoshida et al., 2003). In addition, *myocardin*-deficient mice exhibited no vascular SMC differentiation and died by embryonic day 10.5 (Li et al., 2003), although this may have been secondary to the defect in the extra-embryonic circulation. Moreover, mice lacking the *myocardin* gene in neural crest-derived cells died prior to postnatal day 3 from patent ductus arteriosus, and neural crest-derived SMCs in these mice exhibited a cell-autonomous block in expression of SMC differentiation marker genes (Huang et al., 2008). Taken together, the preceding results provide compelling evidence that myocardin plays a key role in the regulation of expression of SMC differentiation marker genes.

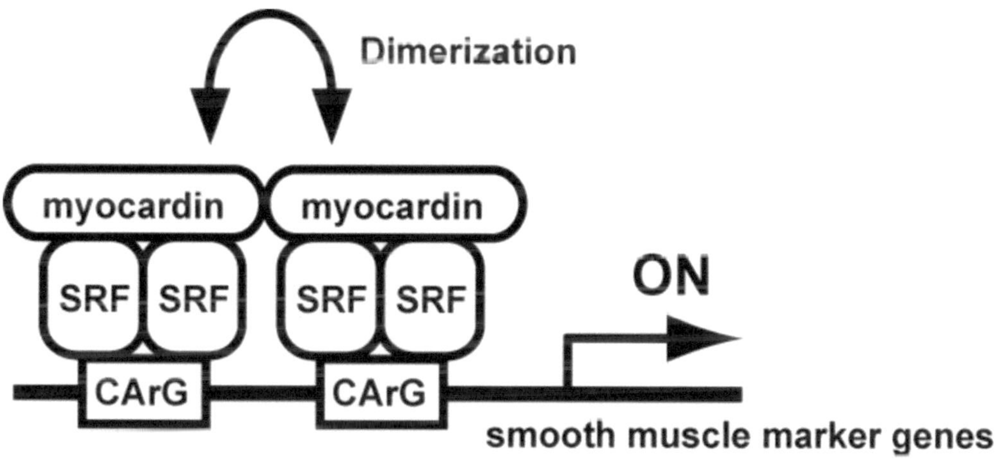

Fig. 1. Myocardin potently induces the transcription of CArG-element containing SMC differentiation marker genes. Myocardin preferentially activates SMC differentiation marker genes which contain multiple CArG elements in their promoter-enhancer regions. Homodimerization of myocardin through the leucine zipper-like domain efficiently activates the transcription. In contrast, myocardin does not induce the transcription of the growth factor-inducible gene, *c-fos*, because it only contains a single CArG element in the promoter.

2.1 Transcriptional mechanism for myocardin-dependent SMC differentiation marker genes

Although myocardin is a powerful transcriptional co-activator of SRF, there are still some questions for the mechanisms whereby myocardin induces SMC differentiation marker genes. One of these questions is: "what *cis*-elements and transcriptional co-activators other than SRF are required for the function of myocardin?" Initial studies (Wang et al., 2001) suggested that myocardin activated the transcription through the formation of complex with SRF and multiple CArG elements, based on the findings that: (1) the single CArG-containing *c-fos* gene had no responsiveness to myocardin; and (2) myocardin could activate an artificial promoter consisting of 4x *c-fos* SREs coupled to the basal promoter. Such a "2-CArG" model, in which multiple CArG elements are required for myocardin-induced transactivation, is strengthened by the results showing that homodimerization of myocardin extraordinary augmented the transcriptional activity of SMC differentiation marker genes (Figure 1) (Wang et al., 2003). However, several SMC-specific genes that only contain single CArG element in their promoter, such as the *telokin* gene and the *cysteine-rich protein-1* (*CRP-1*) gene, have also been shown to be activated by myocardin (Wang et al., 2003; Yoshida et al., 2004b). These results raised a question as to how myocardin distinguishes these single CArG-containing SMC differentiation marker genes from the *c-fos* gene. One hypothesis is that the presence of a ternary complex factor (TCF)-binding site in the *c-fos* promoter regulates the binding of myocardin to SRF. In support of this, it has been shown that one of the TCFs, Elk-1, could compete for SRF binding with myocardin on the SMC promoters (Wang et al., 2004; Yoshida et al., 2007; Zhou et al., 2005). Such a possibility will be discussed in detail in a later section.

An additional possibility is that degeneracy within CArG elements, i.e. conserved base pair substitutions that reduce SRF binding affinity, contributes to the promoter selectivity of myocardin. Consistent with this idea, the majority of SMC differentiation marker genes including *SM α-actin* and *SM-MHC* have degenerate CArG elements in their promoter-enhancer regions (Miano, 2003). For example, both of CArG elements located within 5'-flanking region of the *SM α-actin* gene contain a single G or C substitution within their A/T-rich cores that is 100% conserved between species as divergent as humans and chickens (Shimizu et al., 1995). Results of our previous studies showed that substitution of *SM α-actin* 5' CArGs with the *c-fos* consensus CArGs significantly attenuated injury-induced downregulation of *SM α-actin* expression (Hendrix et al., 2005). In addition, of interest, over-expression of myocardin selectively enhanced SRF binding to degenerate *SM α-actin* CArG elements compared to *c-fos* consensus CArG element in SMCs, as determined by quantitative chromatin immunoprecipitation assays. These results raise a possibility that the degeneracy in the CArG elements is one of the determinants of promoter selectivity of myocardin. However, it should be noted that there is a difference not only in the sequence context of CArG elements, but also in the number of CArG elements between the *SM α-actin* gene versus the *c-fos* gene. Moreover, there is no G or C substitution in the CArG elements of several SMC differentiation marker genes including the *SM22α*, *telokin*, and *CRP-1* genes (Miano, 2003), although previous studies showed that the binding affinity of SRF to *SM22α* CArG-near element was lower than that to the *c-fos* CArG element by electromobility shift assays (EMSA) (Chang et al., 2001). It is interesting to determine whether CArG elements in the *telokin* gene and the *CRP-1* genes also exhibit lower binding affinity to SRF than the *c-fos* consensus CArG element. If this is the case, it is likely that reduced SRF binding to CArG elements, which does not necessarily have G or C substitutions, is one of the mechanisms for target gene selectivity of myocardin. If this is not the case, it is still possible that the degeneracy in CArG elements may explain a part of the promoter selectivity of myocardin, but this mechanism cannot be applicable to all of the SMC differentiation marker genes.

Regarding the mechanism of myocardin-induced transcription of SMC differentiation marker genes, the physical interaction of myocardin with histone acetyltransferase, p300, and class II histone deacetylases, HDAC4 and HDAC5, has been reported (Cao et al., 2005). Indeed, results showed that over-expression of myocardin induced histone H3 acetylation in the vicinity of CArG elements at the *SM α-actin* and *SM22α* promoters in 10T1/2 cells (Cao et al., 2005). In addition, they showed that p300 augmented the stimulatory effect of myocardin on the transcription of the *SM22α* gene, whereas either HDAC4 or HDAC5 repressed the effect of myocardin by co-transfection/reporter assays. Moreover, they demonstrated that p300 and HDACs, respectively, bound to distinct domains of myocardin simultaneously, suggesting that the balance between p300 and HDACs is likely to be one of the determinants of the transcriptional activity of myocardin.

These results are of significant interest in that they provided evidence that transcription of SMC differentiation marker genes is regulated by the recruitment of chromatin modifying enzymes by myocardin. Previous studies showed that SMC differentiation was associated with increased binding of SRF and hyperacetylation of histones H3 and H4 at CArG-containing regions of the *SM α-actin* and *SM-MHC* genes in A404 SMC precursor cells (Manabe & Owens, 2001b). In addition, we showed that over-expression of myocardin selectively enhanced SRF binding to CArG-containing region of the *SM α-actin* gene, but not to that of the *c-fos* gene in the context of intact chromatin in SMCs (Hendrix et al., 2005). Results of studies by another group (Qiu & Li, 2002) also showed that HDACs reduced the transcriptional activity of the *SM22α* gene in a CArG element dependent manner. These findings are consistent with the results showing the association of myocardin with p300 or HDACs (Cao et al., 2005). However, it remains unknown how the association between myocardin and p300 or HDACs regulates the accessibility of SRF to CArG elements, as has been observed during the induction of SMC differentiation in A404 cells (Manabe & Owens, 2001b). It is possible that particular histone modifications by the myocardin-p300 complex enable SRF to bind to CArG-elements within the SMC promoters. It is also possible that the association between myocardin and chromatin modifying enzymes including p300 may alter the binding affinity of myocardin to SRF. Because regulation of SMC differentiation marker genes by platelet-derived growth factor-BB (PDGF-BB) or oxidized phospholipids has been shown to be accompanied by the recruitment of HDACs and thereby changes in acetylation levels at the SMC promoters (Yoshida et al., 2007, 2008a), it is interesting to determine if these changes are caused by the modulation of association between myocardin and these chromatin modifying enzymes.

2.2 Role of the myocardin-related family in SMC differentiation

Two factors were identified as members of the myocardin-related transcription factors: MKL1 (also referred to as MAL, BSAC, and MRTF-A) (Cen et al., 2003; Miralles et al., 2003; Sasazuki et al., 2002; Wang et al., 2002) and MKL2 (also referred to as MRTF-B) (Selvaraj & Prywes, 2003; Wang et al., 2002). It has been shown that expression of *MKL1* mRNA is ubiquitous, whereas expression of *MKL2* mRNA is restricted to several tissues including the brain and the heart (Cen et al., 2003; Selvaraj & Prywes, 2003; Wang et al., 2002). Co-transfection studies revealed that both MKL1 and MKL2 were capable of inducing the transcription of multiple CArG-containing promoters including *atrial natriuretic factor* (*ANF*), *SM22α*, *SM α-actin*, and *cardiac α-actin*. A truncated MKL2 protein that lacks both amino-terminal region and carboxy-terminal region (MKL2ΔNΔC700) behaved as a dominant-negative manner for both MKL1 and MKL2, and over-expression of MKL2ΔNΔC700 inhibited skeletal muscle differentiation in C2C12 skeletal myoblasts (Selvaraj & Prywes, 2003). In addition, MKL1 strongly induced SMC differentiation marker gene expression in undifferentiated embryonic stem cells, even in the absence of myocardin (Du et al., 2004). Moreover, a truncated form of MKL1, which behaved as a dominant-negative form of MKL1 and myocardin, inhibited MKL1-induced transcription of the *SM22α* gene (Du et al., 2004). Taken together, MKL factors appear to be important regulators of SMC differentiation marker gene expression as well as myocardin, and they appear to exhibit the redundant function with myocardin as SRF co-factors. However, the precise roles of MKL factors in SMC differentiation marker gene expression in SMCs are still unclear, because most of these studies analyzing the function of MKL factors have been performed by over-expression experiments. Regarding this point, there are several interesting studies as described below. First, *MKL1* knockout mice were viable, but were unable to effectively nurse their offspring due to a failure in maintenance of the differentiated state of mammary myoepithelial cells during lactation (Li et al., 2006; Sun et al., 2006). Second, conditional knockout of the *MKL2* gene in neural crest-derived cells exhibited a spectrum of cardiovascular defects including abnormal patterning of the branchial arch arteries (Li et al., 2005; Oh et al., 2005). The abnormalities in *MKL2* knockout mice were accompanied by a decrease in SM α-actin expression in SMCs within the branchial arch arteries. Based on the results of these studies, MKL1 is unlikely to play an important role in expression of SMC differentiation marker genes *in vivo*. In addition, role of MKL2 for SMC differentiation in SMCs derived from other origins is still unknown. A biggest issue is how broadly expressed MKL factors regulate SMC-specific/-selective CArG-dependent genes. Recently, several studies suggest the importance of intracellular localization of MKL factors in SMCs and non-SMCs (Hinson et al., 2007; Nakamura et al., 2010; Yoshida et al., 2007). Further studies are required to address this issue.

In summary, it is clear that myocardin plays a critical role in SMC differentiation in concert with the CArG-SRF complex. However, myocardin is not a SMC-specific gene in that it is also expressed in cardiomyocytes, suggesting that myocardin alone is not enough to coordinate expression of SMC differentiation marker genes. It is highly likely that cooperative interaction of the SRF-myocardin complex with other transcription factors is necessary for expression of SMC differentiation marker genes in SMCs. Further studies are needed to clarify these combinatorial mechanisms.

3. Ternary complex factors exhibit dual roles in the transcription of SRF-dependent CArG-Containing genes

TCFs are a subfamily of the Ets domain transcription factors (Buchwalter et al., 2004). TCF was first described as 62 kD nuclear fractions (p62) that form a ternary complex with SRF on the *c-fos* SRE (Shaw et al., 1989). Three members, Elk-1, Sap-1/Elk-4, and Net/Sap-2/Elk-3, have been identified as TCFs. Previous studies demonstrated that TCFs are present on SREs of the *c-fos* gene with SRF dimers both before and after growth factor stimulation, and that after the stimulation with growth factors, TCFs are phosphorylated and activate transcription of the *c-fos* gene (Buchwalter et al., 2004).

Although it has been believed, for a long time, that most of SMC differentiation marker genes lack the TCF-binding site in their promoter regions (Miano 2003), results of recent studies by multiple laboratories including our own (Wang et al., 2004; Yoshida et al., 2007; Zhou et al., 2005) suggest the involvement of Elk-1 in the regulation of SMC differentiation marker genes. They presented evidence that repression of SMC differentiation marker genes including *SM α-actin* and *SM22α* by PDGF-BB was due to the displacement of myocardin from SRF by phosphorylated Elk-1 in cultured SMCs (Figure 2). Indeed, they showed that treatment with PDGF-BB induced phosphorylation of Elk-1 through the activation of the MEK1/2-Erk1/2 pathway and increased the association between Elk-1 and SRF, whereas the association between myocardin and SRF was decreased at the same time. By extensively mapping the domain of myocardin and Elk-1, they found that both factors have a structurally related SRF-binding motif and thereby compete for the common docking region of SRF. These results are very interesting in that phosphorylation of Elk-1 simultaneously exhibits the dual roles in the regulation of CArG-dependent genes: transcriptional activation of the *c-fos* gene versus transcriptional repression of SMC differentiation marker genes.

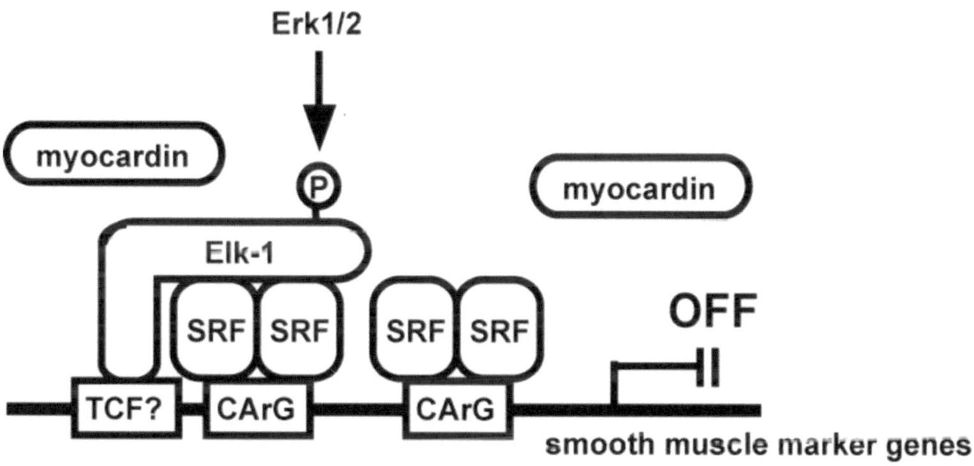

Fig. 2. Phosphorylation of Elk-1 competes for SRF binding with myocardin. The myocardin-SRF-CArG complex activates the transcription of SMC differentiation marker genes in the absence of growth factors as shown in Fig. 1. Activation of the Erk1/2 pathway by growth factors such as PDGF-BB induces phosphorylation of Elk-1. Phosphorylated Elk-1 displaces myocardin from SRF and binds to SRF, thereby suppressing the transcription of SMC differentiation marker genes. It has been reported that phosphorylated Elk-1 is able to bind to the TCF-binding site within the *SM22α* promoter (Wang et al., 2004), although the TCF-binding site is not present within the promoter region of most SMC differentiation marker genes.

However, the mechanisms responsible for these dual effects have not been clearly understood yet. That is, although the binding of Elk-1 on the putative TCF-binding site (5′-TTCCCG-3′) adjacent to the CArG-far element at the *SM22α* promoter was detected by

EMSA and chromatin immunoprecipitation assays (Wang et al., 2004), this sequence is not the consensus binding site for Elk-1 (Treisman et al., 1992). By using "the site selection method" to purify DNA capable of forming ternary complexes from a pool of randomized oligonucleotides, the consensus binding motif for Elk-1 and Sap-1 was determined as 5'-(C/A)(C/A)GGA(A/T)-3' previously (Treisman et al., 1992). The putative TCF-binding site within the *SM22α* gene (sense: 5'-TTCCCG-3' and antisense: 5'-CGGGAA-3') does not match this sequence completely. In addition, although over-expression of Elk-1 downregulated the *SM22α* promoter-luciferase activity through the competition with myocardin, this competition was still observed when the mutational *SM22α*-luciferase construct, in which the putative TCF-binding site was abolished, was used. Furthermore, there is no putative Elk-1 binding site near the CArG elements within the *SM α-actin* promoter (Mack & Owens, 1999). Because chromatin immunoprecipitation assays can detect not only the direct binding of protein to DNA sequence, but also the binding of protein to protein, it is highly possible that the attachment of Elk-1 to the TCF-binding site may not be absolutely required for the competition with myocardin for SRF binding. Nevertheless, the *SM22α* promoter with a mutation in the TCF-binding site has been reported to direct ectopic transcription in the heart in a later embryonic stage, as compared with the wild-type *SM22α* promoter *in vivo* (Wang et al., 2004). Further studies are needed to determine if these findings are applicable to multiple SMC differentiation marker genes.

It is also of interest to determine whether the activation of Elk-1 can recruit histone deacetylases to the promoter regions of SMC differentiation marker genes. Elk-1 contains two transcriptional repression domains, an N-terminal transcriptional repression domain and an R motif located in the C-terminal transcriptional activation domain (Buchwalter et al., 2004). It has been shown that HDAC1 and HDAC2 were recruited to the N-terminal transcriptional repression domain of Elk-1 on the *c-fos* promoter followed by the activation of the MEK1/2-Erk-1/2 pathway, and this recruitment kinetically correlated with the shutoff of the *c-fos* gene expression after growth factor stimulation (Yang et al., 2001; Yang & Sharrocks, 2004). We previously showed that repression of SMC differentiation marker genes after stimulation with PDGF-BB was accompanied by the recruitment of multiple HDACs, HDAC2, HDAC4, and HDAC5 in cultured SMCs (Yoshida et al., 2007). It is possible that the association between Elk-1 and these HDACs on the SMC promoters is one of the mechanisms for repression of SMC differentiation marker gene expression. Moreover, it was reported that SUMO modification of the R motif in Elk-1 could antagonize the MEK1/2-Erk1/2 pathway and repress the transcription of the *c-fos* gene (Yang et al., 2003). Thus, it is also possible that PDGF-BB can induce sumoylation of Elk-1 and exhibit the repressive effects on SMC differentiation marker genes.

In summary, the preceding results indicate that Elk-1 plays dual roles in the transcription of CArG-dependent genes as both an activator and a repressor. However, there are still some questions as discussed above. Clearly, one of the most fascinating questions is to determine if knockdown of Elk-1 abolishes PDGF-BB-induced repression of SMC differentiation marker genes both *in vivo* and *in vitro*.

4. Multiple homeodomain proteins regulate SMC differentiation

Homeodomain proteins are a family of transcription factors with a highly conserved DNA-binding domain that regulate cell proliferation, differentiation, and migration in many cell types during embryogenesis (Gorski & Walsh, 2003). This family is comprised of over 160 genes, and it has been reported that several homeodomain proteins are able to regulate differentiation of SMCs by interacting with the CArG-SRF complex.

One of these factors is Prx-1 (Paired-related homeobox gene-1), which is also known as MHox and Phox (Cserjesi et al., 1992; Grueneberg et al., 1992). Expression of Prx-1 is completely restricted to mesodermally derived cell types during embryogenesis and to cell lines of mesodermal origin including cultured aortic SMCs (Blank et al., 1995; Cserjesi et al., 1992). Previous studies from our laboratory and others showed that Prx-1 was capable of inducing the transcription of the CArG-SRF dependent genes (Grueneberg et al., 1992; Hautmann et al., 1997; Yoshida et al., 2004a). Indeed, we found that angiotensin II increased expression of multiple SMC differentiation marker genes including *SM α-actin*, as well as *Prx-1* expression in cultured SMCs (Hautmann et al., 1997; Turla et al., 1991; Yoshida et al., 2004a). Of major interest, we provided evidence that siRNA-induced suppression of Prx-1 dramatically reduced both basal and angiotensin II-induced transcription of the *SM α-actin* gene (Yoshida et al., 2004a). In addition, Prx-1 increased the SRF binding to degenerate CArG B element within the *SM α-actin* gene by EMSA (Hautmann et al., 1997). Similarly, Prx-1 enhanced the binding of SRF to *c fos* CArG element by EMSA (Grueneberg et al., 1992). However, the formation of a stable higher order complex comprised of Prx-1, SRF, and CArG element was not detected by EMSA. Rather, Prx-1 enhanced both the rate of association and the rate of dissociation between SRF and CArG element, thereby increasing the rate of exchange of SRF on the CArG element. Although further studies are required to clarify these mechanisms in detail, results thus far suggest that Prx-1 plays a key role in the transcription of CArG-dependent genes through regulating the binding of SRF to CArG elements.

Although the preceding results suggest that Prx-1 is involved in the regulation of SMC differentiation marker gene expression (Hautmann et al., 1997; Yoshida et al., 2004a), it also plays a role in proliferation of SMCs. *Prx-1* expression was induced during the development of pulmonary vascular disease in adult rats, and Prx-1 enhanced the proliferation rate of cultured rat A10 SMCs via the induction of tenascin-C expression (Jones et al., 2001). Taken together, results suggest that Prx-1 plays multiple roles in the regulation of differentiation status and the regulation of proliferation status in SMCs. This is consistent with the idea that differentiation and proliferation are not necessarily mutually exclusive processes (Owens & Thompson, 1986; Owens et al., 2004). However, it remains unknown whether Prx-1 exhibits these two roles simultaneously or Prx-1 exhibits distinct roles in a developmental stage-specific manner. Of interest, *Prx-1* knockout mice have been made and shown to exhibit major defects in skeletogenesis and die soon after birth (Martin et al., 1995). Mice null for both *Prx-1* and its homologue, *Prx-2*, showed a vascular abnormality with an abnormal positioning and awkward curvature of the aortic arch and a misdirected and elongated ductus arteriosus (Bergwerff et al., 2000). Moreover, expression of endothelial markers such as Flk-1 and VCAM-1 and von Willebrand factor-positive cells were decreased in the lung of *Prx-1* null newborn mice (Ihida-Stansbury et al., 2004), suggesting that Prx-1 is required for lung vascularization *in vivo*. It will be of interest to directly test the role of Prx-1 in CArG-dependent SMC differentiation marker gene expression in these mice.

Another homeodomain protein related to SMC differentiation is Hex. Hex was originally isolated from hematopoietic tissues by PCR using degenerate oligonucleotide primers corresponding to the conserved homeodomain sequences and has been shown to play an important role in inducing differentiation of vascular endothelial cells (Thomas et al., 1998). In SMCs, Hex protein expression was induced in the neointima after balloon injury of rat aorta, while it was undetectable in normal aorta (Sekiguchi et al., 2001). The expression pattern of Hex was similar to that of SMemb/NMHC-B, a marker of phenotypically modulated SMCs. Hex induced the transcription of the SMemb promoter, and cAMP-responsive element (CRE) located at -481 bp within the promoter was critical for Hex responsiveness. However, Hex failed to bind to CRE directly, thus the precise mechanisms whereby Hex activated the *SMemb* promoter are still unclear. Of interest, subsequent studies showed that Hex also induced expression of a subset of SMC differentiation marker genes including *SM α-actin* and *SM22α,* but not *SM-MHC* and *h1-calponin* (Oyama et al., 2004). Hex induced the transcription of the *SM22α* gene in a CArG-dependent manner, and it enhanced the binding of SRF to CArG-near element within the *SM22α* promoter, as determined by EMSA. In addition, immunoprecipitation assays revealed the physical association between SRF and Hex. As such, the mechanisms whereby Hex induces SMC differentiation marker genes seem to be similar to those of Prx-1. However, results showing that Hex simultaneously activated expression of both SMC differentiation marker genes and those characteristic of phenotypically modulated SMCs are paradoxical, and further studies are clearly needed to precisely define the pathophysiological role of Hex in SMCs.

Nkx-3.2 is also a homeodomain protein that regulates expression of SMC differentiation marker genes (Nishida et al., 2002). It has been demonstrated that a triad of SRF, GATA-6, and Nkx-3.2 formed a complex with their corresponding *cis*-elements and cooperatively transactivated SMC differentiation marker genes including *α1-integrin, SM22α,* and *caldesmon*. Because co-localization of GATA-6, Nkx-3.2, and SRF was exclusively observed in SMCs, SMC-specific gene expression does not appear to be the result of any single transcription factor that is unique to SMCs, but rather is due to unique combinatorial interactions of factors that may be expressed in multiple cell types but only found together in SMCs.

Furthermore, we recently identified Pitx2 as a homeodomain protein which is required for the initial induction of SMC differentiation by using a subtraction hybridization screen (Shang et al., 2008). Over-expression of Pitx2 induced expression of CArG-dependent SMC differentiation marker genes, whereas knockdown of Pitx2 attenuated retinoic acid-induced differentiation of SMCs from undifferentiated SMC precursor cells. Furthermore, *Pitx2* knockout mouse embryos exhibited impaired induction of SMC differentiation markers in the dorsal aorta and branchial arch arteries. We identified three mechanisms for Pitx2-induced transcription of SMC differentiation marker genes (Figure 3). First, Pitx2 bound to its consensus TAATC(C/T) element in the promoter region of SMC differentiation marker genes. Second, Pitx2 physically associated with SRF. Third, Pitx2 mediated exchange of HDACs with p300 to increase acetylation levels of histone H4 at the SMC promoters. These results provide compelling evidence that Pitx2 plays a critical role in the induction of SMC differentiation during the early embryogenesis. Further studies are needed to determine if Pitx2 also contributes to the pathogenesis of vascular diseases including atherosclerosis.

As such, several homeodomain proteins are involved in the regulation of CArG-SRF dependent SMC differentiation marker gene expression, and some of the mechanisms appear to be mediated by common pathways. Further studies are needed to clarify the temporal and spatial roles of each of these homeodomain proteins in SMC differentiation.

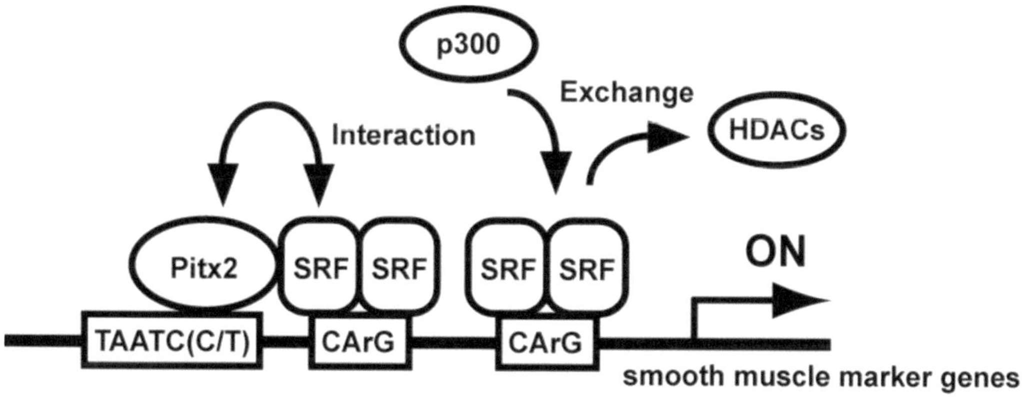

Fig. 3. Pitx2 transactivates SMC differentiation marker genes through three mechanisms. Pitx2 induces expression of SMC differentiation marker genes by: (1) binding to a consensus TAATC(C/T) *cis*-element; (2) interacting with SRF; and (3) mediating exchange of HDACs with p300 at the promoter region of SMC differentiation marker genes. These mechanisms are important for the initial induction of SMC differentiation during the early embryonic development.

5. A number of factors associate with SRF

In addition to the factors described above, there are a number of transcription factors known to interact with SRF. These factors also play key roles in the control of SMC differentiation marker gene expression. In this section, some of these transcription factors will be discussed briefly.

5.1 GATA-6

GATA proteins are a family of zinc finger transcription factors, and play essential roles in development through their interaction with a DNA consensus element, "WGATAR" (Molkentin, 2000). Six GATA transcription factors have been identified in vertebrates, and GATA-4, GATA-5, and GATA-6 are thought to be involved in the formation of the heart, gut, and vessels. During the early murine embryonic development, expression patterns of GATA-6 and GATA-4 were similar, with expression being detected in the precardiac mesoderm, the embryonic heart tube, and the primitive gut (Morrisey et al., 1996). However, during the late development, GATA-6 became the only GATA factor to be expressed in vascular SMCs. Knockout of the *GATA-6* gene in mice resulted in embryonic lethality between embryonic day 6.5 and 7.5, precluding the evaluation of the role of GATA-6 in SMC differentiation and maturation (Morrisey et al., 1998).

As described in a previous section, GATA-6 has shown to interact with SRF and Nkx-3.2 and to induce SMC differentiation marker gene expression (Morrisey et al., 1998; Nishida et al., 2002). *GATA-6* expression in SMCs was rapidly downregulated after vascular injury in rat carotid arteries, and adenovirus-mediated transfer of GATA-6 to the vessel wall after the balloon injury partially inhibited the formation of intimal thickening and reversed the downregulation of SMC differentiation marker genes including *SM α-actin* and *SM-MHC* (Mano et al., 1999). These results suggest the important role of GATA-6 in regulating SMC differentiation. Of interest, results of studies (Yin & Herring, 2005) showed that GATA-6 increased the transcriptional activity of the *SM α-actin* and *SM-MHC* genes, whereas it reduced the transcriptional activity of the *telokin* gene. They found that the GATA-6 binding site was located adjacent to CArG element in the *telokin* promoter and that over-expression of GATA-6 interfered the interaction between myocardin and SRF by mammalian two-hybrid assays. However, it is unclear why GATA-6 has positive and negative effects on CArG-dependent SMC differentiation marker genes. It is possible that these opposite effects are due to the number of CArG elements or the distance between the GATA-6 binding site and the CArG element. Further studies are needed to test these possibilities.

5.2 Klf4

Klf4 is a member of Krüppel-like transcriptional factors that have recently received increased attention. Previously, Klf4 was identified as a binding factor for the transforming growth factor-β1 control element (TCE) found in the promoter region of the *SM α-actin* and *SM22α* genes, based on a yeast one-hybrid screen (Adam et al., 2000). Klf4 exhibited a profound inhibitory effect on expression of SMC differentiation marker genes via a TCE-dependent and a CArG-SRF-dependent manner (Liu et al., 2003, 2005). For example, adenovirus-mediated over-expression of Klf4 repressed endogenous expression of *SM α-actin* and *SM-MHC* genes, as well as expression of *myocardin*, in cultured SMCs as measured by real-time reverse transcription-PCR (Liu et al., 2005). In addition, over-expression of Klf4 completely abolished myocardin-induced activation of SMC differentiation marker genes. Co-immunoprecipitation assays revealed that Klf4 physically interacted with SRF, and chromatin immunoprecipitation assays showed that over-expression of Klf4 markedly reduced the binding of SRF to CArG elements on the *SM α-actin* promoter in intact chromatin of cultured SMCs (Liu et al., 2005). Moreover, PDGF-BB treatment induced *Klf4* mRNA expression in cultured SMCs, and siRNA-induced suppression of Klf4 partially blocked PDGF-BB-induced suppression of SMC differentiation marker genes (Liu et al., 2005). Of significant interest, we demonstrated that conditional knockout of the *Klf4* gene in mice exhibited a delay in suppression of SMC differentiation markers, and an enhanced neointimal formation following vascular injury (Figure 4) (Yoshida et al., 2008b). Additionally, we showed that Klf4, Elk-1, and HDACs cooperatively suppress oxidized phospholipid-induced suppression of SMC differentiation marker genes in cultured SMCs (Yoshida et al., 2008a). Taken together, these results suggest that Klf4 plays a key role in mediating phenotypic switching of SMCs.

5.3 Cysteine-rich LIM-only proteins, CRP1 and CRP2

The members of the cysteine-rich LIM-only protein (CRP) family, CRP1 and CRP2, are expressed predominantly in SMCs and contain two LIM domains in the structure (Henderson et al., 1999; Jain et al., 1996). It is known that the functions of LIM domains are to mediate protein-protein interactions, to target proteins to distinct subcellular locations, and to mediate assembly of multimeric protein complexes. One of the functions of CRP1 and CRP2 is to interact with both the actin crosslinking protein, α-actinin, and the adhesion plaque protein, zyxin, and to regulate the stability and structure of adhesion complexes (Arber & Caroni, 1996; Schmeichel & Beckerle, 1994). In addition to such a cytoplasmic role,

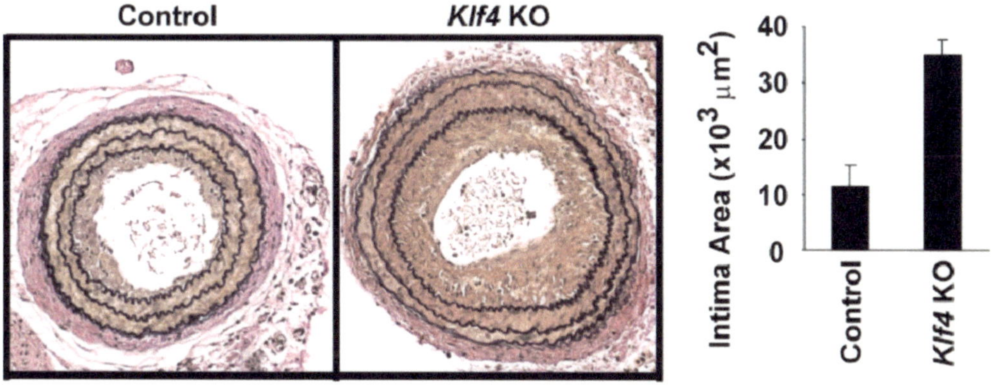

Fig. 4. Conditional knockout of the *Klf4* gene in mice accelerates neointimal formation following vascular injury. Klf4 is a potent repressor of SMC differentiation marker genes. Interestingly, conditional knockout of the *Klf4* gene in mice delays downregulation of SMC differentiation markers, but also accelerates neointimal formation after vascular injury (Yoshida et al., 2008).

it has been reported that CRP1 and CRP2 are also able to function as transcriptional co-factors (Chang et al., 2003). Over-expression of three factors, SRF, GATA-6, and CRP1/CRP2 strongly activated the transcription of SMC differentiation marker genes including *SM α-actin*, *SM-MHC*, *SM22α*, *h1-calponin*, and *h-caldesmon*. The N-terminal LIM domain of CRP1/2 interacted with SRF, and that the C-terminal LIM domain of CRP1/2 interacted with GATA-6, and that SRF and GATA-6 also interacted each other. These results suggest a critical role of CRP1/2 in organizing multiprotein complexes onto the SMC promoters for SMC differentiation. However, it is still unclear how CRP1 and CRP2 are translocated from the cytoplasm to the nucleus and what signaling pathways control their nuclear localization. Moreover, there is a lack of evidence that these factors play a role in control of SMC differentiation marker gene expression *in vivo* in SMCs. Indeed, results of recent studies showed that SMC differentiation in *CRP1* knockout mice or *CRP2* knockout mice appeared to be normal, although neointimal formation was altered after vascular injury (Lilly et al., 2010; Wei et al., 2005). Results raised a question as to the role of CRP1/2 in SMC differentiation.

5.4 PIAS-1

Results of previous studies showed that over-expression of class I basic Helix-Loop-Helix proteins, E2-2, and SRF exhibited a synergistic effect on the transcription of the *SM α-actin* promoter-enhancer in BALBc/3T3 cells (Kumar et al., 2003). However, direct interaction between E2-2 and SRF was undetectable by EMSA using the recombinant proteins. We isolated PIAS-1 (protein inhibitor of activated STAT-1) as an interacting protein for E2-2 by a yeast two-hybrid screen (Kawai-Kowase et al., 2005). We also found that PIAS-1 interacted with SRF, suggesting that PIAS-1 works as a bridging molecule between E2-2 and SRF. Interestingly, PIAS-1 belongs to a family of E3 ligases which promote SUMO modifications of target proteins (Schmidt & Müller, 2002). Indeed, recent studies showed that transcription factors involved in SMC differentiation, such as myocardin and Klf4, were sumoylation targets of PIAS-1. Myocardin sumoylation by PIAS-1 transactivated cardiogenic genes in 10T1/2 fibroblasts (Wang et al., 2007), whereas sumoylation of Klf4 by PIAS-1 promoted transforming growth factor-β induced activation of SM α-actin expression in SMCs (Kawai-Kowase et al., 2009). Further studies are needed to determine effects of *PIAS-1* knockout on SMC differentiation as well as phenotypic switching of SMCs.

6. Conclusion and perspectives

As discussed above, it is clear that the CArG-SRF complex plays a central role in the regulation of SMC differentiation marker gene expression. However, it is also clear that expression of SMC differentiation marker genes is not controlled by the CArG-SRF complex alone, nor by any single transcription factor that is expressed exclusively in SMCs. Rather, SMC-selective gene expression appears to be mediated by complex combinatorial interactions of multiple transcription factors and co-factors, including some that are ubiquitously expressed like SRF and PIAS-1, as well as others that are selective for SMCs like myocardin, Prx-1, CRP-1/2, and GATA-6. In addition to the transcription factors described above, several novel factors, including Fhl2 (Philippar et al., 2004), HERP1 (Doi et al., 2005) and lupaxin (Sundberg-Smith et al., 2008), have also been identified as factors interacting with SRF.

However, our knowledge is immature regarding the overall connection among multiple transcription factors and co-factors that can modify the activity of SRF. Most of studies analyzing the protein-protein interaction thus far have been focused on the relationship among two or three proteins. However, a number of factors should be coordinately regulated and interacted by a single environmental cue. It is of interest to determine whether all of SRF-interacting factors are simultaneously required for SMC differentiation marker gene expression or these factors independently contribute to SMC differentiation marker gene expression in time- and position-specific manner. Thus, in the long term, future studies in the SMC field are needed not only to screen out other key transcription factors, but also to map out the connection networks of these factors.

During the past decade, there is a tremendous progress in our understanding of the roles of chromatin modifying enzymes and chromatin structure in gene transcription in all cell types. Accumulating evidence indicates that the N-terminal tails of histones are the target of numerous modifications, including acetylation, methylation, phosphorylation, ubiqutination, and ADP ribosylation, and that these modifications control gene transcription (Fischle et al., 2003). However, this issue in the SMC field is obviously in its infancy. Thus far, only several transcription factors have been reported to be involved in chromatin remodeling. Clearly, more detailed studies are required to determine the mechanisms whereby SRF and its interacting factors coordinately contribute to chromatin remodeling.

Finally, although much progress has been made in our understanding of the role of transcription factors in the control of SMC differentiation marker gene expression, some of these studies are performed only in cultured SMCs or SM-like systems. Studies of these factors *in vivo* will provide more compelling information to enhance our knowledge about SMC differentiation and development.

7. Acknowledgments

This work was supported in part by Keio Gijuku Academic Development Funds and Takeda Science Foundation.

8. References

Adam, P.J.; Regan, C.P.; Hautmann, M.B. & Owens, G.K. (2000) Positive- and negative-acting Krüppel-like transcription factors bind a transforming growth factor β control element required for expression of the smooth muscle cell differentiation marker SM22α *in vivo*. *J Biol Chem*. 275:37798-37806

Arber, S. & Caroni, P. (1996) Specificity of single LIM motifs in targeting and LIM/LIM interactions in situ. *Genes Dev*. 10:289-300

Arsenian, S.; Weinhold, B.; Oelgeschläger, M.; Rüther, U. & Nordheim, A. (1998) Serum response factor is essential for mesoderm formation during mouse embryogenesis. *EMBO J*. 17:6289–6299

Bergwerff, M.; Gittenberger-de Groot, A.C.; Wisse, L.J.; DeRuiter, M.C.; Wessels, A.; Martin, J.F. et al. (2000) Loss of function of the *Prx1* and *Prx2* homeobox genes alters architecture of the great elastic arteries and ductus arteriosus. *Virchows Arch*. 436:12-19

Blank, R.S.; Swartz, E.A.; Thompson, M.M.; Olson, E.N. & Owens, G.K. (1995) A retinoic acid-induced clonal cell line derived from multipotential P19 embryonal carcinoma cells expresses smooth muscle characteristics. *Circ Res*. 76:742-749

Buchwalter, G.; Gross, C. & Wasylyk, B. (2004) Ets ternary complex transcription factors. *Gene*. 324:1-14

Cao, D.; Wang, Z.; Zhang, C.L.; Oh, J.; Xing, W.; Li, S. et al. (2005) Modulation of smooth muscle gene expression by association of histone acetyltransferases and deacetylases with myocardin. *Mol Cell Biol*. 25:364-376

Cen, B.; Selvaraj, A.; Burgess, R.C.; Hitzler, J.K.; Ma, Z.; Morris, S.W. et al. (2003) Megakaryoblastic leukemia 1, a potent transcriptional coactivator for serum response factor (SRF), is required for serum induction of SRF target genes. *Mol Cell Biol*. 23:6597-6608

Chang, D.F.; Belaguli, N.S.; Iyer, D.; Roberts, W.B.; Wu, S.P.; Dong, X.R. et al. (2003) Cysteine-rich LIM-only proteins CRP1 and CRP2 are potent smooth muscle differentiation cofactors. *Dev Cell*. 4:107-118

Chang, P.S.; Li, L.; McAnally, J. & Olson, E.N. (2001) Muscle specificity encoded by specific serum response factor-binding sites. *J Biol Chem*. 276:17206-17212

Chen, J.; Kitchen, C.M.; Streb, J.W. & Miano, J.M. (2002) Myocardin: a component of a molecular switch for smooth muscle differentiation. *J Mol Cell Cardiol*. 34:1345-1356

Creemers, E.E.; Sutherland, L.B.; Oh, J.; Barbosa, A.C. & Olson, E.N. (2006) Coactivation of MEF2 by the SAP domain proteins myocardin and MASTR. Mol Cell. 23:83-96

Cserjesi, P.; Lilly, B.; Bryson, L.; Wang, Y.; Sassoon, D.A. & Olson, E.N. (1992) MHox: a mesodermally restricted homeodomain protein that binds an essential site in the muscle creatine kinase enhancer. *Development*. 115:1087-1101

Doi, H.; Iso, T.; Yamazaki, M.; Akiyama, H.; Kanai, H.; Sato, H. et al. (2005) HERP1 inhibits myocardin-induced vascular smooth muscle cell differentiation by interering with SRF binding to CArG box. *Arterioscler Thromb Vasc Biol*. 25:2328-2334

Du, K.L.; Ip, H.S.; Li, J.; Chen, M.; Dandre, F.; Yu, W. et al. (2003) Myocardin is a critical serum response factor cofactor in the transcriptional program regulating smooth muscle cell differentiation. *Mol Cell Biol.* 23:2425-2437

Du, K.L.; Chen, M.; Li, J.; Lepore, J.J.; Mericko, P. & Parmacek, M.S. (2004) Megakaryoblastic leukemia factor-1 transduces cytoskeletal signals and induces smooth muscle cell differentiation from undifferentiated embryonic stem cells. *J Biol Chem.* 279:17578-17586

Fischle, W.; Wang, Y. & Allis, C.D. (2003) Histone and chromatin cross-talk. *Curr Opin Cell Biol.* 15:172-183

Gorski, D.H. & Walsh, K. (2003) Control of vascular cell differentiation by homeobox transcription factors. *Trends Cardiovasc Med.* 13:213-220

Grueneberg, D.A.; Natesan, S.; Alexandre, C. & Gilman, M.Z. (1992) Human and *Drosophila* homeodomain proteins that enhance the DNA-binding activity of serum response factor. *Science.* 257:1089-1095

Hautmann, M.B.; Thompson, M.M.; Swartz, E.A.; Olson, E.N. & Owens, G.K. (1997) Angiotensin II-induced stimulation of smooth muscle α-actin expression by serum response factor and the homeodomain transcription factor MHox. *Circ Res.* 81:600-610

Henderson, J.R.; Macalma, T.; Brown, D.; Richardson, J.A.; Olson, E.N. & Beckerle, M.C. (1999) The LIM protein, CRP1, is a smooth muscle marker. *Dev Dyn.* 214:229-238

Hendrix, J.A.; Wamhoff, B.R.; McDonald, O.G.; Sinha, S.; Yoshida, T. & Owens, G.K. (2005) 5' CArG degeneracy in *smooth muscle α-actin* is required for injury-induced gene suppression in vivo. *J Clin Invest.* 115:418-427

Hinson, J.S.; Medlin, M.D.; Lockman, K.; Taylor, J.M. & Mack, C.P. (2007) Smooth muscle cell-specific transcription is regulated by nuclear localization of the myocardin-related transcription factors. *Am J Physiol Heart Circ Physiol.* 292:H1170-H1180

Huang, J.; Cheng, L.; Li, J.; Chen, M.; Zhou, D.; Lu, M.M. et al. (2008) Myocardin regulates expression of contractile genes in smooth muscle cells and is required for closure of the ductus arteriosus in mice. *J Clin Invest.* 118:515-525

Ihida-Stansbury, K.; McKean, D.M.; Gebb, S.A.; Martin, J.F.; Stevens, T.; Nemenoff, R. et al. (2004) Paired-related homeobox gene *Prx1* is required for pulmonary vascular development. *Circ Res.* 94:1507-1514

Jain, M.K.; Fujita, K.P.; Hsieh, C.M.; Endege, W.O.; Sibinga, N.E.; Yet, S.F. et al. (1996) Molecular cloning and characterization of SmLIM, a developmentally regulated LIM protein preferentially expressed in aortic smooth muscle cells. *J Biol Chem.* 271:10194-10199

Jones, F.S.; Meech, R.; Edelman, D.B.; Oakey, R.J. & Jones, P.L. (2001) Prx1 controls vascular smooth muscle cell proliferation and tenascin-C expression and is upregulated with Prx2 in pulmonary vascular disease. *Circ Res.* 89:131-138

Kawai-Kowase, K.; Kumar, M.S.; Hoofnagle, M.H.; Yoshida, T. & Owens, G.K. (2005) PIAS1 activates the expression of smooth muscle cell differentiation marker genes by interacting with serum response factor and class I basic helix-loop-helix proteins. *Mol Cell Biol.* 25:8009-8023

Kawai-Kowase, K.; Ohshima, T.; Matsui, H.; Tanaka, T.; Shimizu, T.; Iso, T. et al. (2009) PIAS1 mediates TGFβ-induced SM α-actin gene expression through inhibition of KLF4 function-expression by protein sumoylation. *Arterioscler Thromb Vasc Biol.* 29:99-106

Kumar, M.S.; Hendrix, J.A.; Johnson, A.D. & Owens, G.K. (2003) Smooth muscle α-actin gene requires two E-boxes for proper expression in vivo and is a target of class I basic helix-loop-helix proteins. *Circ Res.* 92:840-847

Landerholm, T.E.; Dong, X.R.; Lu, J.; Belaguli, N.S.; Schwartz, R.J. & Majesky, M.W. (1999) A role for serum response factor in coronary smooth muscle differentiation from proepicardial cells. *Development.* 126:2053–2062

Li, J.; Zhu, X.; Chen, M.; Cheng, L.; Zhou, D.; Lu, M.M. et al. (2005) Myocardin-related transcription factor B is required in cardiac neural crest for smooth muscle differentiation and cardiovascular development. *Proc Natl Acad Sci USA.* 102:8916-8921

Li, L.; Miano, J.M.; Mercer, B. & Olson, E.N. (1996) Expression of the *SM22α* promoter in transgenic mice provides evidence for distinct transcriptional regulatory programs in vascular and visceral smooth muscle cells. *J Cell Biol.* 132: 849-859

Li, L.; Liu, Z.; Mercer, B.; Overbeek, P. & Olson, E.N. (1997) Evidence for serum response factor-mediated regulatory networks governing *SM22α* transcription in smooth, skeletal, and cardiac muscle cells. *Dev Biol.* 187:311-321

Li, S.; Wang, D.Z.; Wang, Z.; Richardson, J.A. & Olson, E.N. (2003) The serum response factor coactivator myocardin is required for vascular smooth muscle development. *Proc Natl Acad Sci USA.* 100:9366-9370

Li, S.; Chang, S.; Qi, X.; Richardson, J.A. & Olson, E.N. (2006) Requirement of a myocardin-related transcription factor for development of mammary myoepithelial cells. *Mol Cell Biol.* 26:5797-5808

Lilly, B.; Clark, K.A.; Yoshigi, M.; Pronovost, S.; Wu, M.L.; Periasamy, M. et al. (2010) Loss of the serum response factor cofactor, cysteine-rich protein 1, attenuates neointima formation in the mouse. *Arterioscler Thromb Vasc Biol.* 30:694-701

Liu, Y.; Sinha, S. & Owens, G. (2003) A transforming growth factor-β control element required for SM α-actin expression *in vivo* also partially mediates GKLF-dependent transcriptional repression. *J Biol Chem.* 278:48004-48011

Liu, Y.; Sinha, S.; McDonald, O.G.; Shang, Y.; Hoofnagle, M.H. & Owens, G.K. (2005) Kruppel-like factor 4 abrogates myocardin-induced activation of smooth muscle gene expression. *J Biol Chem.* 280:9719-9727

Long, X.; Bell, R.D.; Gerthoffer, W.T.; Zlokovic, B.V. & Miano, J.M. (2008) Myocardin is sufficient for a smooth muscle-like contractile phenotype. *Arterioscler Thromb Vasc Biol.* 28:1505-1510

Mack, C.P. & Owens, G.K. (1999) Regulation of SM α-actin expression in vivo is dependent on CArG elements within the 5' and first intron promoter regions. *Circ Res.* 84:852–861

Madsen, C.S.; Regan, C.P.; Hungerford, J.E.; White, S.L.; Manabe, I. & Owens, G.K. (1998) Smooth muscle-specific expression of the smooth muscle myosin heavy chain gene in transgenic mice requires 5'-flanking and first intronic DNA sequence. *Circ Res.* 82:908-917

Manabe, I. & Owens, G.K (2001a) CArG elements control smooth muscle subtype-specific expression of *smooth muscle myosin* in vivo. *J Clin Invest.* 107: 823-834

Manabe, I. & Owens, G.K. (2001b) Recruitment of serum response factor and hyperacetylation of histones at smooth muscle-specific regulatory regions during differentiation of a novel P19-derived in vitro smooth muscle differentiation system. *Circ Res.* 88:1127-1134

Mano, T.; Luo, Z.; Malendowicz, S.L.; Evans, T. & Walsh, K. (1999) Reversal of GATA-6 downregulation promotes smooth muscle differentiation and inhibits intimal hyperplasia in balloon-injured rat carotid artery. *Circ Res.* 84:647-654

Martin, J.F.; Bradley, A. & Olson, E.N. (1995) The *paired*-like homeo box gene *MHox* is required for early events of skeletogenesis in multiple lineages. *Gene Dev.* 9:1237-1249

Miano, J.M.; Carlson, M.J.; Spencer, J.A. & Misra, R.P. (2000) Serum response factor-dependent regulation of the smooth muscle calponin gene. *J Biol Chem.* 275:9814-9822

Miano, J.M. (2003) Serum response factor: toggling between disparate programs of gene expression. *J Mol Cell Cardiol.* 35:577-593

Miano, J.M.; Ramanan, N.; Georger, M.A.; de Mesy Bentley, K.L.; Emerson, R.L.; Balza, R.O. et al. (2004) Restricted inactivation of serum response factor to the cardiovascular system. *Proc Natl Acad Sci USA.* 101:17132-17137

Miralles, F.; Posern, G.; Zaromytidou, A.I. & Treisman, R. (2003) Actin dynamics control SRF activity by regulation of its coactivator MAL. *Cell.* 113:329-342

Molkentin, J.D. (2000) The zinc finger-containing transcription factors GATA-4, -5, and -6: ubiquitously expressed regulators of tissue-specific gene expression. *J Biol Chem.* 275:38949-38952

Morrisey, E.E.; Ip, H.S.; Lu, M.M. & Parmacek, M.S. (1996) GATA-6: a zinc finger transcription factor that is expressed in multiple cell lineages derived from lateral mesoderm. *Dev Biol.* 177:309-322

Morrisey, E.E.; Tang, Z.; Sigrist, K.; Lu, M.M.; Jiang, F.; Ip, H.S. et al. (1998) GATA6 regulates HNF4 and is required for differentiation of visceral endoderm in the mouse embryo. *Gene Dev.* 12:3579-3590

Nakamura, S.; Hayashi, K.; Iwasaki, K.; Fujioka, T.; Egusa, H., Yatani, H. et al. (2010) Nuclear import mechanism for myocardin family members and their correlation with vascular smooth muscle cell phenotype. *J Biol Chem.* 285:37314-37323

Nishida, W.; Nakamura, M.; Mori, S.; Takahashi, M.; Ohkawa, Y.; Tadokoro, S. et al. (2002) A triad of serum response factor and the GATA and NK families governs the transcription of smooth and cardiac muscle genes. *J Biol Chem.* 277:7308-7317

Norman, C.; Runswick, M.; Pollock, R. & Treisman, R. (1988) Isolation and properties of cDNA clones encoding SRF, a transcription factor that binds to the *c-fos* serum response element. *Cell.* 55:989-1003

Oh, J.; Richardson, J.A. & Olson, E.N. (2005) Requirement of myocardin-related transcription factor-B for remodeling of branchial arch arteries and smooth muscle differentiation. *Proc Natl Acad Sci USA.* 102:15122-15127

Owens, G.K. & Thompson, M.M. (1986) Developmental changes in isoactin expression in rat aortic smooth muscle cells *in vivo*: relationship between growth and cytodifferentiation. *J Biol Chem.* 261:13373-13380

Owens, G.K. (1995) Regulation of differentiation of vascular smooth muscle cells. *Physiol Rev.* 75:487-517

Owens, G.K.; Kumar, M.S. & Wamhoff, B.R. (2004) Molecular regulation of vascular smooth muscle cell differentiation in development and disease. *Physiol Rev.* 84:767-801

Oyama, Y.; Kawai-Kowase, K.; Sekiguchi, K.; Sato, M.; Sato, H.; Yamazaki, M. et al. (2004) Homeobox protein Hex facilitates serum responsive factor-mediated activation of the SM22α gene transcription in embryonic fibroblasts. *Arterioscler Thromb Vasc Biol.* 24:1602-1607

Philippar, U.; Schratt, G.; Dieterich, C.; Müller, J.M.; Galgóczy, P.; Engel, F.B. et al. (2004) The SRF target gene *Fhl2* antagonizes RhoA/MAL-dependent activation of SRF. *Mol Cell*. 16:867-880

Qiu, P. & Li, L. (2002) Histone acetylation and recruitment of serum responsive factor and CREB-binding protein onto SM22 promoter during SM22 gene expression. *Circ Res*. 90:858-865

Sasazuki, T.; Sawada, T.; Sakon, S.; Kitamura, T.; Kishi, T.; Okazaki, T. et al. (2002) Identification of a novel transcriptional activator, BSAC, by a functional cloning to inhibit tumor necrosis factor-induced cell death. *J Biol Chem*. 277:28853-28860

Schmeichel, K.L. & Beckerle, M.C. (1994) The LIM domain is a modular protein-binding interface. *Cell*. 79:211-219

Schmidt, D. & Müller, S. (2002) Members of the PIAS family act as SUMO ligases for c-Jun and p53 and repress p53 activity. *Proc Natl Acad Sci USA*. 99:2872-2877

Sekiguchi, K.; Kurabayashi, M.; Oyama, Y.; Aihara, Y.; Tanaka, T.; Sakamoto, H. et al. (2001) Homeobox protein Hex induces SMemb/nonmuscle myosin heavy chain-B gene expression through the cAMP-responsive element. *Circ Res*. 88:52-58

Selvaraj, A. & Prywes, R. (2003) Megakaryoblastic leukemia-1/2, a transcriptional co-activator of serum response factor, is required for skeletal myogenic differentiation. *J Biol Chem*. 278:41977-41987

Shang, Y.; Yoshida, T.; Amendt, B.A.; Martin, J.F. & Owens, G.K. (2008) Pitx2 is functionally important in the early stages of vascular smooth muscle cell differentiation. *J Cell Biol*. 181:461-473

Shaw, P.E.; Schröter, H. & Nordheim, A. (1989) The ability of a ternary complex to form over the serum response element correlates with serum inducibility of the human *c-fos* promoter. *Cell*. 56:563-572

Shimizu, R.T.; Blank, R.S.; Jervis, R.; Lawrenz-Smith, S.C. & Owens, G.K. (1995) The smooth muscle α-actin gene promoter is differentially regulated in smooth muscle *versus* non-smooth muscle cells. *J Biol Chem*. 270:7631-7643

Sun, Y.; Boyd, K.; Xu, W.; Ma, J.; Jackson, C.W.; Fu, A. et al. (2006) Acute myeloid leukemia-associated *Mkl1* (*Mrtf-a*) is a key regulator of mammary gland function. *Mol Cell Biol*. 26:5809-5826

Sundberg-Smith, L.J.; DiMichele, L.A.; Sayers, R.L.; Mack, C.P. & Taylor, J.M. (2008) The LIM protein leupaxin is enriched in smooth muscle and functions as an serum response factor cofactor to induce smooth muscle cell gene transcription. *Circ Res*. 102:1502-1511

Thomas, P.Q.; Brown, A. & Beddington, R.S. (1998) *Hex*: a homeobox gene revealing peri-implantation asymmetry in the mouse embryo and an early transient marker of endothelial cell precursors. *Development*. 125:85-94

Treisman, R.; Marais, R. & Wynne, J. (1992) Spatial flexibility in ternary complexes between SRF and its accessory proteins. *EMBO J*. 11:4631-4640

Turla, M.B.; Thompson, M.M.; Corjay, M.H. & Owens, G.K. (1991) Mechanisms of angiotensin II- and arginine vasopressin-induced increases in protein synthesis and content in cultured rat aortic smooth muscle cells: evidence for selective increases in smooth muscle isoactin expression. *Circ Res*. 68:288-289

Wang, D.Z.; Chang, P.S.; Wang, Z.; Sutherland, L.; Richardson, J.A.; Small, E. et al. (2001) Activation of cardiac gene expression by myocardin, a transcriptional cofactor for serum response factor. *Cell*. 105:851-862

Wang, D.Z.; Li, S.; Hockemeyer, D.; Sutherland, L.; Wang, Z.; Schratt, G. et al. (2002) Potentiation of serum response factor activity by a family of myocardin-related transcription factors. *Proc Natl Acad Sci USA*. 99:14855-14860

Wang, J.; Li, A.; Wang, Z.; Feng, X., Olson, E.N. & Schwartz, R.J. (2007) Myocardin sumoylation transactivates cardiogenic genes in pluripotent 10T1/2 fibroblasts. *Mol Cell Biol*. 27:622-632

Wang, Z.; Wang, D.Z.; Pipes, G.C.T. & Olson, E.N. (2003) Myocardin is a master regulator of smooth muscle gene expression. *Proc Natl Acad Sci USA*. 100:7129-7134

Wang, Z.; Wang, D.Z.; Hockemeyer, D.; McAnally, J.; Nordheim, A. & Olson, E.N. (2004) Myocardin and ternary complex factors compete for SRF to control smooth muscle gene expression. *Nature*. 428:185-189

Wei, J.; Gorman, T.E.; Liu, X.; Ith, B.; Tseng, A.; Chen, Z. et al. (2005) Increased neointima formation in cysteine-rich protein 2-deficient mice in response to vascular injury. *Circ Res*. 97:1323-1331

Yang, S.H.; Vickers, E.; Brehm, A.; Kouzarides, T. & Sharrocks, A.D. (2001) Temporal recruitment of the mSin3A-histone deacetylase corepressor complex to the ETS domain transcription factor Elk-1. *Mol Cell Biol*. 21:2802-2814

Yang, S.H.; Jaffray, E.; Hay, R.T. & Sharrocks, A.D. (2003) Dynamic interplay of the SUMO and ERK pathways in regulating Elk-1 transcriptional activity. Mol Cell. 12:63-74

Yang, S.H. & Sharrocks, A.D. (2004) SUMO promotes HDAC-mediated transcriptional repression. *Mol Cell*. 13:611-617

Yin, F. & Herring, B.P. (2005) GATA-6 can act as a positive or negative regulator of smooth muscle-specific gene expression. *J Biol Chem*. 280:4745-4752

Yoshida, T.; Sinha, S.; Dandré, F.; Wamhoff, B.R.; Hoofnagle, M.H.; Kremer, B.E. et al. (2003) Myocardin is a key regulator of CArG-dependent transcription of multiple smooth muscle marker genes. *Circ Res*. 92:856-864

Yoshida, T.; Hoofnagle, M.H. & Owens, G.K. (2004a) Myocardin and Prx1 contribute to angiotensin II-induced expression of smooth muscle α-actin. *Circ Res*. 94:1075-1082

Yoshida, T.; Kawai-Kowase, K. & Owens, G.K. (2004b) Forced expression of myocardin is not sufficient for induction of smooth muscle differentiation in multipotential embryonic cells. *Arterioscler Thromb Vasc Biol*. 24:1596-1601

Yoshida, T. & Owens, G.K. (2005) Molecular determinants of vascular smooth muscle cell diversity. *Circ Res*. 96:280-291

Yoshida, T.; Gan, Q.; Shang, Y. & Owens, G.K. (2007) Platelet-derived growth factor-BB represses smooth muscle cell marker genes via changes in binding of MKL factors and histone deacetylases to their promoters. *Am J Physiol Cell Physiol*. 292:C886-C895

Yoshida, T.; Gan, Q. & Owens, G.K. (2008a) Krüppel-like factor 4, Elk-1, and histone deacetylases cooperatively suppress smooth muscle cell differentiation markers in response to oxidized phospholipids. *Am J Physiol Cell Physiol*. 295:C1175-C1182

Yoshida, T.; Kaestner, K.H. & Owens, G.K. (2008b) Conditional deletion of Krüppel-like factor 4 delays downregulation of smooth muscle cell differentiation markers but accelerates neointimal formation following vascular injury. *Circ Res*. 102:1548-1557

Zhou, J.; Hu, G. & Herring, B.P. (2005) Smooth muscle-specific genes are differentially sensitive to inhibition by Elk-1. *Mol Cell Biol*. 25:9874-9885

3

Trans Fatty Acids and Human Health

Sebastjan Filip and Rajko Vidrih
Biotechnical Faculty,
Department of Food Science and Technology,
University of Ljubljana,
Slovenia

1. Introduction

According to various studies, fats of animal and vegetable origins satisfy 22% to 42% of the daily energy demands of human beings (Srinivasan et al., 2006; Wagner et al., 2008; Willet, 2006). Some fats, and especially those that are hydrogenated, contain *trans* fatty acids (TFAs), i.e. unsaturated fatty acids with at least one double bond in a *trans* configuration (Craig-Schmidt, 2006). This *trans*-double-bond configuration results in a greater bond angle than for the *cis* configuration, thus producing a more extended fatty-acid carbon chain that is more similar to that of the saturated fatty acids (SFAs), rather than to that of the *cis*-unsaturated double-bond-containing fatty acids (Fig. 1) (Moss, 2006; Oomen et al., 2001).

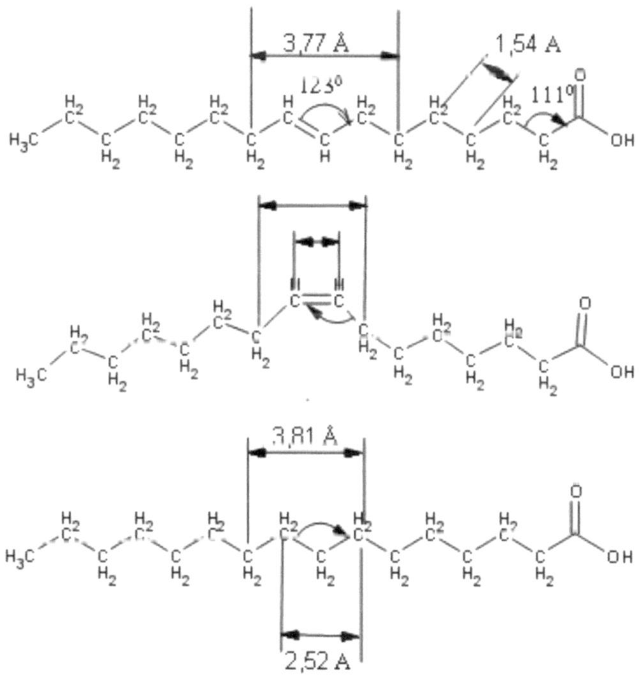

Fig. 1. Structure of different isomers of C16 (Willett, 2006)

Fat is a thus major source of energy for the body, and it also aids in the absorption of vitamins A, D, E and K, and of the carotenoids. Both animal-derived and plant-derived food products contain fat, and when eaten in moderation, fat is important for correct growth and development, and for the maintenance of good health. As a food ingredient, fat provides taste, consistency and stability, and helps us to feel 'full'. In addition, parents should be aware that fats are an especially important source of calories and nutrients for infants and toddlers (up to 2 years of age), who have the highest energy needs per unit body weight of any age group.

However, SFAs and TFAs raise low-density lipoprotein (LDL; or 'bad') cholesterol levels in the blood, thereby increasing the risk of heart disease. Indeed, prospective epidemiological studies and case-control studies support a major role for TFAs in the risk of cardiovascular disease, and therefore dietary cholesterol can also contribute to heart disease (see below). Unsaturated fats, which can be mono-unsaturated or polyunsaturated, do not raise LDL cholesterol and are beneficial to health when consumed in moderation.

Hydrogenated oils tend to have a higher TFA content than oils that do not contain hydrogenated fats. In the partially hydrogenated soybean oil, which is the major source of TFAs worldwide, the main isomer is *trans*-10 C18:1. In the European countries with the highest TFA intake (The Netherlands and Norway), consumption of partially hydrogenated fish oils was common until the mid-1990s, after which they largely disappeared from the dietary fat intake. These partially hydrogenated fish oils included a variety of very-long-chain TFAs. Recent findings from Asian countries (India and Iran) have indicated a very high intake of TFAs from partially hydrogenated soybean oil (4% of energy). Thus, TFAs appear to be a particular problem in developing countries where soybean oil is used.

Formation of these *trans* double bonds thus impacts on the physical properties of a fatty acid. Fatty acids that contain a *trans* double bond have the potential for closer packing and alignment of their acyl chains, which will result in decreased molecular mobility (Willett, 2006). Therefore, the oil fluidity will be reduced when compared to that of fatty acids that contain a *cis* double bond. Partial hydrogenation of unsaturated oils results in the isomerisation of some of the remaining double bonds and the migration of others, producing an increase in the TFA content and a hardening of the fat. It has been shown that foods that contain hydrogenated oils tend to have a higher TFA content than those that do not contain hydrogenated oils (Moss, 2006; Oomen et al., 2001). Nevertheless, the hydrogenation of oils, such as corn oil, can result in both *cis* and *trans* double bonds, which are generally located anywhere between carbon 4 and carbon 16 of the fatty acids. One of the major TFAs is elaidic acid (*trans*-9 C18:1), although during hydrogenation of polyunsaturated fatty acids (PUFAs), small amounts of several other TFAs are produced, including: *trans*-9,*cis*-12 C18:2; *cis*-9,*trans*-12 C18:2; *cis*-9,*cis*-12,*trans*-15 C18:3; and *cis*-5,*cis*-8,*cis*-11,*cis*-14,*trans*-17 C20:5 (Craig-Schmidt, 2006; Wagner et al., 2008). Conversely, one way to produce 'zero' levels of TFAs is through the *trans*-esterification reaction between vegetable oils and solid fatty acids, like C8:0, C12:0, C14:0 and C16:0.

Correlations between high intake of industrially produced TFAs (IP-TFAs) and increased risk of coronary heart disease (CHD) have been reported (Stender et al., 2006; Tarrago-Trani et al., 2006), and lowering the intake of TFAs can also reduce the incidence of CHD (Willett, 2006). Estimates based on changes in plasma concentrations of LDL and high-density lipoprotein (HDL) indicate around a 4% reduction in CHD incidence, while based on epidemiological associations, when TFA intake is lowered by 2% (5 g/day), the estimates indicate a >20% reduction in CHD incidence (Katan, 2006; Moss, 2006). In The Netherlands, a major reduction in the TFA content of retail foods was achieved in the 1990s through the efforts of the industry and with minimal government intervention. Society pressure is also now helping to reduce the TFA content of 'fast foods'. This illustrates the feasibility of reducing TFAs in fast foods without increasing the saturated fats, with the daily intake kept as low as possible, to minimise the health risks (Stender et al., 2006).

Comparison of the different recommendations for macronutrients in some European countries, for the World Health Organisation/ Food and Agriculture Organisation of the United Nations (WHO/FAO), and in the USA and Canada, are given in Table 1. Most of the recommendations are the same, or are in similar ranges. The recommendations for protein, however, are expressed differently, either as grams per day or grams per kilogram per day, and usually without any indication of a representative weight at each age to allow conversion of one to the other. The Joint FAO/WHO/United Nations University (UNU) Expert Consultation of 1985 (WHO, 1985) defined the protein requirement of an individual as "the lowest level of dietary protein intake that will balance the losses of nitrogen from the body in persons maintaining an energy balance at modest levels of physical activity". The human body can synthesise both SFAs and mono-unsaturated fatty acids (MUFAs) from acetate, whereas PUFAs (in both the n–6 linoleic acid and n–3 linolenic acid series) are required in the diet, and they are therefore known as essential fatty acids. These essential fatty acids are important for various cell-membrane functions, such as fluidity, permeability, activity of membrane-bound enzymes and receptors, and signal transduction. Linoleic and linolenic acids can be elongated and desaturated in the body, and transformed into biologically active substances, like prostaglandins, prostacyclins and leukotrienes. These substances participate in the regulation of blood pressure, renal function, blood coagulation, inflammatory and immunological reactions, and many other functions (Nordic Nutrition Recommendations, 2004). The DACH Reference Values for Nutrient Supply (DACH, 2000) for total fat intake in adults (not more than 30% of the energy intake) are related to light work, heavy muscle work (not more than 35% of energy intake) and extremely heavy work (not more than 40% of energy intake). SFAs should not exceed 10% of energy intake. PUFAs should provide about 7%, and up to 10% if SFAs provide more than 10% of energy intake. MUFAs should constitute the rest. TFAs should contribute not more than 1% of the daily energy. The ratio of n–6 linoleic acid to n–3 linolenic acid should be about 5:1 (WHO/FAO, 2002). These fatty acids compete for the metabolic enzymes, and it is therefore important to maintain a balance between them (Nordic Nutrition Recommendations, 2004). The Nordic Nutrition Recommendations indicate the limiting of the intake of SFAs plus TFAs to about 10% of the daily energy and the total fat intake to 30% of the daily energy (25%-30%) (Filip et al., 2010). The recommendations for carbohydrate intake are from 50%of the daily energy in the DACH (2000) reference values, to 55% (50%-60%) in the Nordic Nutrition Recommendations (2004), 55%-75% by WHO/FAO, and 45%-65% in the USA/ Canada recommendations, as detailed in Table 1.

Component	NNR (2004)	DACH (2000)	WHO/FAO (2002)	Euro Diet (2000)	USA/Canada AMDR (2002)
Total energy from fat (%)	30 (25-35)	30	15-30	<30	20-35
SFAs (%)	≤10	10	<10	<10	Minimise
PUFAs (%)	5 (10)	7-10	6-10	-	-
n-6 FAs (%)	4 (9)	2.5	5-8	4-8	5-10 (linoleic)
n-3 FAs (%)	1	0.5	1-2	2 (linolenic)	0.6-1.2
TFAs (%)	Included in SFAs	1	<1	<2	Minimise
MUFAs (%)	10-15	The rest of the total			-
Total energy from carbohydrates (%)	55 (50-60)	50	55-75	>55	45-65
Energy from sugars (%)	<10	30	<10		<25
Fibre (g/day)	25-35 (3 g/MJ) (12.5 g/1000 kcal)				25-38 (14 g/1000 kcal)
Energy from proteins (%)	15 (10-20)	8-10	10-15	-	10-35
Cholesterol (mg/day)	300		<300		Minimise
Salt (sodium) (g/day)	5-6 (2.3-2.7)		<5 (2)		

NNR, Nordic Nutrition Recommendations; DACH, Austria-Germany-Switzerland Reference Values for Nutrient Supply; WHO, World Health Organisation; FAO, Food and Agriculture Organisation of the United Nations; AMDR; acceptable macronutrient distribution; FAs, fatty acids; SFAs, saturated fatty acids; PUFAs, polyunsaturated fatty acids; TFA, *trans* fatty acids; MUFAs, mono-unsaturated fatty acids.

Table 1. Comparison of reference daily intakes for adults according to different recommendations around the World (Pavlovic et al., 2007)

As indicated above, prospective epidemiological studies and case-control studies using adipose-tissue analyses have confirmed a major role for TFAs in the risk of CHD. The magnitude of the association with CHD is considerably stronger than for SFAs, and it is stronger than that predicted for the effects of TFAs on LDL and HDL cholesterol (Katan, 2006; Tarrago-Trani et al., 2006). In this context, it needs to be considered that data for the Russian Federation show that every year 1,005 people per 100,000 of the population between 25 and 64 years of age die because of circulatory system diseases (WHO, 2008). As a consequence influence of TFAs on CHD, in 2003, the United States FDA issued a ruling that required food manufacturers to list the TFAs in the nutritional facts labels of all packaged food products (FDA, 2003), with the food industry being given until 1 January, 2006 to comply. Along with these growing health concerns about TFAs, this mandate led to marked changes in the fat and oil industries, with newer technologies developed to reduce the TFA contents of fats and oils used in the manufacture of food products. Conversely, given the labelling mandate and these technological advances, it is possible that food products traditionally considered to be sources of TFAs are now much lower in, or indeed do not contain, TFAs (Borra et al., 2007). Then in late 2006, New York City became the first major city in the United States to pass a regulation limiting IP-TFAs in restaurants. This has served as a model for others to follow, with these regulations including: a maximum level per serving size of 0.5 g TFAs; a distinction between frying and baking, with a phased-in implementation; a help centre to assist restaurants to make the switch to more healthy options; and plans to evaluate the regulation and its impact on CHD (Borra et al., 2007).

Accurate quantification of C18:1 TFAs in food products is thus an important issue, with policies recently implemented in different countries to limit their consumption and their occurrence in food products because of their relationship with CHD (Carriquiry et al., 2008; Chen et al., 2007).

2. History

Margarine was invented in 1869 by Hippolyte Mège Mouriès, a French food research chemist, in response to a request by Napoleon III for a wholesome alternative to butter. It is not entirely clear whether the primary aim was the betterment of the working classes or the economics of the food supply to the French army. In the laboratory, Mège Mouriès solidified purified fat, after which the resulting substance was pressed in a thin cloth, which formed stearine and discharged oil. This oil formed the basis of the butter substitute. For the new product, Mège Mouriès used margaric acid, a fatty-acid component isolated in 1813 by the Frenchman Michel Eugène Chevreuil. While analysing the fatty acids that are the building blocks of fats, he singled out this one and named it margaric acid, because of the lustrous pearly drops that reminded him of the Greek word for pearls, i.e. margarites (Chen et al., 2008; Craig-Schmidt, 2006).

In 1871, Mège Mouriès sold this know-how to the Dutch firm Jurgens, which is now part of Unilever. In the early days, margarine contained two types of fat: a large proportion of animal fat and a small proportion of vegetable fat. As time passed, the small vegetable-fat element increased, through two specific stages in the process. First, by improving the process of refining vegetable oils, use could be made of a greater variety of liquid oils and a higher proportion of solid vegetable fats. Secondly, through the development of processes for turning liquid oils into solid fats on a commercial scale, use could be made of larger quantities of liquid vegetable oils (Filip, 2010).

During the early years of this period, in the late 1800s, TFA intake from partially hydrogenated vegetable oils was minimal. Indeed, it was not until the late 1800s that the process of partial hydrogenation of oils was invented in Europe. These partially hydrogenated oils apparently entered the United States food supply by 1920. Although the rate of increase before 1950 is not completely clear, by 1950 the amount of IP-TFAs in the food supply was quite substantial. Partly because of economic effects during World War II, margarine production rose rapidly as a replacement for butter (Chen et al., 2007). Then during the 1960s, margarine became viewed as a healthy alternative to butter because of its absence of cholesterol and its low content of SFAs. Thus, consumption increased further, and so margarine, which was heavily hydrogenated at that time, became widespread in the food supply and was the major source of IP-TFAs. This phenomenon is illustrated in Figure 2. The total TFAs consumption was approximately 2% to 3% of the food energy. Since then, the sources of TFAs have changed, from mainly margarine to mainly deep-fried fast foods and commercially baked products, although per capita, the intake has remained roughly the same (Willett, 2006).

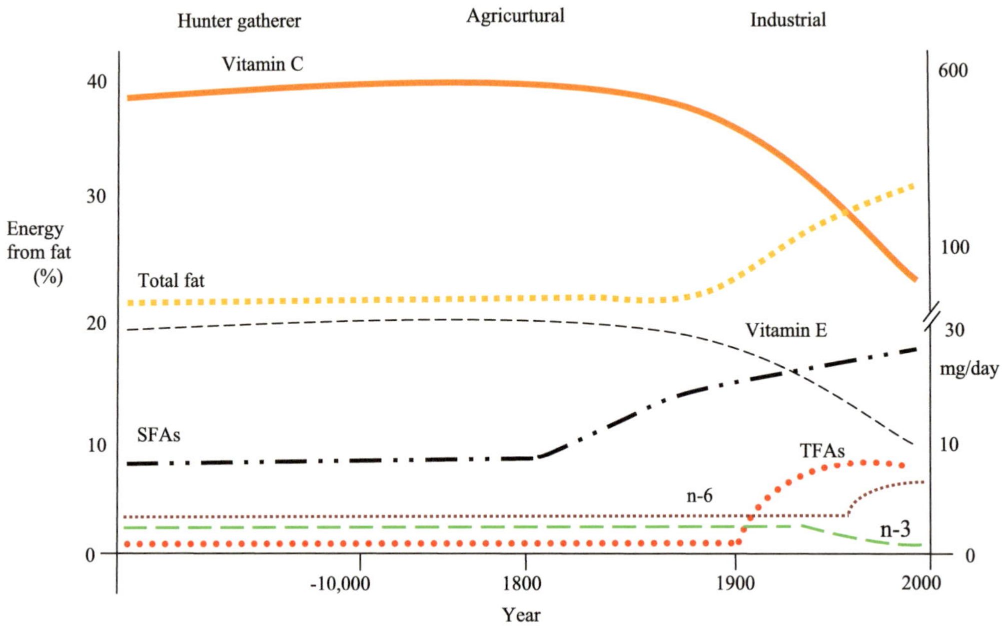

Fig. 2. Relative food energy supplied by the different fatty acids, and the predicted changes for the food industry and fat hydrogenation (Simopoulos, 2004)

After World War II, the process of making hydrogenated and hardened fats from cheaper sources of vegetable oils was widely adopted. Margarines were developed and marketed as alternatives to butter, and vegetable shortening increasingly replaced animal fats in cooking (Albers et al., 2008). However, as early as 1975, at what is now the University of Glamorgan in South Wales, a group of scientists led by Leo Thomas suspected that deaths from CHD were connected with this eating of partially hydrogenated fats. It is now generally accepted that TFAs are actually worse for health than the SFAs that they were designed to replace (Blake, 2009).

3. Studies of *trans* fatty acids

Increases in 'civilization diseases' in the developed world led scientists to investigate why this was happening. While there is enough food that is also cheaper and more accessible than ever before in the developed world, we are witnessing more and more overweight and obese populations. Modern populations have worse nutrition habits than ever before, except for some specific small social groups e.g. through religion, ecology and ethnic aspects (WHO, 2008). Obesity is a severe health issue that is characterised by fat accumulation and defined by means of the body mass index (BMI), as body weight [kg]/ (height [m])^2. According to this index, different obesity levels have been described, ranging from overweight (BMI, 25.0-29.9), through obese (BMI, 30.0-40.0) to the most detrimental stage, morbid obesity (BMI, ≥40) (Garaulet et al., 2011). The relevance of this classification is that as the BMI increases, the morbidity and mortality risks also increase (Bray, 2003). Furthermore, regional fat accumulation is an important factor in the development of obesity-related alterations. It has been suggested that excess visceral fat is more detrimental than excess subcutaneous fat, because visceral deposits release free fatty acids directly into the portal vein (Bray, 2003). The fatty acid pattern carried to the portal circulation is of great importance, because different fatty acids show distinct atherogenicities, depending on the chain length and degree of unsaturation. Here, SFAs have been associated with increased cardio-metabolic risk, while n-3 and n-9 unsaturated fatty acids have been proposed as protective agents against these alterations (Garaulet et al., 2011).

3.1 Studies in animals

In milk fat, TFAs are produced by anaerobic fermentation of PUFAs in the rumen of lactating cows (Destaillats et al., 2007; Fournier et al., 2006). This fermentation process is called biohydrogenation, and it results in TFAs that can be further metabolised in the mammary gland. Accurate estimations of fatty-acid compositions are vital not only for the definition of the nutrient composition of foods, but also to accurately determine treatment effects that can alter the fatty-acid composition of the foods (Ascherio, 2002; Burdge et al., 2005; Kummerow et al., 2004; Murrieta et al., 2003; Triantafillou et al., 2003).

There is a considerable overlap of TFA isomers in fats of ruminant origin and in partially hydrogenated vegetable oils, as they have many isomers in common. However, there are considerable differences in the amounts of individual TFAs in these sources. While there is evidence of unfavourable effects of TFAs from hydrogenated vegetable oils on LDL and other risk factors for atherosclerosis, at present it is not certain which of the component(s) of the TFAs created by chemical hydrogenation are responsible for these a negative metabolic effects (Ascherio, 2002). Prospective studies addressing the effects of TFA intake on CHD risk, where estimates of TFA intake were based on dietary protocols, have mostly been carried out in populations with a relatively low intake of dairy or ruminant TFAs (Pfeuffer & Schrezenmeir, 2006). Nevertheless, the biggest effects of fatty-acid composition and the nutritive quality of foods of animal origin, like meat and milk products, depend on the feed quality and the health of the animals.

3.2 Studies in humans

These TFA-containing fats can be incorporated into both foetal and adult tissues, although the transfer rate through the placenta continues to be a contradictory subject. In preterm infants and healthy term babies, the *trans* isomers have been inversely correlated with infant birth mass (Koletzko & Müller, 1990). Maternal milk reflects precisely the mother's daily dietary intake of TFAs, with presence of 2% to 5% total TFAs in human milk. The levels of linoleic acid in human milk are increased by a high *trans* diet, although long-chain polyunsaturated TFAs remain mostly unaffected (Koletzko, 1992; Koletzko & Desci, 1994). Alterations in the maternal dietary intake of PUFAs cause similar changes in the PUFA content of their milk. Several investigations have shown that supplementation of the consumed fat with fish oils increases the amounts of C20:5n-3 and C22:6n-3 in the milk and in the maternal and infant erythrocyte lipids. Likewise, infant tissues incorporate the TFAs from the maternal milk, increasing the levels of linoleic acid and decreasing arachidonic acid and docosahexaenoic acid. This suggests an inhibitory effect of TFAs on the liver n-6 fatty-acid-desaturase activity (Jensen et al., 1992).

As opposed to blood and liver, the brain appears to be protected from TFA accumulation in experimental animals, although no data have yet been reported for newborn humans (Larqué, 2001). A significant interaction between diet and pregnancy was shown for the activities of Δ6-desaturase and glucose 6-phosphatase in liver microsomes: dietary TFAs decreased the activities of both of these enzymes, although only in pregnant rats (Larqué et al., 2000; Larqué & Zamora, 2000; Larqué et al., 2003). In Spain, TFAs in human milk were investigated by Boatella et al. (Boatella et al., 1993), and they showed that the average content of TFAs in 38 samples was 0.98% of the milk fatty acids. This value is lower than that for human milk from other developed countries, where consumption of hydrogenated fats is higher. In a study by Chen et al. (Chen et al., 1995) on TFAs in human milk in Canada, the mean total TFA content was 7.19% (±3.03%) of the total milk fatty acids, with a range from 0.10% to 17.15%.

The compelling data linking dietary TFAs to increased risk of CHD have originated from large, prospective, population-based studies, which included from 667 to 80,082 men and women across different age groups who were monitored for six to 20 years. This link has also been seen in controlled feeding trials (Oomen et al., 2001). Among these studies, there are: the United States Health Professional's follow-up study; the Finnish alpha-tocopherol, β-carotene Cancer Prevention Study; the United States nurse's health study (with 14-year and 20-year follow-up) (Willett, 2006); and the Dutch Zutphen elderly study (Oomen et al., 2001). These studies are consistent in their finding of a strong positive association between TFA intake and the risk of CHD. Interestingly, a weaker correlation between SFA intake and the risk of CHD also has been reported (Willettt, 2006).

The Zutphen elderly study included 667 men from 64 to 84 years of age who were free of CHD at baseline (Oomen et al., 2001). Dietary surveys were used to establish the food consumption patterns of the participants. Information on risk factors and diet were obtained in 1985, 1990 and 1995. After a 10-year follow-up, from 1985-1995, there were 98 cases of fatal or non-fatal CHD. The findings showed that over this period, the mean TFA intake decreased from 4.3% to 1.9% of the food energy. After adjustments for age, BMI, smoking and dietary covariates, TFA intake at baseline was positively associated with 10-year risk of CHD. Thus, a high intake of TFAs, which included all types of isomers, contributed to the risk of CHD. A substantial decrease in TFA intake, which was mainly due to the lowering of the TFA content in edible fats in the Dutch industry, therefore had a large impact on public health (Craig-Schmidt, 2006; Larqué et al., 2001).

In multiple and rigorous randomised trials, the intake of TFAs has been consistently shown to have adverse effects on blood lipids, and most notably on the LDL/HDL cholesterol ratio, which is a strong marker of cardiovascular risk. When a mixture of TFA isomers obtained by partial hydrogenation of vegetable oils is used to replace oleic acid, there is a dose-dependent increase in the LDL/HDL ratio. The relationship between the levels of TFAs as the percentage of energy and the increase in the LDL/HDL ratio appears to be approximately linear, with no evidence of a threshold at low levels of TFA intake, and with a slope that is twice as steep as that observed by replacing oleic acid with a SFA (Borra et al., 2007; Mensink & Nestel, 2009). Studies comparing animal and vegetable TFAs have shown similar effects on the total/HDL cholesterol ratio. The effects of TFAs on lipoproteins from both sources appeared at doses exceeding 2% of energy (Mensink & Nestel, 2009). The average impact of TFA-induced changes in the LDL/HDL ratio corresponds to tens of thousands of premature deaths in the United States alone (Mensink & Nestel, 2009). Although dramatic, this effect is substantially smaller than the increase in cardiovascular mortality associated with TFA intake in epidemiological studies, suggesting that other mechanisms are likely to contribute to the toxicity of TFAs (Ascherio, 2006). Thus, although there is accumulating evidence linking inflammatory proteins and other biomarkers to CHD, lipid concentrations in the blood remain one of the strongest and most consistent predictors of risk. Therefore, the LDL/HDL cholesterol ratio is probably the best marker to date for estimating the effects of TFAs on plasma lipids, which are most likely relevant to CHD incidence and mortality (Larqué & Zamora, 2001).

Further rigorous randomised trials to establish the effects of hydrogenated fats and TFA intake on individual lipoprotein classes started in 1990, when a report from The Netherlands suggested that a diet enriched in elaidic acid (*trans*-9 C18:1) increases the total and LDL cholesterol concentrations and decreased HDL cholesterol concentrations, compared to a diet enriched in oleic acid. In contrast, enrichment of the diet with SFAs increases LDL cholesterol, but has no effect on HDL cholesterol, thus resulting in a smaller adverse change than in the case of elaidic acid (Mensink & Katan, 1993; Mensink & Nestel, 2009).

3.3 Studies of antioxidant effects

In one study (Filip et al., 2011), the effects of natural antioxidants on formation of TFAs during heat treatment of sunflower oil was investigated. The data from the fatty acid analyses are summarized in Table 2. Here, the non-treated control sunflower oil had a 7.5% palmitic acid content, with 4.5% stearic acid, 25.0% oleic acid, and 60.5% linoleic acid, as is usual for the common (not high in oleic acid) sunflower oils; these data compare well with those of other studies (Sánchez-Gimeno et al., 2008; Bansal, Zhou, Tan, Neo, & Lo, 2009). This sunflower oil was purchased directly from a supplier of oils that are used mainly by small food enterprises (Zvijezda d.d., Zagreb, Croatia). The natural antioxidant extract of rosemary (*Rosmarinus officinalis* L.) that was added to this sunflower oil (SOR) was purchased directly from Vitiva d.d., Markovci, Slovenia (INOLENS4®; Product N° 301770; Batch N°. LAB. 09-779004), and had a carnosic acid content of 4.30%. Similarly, the lutein added to this sunflower oil (SOL) was from pelargonium (2.2% mixture), as obtained from Etol, d.o.o., Celje, Slovenia (NovaSoL® Lutein; Aquanova AG, Birkenweg 8-10, Germany).

The initial levels of the total TFAs in the samples was 0.91% (±0.01%). This compares with the range from 0.15% to 6.03% reported by Bansal et al. (2009) for TFAs in refined oils (soybean, corn, sunflower, high oleic sunflower, low erucic rapeseed and high erucic rapeseed oils). The aim in this study with the sunflower oil was to evaluate the effects of heat on this TFA composition of the oil when subjected to treatment representative of deep-fat frying (185 ±5°C). Since sunflower oil is in common use for deep-fat frying, it is particularly important to know what species and levels of TFA isomers appear during such heat treatment (Filip et al., 2011; Martin et al., 2007).

In this study, we focussed mainly on these effects of heat on the TFAs with 18 carbon atoms, which were the most represented. Prior to the treatment, the content of *trans* C 18:1, t-9 was 0.67% (±0.08%). At the end of the heat treatment (120 h at 185 ±5°C), in the control sunflower oil the *trans* C 18:1, t-9 increased to 1.12% (±0.14%), in SOR, to 0.99% (±0.04%), and in SOL, to 0.91% (±0.01%). Within each treatment, these increases were significantly different from the

Component	Time (h)					
	0	24	48	72	96	120
Sunflower oil (control)						
SFAs (%)	12.43 ±0.13^{b}	12.54 ±0.12^{b}	12.77 ±0.58^{b}	14.02 ±0.49^{ab}	14.62 ±2.63^{b}	14.76 ±0.35^{a}
MUFAs (%)	26.13 ±0.68^{d}	28.56 ±1.22^{c}	29.40 ±1.06^{cb}	29.84 ±0.85^{abc}	31.18 ±0.96^{ab}	31.59 ±0.35^{a}
PUFAs (%)	61.44 ±0.75^{a}	58.50 ±1.23^{b}	57.83 ±1.33^{b}	56.14 ±1.15^{bc}	56.20 ±3.01^{bc}	53.64 ±2.08^{c}
n6 PUFAs (%)	61.13 ±0.76^{a}	58.20 ±1.23^{b}	57.82 ±1.34^{b}	55.64 ±1.17^{bc}	55.66 ±3.03^{bc}	53.05 ±2.08^{c}
n3 PUFAs (%)	0.31 ±0.02^{b}	0.30 ±0.00^{b}	0.31 ±0.02^{b}	0.34 ±0.01^{a}	0.35 ±0.02^{a}	0.36 ±0.01^{a}
n6/n3	199.93 ±15.84^{a}	192.92 ±4.71^{a}	185.41 ±11.56^{a}	163.68 ±7.73^{b}	159.78 ±16.01^{b}	149.37 ±6.99^{b}
TFAs (%)	0.91 ±0.03^{d}	0.99 ±0.06^{d}	1.25 ±0.07^{c}	1.46 ±0.15^{b}	1.56 ±0.09^{b}	1.71 ±0.07^{a}
Sunflower oil with rosemary extract (SOR; 1.0g/kg oil)						
SFAs (%)	12.39 ±0.57c	12.70 ±0.48c	12.74 ±0.41c	13.80 ±0.29^{b}	14.02 ±0.70^{ab}	14.68 ±0.61^{a}
MUFAs (%)	25.72 ±1.92bc	25.37 ±1.67c	28.73 ±0.81ab	25.69 ±3.46^{bc}	28.87 ±0.40^{ab}	30.25 ±2.24^{a}
PUFAs (%)	61.88 ±1.67a	61.93 ±1.43a	58.53 ±0.57bc	60.51 ±3.33^{ab}	57.11 ±0.55^{cd}	55.07 ±1.71^{d}
n6 PUFAs (%)	61.58 ±1.66a	61.62 ±1.43a	58.13 ±0.56bc	60.07 ±3.32^{ab}	56.56 ±0.57^{cd}	54.45 ±1.72^{d}
n3 PUFAs (%)	0.31 ±0.02b	0.31 ±0.01b	0.31 ±0.01b	0.33 ±0.01^{a}	0.33 ±0.01^{a}	0.35 ±0.01^{a}
n6/n3	201.53 ±10.73a	198.56 ±6.72a	186.36 ±5.67b	179.91 ±9.26^{bc}	169.54 ±7.89^{c}	154.65 ±3.96^{d}
TFAs (%)	0.91 ±0.09d	0.82 ±0.02d	1.02 ±0.05c	1.24 ±0.20^{c}	1.35 ±0.10^{b}	1.55 ±0.16^{a}
Sunflower oil with lutein (SOL; 0.1g/kg oil)						
SFAs (%)	12.51 ±0.72^{c}	12.36 ±0.35^{c}	13.06 ±0.36^{bc}	13.21 ±0.65^{bc}	13.91 ±0.54^{ab}	14.84 ±0.96^{a}
MUFAs (%)	26.25 ±2.60^{b}	25.05 ±0.64^{b}	28.22 ±2.49^{b}	27.55 ±2.79^{b}	28.07 ±0.85^{b}	32.79 ±1.63^{a}
PUFAs (%)	61.24 ±2.82^{ab}	62.59 ±0.72^{a}	58.72 ±2.47^{b}	59.24 ±3.15^{b}	58.02 ±1.37^{b}	52.37 ±0.74^{c}
n6 PUFAs (%)	60.93 ±2.83^{ab}	62.29 ±0.72^{a}	58.31 ±2.48^{bc}	58.80 ±3.15^{bc}	57.51 ±1.40^{c}	51.80 ±0.73^{d}
n3 PUFAs (%)	0.31 ±0.02^{b}	0.31 ±0.01^{b}	0.32 ±0.01^{ab}	0.33 ±0.02^{ab}	0.33 ±0.02^{ab}	0.35 ±0.03^{a}
n6/n3	199.10 ±16.69^{ab}	203.99 ±5.54^{a}	180.24 ±9.67^{bc}	177.99 ±19.87^{c}	174.65 ±12.92^{c}	149.07 ±10.26^{d}
TFAs (%)	0.91 ±0.06^{c}	0.84 ±0.03^{c}	1.01 ±0.02^{b}	1.23 ±0.16^{b}	1.28 ±0.11^{b}	1.43 ±0.04^{a}

SFAs, saturated fatty acids; MUFAs, mono-unsaturated fatty acids; PUFAs, polyunsaturated fatty acids; TFAs, trans fatty acids; $^{a, b, c, d}$ Values followed by a different letter are significantly different along each row according to the Duncan test (P <0.05);

Table 2. Effect of cooking heat (185 ±5°C) on the fatty acids composition of sunflower oil, with the addition of the natural antioxidants of a rosemary extract (SOR) and of lutein (SOL) (Filip et al., 2011) start to the end of the treatment (P <0.001), and also the decreases in *trans* C 18:1, t-9 production with the addition of rosemary oil and lutein were statistically significant in comparison with the control (SOR vs. sunflower oil: 0.32% vs. 0.45%; SOL vs. sunflower oil: 0.24% vs. 0.45%; P <0.001 for both). These data are consistent with an earlier report where there were reductions in *trans*-isomerisation and polar compounds in model oils when α-tocopherol (1%) was added as an antioxidant (Tsuzuki et al., 2008).

When the content of the total TFAs is expressed as the sum of the unsaturated FAs with at least one *trans* double bond, these increased significantly from the initial control sunflower oil of 0.91% (±0.03%), to 1.71% (±0.07%) at 120 h, with significantly lower increases for SOR and SOL, to 1.55% (±0.16%) and 1.43% (±0.04%), respectively (Table 2). Indeed, these differences among treatments were statistically significant (P <0.001) at each step of the heat treatment (24, 48, 72, 96, 120 h). These data relating particularly to the increases in TFAs are comparable to those of Gamel et al. (1999), where they looked at the effects of phenol extracts on TFA formation during frying. A linear relationship between the amounts of elaidic acid and the number of frying cycles has also been reported (Bansal et al., 2009).

According to the nutritional recommendations of the various health authorities, the content of SFAs should not exceed 30% in dietary fats. Sunflower oil thus fits into this recommendation, even though its content in the control sunflower oil increased from 12.43% (±0.13%) to 14.76% (±0.35%), and in the SOR and SOL to 14.68% (±0.61%) and 14.84% (±0.96%), respectively (Table 2).

The initial PUFA:SFA ratio here was 4.94 (±0.10), and after the full time of the heat exposure for the control sunflower oil, this was significantly decreased to 3.64 (±0.14) (P ≤0.05). Meanwhile, , for the SOR and SOL at 120 h of heat treatment, the PUFA:SFA ratio decreased to 3.75 (±0.09; P <0.001) and 3.54 (±0.18; P <0.001). As higher PUFA/SFA ratios are more nutritionally appropriate, these data confirm that the heat treatments of this sunflower oil also worsened this nutritional factor.

4. *Trans* fatty acids and legislation

Governments are increasingly recognising that the risks to consumers from the increased consumption of TFAs cannot be ignored. In 2003, Denmark became the first country to introduce laws to control the sale of foods containing TFAs. This started with the publication of a study in The Lancet by Willett in 1993. Then the Danish Nutrition Council, which was established in 1992, was the driving force behind the campaign that convinced Danish politicians that IP-TFAs can be removed from foods without any effects on their taste, price or availability. The Nutrition Council argued that as no positive health effects of IP-TFAs had ever been reported, then just the suspicion that a high intake has harmful effects on health justified the ban (Astrup, 2006; Mjøs, 2003). The Danish success story might be interesting for other countries, where this unnecessary health hazard could also be eliminated from the foods.

Then in January 2006, it became law in the United States that the contents of TFAs have to be specifically listed on food labels. There is a complication to this, however, because there were two reasons why the consumers might not see a TFA content on the label of a food product. First, although products entering interstate commerce on or after 1 January, 2006, had to be labelled, the FDA realized that it would take some time for food products to move through the distribution chain to a store shelf. Then, foods that contain less than 0.5 g TFAs per serving can be labelled as being free from TFAs. Furthermore, in Europe, the declaring of TFAs on food labels is still not obligatory in many countries. At the same time, these regulations only applied to food that was labelled; food sold in restaurants and canteens was not covered by this law (FDA, 2003; Moss, 2006; Stender et al., 2006). Thus many still feel that foods that contain more than 4 g/100 g SFAs and TFAs together should not be claimed to be healthy food. Indeed, Danish law prohibits the sale of foods that contain more than 2 g TFAs per 100 g of fat, excluding food that naturally contains more TFAs (Filip et al., 2010). Denmark decided to impose this maximum level of IP-TFAs as labelling was deemed insufficient to protect consumers, and especially for risk groups like children and adults with a high intake of fast foods (Garchés & Mancha, 1993; Leth et al., 2006).

Then, in December 2006, the Board of Health of New York City banned many TFAs from restaurants in the city, prompting similar moves in Philadelphia, Montgomery County in Maryland, and the Boston suburb of Brooklyn. The first phase of the regulation applies to oils, shortening and margarine, used in cooking and as spreads, and for recipes that contain more than 0.5 g TFA per serving. Since 1 July, 2007, New York City officials have also called for restaurants to clearly display calorie counts next to their menu items, in a bid to increase consumer awareness of the nutritional content of their food. By 1 July, 2008, the ban had been extended to include TFAs used in baked goods, including bread and cakes, in prepared foods, salad dressings and oils used for deep frying, and in dough and cake batter. Similar bans are being proposed in Chicago and in the state of Illinois; other cities may follow suit, most likely in California (Albers et al., 2008; Blake, 2009).

The American Heart Association recommends a healthy dietary pattern and lifestyle to combat heart disease, limiting TFA consumption to less than 1% (or approximately 2 g on a 2,000-calorie diet), and saturated fat consumption to less than 7% of the total daily calories (Borra et al., 2007). This is consistent with the TFA recommendations made by the American Dietetic Association and the Dietitians of Canada (ADA, 2007).

The benefits of adding TFAs on food Nutrition Facts labels in the United States means that consumers now know the levels of SFAs, TFAs and cholesterol in the foods that they choose to eat. This enables them to make heart-healthy food choices, to help them to reduce their risk of CHD. This labelling is also of particular interest to those concerned about high blood cholesterol. However, to gain the full benefit of this system, all of the consumers need be aware of the risk posed by consuming too high levels of SFAs, TFAs and cholesterol.

At the same time, about half of the convenience products on the Austrian market that have been tested contained less than 1% TFAs, and one third less than 5% (Wagner et al., 2008). However, almost 5% of the products tested contained more than 20% TFAs. A similar level was seen for fast food products, with the highest TFA levels of 8.9%, while the total TFAs of household fats were significantly lower (1.45% ±1.99%) than fats for industrial use (7.83% ±10.0%; $P < 0.001$). Compared to investigations in Austria (and Germany) around 10 years ago, the TFA contents of foods have decreased significantly. About half of the investigated products contained less than 1% of TFAs or total fatty acids, although very high levels of TFAs (>15%) are still detected, and an intake of more than 5 g TFA per portion is possible, which has been shown to significantly increase the risk of CHD (Oomen et al., 2001; Wagner et al., 2008; Wilett, 2006).

5. Analytical methods for *trans* fatty acid determination

The fatty acid composition of food is usually determined using gas-liquid chromatography of the corresponding fatty acid methyl esters (FAMEs) (Baggio et al., 2005; Bondia-Pons et al., 2004; Chen et al., 1999; Ratnayake, 1995; Ulberth & Henninger; 1992). Usually, the FAMEs can be conveniently prepared by heating lipids with a large excess of either acid-catalysed or base-catalysed reagents. However, most of the analytical methods are time consuming and impractical for the processing of large numbers of samples, because the lipids have to be extracted prior to preparation of the FAMEs. For this reason, some procedures have been developed that can be used to prepare FAMEs directly from fresh tissue (Park & Goins, 1994; Garchés & Mancha, 1993).

6. Consumption of *trans* fatty acids

Vaccenic acid (*trans*-11 C18:1) accounts for over 60% of the natural TFAs, whereas with IP-TFAs, a broad mixture of TFAs is produced, with elaidic acid (*trans*-9 C18:1) as the main product (Oomen et al., 2001). In recent years, new technologies have been developed to reduce the TFA content in fats and oils used in the manufacture of food products. As indicated above, the content of TFAs in Danish food has been monitored for the last 30 years. In margarine and shortening, the TFA content has steadily declined, from about 10 g per 100 g of margarine in the 1970s, to practically no TFAs in margarine in 1999, to efficiently reduce the health risk related to TFAs.

In North America, the daily TFA intake has been estimated using food frequency questionnaires, and it was found to be 3-4 g per person (ADA, 2007), while by extrapolation of human milk data, it was said to be greater than 10 g per person (Chardigny et al., 1995). The data also show that the levels of TFAs can vary considerably among foods within any specific category, reflecting the differences in the fats and oils used in the manufacturing or preparation processes. For example, the range of TFAs in 17 brands of crackers was from 23% to 51% of the total fatty acids, which represents differences of 1 g to 13 g TFAs per 100 g of crackers. These data thus show that the wide variability in the TFA content of different foods can result in large errors in the estimation of the TFA intake of individuals, and potentially, of groups (Innis, 2006).

TFA consumption in European countries varies considerably. The diet in northern European countries traditionally contains more TFAs than that in the Mediterranean countries, where olive oil is commonly used. The diet in France has always been relatively low in TFAs, because France has traditionally used predominantly ruminant fats, as compared to hydrogenated vegetable oils. A more recent decrease in dietary TFAs has been seen due to the modification of commercial fats and changes in consumer choice (Larqué et al., 2001). In the TRANSFAIR study (Poppel et al., 1998), which was based on a market basket analysis of diets across 14 European countries, the mean daily intake of TFAs in European countries ranged from the lowest in Greece (1.4 g TFA per day) to the highest in Iceland (5.4 g TFA per day) (Fig. 3).

The lover daily intake of TFAs was recorded in Greece where 1.4 g of TFAs are consumed per day what represent 0.6 % of daily energy intake. The highest daily intake of TFAs was recorded in Iceland where 5.4 g of TFAs are consumed per day what represent 2.0 % of daily energy intake. As shown by researches (Innis et al., 1999; Leth et al., 2006; Poppel et al., 1998) the lowest TFA intake is more often in countries with Mediterranean type of nutrition habits (Mediterranean diet).

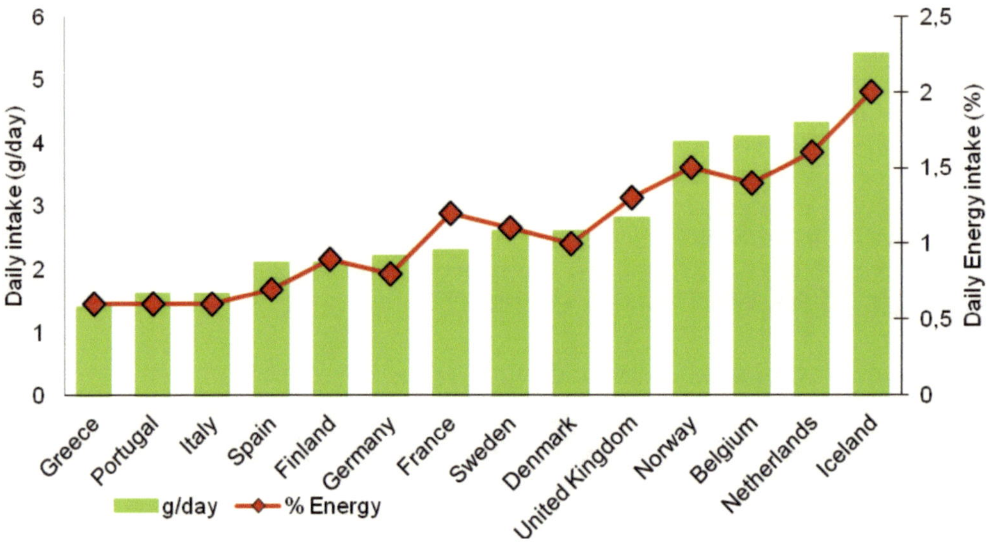

Fig. 3. Mean daily intake of TFAs across the European countries (Innis et al., 1999; Leth et al., 2006; Poppel et al., 1998)

6.1 Dairy products and *trans* fatty acids

Milk fat is also the most abundant source of conjugated linoleic acids (CLAs), which are a group of geometrical and positional isomers of linoleic acid (LA *cis*-9,*cis*-12 C18:2). The major isomer of the CLAs in milk fat is *cis*-9, *trans*-11, and it represents 80 g to 90 g per 100 g of the total CLAs (Chardigny et al., 1995; Ledoux et al., 2005; Seçkim et al., 2005). Some of these fatty acids have biological, physiological and nutritional properties that are very interesting for consumer health, as especially seen for butyric acid and CLAs (Pandya & Ghodke, 2007). The CLAs are synthesised in ruminants both from dietary linoleic acid (*cis*-9,*cis*-12 C18:2) in the rumen by the microbial flora, and from vaccenic acid (*trans*-11 C18:1) in the mammary glands during *de-novo* synthesis (Bauman & Griinari, 2001).

6.2 Industrially produced fat and *trans* fatty acids

Brát and Pokorný (Brát & Pokorný, 2000) investigated a series of 20 margarines, nine cooking fats, and butter that were available on the Czech market. They used the American Oil Chemistry Society standard analysis methods, with capillary gas chromatography. The margarines contained 15.2% to 54.1% cooking fats, and 16.5% to 59.1% SFAs, which was less than the butter. The content of linoleic acid varied between 3.7% and 52.4% in the margarines; small amounts of linolenic acid were present in most samples, while oleic acid prevailed in the cooking fats. Monoenoic TFAs were present only in trace amounts in 10 samples, and *trans*-polyenoic acids were present only in small amounts. Most cooking fats had a high content of TFAs. They summarised these data by indicating that the number of *trans*-free margarines had rapidly increased over a few years.

More recently, Cenčič-Kodba (Cenčič-Kodba, 2007) examined 13 margarines and fatty food samples in Slovenia, which were selected according to the frequency of use among the population group in the community. All of the fried food and bakery food samples included in this study contained TFAs, the levels of which varied from less than 0.5% to 6.8%. The highest TFA content in the margarines was 5.2%, with 0.3% as the lowest, and a mean margarine TFA content of 2.3%. The main TFAs were the *trans* isomers of mono-unsaturated octadecenoic acid (C18:1).

Similarly, the findings of Larqué et al. (Larqué et al., 2003) suggest that Spanish margarines have moved to becoming products with a potentially healthier distribution of fatty acids. Even so, the great variability shown in the fatty-acid compositions of margarines and the poor labelling continue to highlight the importance of greater consumer information to avoid detrimental changes to the traditional Mediterranean diet in Spain.

7. Conclusions and future trends

It can be concluded at present that the reduction of TFAs in the food supply is a complex issue that has involved, and still involves, interdependent and interrelated stakeholders. Any further actions taken to reduce TFAs need to be carefully considered, regarding both the intended and unintended consequences related to nutrition and public health. As shown above, the WHO (WHO/FAO, 2002) has already included TFA levels in their recommended daily food intake (Table 1). Many different options of alternative oils and fats can now be used to replace TFAs, as many of these are already available, while others are still being developed. However, decisions on which alternatives to use are complicated and often time consuming, and they involve considerations of health effects, food availability, quality and taste, research and development investments, supply-chain management, operational modifications, consumer acceptance, and cost (Borra et al., 2007; FDA, 2003).

As industry responses are now well underway following the policy actions over the past few years, it is possible to take a present-day 'snapshot' of industry activities that provide preliminary answers to these considerations. The first results of most of the anti-*trans* fat campaigns can be seen as modifications that have been made to the fatty-acid compositions of industrial fats. In these fats, there are significantly higher levels of SFAs and possibly a higher index of atherogenicity. Several major food companies have announced efforts to remove TFAs from their leading brands over the past two decades, starting with Unilever in the 1990s, and then more recently with Nestlé in 2002, Kraft in 2003, Campbell's in 2004 (for Goldfish crackers), Kellogg's in 2005, and Frito-Lay in 2006 (for chips). It is of note that the earliest announcements came from European firms, where the use of partially hydrogenated soy was not as common as it was in the United States, and thus this reformulation process has not been as onerous.

The announcements over the last three years or so have reflected the attention brought to this issue through lawsuits and debates about nutritional labelling regulations. Many companies even chose to implement the disclosure of these *trans*-fat contents earlier than the January 1, 2006, deadline, particularly when they were able to advertise 'zero' *trans* fats on their products (Crisco, 2008).

One aspect for producing such zero TFAs lies in the transesterification reactions between vegetable oils and the SFAs of C8:0, C12:0, C14:0 and C16:0. These reactions can be catalysed by an immobilised sn-1,3 specific *Rhizomucor miehei* lipase. When considering a TFA-free or low TFA fat that is suitable for use as a confectionery fat, a non-hydrogenated vegetable fat composed of an inter-esterified fat can be used: this can be obtained by subjecting a blend of at least one fat rich in lauric acid and at least one fat without lauric acid to inter-esterification (Farmani et al., 2007).

For all of the products introduced in 2005 and 2006 that have claimed to contain no *trans* fats, the most commonly used oil ingredients have been canola, sunflower and soybean oils. Palm oil, which is high in saturated fat, also appears among the commonly used ingredients, but not as an alternative to reducing TFAs. Eleven percent of food producers in the United States still use partially hydrogenated oils as ingredient, because the regulations allow 0.5 g per serving of *trans* fats in products that claim to contain 'no *trans* fat', while the use of small amounts of partially hydrogenated oils has facilitated the reformulation of some products (Unnevehr & Jagmanaite, 2008).

Between 2006 and 2007, consumer awareness of *trans* fats increased and attained levels similar to those for saturated fats. This increased awareness has been associated with improved self-reporting behaviour in consumer shopping for groceries (Eckel et al., 2009). However, food labels and food claims that accompany packed foods are still largely incomprehensible for consumers, and therefore they appear to be of very little use at present. Moreover, in Europe, consumers still cannot identify the content of TFAs in the labelling of food products, particularly as the only legislation that restricts the content of TFAs in Europe is in Denmark.

At the same time, we have to be aware that indicators are showing that the world population is still increasing and is expected to reach nearly 8.9 thousand million (8,900,000,000) by the year 2050 (UN, 2004). Knowing of some of the problems that are associated with this increasing population, we are now combating the need that will arise for more and more potential food products to be used for biofuels (Fink & Medved, 2011). Thus, in the future, it will become increasingly difficult to assure food security and food safety, as well as the nutritional quality of food. Indeed, it is the nutritional quality of food and its distribution all over the World that are the main factors that will have a huge impact on human health. In this way, human health is more than just of personal value, as it is also part of the welfare of the whole of our society.

8. References

ADA (2007). American Dietetic Association. Position of the American Dietetic Association and Dietitians of Canada: Dietary fatty acids. Journal of the American Dietetic Association, Vol. 107, No.9, (September 2007), pp.1599.e1-1599.e15, ISSN 0002-8223

Albers, M.J., Harnack, L.J., Steffen, L.M., & Jacobs, D.R. (2008). 2006 marketplace survey of trans-fatty acid content of margarines and butters, cookies and snack cakes, and savoury snacks. *Journal of American Dietetic Association,* Vol. 108, No. 2, (February 2008), pp. 367-370, ISSN 0002-8223

Ascherio, A. (2002). Epidemiological studies on dietary fats and coronary heart disease. *The American Journal of Medicine,* Vol. 113, No. 9B, (December 2002), pp. 9-12, ISSN 0002-9343

Ascherio, A. (2006). Trans fatty acids and blood lipids. *Atherosclerosis Supplements,* Vol. 7, No. 2, (May 2006), pp. 25-27, ISSN 1567-5688

Astrup, A. (2006). The trans fatty acid story in Denmark. *Atherosclerosis Supplements,* Vol. 7, No. 2 (May 2006), pp. 43-46, ISSN 1567-5688

Baggio, S.R., Miguel, A.M.R., & Bragagnolo, N. (2005). Simultaneous determination of cholesterol oxides, cholesterol and fatty acids in processed turkey meat products. *Food Chemistry,* Vol. 89, No. 3, (February 2005), pp. 475-484, ISSN 0308-8146

Bansal ,G., Zhou, W., Tan, T.W., Neo, F.L., & Lo, H.L. (2009). Analysis of trans fatty acids in deep frying oils by three different approaches. *Food Chemistry,* Vol. 116, No. 2, (September 2009), pp. 535-541, ISSN 0308-8146

Bauman, D.E., & Griinari, J.M. (2001). Regulation and nutritional manipulation of milk fat: Low-fat milk syndrome. *Livestock Production Science,* Vol. 70, No. 1-2, (July 2001), pp. 15-29, ISSN 0301-6226

Blake, T. (2009) Trans Fats, BBC. (http://www.bbc.co.uk/food/food_matters/transfats.shtml).

Boatella, J., Rafecas, M., Codony, R., Gibert, A., Rivero, M., Tormo, R., Infante, D., & Sánchez-Valverde, F. (1993). Trans fatty acid content of human milk in Spain. *Journal of Pediatric Gastroenterology and Nutrition,* Vol. 16, No. 4, (May 1993), pp. 432-434, ISSN 0277-2116

Bondia-Pons, I., Castellote, A.I., & López-Sabater, M.C. (2004). Comparison of conventional and fast gas chromatography in human-plasma fatty-acid determination. *Journal of Chromatography B,* Vol. 809, No. 2, (October 2004), pp. 339-344, ISSN 1570-0232

Borra, S., Kris-Etherton, P.M., Dausch, J.G., & Yin-Piazza, S. (2007). An update of trans-fat reduction in the American diet. *Journal of American Dietetic Association,* Vol. 107, No. 12, pp. 2048-2050, ISSN 0002-8223

Brát, J., & Pokorný, J. (2000). Fatty acid composition of margarines and cooking fats available on the Czech market. *Journal of Food Composition and Analalysis,* Vol. 13, No. 4, (August 2000), pp. 337-343, ISSN 0889-1575

Bray, G.A. (2001). Risk of obesity. *Endocrinology and Metabolism Clinics of North America,* Vol. 32, No. 4, (December 2003), pp. 787-804, ISSN 0889-8529

Burdge, G.C., Derrick, P.R., Russell, J.J., Tricon, S., Kew, S., Banerjee, T., Grimble, R.F., Williams, C.M., Yaqoob, P., & Calder, P.C. (2005). Incorporation of cis-9, trans-11 or trans-10, cis-12 conjugated linoleic acid in human erythrocytes *in vivo*. *Nutrition Research,* Vol. 25, No. 1, (January 2005), pp. 13-19, ISSN 0271-5317

Carriquiry, M., Weber, W.J., Baumgard, L.H., & Crooker, B.A. (2008). *In vitro* biohydrogenation of four dietary fats. *Animal Feed Science and Technology,* Vol. 141, No. 3-4, (April 2008), pp. 339-355, ISSN 0377-8401

Cenčič-Kodba, Z.: Content of Trans Fatty Acids in Margarines and Selected Fatty Foods Marketed in Slovenia. In: 3rd Slovenian Congress on Food and Nutrition, Food Processing - Innovation - Nutrition - Healthy Consumers, P. Raspor, T. Buzeti, L. Gašperlin, M. Jevšnik, B. Kovač, A. Krumpak, P. Medved, S. Oštir, P. Plahuta, M. Simčič, S. Smole-Možina (Eds.), Slovenian Nutrition Society, Ljubljana, Slovenia (2007) p. 119.

Chardigny, J.M., Wolff, R.L., Mager, E., Sébédio, J.L., Martine, L., & Juanéda, P. (1995). Trans mono- and polyunsaturated fatty acids in human milk. *European Journal of Clinical Nutrition,* Vol. 49, No. 7, (July 1995), pp. 523-531, ISSN 0954-3007

Chen, J., Cao, Y., Gao, H., Yang, L., & Chen, Z.Y. (2007). Isomerization of conjugated linolenic acids during methylation. *Chemistry and Physics of Lipids,* Vol. 150, No. 2, (December 2007), pp. 136-142, ISSN 0009-3084

Chen, S.H., Chen, K.C., & Lien, H.M. (1999). Determination of fatty acids in vegetable oil by reversed-phase liquid chromatography with fluorescence detection. *Journal of Chromatography A,* Vol. 849, No. 2, (July 1999) pp. 357-369, ISSN 0021-9673

Chen, Z.Y., Pelletier, G., Hollywood, R., & Ratnayake, W.M.N. (1995). Trans fatty acid isomers in Canadian human milk. *Lipids,* Vol. 30, No. 1, (1995), pp. 15-21, ISSN 0024-4201

Craig-Schmidt, M.C. (2006). Worldwide consumption of trans fatty acids. *Atherosclerosis Supplements,* Vol. 7, No. 2, (May 2006), pp. 1-4, ISSN 1567-5688

Crisco® Shortening products reformulated to contain zero gram trans fat per serving (2008) (http://www.crisco.com/Promotions_News/Press_Releases/2007/zero_grams_ttr an_fat)

DACH (2000) Referenzwerte für die Nährstoffzufuhr, Deutsche Gesellschaft für Ernährung eV (DGE), Österreichische Gesellschaft für Ernährung (ÖGE), Schweizerische Gesellschaft für Ernährungsforchung (SGE), Schweizerische Vereinigung für Ernährung (SVE). English version published 2002.

Destaillats, F., Golay, P.A., Joffre, F., de Wispelaere, M., Hug, B., Giuffrida, F., Fauconnot, L., & Dionisi, F. (2007). Comparison of available analytical methods to measure trans-octadecenoic acid isomeric profile and content by gas-liquid chromatography in milk fat. *Journal of Chromatography A,* Vol. 1145, No. 1-2, (March 2007), pp. 222-228, ISSN 0021-9673

Diet, nutrition and the prevention of chronic diseases. WHO Technical Report Series 916, Geneva, Switzerland (2003)

Eckel, R.H., Kris-Etherton, P., Lichtenstein, A.H., Wylie-Rosett, J., Groom, A., Stitzel, K.F., & Yin-Piazza, S. (2009). Americans' awareness, knowledge, and behaviors regarding fats: 2006-2007. *Journal of American Dietetic Association,* Vol. 109, No. 2, (February 2009), pp. 288-296, ISSN 0002-8223

Farmani, J., Hamedi, M., Safari, M., & Madadlou, A. (2007). Trans-free Iranian vanaspati through enzymatic and chemical trans esterification of triple blends of fully hydrogenated soybean, rapeseed and sunflower oils. *Food Chemistry,* Vol. 102, No. 3, (February 2007), pp. 827-833, ISSN 0308-8146

FDA (2003). Federal Register, Food Labelling Trans Fatty Acids in Nutrition Labelling; Consumer research to consider nutrient content and health claims and possible footnote or disclosure statements, final rule and proposed rule, Food and Drug Administration, Vol. 58, (July 2003), pp. 41433-41506.

Filip, S., Fink, R., Hribar, J., & Vidrih, R. (2010). Trans fatty acids in food and their influence on human health. *Food Technology and Biotechnology,* Vol. 48, No. 2, (April-June 2010), pp. 135-142, ISSN 1330-9862

Filip, S., Hribar, J., & Vidrih, R. (2011). Influence of natural antioxidants on the formation of trans fatty acids during heat treatment of sunflower oil. *European Journal of Lipid Science and Technology,* Vol. 113, No. 2, (February 2011), pp. 224-230, ISSN 1438-9312

Fink, R., & Medved, S. (2011). Global prospective on first generation liquid biofuel production. *Turkish Journal of Agriculture and Forestry,* Vol. 35, No. 5, (September 2011), pp. 453-459, ISSN 1303-6173

Fournier, V., Juanéda, P., Destaillats, F., Dionisi, F., Lambelet, P., Sébédio, L.L., & Berdeaux, O. (2006). Analysis of eicosapentaenoic and docosahexaenoic acid geometrical isomers formed during fish-oil deodorisation. *Journal of Chromatography A*, Vol. 1129, No. 1, (September 2006), pp. 21-28, ISSN 0021-9673

Gamel, T.H., Kiritsakis, A., & Petrakis, C. (1999). Effect of phenolic extracts on trans fatty acid formation during frying. *Grasas y Aceites*, Vol. 50,No. 6, (July 1999), pp. 421-425, ISSN 0017-3495

Garaulet, M., Hernandez-Morante, J.J., Tebar, F.J., & Zamora, S. (2011).Relation between degree of obesity and site-specific adipose tissue fatty acid composition in Mediterranean population. *Nutrition*, Vol. 27, No. 2, (February 2011), pp. 170-176, ISSN 0899-9007

Garchés, R., & Mancha, M. (1993). One-step lipid extraction and fatty acid methyl esters preparation from fresh plant tissues. *Analytical Biochemistry*, Vol. 211, No. 15, (May 1993), pp. 139-143, ISSN 0003-2697

Innis, S.M. (2006). *Trans* fatty intakes during pregnancy, infancy and early childhood. Atherosclerosis Supplements, Vol.7, No.2, (May 2006), pp. 17-20, ISSN1567-5688

Katan, M.B. (2006). Regulation of trans fats: The gap, the Polder and McDonald's French fries. *Atherosclerosis Supplements*, Vol. 7, No. 2, (May 2006), pp. 63-66, ISSN 1567-5688

Koletzko, B., & Decsi, T. (1994). Fatty acid composition of plasma lipid classes in healthy subjects from birth to young adulthood. *European Journal of Pediatrics*, Vol. 153, No. 7, (July 1994), pp. 520-525, ISSN 0340-6199

Koletzko, B., & Müller, J. (1990). Cis- and trans-isomeric fatty acids in plasma lipids of newborn infants and their mothers. *Biology of the Neonate*, Vol. 57, No. 3-4, pp. 172-178, ISSN 0006-3126

Koletzko, B. (1992). Trans fatty acids may impair biosynthesis of long-chain polyunsaturates and growth in man. *Acta Paediatrica*, Vol. 81, No. 4, (April 1992), pp. 302-306, ISSN 0803-5253

Kummerow, F.A., Zhou, Q., Mahfouz, M.M., Smiricky, M.R., Grieshop, C.M., & Schaeffer, D.J. (2004). Trans fatty acids in hydrogenated fat inhibited the synthesis of the polyunsaturated fatty acids in the phospholipid of arterial cells. *Life Science*, Vol. 74, No. 22, (April 2004), pp. 2707-2723, ISSN 0024-3205

Larqué, E., Garaulet, M., Pérez-Llamas, F., Zamora, S., & Tebar, F.J. (2003a). Fatty acid composition and nutritional relevance of most widely consumed margarines in Spain. *Grasas y Aceites*, Vol. 54, No. 1, (March 2003), pp. 65-70, ISSN 0017-3495

Larqué, E., García-Ruiz, P.A., Perez-Llamas, F., Zamora, S., & Gil, A. (2003b). Dietary trans fatty acids alter the compositions of microsomes and mitochondria and the activities of microsome Δ6-fatty acid desaturase and glucose 6-phosphatase in livers of pregnant rats. *The Journal of Nutrition*, Vol. 133, No. 8, (August 2003), pp. 2526-2531, ISSN 0022-3166

Larqué, E., Pérez-Llamas, F., Puerta, V., Girón, M.D., Suárez, M.D., Zamora, S., & Gil, A. (2000a). Dietary trans fatty acids affect docosahexaenoic acid concentrations in plasma and liver but not brain of pregnant and fetal rats. *Pediatric Research*, Vol. 47, No. 2, (February 2000), pp. 278-283, ISSN 0031-3998

Larqué, E., Zamora, S., & Gil, A. (2000b). Dietary trans fatty acids affect the essential fatty-acid concentration of rat milk. *The Journal of Nutrition,* Vol. 130, No. 4, (April 2000), pp. 847-851, ISSN 0022-3166

Larqué, E., Zamora, S., & Gil, A. (2001). Dietary trans fatty acids in early life: A review. *Early Human Devevelopment,* Vol. 65, No. 1, (October 2001), pp. 31-41, ISSN 0378-3782

Ledoux, M., Chardigny, J.M., Darbois, M., Soustre, Y., Sébédio, J.L., & Laloux, L. (2005). Fatty acid composition of French butters, with special emphasis on conjugated linoleic acid (CLA) isomers. *Journal of Food Composition Analysis,* Vol. 18, No. 5, (August 2005), pp. 409-425, ISSN 0889-1575

Leth, T. Jensen, H.G., Mikkelsen, A.A., & Bysted, A. (2006). The effect of the regulation on trans fatty acid content in Danish food. *Atheroscleroossis Supplements,* Vol. 7, No. 2, (May 2006), pp. 53-56, ISSN 1567-5688

Margarine IMACE- International Margarine Association of the Countries of Europe. (2009). (http://www.imace.org/margarine/history.htm).

Marinka, J., Polak, T., Filip, S., & Vidrih, R. (2011). Quantitative comparison of the fatty acid composition of dairy and artificial creams and their nutrition value in human diet. *Milchwissenschaft,* Vol. 66, No. 2, (April 2011), pp. 186-189, ISSN 0026-3788

Mensink, P.R., & Katan, B.M. (1993). Trans monounsaturated fatty acids in nutrition and their impact on serum lipoprotein levels in man. *Progres in Lipid Research,* Vol. 32, No. 1, (1993), pp. 111-122, ISSN 0163-7827

Mensink, R.P., & Nestel, P. (2009). Trans fatty acids and cardiovascular risk markers: Does the source matter? *Current Opinion in Lipidology,* Vol. 20, No. 1, (February 2009), pp. 1-2, ISSN 0957-9672

Mjøs, S.A. (2003). Identification of fatty acids in gas chromatography by application of different temperature and pressure programmes on a single capillary column. *Journal of Chromatography A,* Vol. 1015, No. 1-2, (October 2003), pp. 151-161, ISSN 0021-9673

Moss, J. (2006). Labelling of trans fatty acid content in food, regulations and limits - The FDA view. *Atherosclerosis Supplements,* Vol. 7, No. 2, (May 2006), pp. 57-95, ISSN 1567-5688

Murrieta, C.M., Hess, B.W., & Rule, D.C. (2003). Comparison of acidic and alkaline catalysts for preparation of fatty-acid methyl esters from ovine muscle with emphasis on conjugated linoleic acid. *Meat Science,* Vol. 65, No. 1, (September 2003), pp. 523-529, ISSN 0309-1740

Nordic Nutrition Recommendations 2004: Integrating Nutrition and Physical Activity. NORD 2004. Copenhagen, Nordic Councilof Ministries, 2004.

Oomen, C.M., Ocké, M.C., Feskens, E.J.M., van Erp-Baart, M.A.J., Kok, F.J., & Kromhout, D. (2001). Association between trans fatty acid intake and 10-year risk of coronary heart disease in the Zutphen Elderly Study: prospective population-based study, *The Lancet,* Vol. 357, No. 10, (March 2001), pp. 746-751, ISSN 0140-6736

Pandya,A.J., & Ghodke, K.M. (2007). Goat and sheep milk products other than cheeses and yoghurt. *Small Ruminant Research,* Vol. 68, No. 1-2, (March 2007), pp. 193-206, ISSN 0921-4488

Park, W.P., & Goins, E.R. (1994). *In-situ* preparation of fatty acid methyl esters for analysis of fatty acid composition in foods. *Journal of Food Science,* Vol. 59, No. 6, (1994), pp. 1262-1266, ISSN 1750-3841

Pavlovic, M., Prentice, A., Thorsdottir, I., Wolfram, G., & Branca, F. (2007). Challenges in harmonizing energy and nutrient recommendations in Europe. *Annals of Nutrition and Metabolism,* Vol. 51, No. 2, (June 2007), pp. 108-114, ISSN 0250-6807

Pfeuffer, M., & Schrezenmeir, J. (2006). Impact of trans fatty acids of ruminant origin compared with those from partially hydrogenated vegetable oils on CHD risk. *International Dairy Journal,* Vol. 16, No. 11, (November 2006), pp. 1383-1388, ISSN 0958-6946

Poppel, G., van Erp-Baart, M.A., Leth T., Gevers, E., van Amelsvoort, J., Lanzmann-Petithory, D., Kafatos, A., & Aro, A. (1998). Trans fatty acids in foods in Europe: The TRANSFAIR study. *Journal of Food Composition and Analysis,* Vol. 11, No. 2, (June 1998), pp. 112-136, ISSN 0889-1575

Position of the American Dietetic Association and Dietitians of Canada: Dietary Fatty Acids, *Journal of American Dietetic Association,* Vol. 107, No. 9, (September 2007), pp. 1599.e1-1599.e15, ISSN 0002-8223

Ratnayake, W.M.N. (1995). Determination of trans unsaturation by infrared spectrophotometry and determination of fatty-acid composition of partially hydrogenated vegetable oils and animal fats by gas chromatography/ infrared spectrophotometry: Collaborative study. *Journal of AOAC International,* Vol. 78, No. 3, (1995), pp. 783-802, ISSN 1060-3271

Salobir, K. (2001). Nutritional functionality of fats. In: 21st Food Technology Days 2001, Functional Foods, B. Žlender, L. Gašperlin (Eds.) Biotechnical Faculty, Ljubljana, Slovenia, pp. 121-136.

Seçkim, A.K., Gursoy, O., Kinik, O., & Akbulut, N. (2005). Conjugated linoleic acid (CLA) concentration, fatty acid composition and cholesterol content of some Turkish dairy products. *LWT-Food Science and Technology,* Vol. 38, No. 8, (December 2005), pp. 909-915, ISSN 0023-6438

Simopoulos, A.P. (2004). Omega-3 fatty acids and antioxidants in edible wild plants. *Biological Research,* Vol. 37, No. 2, (2004), pp. 263–277, ISSN 0716-9760

Srinivasan, S.C., Irz, X., & Shankar, B. (2006). An assessment of the potential consumption impact of WHO dietary norms in OECD countries. *Food Policy,* Vol. 31, No. 1, (February 2006), pp. 53-77, ISSN 0306-9192

Stender, S., Dyerberg, J., Bysted, A., Leth, T., & Astrup, A. (2006). A trans world journey. *Atherosclerosis Supplements,* Vol. 7, No. 2, (May 2006), pp. 47-52, ISSN 1567-5688

Tarrago-Trani, M.T., Phillips, K.M., Lemar, L.E., & Holden, J.M. (2006). New and existing oils and fats used in products with reduced trans fatty acid content, *Journal of American Dietetic Association,* Vol. 106, No. 6, (June 2006), pp. 867-880, ISSN 0002-8223

Triantafillou, D., Zografos, V., & Katsikas, H. (2003). Fatty acid content of margarines in the Greek market (including trans-fatty acids): A contribution to improving consumer's information. *International Journal of Food Sciences and Nutrition,* Vol. 54, No. 2, (March 2003), pp. 135-141, ISSN 0963-7486

Tsuzuki, W., Nagata, R., Yunoki, R., Nakajima, M., & Nagata, T. (2008). *cis/trans*-Isomerization of triolein, trilinolein and trilinolenin induced by heat treatment. *Food Chemistry,* Vol. 108, No. 1, (May 2008), pp. 75-80, ISSN 0308-8146

Ulberth, F., & Henninger, M. (1992). Simplified method for the determination of trans monoenes in edible fats by TLC-GLC. *Journal of American Oil Chemist's Society* Vol. 69, No. 8, (August 1992), pp. 829-831, ISSN 0003-021X

UN (2004). World Population to 2300. United Nations. Department of Economic and Social Affairs, Population Division, New York, USA (2004), pp. 4-10.

Unnevehr, L.J., & Jagmanaite, E. (2008). Getting rid of trans fats in the US diet: Policies, incentives and progress. *Food Policy,* Vol. 33, No. 6, (December 2008), pp. 497-503, ISSN 0306-9192

Wagner, K.H., Plasse, E., Proell, C., & Kanzler, S. (2008). Comprehensive studies on the trans fatty acid content of Austrian foods: Convenience products, fast food and fats. *Food Chemistry,* Vol. 108, No. 3, (June 2008), pp. 1054-1060, ISSN 0308-8146

Willett, W.C. (2006). Trans fatty acids and cardiovascular disease - Epidemiological data. *Atherosclerossis Supplements,* Vol. 7, No. 2, (May 2006), pp. 5-8, ISSN 1567-5688

WHO (2008). Atlas of Health in Europe, WHO , Copenhagen, Denmark, pp.125, ISBN 978-92-890-1411

WHO/FAO (2002). Human Vitamin and Mineral Requirements. Report of a Joint WHO/FAO Expert Consultation.

WHO (1985). Energy and protein requirements. World health organization, Technical report series 724, (Geneva 1985), ISSN 0512-3054

4

Control and Coordination of Vasomotor Tone in the Microcirculation

Mauricio A. Lillo, Francisco R. Pérez, Mariela Puebla, Pablo S. Gaete and Xavier F. Figueroa
Departamento de Fisiología, Facultad de Ciencias Biológicas, Pontificia Universidad Católica de Chile, Santiago, Chile

1. Introduction

The blood vascular system consists in a complex network of vessels that is mainly intended to provide oxygen and nutrients to all individual cells of peripheral tissues and help to dispose metabolic wastes. Several distinct functional compartments can be distinguished in the vascular network: arteries, arterioles, capillaries, venules and veins. Conduit arteries (diameter, 1 to several millimeters) carry blood away from the heart through a divergent arborescence that reaches and penetrates into the tissues via the feed arteries (diameter, 100 to 500 μm) (Davis *et al.*, 1986; Segal, 2000, 2005). These muscular vessels give rise to the arterioles (diameter, < 100 μm), which control and coordinate the blood flow distribution in such a way that each capillary is correctly supplied at the proper pressure (Mulvany, 1990; Segal, 2005). This part of the vascular network composed of arterioles, capillaries and venules is embedded within the organ irrigated and is called microcirculation (Davis *et al.*, 1986; Segal, 2005; Lockhart *et al.*, 2009). Finally, veins carry blood back to the heart through a convergent arborescence.

In general, the vascular wall of arteries consists of an outer tunica adventitia, a central tunica media, and an inner tunica intima. The adventitia mainly contains connective tissue, fibroblasts, mast cells, macrophages, and nerve axons. Although the amount of the wall taken up by adventitia varies with the vascular territory, it is directly proportional to the size of the vessel (Gingras *et al.*, 2009). The media is comprised of circumferentially arranged smooth muscle cells and is bounded on the luminal side by a well-defined internal elastic lamina. An external elastic lamina may also be present between the media and the adventitia or even within the media in larger vessels such as the aorta, but this structure is fragmented in small arteries and absent in arterioles (Mulvany, 1990; London *et al.*, 1998). The number of smooth muscle cell layers decreases with decreasing vessel diameter and, in arterioles, only an unbroken monolayer of smooth muscle cells is found (Davis *et al.*, 1986; Mulvany, 1990; Segal, 2005). In contrast, the structure of the intima is similar in all blood vessels and is formed by a smooth, continuous single layer of endothelial cells that lines the inner surface of the vessels (Mulvany, 1990). These cells are very thin (2 μm thick) and elongated (10 to 20 μm wide and 100 to 150 μm long, in arterioles), and are oriented parallel to the longitudinal axis of the vessel (Haas & Duling, 1997).

Correct supply of blood to the tissues relies on the ability of the vascular system to adjust the resistance of each vessel by controlling its lumen diameter, which is, in turn, a function of the level of tone of the vascular smooth muscle (i.e. vasomotor tone). As blood vessels are complex structures that must work as an unit, control of vasomotor tone depends on the fine synchronization of function of the different cellular components of the vessel wall, mainly smooth muscle cells and endothelial cells (Segal, 2000; Figueroa *et al.*, 2004; Segal, 2005; Figueroa & Duling, 2009). Such synchronization and coordination is accomplished by an intricate system of radial and longitudinal cell-to-cell communication (Beach *et al.*, 1998; Figueroa *et al.*, 2004; Rummery & Hill, 2004; Segal, 2005; Figueroa & Duling, 2009; Bagher & Segal, 2011). In addition, arterioles in the microcirculation form a complex network, and then, the changes in the luminal diameter of different arteriolar segments must also be coordinated to regulate blood flow distribution and peripheral vascular resistance (Figueroa *et al.*, 2004; Rummery & Hill, 2004; Segal, 2005; Figueroa & Duling, 2008). It has typically been assumed that most of the total resistance to blood flow resides on the arterioles. However, it has become apparent that as much as 50% of the precapillary resistance lies proximal to the arterioles (Davis *et al.*, 1986; Mulvany, 1990; Segal, 2000), which situates the feed arteries at a key point for controlling vascular function and highlights the importance of the functional communication between arterioles and feed arteries in the regulation of blood flow distribution.

It is widely recognized that the endothelium plays a critical role controlling function of the vessel wall by the release of paracrine molecules such as nitric oxide (NO), prostaglandins (PGs) and also by the activation of the signaling mechanism known as endothelium-derived hyperpolarizing factor (EDHF) (Moncada *et al.*, 1991; Busse *et al.*, 2002; Feletou & Vanhoutte, 2007; Vanhoutte *et al.*, 2009). However, another mechanism of communication that has emerged as a key pathway to command and coordinate the vascular wall function is the direct cell-to-cell communication via gap junctions (Sandow *et al.*, 2003; Figueroa *et al.*, 2004, 2006). In addition, it is important to note that K^+ channels expressed in the endothelium and smooth muscle cells play a central role in the control of vasomotor tone by paracrine or gap junction-mediated signaling mechanisms (Jackson, 2005).

2. Membrane potential and vascular K^+ channels

In contrast to endothelial cells, Ca^{2+} is a signal for contraction in smooth muscle cells. In smooth muscle cells of blood vessels the L-type voltage-dependent Ca^{2+} channels play a central role controlling the vasomotor tone (Jackson, 2000). Changes in membrane potential modulate the opening of these Ca^{2+} channels. Thereby, depolarization produces a Ca^{2+} influx that leads to vasoconstriction and, on the contrary, hyperpolarization leads to a reduction in intracellular Ca^{2+} concentration and, subsequently, vasodilation (Jackson, 2000, 2005). In this context, K^+ channels play a pivotal role in vascular function by controlling the membrane potential of both endothelial and smooth muscle cells. The main K^+ channels expressed in resistance vessels, from a functional point of view, are: the ATP-sensitive K^+ channels (K_{ATP}), inward rectifying K^+ channels (K_{ir}) and Ca^{2+}-activated K^+ channels (K_{Ca}) of small (SK_{Ca}), intermediate (IK_{Ca}) and large (BK_{Ca}) conductance (Jackson, 2000, 2005). K_{ATP} and K_{ir} are expressed in both endothelial and smooth muscle cells (Quayle *et al.*, 1996; Jackson, 2000, 2005; Ko *et al.*, 2008), whereas BK_{Ca} are mostly found in smooth muscle cells (Jackson, 2005; Ko *et al.*, 2008), but, on occasion, these K^+ channels have also been described in endothelial cells (Papassotiriou *et al.*, 2000; Wang *et al.*, 2005). In contrast, SK_{Ca} and IK_{Ca} are expressed exclusively in endothelial cells (Jackson, 2000; Kohler *et al.*, 2000; Nilius & Droogmans, 2001; Eichler *et al.*, 2003; Taylor *et al.*, 2003; Brahler *et al.*, 2009).

All these K^+ channels play critical roles in the regulation of vascular function. K_{ATP} channels are opened at rest, and then, are very relevant in the control of smooth muscle membrane potential and vasomotor tone in basal unstimulated conditions (Jackson, 1993, 2000). Interestingly, K_{ir} are typically closed at resting conditions, but are activated by hyperpolarization of membrane potential and by increments in extracellular K^+ concentration ($[K^+]_o$) smaller than 20 mM (Jackson, 2005; Jantzi *et al.*, 2006; Smith *et al.*, 2008). Although BK_{Ca} channels are involved in the response to several vasomotor stimuli, the most relevant function of these K^+ channels is the tonic control of vasomotor tone by buffering the smooth muscle cell depolarization. The increase in intracellular Ca^{2+} concentration associated to smooth muscle depolarization activates local Ca^{2+} transients (i.e. Ca^{2+} sparks) that result from the opening of tightly clustered ryanodine receptor channels located at extensions of sarcoplasmic reticulum. Ca^{2+} sparks activate a BK_{Ca}-dependent hyperpolarizing current that opposes the smooth muscle depolarization, and thereby, regulates the magnitude of the vasoconstriction (Jaggar *et al.*, 1998; Gollasch *et al.*, 2000; Gordienko *et al.*, 2001; Lohn *et al.*, 2001). SK_{Ca} and IK_{Ca} channels play a central role in the endothelial cell control of vasomotor tone and peripheral vascular resistance (Busse *et al.*, 2002; Eichler *et al.*, 2003; Taylor *et al.*, 2003; Si *et al.*, 2006; Brahler *et al.*, 2009). However, probably the most recognized function of these K^+ channels is their participation in the EDHF signaling (see below) (Busse *et al.*, 2002; Vanhoutte, 2004).

3. Paracrine signaling in the vessel wall

One of the most well-characterized mode of communication in the vessel wall is the production of paracrine signals by endothelial cells such as PGs, NO and EDHF (Vanhoutte, 2004; Vanhoutte *et al.*, 2009). The role of these signaling pathways in vascular physiology has been extensively studied and there are several recent reviews that address their involvement in vascular function in normal conditions and disease (Feletou & Vanhoutte, 2009; Vanhoutte *et al.*, 2009; Rafikov *et al.*, 2011). In this section, we will address the most relevant aspects of these signals in relation to the control of vasomotor tone in physiological conditions.

3.1 Prostaglandins

PGs are a family of bioactive lipids derived from arachidonic acid (AA or 5,8,11,14-eicosatetraenoic acid), which, in turn, is generated by the enzyme phospholipase A_2 (PLA_2) from phospholipids of the cell membrane in a Ca^{2+}-dependent manner (Simmons *et al.*, 2004; Fortier *et al.*, 2008). The metabolism of PGs is complex and depends on the hydrolysis of AA by the enzymes cyclooxygenase-1 (COX-1) or cyclooxygenase-2 (COX-2) to form the unstable endoperoxide derivative, prostaglandin G_2 (PGG_2), and subsequently, prostaglandin H_2 (PGH_2) (Simmons *et al.*, 2004). PGH_2 is the parent compound of all PGs, which are synthesized by specific enzymes: prostaglandin I_2 synthase (PGIS), prostaglandin E_2 synthase (PGES-1), prostaglandin D_2 synthase (PGDS), prostaglandin $F_{2}\alpha$ synthase (PGES-2), and thromboxane A_2 synthase (TBXAS-1) that catalyze the production of prostacyclins (PGI_2), PGE_2, PGD_2, $PGF_2\alpha$ and thromboxane A2 (TXA_2), respectively (Simmons *et al.*, 2004; Gryglewski, 2008). The presence of the different PG synthases varies from tissue to tissue. Finally, PGs are released to the extracellular space and exert their physiological effects by acting on specific membrane receptors (Norel, 2007), as depicted in Figure 1. Then, the production of prostanoids is triggered by an increase in intracellular Ca^{2+} concentration and the key reaction of this complex enzymatic cascade is catalyzed by the enzymes COXs (Figure 1).

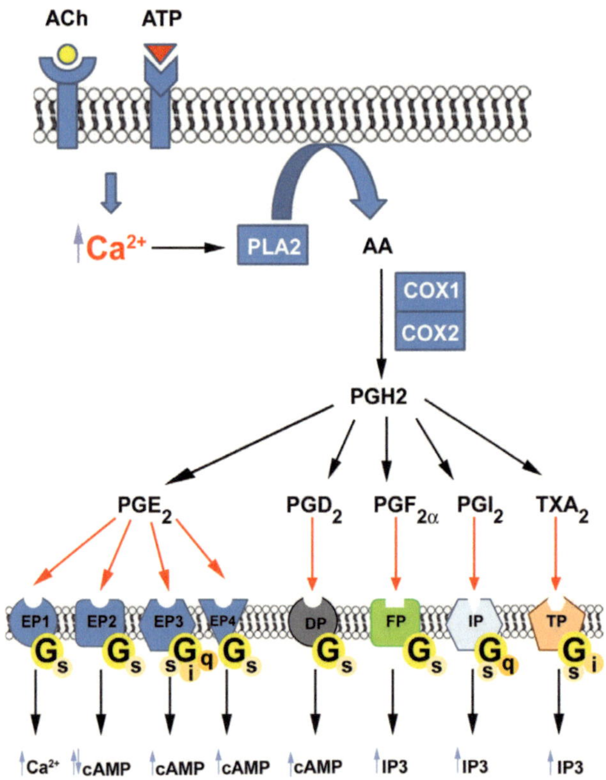

Fig. 1. Biosynthetic pathway of prostaglandins (PGs). An increase in intracellular Ca^{2+} concentration activates the production of arachidonic acid (AA) by phospholipase A2 (PLA2) from cell membrane phospholipids. The enzymes cyclooxygenase-1 (COX-1) or cyclooxygenase-2 (COX-2) convert AA into the endoperoxide PGH2, which is then metabolized by several synthases to PGs PGD_2, PGE_2, $PGF_2\alpha$, TXA_2 and PGI_2 (prostacyclin). Each PG acts on specific membrane receptors located in endothelial and/or smooth muscle cells. The transduction pathways activated by PGs are also depicted in the figure.

COX-1 and COX-2 are very similar and show a 60% homology. However, COX-1 is expressed constitutively, whereas the expression of COX-2 is inducible, since the levels of this COX isoform are very low in normal conditions and its expression increases in response to pro-inflammatory stimuli (Simmons *et al.*, 2004). Consistent with this, in normal physiological conditions, vascular endothelial and smooth muscle cells express COX-1 (Vanhoutte, 2009). In these cells, COX-1 mainly leads to the production of PGI_2, which induces the relaxation of smooth muscle cells by the stimulation of IP receptors (Figure 1) (Gryglewski, 2008; Vanhoutte, 2009). In contrast to COX-1, expression of COX-2 in normal blood vessels is very low (Crofford *et al.*, 1994; Schonbeck *et al.*, 1999). However, Topper et al. (Topper *et al.*, 1996) found that laminar shear stress, but not turbulent flow, up-regulates the levels of COX-2 expression in cultures of vascular endothelial cells. Laminar shear stress is a highly relevant stimulus that is involved in the tonic control of vasomotor tone, which highlights the participation of COXs and PGs in the regulation of vascular function.

3.2 Nitric oxide

Probably, the most relevant intercellular communication signal in vascular physiology is the endothelium-dependent NO production. NO is a potent vasodilator synthesized by the enzyme NO synthase (NOS) (Moncada *et al.*, 1991). The substrates for NOS-mediated NO production are the amino acid L-arginine, molecular oxygen and nicotinamide adenine dinucleotide phosphate (NADPH). Three isoforms of NOS have been described: endothelial NOS (eNOS), neuronal NOS (nNOS) and inducible NOS (iNOS) (Moncada *et al.*, 1991; Alderton *et al.*, 2001). The enzyme expressed in endothelial cells (eNOS) is the main NOS isoform found in the vascular system in normal conditions. The NO released by endothelial cells elicits the relaxation of the underlying vascular smooth muscle cells mainly through the initiation of the signaling cascade cGMP/PKG by activation of soluble guanylate cyclase, which has been ascribed as the primary receptor of NO (Moncada *et al.*, 1991). Although certainly the cGMP-dependent signaling pathway has several targets in the vessel wall, the relaxation induced by NO is mainly associated with a reduction in the Ca^{2+} sensitivity of smooth muscle contractile machinery (Bolz *et al.*, 1999; Bolz *et al.*, 2003).

Consistent with the importance of NO in vascular function, the activity of eNOS is finely regulated at transcriptional and posttranscriptional level (Fleming & Busse, 2003). Although eNOS was initially characterized as a Ca^{2+}-dependent enzyme and binding of the complex Ca^{2+}-calmodulin plays a central role in the activation of eNOS, NO production is also modulated by phosphorylation and protein-protein interactions (Mount *et al.*, 2007; Rafikov *et al.*, 2011). In this context, the sub-cellular targeting of eNOS is a key process in the regulation of NO production. Two functional pools of eNOS have been identified in vascular endothelial cells: one associated to Golgi complex and other located at caveolae, a subset of invaginated plasmalemmal rafts where the function of key signaling proteins is coordinated (Govers & Rabelink, 2001; Goligorsky *et al.*, 2002; Michel & Vanhoutte, 2010), which provides eNOS with a special proximity to signaling molecules, such as calmodulin, Ca^{2+} channels, BK_{Ca} channels and plasma membrane Ca^{2+} pumps (Darby *et al.*, 2000; Wang *et al.*, 2005). Although both pools of eNOS have been demonstrated to be functional, it is widely recognized that the integrity of caveolae is critical for the control of Ca^{2+}-mediated activation of NO production. In caveolae, eNOS is found in an inhibitory association with caveolin-1, an integral membrane protein of this signaling microdomain, and the interaction of eNOS with calcium-calmodulin releases the enzyme from its inhibitory association with caveolin-1 (Govers & Rabelink, 2001; Goligorsky *et al.*, 2002; Michel & Vanhoutte, 2010).

The eNOS localization at caveolae seems to be essential for the regulation of eNOS function by controlling L-arginine substrate supply. Typically, regulation of L-arginine availability has been under-appreciated, since intracellular L-arginine concentration is saturating from the perspective of eNOS kinetics (Km = ~5 μM) (Harrison, 1997). However, several reports indicate that increments in extracellular L-arginine levels can enhance NO production in endothelial cells (Zani & Bohlen, 2005; Kakoki *et al.*, 2006), despite a saturating intracellular L-arginine concentration, which was termed as the "Arginine Paradox" (McDonald *et al.*, 1997). This control of NO production by substrate suggests that intracellular L-arginine is not fully available for eNOS, whereas extracellular L-arginine is preferentially delivered to the enzyme. Consistent with this notion, NO production seems to be coupled to L-arginine uptake, because the main carrier that transports 60 - 80% of L-arginine across the plasma membrane of endothelial cells, the cationic amino acid transporter-1 (CAT-1), was found to co-localize with eNOS in caveolae (McDonald *et al.*, 1997) (Figure 2). Interestingly, it was reported that eNOS interacts directly with CAT-1 in bovine aortic endothelial cells (BAECs), and apparently, the eNOS-CAT-1 association in addition to facilitate the delivery of extracellular L-arginine for NO generation, also enhances the eNOS enzymatic activity by increasing the activating phosphorylation of the enzyme at serine 1179 and 635, and by decreasing the association of eNOS with caveolin-1 (Li *et al.*, 2005).

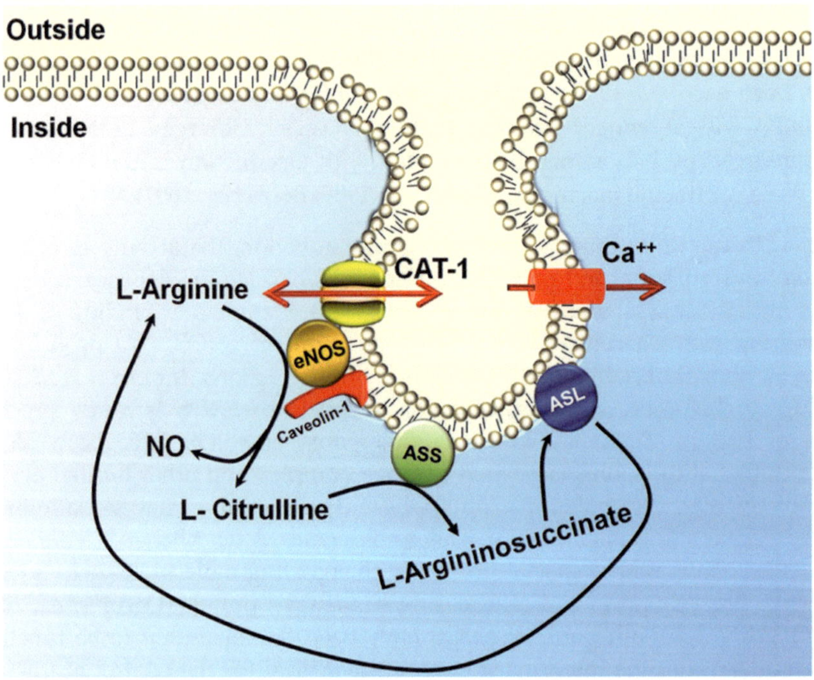

Fig. 2. Local control of eNOS activity by L-arginine. eNOS synthesizes nitric oxide (NO) and the byproduct L-citrulline from L-arginine. The eNOS localization at signaling microdomains known as caveolae provides to this enzyme with a direct, local source of L-arginine. In caveolae, eNOS is in direct association with the main carrier of L-arginine in endothelial cells, the cationic amino acid transporter-1 (CAT-1), and is also associated with the enzymes argininosuccinate synthase (ASS) and argininosuccinate lyase (ASL) that regenerate L-arginine from L-citrulline.

Another mechanism that has emerged as an important source of L-arginine supply for NO production is the regeneration of L-arginine from the other product of the eNOS-catalyzed reaction, L-citrulline. This regeneration is catalyzed by the enzymes argininosuccinate synthase (ASS) and argininosuccinate lyase (ASL), which are mostly expressed in caveolae in endothelial cells (Flam *et al.*, 2001; Solomonson *et al.*, 2003) (Figure 2). Interestingly, addition of exogenous L-citrulline results in a larger increase in endothelial NO production than that observed with exogenous L-arginine, without a proportional increase in intracellular L-arginine (Solomonson *et al.*, 2003), suggesting that recycling of L-citrulline to L-arginine is channeled directly to synthesize NO (Figure 2). In addition, it was estimated that under maximum stimulation of NO production with bradykinin, but not in unstimulated conditions, approximately 80% of the eNOS-catalyzed L-arginine was supplied by the recycling of L-citrulline (Solomonson *et al.*, 2003). These findings indicate that eNOS activation is functionally coupled with the L-citrulline recycling system (ASS and ASL) in caveolae (Figure 2). Therefore, NO production seems to be regulated by a complex interaction between different pools of L-arginine, where direct channeling to eNOS of the L-arginine regenerated from L-citrulline by the coordinated action of the enzymes ASS and ASL is likely to play a central role (Figure 2).

3.3 Endothelium-derived hyperpolarizing factor

Although the development of knockout animals has demonstrated the importance of the multiple functions of NO along the whole vascular system, it has become apparent that the relevance of NO in the control of vasomotor tone depends on vessel size. Accordingly, NO is the primary endothelium-dependent vasodilator signal in large, conduit vessels (Shimokawa *et al.*, 1996). However, an additional vasodilator component has also been identified in small resistance arteries and arterioles (Suzuki *et al.*, 1992; Murphy & Brayden, 1995). In these vessels, blockade of NO and PG production only attenuates the response to endothelium-dependent vasodilators such as acetylcholine (ACh) or bradykinin (Vanhoutte, 2004). The relaxant pathway resistant to NOS and COX blockers is associated with smooth muscle hyperpolarization, and thereby, it was attributed to the release of an endothelium-derived hyperpolarizing factor (EDHF). The chemical nature of EDHF remains controversial and seems to depend on vessel size, vascular territory, and species (Vanhoutte, 2004). In this context, several EDHF candidates have been proposed, such as K^+ ions (Edwards *et al.*, 1998), epoxyeicosatrienoic acids (EETs) (Archer *et al.*, 2003; Fleming, 2004), hydrogen peroxide (Shimokawa & Morikawa, 2005), and C-type natriuretic peptide (CNP) (Chauhan *et al.*, 2003; Ahluwalia & Hobbs, 2005). However, in most cases, the EDHF-mediated smooth muscle hyperpolarization and vasodilation has been shown to be sensitive to simultaneous blockade of SK_{Ca} and IK_{Ca} (Doughty *et al.*, 1999; Ghisdal & Morel, 2001; Crane *et al.*, 2003; Eichler *et al.*, 2003; Hilgers *et al.*, 2006). Interestingly, these K^+ channels have been reported to be located in two different subcellular domains. While SK_{Ca} channels are found in caveolae (Absi *et al.*, 2007; Rath *et al.*, 2009), IK_{Ca} channels were proposed to be expressed in the abluminal side of endothelial cells (Figure 3), facing Na^+ pumps and K_{ir} channels situated in smooth muscle cells (Edwards *et al.*, 1998; Dora *et al.*, 2008). Then, the opening of IK_{Ca} channels may increase the K^+ ion concentration in the myoendothelial space, which may couple endothelial cell IK_{Ca} signaling to Na^+ pump- and K_{ir} channel-mediated smooth muscle hyperpolarization (Edwards *et al.*, 1998; Dora *et al.*, 2008) (Figure 3).

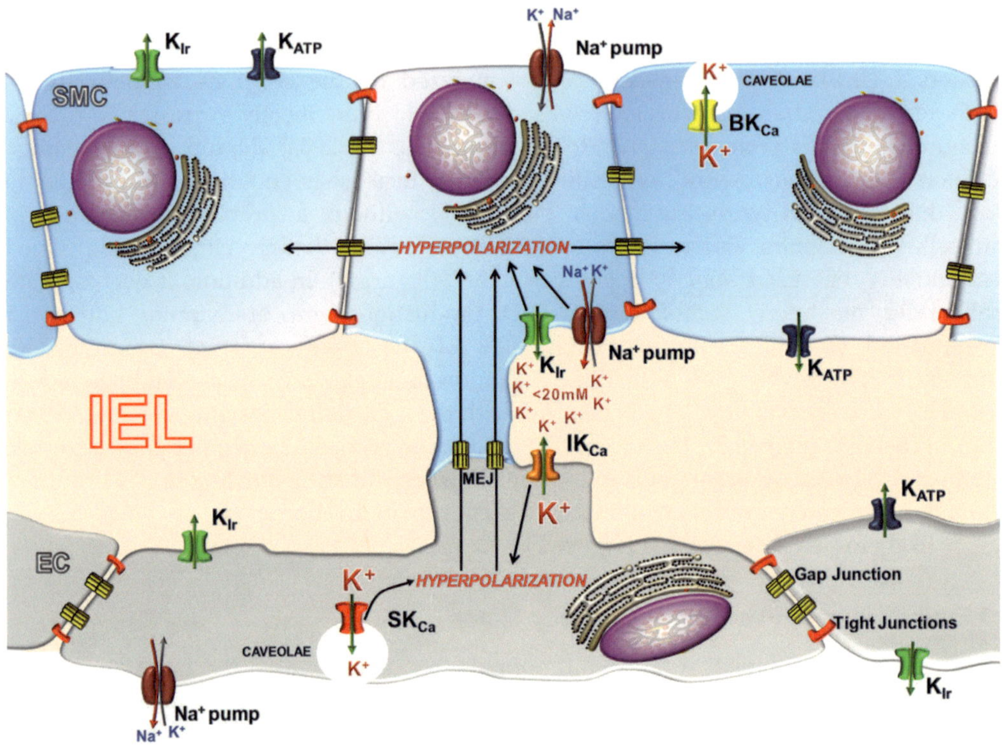

Fig. 3. K^+ channel distribution and endothelium-dependent vasodilation. Ca^{2+}-activated K^+ channels of small (SK_{Ca}) and intermediate (IK_{Ca}) conductance may contribute to the vasodilation associated with an endothelium-mediated smooth muscle hyperpolarization (response typically attributed to an endothelium-derive hyperpolarizing factor, EDHF) by two pathways. First, the hyperpolarization induced by activation of SK_{Ca} and IK_{Ca} is transmitted electrotonically to the underlying smooth muscle cells (SMC) through the gap junctions located at discrete points of contact between endothelial and smooth muscle cells, structure known as myoendothelial junctions (MEJ). In addition, the small increase in extracellular K^+ concentration (<20 mM) resulting from the opening of the IK_{Ca} found at the abluminal side of endothelial cells (EC) may activate inward rectifying K^+ channels (K_{ir}) and Na^+ pump in smooth muscle cells. Between SMC and EC is found the internal elastic lamina (IEL).

Notwithstanding the smooth muscle hyperpolarization is considered to be the hallmark of EDHF action (Vanhoutte, 2004), it is important to note that hyperpolarization of the vessel wall is not a unique characteristic of EDHF. In several vessel preparations, in addition to a reduced Ca^{2+} sensitivity of the contractile machinery, the NO-dependent vasodilation has also been associated with smooth muscle hyperpolarization (Cohen *et al.*, 1997; Lang & Watson, 1998). Furthermore, consistent with a NO-mediated hyperpolarization, NO has been reported to activate BK_{Ca}, K_{ir} and K_{ATP} channels on the smooth muscle cells and endothelial cells directly or through the activation of cGMP production (Bolotina *et al.*, 1994; Abderrahmane *et al.*, 1998; Lee & Kang, 2001; Si *et al.*, 2002; Schubert *et al.*, 2004). Therefore, NO and EDHF are not only complementary, but also additive and the effect of both vasodilator components may be confounded. In this context, it is interesting to note that, as mentioned above, the EDHF-mediated response is typically studied in presence of NOS and COX blockers. However, NOS inhibition with analogues of L-arginine is a slow, time-dependent process and, on occasion, blockade of NO production with these drugs has been observed to be incomplete (Vanheel & Van de Voorde, 2000; Figueroa *et al.*, 2001; Chauhan *et al.*, 2003; Stoen *et al.*, 2003; Stankevicius *et al.*, 2006), and then, the residual NO production observed in presence of NOS inhibitors may contribute to the vasodilation associated with the smooth muscle hyperpolarization attributes to EDHF. In addition, the findings reported recently by Gaete et al. (Gaete *et al.*, 2011) are another important point to take into account in the interaction between EDHF and NO. In this work Gaete et al., demonstrated that SK_{Ca} and IK_{Ca} channels control the Ca^{2+}-dependent NO release, and thereby, the inactivation of these K^+ channels is associated with an increase in NAD(P)H oxidase-mediated superoxide production, which leads to the inhibition of eNOS primarily by its phosphorylation at threonine 495 (Gaete *et al.*, 2011). These findings highlight the relevance of these K^+ channels in the control of vascular function and indicate that the participation of superoxide in the EDHF-mediated response associated to SK_{Ca} and IK_{Ca} channels must be evaluated.

Furthermore, the regulation of NO and EDHF is different depending on gender. In male animals, NO is the major endothelium-dependent vasodilator signal, but in female EDHF prevails over NO or PGI_2 (Scotland *et al.*, 2005). In this context, it is interesting to note that estrogen enhances the EDHF-mediated vasodilation in response to flow (Huang *et al.*, 2001), which suggests that the EDHF-dependent signaling pathway may be more important in the control of blood pressure in female than in male animals. This idea was confirmed using an eNOS/COX-1 double knockout. Deletion of eNOS and COX-1 did not alter the mean arterial blood pressure in female mice, whereas the double knockout resulted in hypertension in male mice (Scotland *et al.*, 2005). In these animals, the endothelium-dependent relaxation was intact in resistance vessels of female mice and was mediated by the smooth muscle hyperpolarization (Scotland *et al.*, 2005), strongly supporting that EDHF plays a predominant role in the tonic control of blood pressure in female. These data suggest that EDHF rather than NO may underlie the higher resistance of premenopausal females to cardiovascular diseases such as hypertension.

4. Gap junction communication in the vascular function

Gap junctions are intercellular channels that directly connect the cytoplasm of neighboring cells, allowing the passage of current or molecules smaller than ~1.4 nm of diameter such as metabolites (e.g., ADP, glucose, glutamate and glutathione) or second messengers (e.g., Ca^{2+}, cAMP and IP_3) (Evans & Martin, 2002; Saez *et al.*, 2003). These intercellular channels are made up by a protein family known as connexins (Cx), which are named according to their predicted molecular mass expressed in kDa. Connexin proteins have four transmembrane domains with the N- and C-termini located on the cytoplasmic membrane face. The radial arrangement of six connexins around a central pore makes a connexon or hemichannel, and the association in the plasma membrane of two hemichannels provided by adjacent cells forms an intercellular gap junction channel (Evans & Martin, 2002; Saez *et al.*, 2003). It is noteworthy that independent hemichannels can also remain unpaired and functional, which have been recognized to release paracrine signals such as ATP, PGE_2 or NAD^+ (Goodenough & Paul, 2003; Cherian *et al.*, 2005; Saez *et al.*, 2005). The importance of this mode of communication in the vasculature is just starting to be evaluated and, consistent with the participation of vascular hemichannels in paracrine signaling, human microvascular endothelial cell (HMEC-1) monolayers were found to release ATP through Cx43-formed hemichannels (Faigle *et al.*, 2008).

At least twenty connexin isoforms have been described in mammals and one cell type may express more than one connexin (Saez *et al.*, 2003). However, the expression of several connexins in one cell does not seem to be redundant, because gap junctions are not just simple channels that offer a low-resistance intercellular pathway, but connexins mediate highly specific cell-to-cell signaling pathways, and the molecular selectivity as well as subcellular localization differs among connexins (Saez *et al.*, 2003; Figueroa *et al.*, 2004; Locke *et al.*, 2005). Thus, although these proteins may have some overlap in function, they work in concert (Simon & Goodenough, 1998; Figueroa *et al.*, 2004, 2006; Haefliger *et al.*, 2006) and, consequently, it has been observed that many times the function of one connexin cannot be replaced by other connexin isoform (White, 2003; Haefliger *et al.*, 2006; Zheng-Fischhofer *et al.*, 2006; Wolfle *et al.*, 2007). In addition, hemichannels can be composed by one or a mixture of connexin proteins, which provides an additional mechanism for fine regulation of gap junction-mediated signaling processes (White & Bruzzone, 1996; He *et al.*, 1999; Beyer *et al.*, 2000; Cottrell *et al.*, 2002; Moreno, 2004).

Five connexin proteins have been found to be expressed in the vasculature: Cx32, Cx37, Cx40, Cx43, and Cx45 (Severs *et al.*, 2001; Figueroa *et al.*, 2004; Haefliger *et al.*, 2004; Okamoto *et al.*, 2009). The expression of connexins in the different cell types of the vessel wall is not uniform and vary with vessel size, vascular territory, and species (van Kempen *et al.*, 1995; van Kempen & Jongsma, 1999; Hill *et al.*, 2002). In most cases, Cx45 is only observed in smooth muscle cells and has mainly been detected in brain vessels (Kruger *et al.*, 2000; Li & Simard, 2001). In contrast, the expression of Cx32 and Cx37 seems to be restricted to the endothelium (Gabriels & Paul, 1998; van Kempen & Jongsma, 1999; Severs *et al.*, 2001; Okamoto *et al.*, 2009), but Cx37 has also been detected in smooth muscle cells (Rummery *et al.*, 2002). Although Cx40 and Cx43 may be expressed in both cell types (Little *et al.*, 1995; Gabriels & Paul, 1998; van Kempen & Jongsma, 1999; Severs *et al.*, 2001), Cx40 is located predominately in endothelial cells (Gabriels & Paul, 1998; van Kempen & Jongsma, 1999) and Cx43 is the most prominent gap junction protein found in smooth muscle cells (van Kempen & Jongsma, 1999). It should be noted, however, that in mouse, Cx40 is expressed exclusively in the endothelium (de Wit *et al.*, 2000; Figueroa *et al.*, 2003; Figueroa & Duling, 2008).

In addition to connexins, another family of three members of membrane proteins named pannexins (Panxs 1-3) has been documented (Bruzzone *et al.*, 2003). Apparently, pannexins only form hemichannels, and then, the main function of pannexin-based channels is paracrine or autocrine communication (Locovei *et al.*, 2006). Although connexins and pannexins share a similar membrane topology, their amino acid sequences present only a 16% homology (Bruzzone *et al.*, 2003). Only the expression of Panx-1 has been identified in blood vessels at the moment and recently this pannexin was found to be involved in the activation of the vasoconstrictor response mediated by α1-adrenoceptor stimulation (Billaud *et al.*, 2011).

4.1 Gap junctions in vascular smooth muscle

Coordination of vasomotor signals among smooth muscle cells is critical for the function of blood vessels. As mentioned above, the contractile state of smooth muscle cells depends on the cytoplasmic Ca^{2+} concentration and Ca^{2+} sensitivity of the contractile apparatus. Intracellular Ca^{2+} concentration is controlled by the smooth muscle cell membrane potential. Then, gap junctions play a central role integrating the smooth muscle cell function because these intercellular channels synchronize changes in both membrane potential and intracellular Ca^{2+} between adjacent smooth muscle cells (Christ *et al.*, 1991; Christ *et al.*, 1992; Christ *et al.*, 1996).

In addition, gap junction communication of vascular smooth muscle cells seems to be involved in the development of myogenic vasomotor tone in resistance arteries (Lagaud *et al.*, 2002; Earley *et al.*, 2004). Interestingly, the participation of gap junction in this process is not related to synchronization of Ca^{2+} signaling, but rather to earlier signaling events such as coordination of the smooth muscle cell-depolarization or directly the mechanosensitivity of the vascular smooth muscle. This notion is supported by the fact that the gap junctions and connexin hemichannels inhibitors Gap27 (a connexin mimetic peptide) or 18α-glycyrrhetinic acid, in addition to block Ca^{2+} influx and vasoconstriction in mesenteric resistance arteries, also prevented the pressure-induced smooth muscle cell depolarization (Earley *et al.*, 2004). It is important to note that Gap27 and 18α-glycyrrhetinic acid are two well-known gap junction blockers, but they also block connexin-formed hemichannels, which indicates that hemichannels may also be involved in the development of the myogenic response. In any case, the involvement of Cx43-based channels in the control of vasomotor tone is consistent with the finding that tensile stretch increased the expression of this connexin as well as gap junction intercellular communication in vascular smooth muscle cells (Cowan *et al.*, 1998). Interestingly, this response was mediated by the formation of reactive oxygen species (Cowan *et al.*, 1998; Cowan *et al.*, 2003), which has been reported to contribute to the initiation of the myogenic constriction in mouse-tail arterioles (Nowicki *et al.*, 2001).

Cx43 has also been involved in the regulation of cell proliferation and migration in the vasculature (Polacek *et al.*, 1997; Yeh *et al.*, 1997; Kwak *et al.*, 2001), which can be appreciated in Cx43-deficient smooth muscle cells. Damage of carotid artery by vascular occlusion or wire injury resulted in an increase in neointima and adventitia formation in smooth muscle cell Cx43 specific knockout mice as compared to wild type animals (Liao *et al.*, 2007), suggesting an accelerated growth of smooth muscle cell with the Cx43 deletion, which was further confirmed using cultured cells. Nevertheless, in apparent opposition to these findings, Chadjichristos et al. (Chadjichristos *et al.*, 2006) show that in heterozygous Cx43 knockout mice the neointimal formation was reduced. However, in those animals, Cx43 was reduced from all cell types expressing Cx43 and the experiments included a high-fat diet, which may have influenced the result by either vascular adaptive response to the diet or complex interactions between different cell types. Although the participation of Cx43 in neointimal formation demands further investigation, these data highlight the relevance of Cx43 in the feedback control pathways necessary for vascular morphogenesis.

4.2 Gap junctions in vascular endothelium

The endothelium plays a key role in the tonic control of blood pressure and the development of knockout animals of vascular connexins has disclosed that gap junction communication of endothelial cells is essential in the coordination and integration of microvascular function. Vascular endothelial cells-specific deletion of Cx43 (VEC Cx43-/-) results in hypotension (Liao *et al.*, 2001) and, in contrast, ablation of Cx40 produces a hypertension associated with an irregular vasomotion (de Wit *et al.*, 2000; de Wit *et al.*, 2003; Figueroa & Duling, 2008) and a dysregulation of renin production (Krattinger *et al.*, 2007; Wagner *et al.*, 2007). Although deletion of Cx37 does not appear to alter vascular function or blood pressure (Figueroa & Duling, 2008), several polymorphisms of this connexin have been associated with myocardial infarction, coronary artery disease and atherosclerosis (Boerma *et al.*, 1999; Yamada *et al.*, 2002; Hirashiki *et al.*, 2003; Yamada *et al.*, 2004). In mice, Cx40 and Cx37 are primarily expressed in the endothelium, which emphasizes the importance of the endothelial cell-gap junction communication in the control of cardiovascular homeostasis.

Although the mechanistic bases of the hypotension observed in VEC Cx43-/- are still unknown, the plasma levels of angiotensin I and II as well as NO were elevated in these animals (Liao *et al.*, 2001), suggesting that a dysregulation of NO production may have been the responsible of the hypotension with the subsequent activation of the renin-angiotensin system. Also, it is interesting to note that shear stress up-regulates the expression of Cx43 in cultured endothelial cells (DePaola *et al.*, 1999; Bao *et al.*, 2000) and in the endothelium of rat cardiac valves (Inai *et al.*, 2004), which suggests that Cx43 may be involved in the response to mechanical stimuli.

4.3 Gap junctions in smooth muscle-endothelium communication

Smooth muscle cells and endothelial cells have also been found to be electrically and metabolically connected by gap junctions located at discrete points of contact between the two cell types at the myoendothelial junction (MEJ) (Beny & Pacicca, 1994; Little *et al.*, 1995; Emerson & Segal, 2000; Sandow *et al.*, 2003). This heterocellular communication seems to play a pivotal role in the Ca^{2+}-mediated responses induced by endothelium-dependent vasodilators, such as ACh. As mentioned above, these vasodilator responses are typically paralleled by hyperpolarization of the underlying smooth muscle cells (Emerson & Segal, 2000; Goto *et al.*, 2002; Griffith, 2004), which has been attributed to the release of an EDHF (Vanhoutte, 2004; Feletou & Vanhoutte, 2009). However, the direct electrotonic transmission of a hyperpolarizing current from the endothelial cells to the smooth muscle cells via myoendothelial gap junctions may explain the EDHF pathway (Busse *et al.*, 2002; Dora *et al.*, 2003; Griffith, 2004). In this perspective, the increase in endothelial cell intracellular Ca^{2+} concentration activates SK_{Ca} and IK_{Ca} channels leading to the endothelium-dependent hyperpolarization of smooth muscle cells via gap junctions located at the MEJ (Busse *et al.*, 2002; Crane *et al.*, 2003; Eichler *et al.*, 2003; Feletou *et al.*, 2003) (Figure 3). Consistent with this hypothesis, the EDHF-dependent vasodilation has been reported to be prevented by connexin-mimetic peptides that are thought to specifically block gap junctions (De Vriese *et al.*, 2002; Karagiannis *et al.*, 2004; Chaytor *et al.*, 2005) as well as endothelial cell-selective loading of antibodies directed against the carboxyl-terminal region of Cx40 (Mather *et al.*, 2005). Interestingly, the gap junction-mediated EDHF signal might be controlled by NO through S-nitrosylation. Cx43-based channels can be activated by S-nitrosylation (Retamal *et al.*, 2006). Cx43 and eNOS has been found to be express at MEJ and the activation of NO production in this microdomains leads to a S-nitrosylation-associated opening of Cx43-formed myoendothelial gap junction (Straub *et al.*, 2011), which support the idea that EDHF and NO are not parallel, independent vasodilator components, but in contrast, they work in concert.

Flow (i.e. shear stress) is one of the most important stimuli involved in the tonic regulation of vasomotor tone. Although the response to shear stress is thought to be mediated primarily by NO, shear stress has also been reported to activate an EDHF-dependent vasodilator response (Watanabe *et al.*, 2005), which suggests that a gap junction-mediated EDHF pathway may be involved in the tonic control of peripheral vascular resistance. Consistent with this idea, intrarenal infusion of connexin-mimetic peptides homologous to the second extracellular loop of Cx43 (^{43}Gap 27) or Cx40 (^{40}Gap 27) not only decreased basal renal blood flow, but also increased mean arterial blood pressure of rats, either in presence or absence of NOS and COX blockers (De Vriese *et al.*, 2002), suggesting that connexin-mimetic peptides induced vasoconstriction by disrupting or reducing the response to a tonic vasodilator stimulus such as shear stress.

5. Conduction of vasomotor responses

Longitudinal conduction of vasomotor responses provides an essential means of coordinating changes in diameter and flow distribution among vessels of the microcirculation. Vasomotor signals spread along the vessel length through gap junctions connecting cells of the vessel wall, and thereby, participate in the minute-to-minute coordination of vascular resistance by integrating function of proximal and distal vascular segments in the microcirculation (de Wit *et al.*, 2000; Figueroa *et al.*, 2004, 2006). Although vasoconstrictor responses are thought to be conducted by smooth muscle cells (Welsh & Segal, 1998; Bartlett & Segal, 2000; Budel *et al.*, 2003), the cellular pathway for conduction of vasodilator signals is more controversial and may be either exclusively by the endothelium (Emerson & Segal, 2000; Segal & Jacobs, 2001) or by both smooth muscle and endothelial cells (Bartlett & Segal, 2000; Budel *et al.*, 2003). The cellular pathway for conduction of vasomotor responses has been studied by selectively damaging a short segment of endothelial cells or smooth muscle cells by injection of an air bubble via a side branch (Bartlett & Segal, 2000; Figueroa *et al.*, 2007) or with a light-dye (fluorescein-conjugated dextran) treatment (Emerson & Segal, 2000). In feed arteries, selective damage of the endothelium completely blocked the ACh-induced conducted vasodilation (Emerson & Segal, 2000; Segal & Jacobs, 2001), but in arterioles, either damage of the endothelium or the smooth muscle did not affect the ACh-induced conducted responses (Bartlett & Segal, 2000; Budel *et al.*, 2003), which led to the proposal that the cellular pathway for conduction of vasodilations depends on the functional location of the vessel in the microvascular network (Segal, 2005). However, the cellular pathway of vasodilator signals may also depend on the stimulus that initiated the response, because, in contrast to ACh, selective damage of the endothelium blocked the vasodilation induced by bradykinin in arterioles (Welsh & Segal, 1998; Budel *et al.*, 2003).

Direct measurements of membrane potential have shown that conducted vasomotor responses are associated with rapid propagation (milliseconds) of an electrical signal along the vessel length (Xia & Duling, 1995; Welsh & Segal, 1998; Emerson & Segal, 2000). Because many observations have revealed an exponential decay of the conducted electrical signal, it was proposed that longitudinal spread of vasomotor responses reflects the passive, electrotonic conduction of changes in membrane potential via gap junctions connecting cells of the vessel wall (Pacicca *et al.*, 1996; Welsh & Segal, 1998; Gustafsson & Holstein-Rathlou, 1999). Therefore, the decay of the conducted vasomotor responses along the vessel length should be consistent with the length constant estimated from electrotonic potentials produced by current injection into the smooth muscle or endothelial cells of arterioles, which is between 0.9 and 1.6 mm (Hirst & Neild, 1978; Hirst *et al.*, 1997; Emerson *et al.*, 2002).

Conduction of vasoconstrictor responses typically behaves as predicted by the electrotonic model. However, a simple electrotonic model often fails to predict conduction of vasodilator signals initiated by endothelium-dependent stimuli, such as ACh or bradykinin. These signals have been reported to propagate for many millimeters without showing noticeable decay in magnitude (Emerson & Segal, 2000; Figueroa & Duling, 2008). In addition, the electrical length constant of ACh-induced hyperpolarization has been shown to be longer than that measured for current injection (Emerson *et al.*, 2002) and the hyperpolarizing signal activated by ACh has been also reported to increase during the first 1000 μm of longitudinal conduction (Crane *et al.*, 2004). The lack of decay of these responses suggests that a regenerative, energy-dependent mechanism underlies the conduction process, similar to that described in neurons. Consistent with this idea, electrical stimulation also activates a conducted, non-decremental endothelium-dependent vasodilation that was hypothesized to be mediated by a complex interplay between voltage-gated Na^+ channels (Na_v) and T type, voltage-gated Ca^{2+} channels (T-Ca_v) (Figueroa *et al.*, 2007). In this hypothetic model, Na_v channels underlie the conduction of the signal and T-Ca_v mediates the vasodilation. Interestingly, deletion of Cx40 selectively eliminates the regenerative component of the conducted vasodilation induced by ACh (Figueroa & Duling, 2008), bradykinin (de Wit *et al.*, 2000) or electrical stimulation (Figueroa *et al.*, 2003), leaving a decaying component consistent with the electrotonic model (Figueroa & Duling, 2008), which suggests that Cx40-based gap junctions provide the pathway for the intercellular propagation of the regenerative conducted component of vasodilator signals. Deletion of Cx37 did not affect conduction of vasodilator responses (Figueroa & Duling, 2008) and replacement of Cx40 by Cx45 did not restore the non-decremental component of the conducted vasodilation activated by ACh or bradykinin (Wolfle *et al.*, 2007), supporting the idea that individual connexins have different functions.

The opening of K_{ir} channels induced by the smooth muscle hyperpolarization may be an alternative hypothesis to explain the extended conduction of vasodilator responses. An intrinsic biophysical property of K_{ir} channels is that they increase their activity upon cell hyperpolarization and it has been proposed that the activation of these K^+ channels in the smooth muscle cells amplify the hyperpolarizing current initiated by ACh, thereby facilitating the conduction of this signal (Jantzi *et al.*, 2006). However, as mentioned above, current-induced hyperpolarization decays faster than the response induced by ACh (Emerson *et al.*, 2002), which argues against the participation of K_{ir} alone in the non-decremental component of the conducted vasodilation, and suggests that further investigation is needed to elucidate the mechanisms involved in the conduction of vasomotor responses.

6. Neurovascular coupling

The brain has a very high metabolic demand and its activity depends on the communication between brain cells and local microvessels (i.e. neurovascular unit). Then, the function of cerebral microcirculation must be coupled to neuronal activity, which is known as neurovascular coupling (Hawkins & Davis, 2005; Leybaert, 2005). In this case, however, vasomotor signals seem to be conducted by astrocytes as opposed to smooth muscle or endothelium (Anderson & Nedergaard, 2003; Zonta *et al.*, 2003; Mulligan & MacVicar, 2004; Koehler *et al.*, 2006; Metea & Newman, 2006; Takano *et al.*, 2006). Tight spatial and temporal coupling between neuronal activity and blood flow is essential for brain function (Anderson & Nedergaard, 2003; Hawkins & Davis, 2005; Leybaert, 2005) and astrocytes are found in a strategic location between neurons and the microvasculature, with the astrocytic endfeet ensheathing the vessels. This spatial organization places the astrocytes in a key position to orchestrate the neurovascular coupling and an increasing body of evidence shows that the astrocyte transduces and conducts to the local microvasculature vasomotor signals generated by an increase in synaptic activity (Anderson & Nedergaard, 2003; Zonta *et al.*, 2003; Mulligan & MacVicar, 2004; Metea & Newman, 2006; Takano *et al.*, 2006) (Figure 4). As a result, astrocytes couple neuronal activation to vasodilation of local parenchymal arterioles (Figure 4), which, in turn, leads to an increase in blood-borne energy substrate that rapidly matches the enhanced metabolic demand (Anderson & Nedergaard, 2003; Hawkins & Davis, 2005; Leybaert, 2005).

Calcium seems to be the intracellular vasomotor signal of the astrocyte-mediated neurovascular coupling. Astrocytes express receptors for several neurotransmitters such as glutamate, GABA and ATP (Anderson & Nedergaard, 2003; Leybaert, 2005; Koehler *et al.*, 2009), which can initiate Ca^{2+} signals (Figure 4). Then, the increase in neuronal activity results in an astrocytic calcium signaling that propagates through the astrocytic processes into the endfeet (Anderson & Nedergaard, 2003; Zonta *et al.*, 2003; Filosa *et al.*, 2004; Mulligan & MacVicar, 2004; Straub *et al.*, 2006). The increase in cytosolic calcium concentration in the endfeet ultimately causes the release of vasoactive factors and arteriolar dilation (Anderson & Nedergaard, 2003; Zonta *et al.*, 2003; Mulligan & MacVicar, 2004; Filosa *et al.*, 2006; Straub *et al.*, 2006) (Figure 4). Interestingly, astrocytes express gap junctions (Martinez & Saez, 2000; Saez *et al.*, 2003; Retamal *et al.*, 2006) and a calcium signal may propagate between neighboring astrocytes in a wave-like manner (Cornell-Bell *et al.*, 1990; Nedergaard, 1994; Cai *et al.*, 1998; Nedergaard *et al.*, 2003), coordinating the neurovascular coupling in the local cerebral microcirculation (Anderson & Nedergaard, 2003; Zonta *et al.*, 2003; Filosa *et al.*, 2004; Mulligan & MacVicar, 2004). Some of the Ca^{2+}-dependent vasodilator mechanisms that may be activated at the astrocytic endfeet facing the vessel wall are the production of epoxyeicosatrienoic acid (EETs) by the cytochrome P450 epoxygenase and PGs by the COX enzyme (Anderson & Nedergaard, 2003; Zonta *et al.*, 2003; Zonta *et al.*, 2003; Filosa *et al.*, 2004; Straub *et al.*, 2006; Koehler *et al.*, 2009), and also ATP release (Shi *et al.*, 2008) via connexin or pannexin hemichannels (Figure 4). In addition, astrocytic endfeet express BK_{Ca} and Girouard et al. (Girouard *et al.*, 2010) recently showed in mouse cortical brain slices that these K^+ channels play a central role in neurovascular coupling through the release of K^+ ion into the perivascular space (Figure 4). The small increase in local $[K^+]_o$ (<20 mM) activates the K_{ir} channels located in the smooth muscle cell membrane facing the endfeet, which leads to hyperpolarization, and subsequently, vasodilation (Girouard *et al.*, 2010) (Figure 4). It is noteworthy that a higher increase in $[K^+]_o$ would produce smooth muscle cell depolarization and vasoconstriction (Girouard *et al.*, 2010).

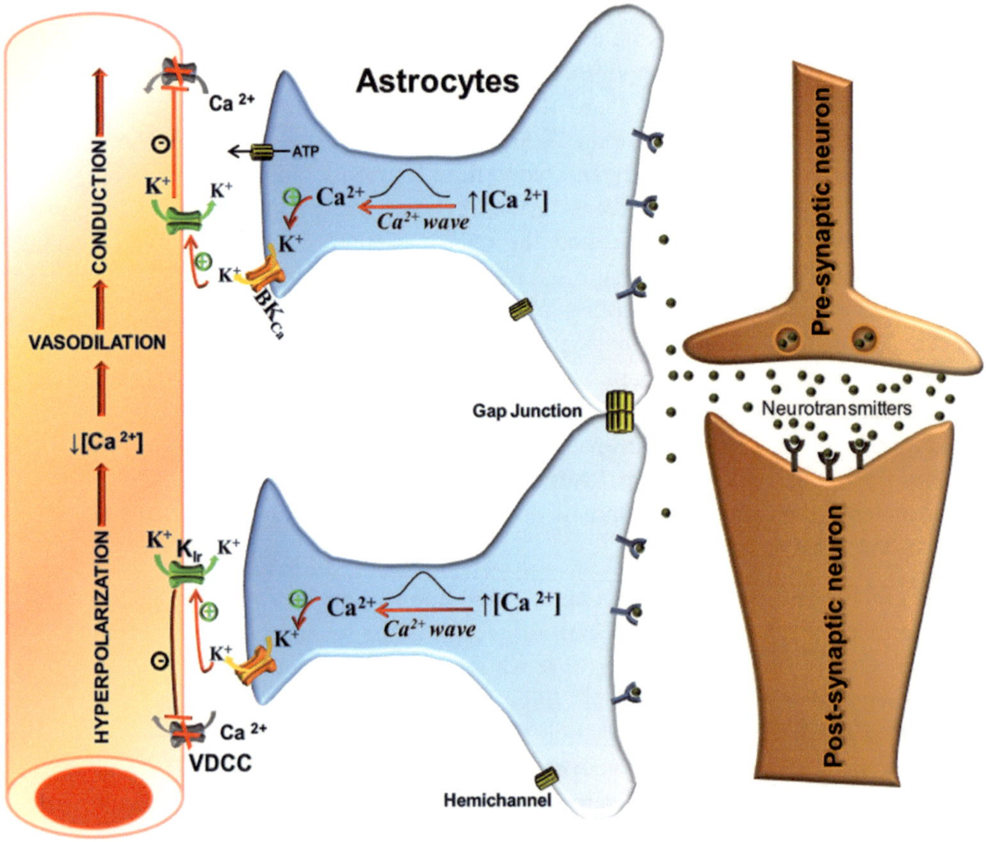

Fig. 4. Astrocytes-mediated neurovascular coupling. Neurotransmitters may exit the synaptic cleft and activate receptors on astrocytes, which couple neuronal activity with astrocyte signaling. The activation of astrocyte receptors triggers a Ca^{2+} wave that reaches the astrocytic endfeet, leading to the opening of large conductance Ca^{2+}-activated K^+ channels (BK_{Ca}). The K^+ ion release via BK_{Ca} elicits a small increase in extracellular K^+ concentration (<20 mM) in the perivascular space that activates the K_{ir} channels located in the smooth muscle cell membrane facing the endfeet, which, in turn, leads to hyperpolarization, and subsequently, vasodilation. The vessel wall hyperpolarization-mediated vasodilation is conducted to upstream arterioles, coupling function of proximal and distal vessels.

As described in the peripheral microcirculation (Segal & Kurjiaka, 1995; Segal, 2000), local vasodilation of cerebral arterioles must be communicated to upstream vascular segments to produce a functional increase of blood flow supply and effectively match the local metabolic demand (Cox *et al.*, 1993; Iadecola *et al.*, 1997). Although vasomotor responses have been observed to be conducted by the wall of cerebral arterioles (Dietrich *et al.*, 1996; Horiuchi *et al.*, 2002), it seems to be that astrocytes also play a central role in integrating function of local arterioles with upstream cerebral vessels involved in the neurovascular coupling. Pial arterioles are important upstream vessels of the parenchymal cerebral arterioles. It is important to note that pial arterioles overlie a thick layer of astrocytic processes, known as the glia limitans, which isolate these arterioles from the neurons that are located right below. Vasodilation of pial arterioles associated with neuronal activation was blocked by either selective elimination of astrocytes with L-α aminoadipic acid treatment or the inhibition of Cx43-based channels with the specific connexin mimetic peptide gap-27 (Xu *et al.*, 2008). In astrocytes, Cx43 may be found forming unpaired hemichannels or gap junction intercellular channels (Stout *et al.*, 2002; Saez *et al.*, 2003; Retamal *et al.*, 2006). Thus, astrocytic Cx43-based channels could be involved in the coordination of calcium waves between astrocytes, or in the release of vasoactive factors such as ATP that can be metabolized to the potent vasodilator, adenosine (Shi *et al.*, 2008)

7. Conclusion

Control of vasomotor tone relies on a complex interplay between NO, PGs, K^+ channels and gap junction communication. It is typically thought that NO is the most relevant endothelium-dependent vasodilator signal, but, in resistance vessels and arterioles, K^+ channels and gap junction communication between the cells of the vessel wall have emerged as major players in the tonic control and coordination of vascular function. While several K^+ channels (e.g. BK_{Ca}, K_{ir} and K_{ATP} channels) may contribute to the vasodilator response induced by NO, the endothelial cell K^+ channels, SK_{Ca} and IK_{Ca}, seem to be involved in the fine regulation of eNOS activation. In addition, it has become apparent that NO production is also modulated by a delicate caveolar control of L-arginine supply. Although myoendothelial gap junction communication probably contributes to the EDHF signaling mediated by SK_{Ca} and IK_{Ca} channels, the strategic spatial organization of IK_{Ca} and K_{ir} may also be involved in the intercellular transmission of an endothelium-initiated smooth muscle hyperpolarization. A similar organization, but between BK_{Ca} and K_{ir} channels, is observed in the astrocyte-mediated neurovascular coupling. Connexin- and pannexin-based hemichannels are an attractive signaling mechanism that may be involved in the control of vascular function, but the study of hemichannels in resistance vessels is just beginning.

8. Acknowledgment

This work was supported by Grant Anillos ACT-71 from Comisión Nacional de Investigación Científica y Tecnológica - CONICYT and Grant #1100850 and #1111033 from Fondo Nacional de Desarrollo Científico y Tecnológico - FONDECYT.

9. References

Abderrahmane A, Salvail D, Dumoulin M, Garon J, Cadieux A & Rousseau E. (1998). Direct activation of K(Ca) channel in airway smooth muscle by nitric oxide: involvement of a nitrothiosylation mechanism? *Am J Respir Cell Mol Biol* 19, 485-497.

Absi M, Burnham Mp, Weston Ah, Harno E, Rogers M & Edwards G. (2007). Effects of methyl beta-cyclodextrin on EDHF responses in pig and rat arteries; association between SK(Ca) channels and caveolin-rich domains. *Br J Pharmacol* 151, 332-340.

Ahluwalia A & Hobbs AJ. (2005). Endothelium-derived C-type natriuretic peptide: more than just a hyperpolarizing factor. *Trends Pharmacol Sci* 26, 162-167.

Alderton Wk, Cooper Ce & Knowles RG. (2001). Nitric oxide synthases: structure, function and inhibition. *Biochem J* 357, 593-615.

Anderson Cm & Nedergaard M. (2003). Astrocyte-mediated control of cerebral microcirculation. *Trends Neurosci* 26, 340-344; author reply 344-345.

Archer SL, Gragasin FS, Wu X, Wang S, Mcmurtry S, Kim DH, Platonov M, Koshal A, Hashimoto K, Campbell WB, Falck JR & Michelakis ED. (2003). Endothelium-derived hyperpolarizing factor in human internal mammary artery is 11,12-epoxyeicosatrienoic acid and causes relaxation by activating smooth muscle BK(Ca) channels. *Circulation* 107, 769-776.

Bagher P & Segal SS. (2011). Regulation of blood flow in the microcirculation: role of conducted vasodilation. *Acta Physiol (Oxf)* 202, 271-284.

Bao X, Clark CB & Frangos JA. (2000). Temporal gradient in shear-induced signaling pathway: involvement of MAP kinase, c-fos, and connexin43. *Am J Physiol Heart Circ Physiol* 278, H1598-1605.

Bartlett IS & Segal SS. (2000). Resolution of smooth muscle and endothelial pathways for conduction along hamster cheek pouch arterioles. *Am J Physiol Heart Circ Physiol* 278, H604-612.

Beach JM, McGahren ED & Duling BR. (1998). Capillaries and arterioles are electrically coupled in hamster cheek pouch. *Am J Physiol* 275, H1489-1496.

Beny JL & Pacicca C. (1994). Bidirectional electrical communication between smooth muscle and endothelial cells in the pig coronary artery. *Am J Physiol* 266, H1465-1472.

Beyer EC, Gemel J, Seul KH, Larson DM, Banach K & Brink PR. (2000). Modulation of intercellular communication by differential regulation and heteromeric mixing of co-expressed connexins. *Braz J Med Biol Res* 33, 391-397.

Billaud M, Lohman AW, Straub AC, Looft-Wilson R, Johnstone SR, Araj CA, Best AK, Chekeni FB, Ravichandran KS, Penuela S, Laird DW & Isakson BE. (2011). Pannexin1 regulates alpha1-adrenergic receptor- mediated vasoconstriction. *Circ Res* 109, 80-85.

Boerma M, Forsberg L, Van Zeijl L, Morgenstern R, De Faire U, Lemne C, Erlinge D, Thulin T, Hong Y & Cotgreave IA. (1999). A genetic polymorphism in connexin 37 as a prognostic marker for atherosclerotic plaque development. *J Intern Med* 246, 211-218.

Bolotina VM, Najibi S, Palacino JJ, Pagano PJ & Cohen RA. (1994). Nitric oxide directly activates calcium-dependent potassium channels in vascular smooth muscle. *Nature* 368, 850-853.

Bolz SS, de Wit C & Pohl U. (1999). Endothelium-derived hyperpolarizing factor but not NO reduces smooth muscle Ca2+ during acetylcholine-induced dilation of microvessels. *Br J Pharmacol* 128, 124-134.

Bolz SS, Vogel L, Sollinger D, Derwand R, de Wit C, Loirand G & Pohl U. (2003). Nitric oxide-induced decrease in calcium sensitivity of resistance arteries is attributable to activation of the myosin light chain phosphatase and antagonized by the RhoA/Rho kinase pathway. *Circulation* 107, 3081-3087.

Brahler S, Kaistha A, Schmidt VJ, Wolfle SE, Busch C, Kaistha BP, Kacik M, Hasenau AL, Grgic I, Si H, Bond CT, Adelman JP, Wulff H, de Wit C, Hoyer J & Kohler R. (2009). Genetic deficit of SK3 and IK1 channels disrupts the endothelium-derived hyperpolarizing factor vasodilator pathway and causes hypertension. *Circulation* 119, 2323-2332.

Bruzzone R, Hormuzdi SG, Barbe MT, Herb A & Monyer H. (2003). Pannexins, a family of gap junction proteins expressed in brain. *Proc Natl Acad Sci U S A* 100, 13644-13649.

Budel S, Bartlett IS & Segal SS. (2003). Homocellular conduction along endothelium and smooth muscle of arterioles in hamster cheek pouch: unmasking an NO wave. *Circ Res* 93, 61-68.

Busse R, Edwards G, Feletou M, Fleming I, Vanhoutte PM & Weston AH. (2002). EDHF: bringing the concepts together. *Trends Pharmacol Sci* 23, 374-380.

Cai S, Garneau L & Sauve R. (1998). Single-channel characterization of the pharmacological properties of the K(Ca2+) channel of intermediate conductance in bovine aortic endothelial cells. *J Membr Biol* 163, 147-158.

Chadjichristos CE, Matter CM, Roth I, Sutter E, Pelli G, Luscher TF, Chanson M & Kwak BR. (2006). Reduced connexin43 expression limits neointima formation after balloon distension injury in hypercholesterolemic mice. *Circulation* 113, 2835-2843.

Chauhan S, Rahman A, Nilsson H, Clapp L, MacAllister R & Ahluwalia A. (2003). NO contributes to EDHF-like responses in rat small arteries: a role for NO stores. *Cardiovasc Res* 57, 207-216.

Chauhan SD, Nilsson H, Ahluwalia A & Hobbs AJ. (2003). Release of C-type natriuretic peptide accounts for the biological activity of endothelium-derived hyperpolarizing factor. *Proc Natl Acad Sci U S A* 100, 1426-1431.

Chaytor AT, Bakker LM, Edwards DH & Griffith TM. (2005). Connexin-mimetic peptides dissociate electrotonic EDHF-type signalling via myoendothelial and smooth muscle gap junctions in the rabbit iliac artery. *Br J Pharmacol* 144, 108-114.

Cherian PP, Siller-Jackson AJ, Gu S, Wang X, Bonewald LF, Sprague E & Jiang JX. (2005). Mechanical strain opens connexin 43 hemichannels in osteocytes: a novel mechanism for the release of prostaglandin. *Mol Biol Cell* 16, 3100-3106.

Christ GJ, Moreno AP, Melman A & Spray DC. (1992). Gap junction-mediated intercellular diffusion of Ca2+ in cultured human corporal smooth muscle cells. *Am J Physiol* 263, C373-383.

Christ GJ, Moreno AP, Parker ME, Gondre CM, Valcic M, Melman A & Spray DC. (1991). Intercellular communication through gap junctions: a potential role in pharmacomechanical coupling and syncytial tissue contraction in vascular smooth muscle isolated from the human corpus cavernosum. *Life Sci* 49, PL195-200.

Christ GJ, Spray DC, el-Sabban M, Moore LK & Brink PR. (1996). Gap junctions in vascular tissues. Evaluating the role of intercellular communication in the modulation of vasomotor tone. *Circ Res* 79, 631-646.

Cohen RA, Plane F, Najibi S, Huk I, Malinski T & Garland CJ. (1997). Nitric oxide is the mediator of both endothelium-dependent relaxation and hyperpolarization of the rabbit carotid artery. *Proc Natl Acad Sci U S A* 94, 4193-4198.

Cornell-Bell AH, Finkbeiner SM, Cooper MS & Smith SJ. (1990). Glutamate induces calcium waves in cultured astrocytes: long range glial signaling. *Science* 247, 470-473.

Cottrell GT, Wu Y & Burt JM. (2002). Cx40 and Cx43 expression ratio influences heteromeric/ heterotypic gap junction channel properties. *Am J Physiol Cell Physiol* 282, C1469-1482.

Cowan DB, Jones M, Garcia LM, Noria S, del Nido PJ & McGowan FX, Jr. (2003). Hypoxia and stretch regulate intercellular communication in vascular smooth muscle cells through reactive oxygen species formation. *Arterioscler Thromb Vasc Biol* 23, 1754-1760.

Cowan DB, Lye SJ & Langille BL. (1998). Regulation of vascular connexin43 gene expression by mechanical loads. *Circ Res* 82, 786-793.

Cox SB, Woolsey TA & Rovainen CM. (1993). Localized dynamic changes in cortical blood flow with whisker stimulation corresponds to matched vascular and neuronal architecture of rat barrels. *J Cereb Blood Flow Metab* 13, 899-913.

Crane GJ, Gallagher N, Dora KA & Garland CJ. (2003). Small- and intermediate-conductance calcium-activated K+ channels provide different facets of endothelium-dependent hyperpolarization in rat mesenteric artery. *J Physiol* 553, 183-189.

Crane GJ, Neild TO & Segal SS. (2004). Contribution of active membrane processes to conducted hyperpolarization in arterioles of hamster cheek pouch. *Microcirculation* 11, 425-433.

Crofford LJ, Wilder RL, Ristimaki AP, Sano H, Remmers EF, Epps HR & Hla T. (1994). Cyclooxygenase-1 and -2 expression in rheumatoid synovial tissues. Effects of interleukin-1 beta, phorbol ester, and corticosteroids. *J Clin Invest* 93, 1095-1101.

Darby PJ, Kwan CY & Daniel EE. (2000). Caveolae from canine airway smooth muscle contain the necessary components for a role in Ca(2+) handling. *Am J Physiol Lung Cell Mol Physiol* 279, L1226-1235.

Davis MJ, Ferrer PN & Gore RW. (1986). Vascular anatomy and hydrostatic pressure profile in the hamster cheek pouch. *Am J Physiol* 250, H291-303.

De Vriese AS, Van de Voorde J & Lameire NH. (2002). Effects of connexin-mimetic peptides on nitric oxide synthase- and cyclooxygenase-independent renal vasodilation. *Kidney Int* 61, 177-185.

de Wit C, Roos F, Bolz SS, Kirchhoff S, Kruger O, Willecke K & Pohl U. (2000). Impaired conduction of vasodilation along arterioles in connexin40-deficient mice. *Circ Res* 86, 649-655.

de Wit C, Roos F, Bolz SS & Pohl U. (2003). Lack of vascular connexin 40 is associated with hypertension and irregular arteriolar vasomotion. *Physiol Genomics* 13, 169-177.

DePaola N, Davies PF, Pritchard WF, Jr., Florez L, Harbeck N & Polacek DC. (1999). Spatial and temporal regulation of gap junction connexin43 in vascular endothelial cells exposed to controlled disturbed flows in vitro. *Proc Natl Acad Sci U S A* 96, 3154-3159.

Dietrich HH, Kajita Y & Dacey RG, Jr. (1996). Local and conducted vasomotor responses in isolated rat cerebral arterioles. *Am J Physiol* 271, H1109-1116.

Dora KA, Gallagher NT, McNeish A & Garland CJ. (2008). Modulation of endothelial cell KCa3.1 channels during endothelium-derived hyperpolarizing factor signaling in mesenteric resistance arteries. *Circ Res* 102, 1247-1255.

Dora KA, Sandow SL, Gallagher NT, Takano H, Rummery NM, Hill CE & Garland CJ. (2003). Myoendothelial gap junctions may provide the pathway for EDHF in mouse mesenteric artery. *J Vasc Res* 40, 480-490.

Doughty JM, Plane F & Langton PD. (1999). Charybdotoxin and apamin block EDHF in rat mesenteric artery if selectively applied to the endothelium. *Am J Physiol* 276, H1107-1112.

Earley S, Resta TC & Walker BR. (2004). Disruption of smooth muscle gap junctions attenuates myogenic vasoconstriction of mesenteric resistance arteries. *Am J Physiol Heart Circ Physiol* 287, H2677-2686.

Edwards G, Dora KA, Gardener MJ, Garland CJ & Weston AH. (1998). K+ is an endothelium-derived hyperpolarizing factor in rat arteries. *Nature* 396, 269-272.

Eichler I, Wibawa J, Grgic I, Knorr A, Brakemeier S, Pries AR, Hoyer J & Kohler R. (2003). Selective blockade of endothelial Ca2+-activated small- and intermediate-conductance K+-channels suppresses EDHF-mediated vasodilation. *Br J Pharmacol* 138, 594-601.

Emerson GG, Neild TO & Segal SS. (2002). Conduction of hyperpolarization along hamster feed arteries: augmentation by acetylcholine. *Am J Physiol Heart Circ Physiol* 283, H102-109.

Emerson GG & Segal SS. (2000). Electrical coupling between endothelial cells and smooth muscle cells in hamster feed arteries: role in vasomotor control. *Circ Res* 87, 474-479.

Emerson GG & Segal SS. (2000). Endothelial cell pathway for conduction of hyperpolarization and vasodilation along hamster feed artery. *Circ Res* 86, 94-100.

Evans WH & Martin PE. (2002). Gap junctions: structure and function (Review). *Mol Membr Biol* 19, 121-136.

Faigle M, Seessle J, Zug S, El Kasmi KC & Eltzschig HK. (2008). ATP release from vascular endothelia occurs across Cx43 hemichannels and is attenuated during hypoxia. *PLoS One* 3, e2801.

Feletou M & Vanhoutte PM. (2007). Endothelium-dependent hyperpolarizations: past beliefs and present facts. *Ann Med* 39, 495-516.

Feletou M & Vanhoutte PM. (2009). EDHF: an update. *Clin Sci (Lond)* 117, 139-155.

Feletou M, Vanhoutte PM, Weston AH & Edwards G. (2003). EDHF and endothelial potassiun channels: IKCa and SKCa. *Br J Pharmacol* 140, 225; author reply 226.

Figueroa XF, Alvina K, Martinez AD, Garces G, Rosemblatt M, Boric MP & Saez JC. (2004). Histamine reduces gap junctional communication of human tonsil high endothelial cells in culture. *Microvasc Res* 68, 247-257.

Figueroa XF, Chen CC, Campbell KP, Damon DN, Day KH, Ramos S & Duling BR. (2007). Are voltage-dependent ion channels involved in the endothelial cell control of vasomotor tone? *Am J Physiol Heart Circ Physiol* 293, H1371-1383.

Figueroa XF & Duling BR. (2008). Dissection of two Cx37-independent conducted vasodilator mechanisms by deletion of Cx40: electrotonic versus regenerative conduction. *Am J Physiol Heart Circ Physiol* 295, H2001-2007.

Figueroa XF & Duling BR. (2009). Gap junctions in the control of vascular function. *Antioxid Redox Signal* 11, 251-266.

Figueroa XF, Isakson BE & Duling BR. (2004). Connexins: gaps in our knowledge of vascular function. *Physiology (Bethesda)* 19, 277-284.

Figueroa XF, Isakson BE & Duling BR. (2006). Vascular gap junctions in hypertension. *Hypertension* 48, 804-811.

Figueroa XF, Martınez AD, Gonzalez DR, Jara PI, Ayala S & Boric MP. (2001). In vivo assessment of microvascular nitric oxide production and its relation with blood flow. *Am J Physiol Heart Circ Physiol* 280, H1222-1231.

Figueroa XF, Paul DL, Simon AM, Goodenough DA, Day KH, Damon DN & Duling BR. (2003). Central role of connexin40 in the propagation of electrically activated vasodilation in mouse cremasteric arterioles in vivo. *Circ Res* 92, 793-800.

Filosa JA, Bonev AD & Nelson MT. (2004). Calcium dynamics in cortical astrocytes and arterioles during neurovascular coupling. *Circ Res* 95, e73-81.

Filosa JA, Bonev AD, Straub SV, Meredith AL, Wilkerson MK, Aldrich RW & Nelson MT. (2006). Local potassium signaling couples neuronal activity to vasodilation in the brain. *Nat Neurosci* 9, 1397-1403.

Flam BR, Hartmann PJ, Harrell-Booth M, Solomonson LP & Eichler DC. (2001). Caveolar localization of arginine regeneration enzymes, argininosuccinate synthase, and lyase, with endothelial nitric oxide synthase. *Nitric Oxide* 5, 187-197.

Fleming I. (2004). Cytochrome P450 epoxygenases as EDHF synthase(s). *Pharmacol Res* 49, 525-533.

Fleming I & Busse R. (2003). Molecular mechanisms involved in the regulation of the endothelial nitric oxide synthase. *Am J Physiol Regul Integr Comp Physiol* 284, R1-12.

Fortier MA, Krishnaswamy K, Danyod G, Boucher-Kovalik S & Chapdalaine P. (2008). A postgenomic integrated view of prostaglandins in reproduction: implications for other body systems. *J Physiol Pharmacol* 59 Suppl 1, 65-89.

Gabriels JE & Paul DL. (1998). Connexin43 is highly localized to sites of disturbed flow in rat aortic endothelium but connexin37 and connexin40 are more uniformly distributed. *Circ Res* 83, 636-643.

Gaete P, Lillo M, Ardiles N, Pérez F & Figueroa X. (2011). Ca^{2+}-activated K^+ channels of small and intermediate conductance control eNOS activation through NAD(P)H oxidase. *Free Radic. Biol. Med.,* doi:10.1016/j.freeradbiomed.2011.11.036

Ghisdal P & Morel N. (2001). Cellular target of voltage and calcium-dependent K(+) channel blockers involved in EDHF-mediated responses in rat superior mesenteric artery. *Br J Pharmacol* 134, 1021-1028.

Gingras M, Farand P, Safar ME & Plante GE. (2009). Adventitia: the vital wall of conduit arteries. *J Am Soc Hypertens* 3, 166-183.

Girouard H, Bonev AD, Hannah RM, Meredith A, Aldrich RW & Nelson MT. (2010). Astrocytic endfoot Ca2+ and BK channels determine both arteriolar dilation and constriction. *Proc Natl Acad Sci U S A* 107, 3811-3816.

Goligorsky MS, Li H, Brodsky S & Chen J. (2002). Relationships between caveolae and eNOS: everything in proximity and the proximity of everything. *Am J Physiol Renal Physiol* 283, F1-10.

Gollasch M, Lohn M, Furstenau M, Nelson MT, Luft FC & Haller H. (2000). Ca2+ channels, Ca2+ sparks, and regulation of arterial smooth muscle function. *Z Kardiol* 89 Suppl 2, 15-19.

Goodenough DA & Paul DL. (2003). Beyond the gap: functions of unpaired connexon channels. *Nat Rev Mol Cell Biol* 4, 285-294.

Gordienko DV, Greenwood IA & Bolton TB. (2001). Direct visualization of sarcoplasmic reticulum regions discharging Ca(2+)sparks in vascular myocytes. *Cell Calcium* 29, 13-28.

Goto K, Fujii K, Kansui Y, Abe I & Iida M. (2002). Critical role of gap junctions in endothelium-dependent hyperpolarization in rat mesenteric arteries. *Clin Exp Pharmacol Physiol* 29, 595-602.

Govers R & Rabelink TJ. (2001). Cellular regulation of endothelial nitric oxide synthase. *Am J Physiol Renal Physiol* 280, F193-206.

Griffith TM. (2004). Endothelium-dependent smooth muscle hyperpolarization: do gap junctions provide a unifying hypothesis? *Br J Pharmacol* 141, 881-903.

Gryglewski RJ. (2008). Prostacyclin among prostanoids. *Pharmacol Rep* 60, 3-11.

Gustafsson F & Holstein-Rathlou N. (1999). Conducted vasomotor responses in arterioles: characteristics, mechanisms and physiological significance. *Acta Physiol Scand* 167, 11-21.

Haas TL & Duling BR. (1997). Morphology favors an endothelial cell pathway for longitudinal conduction within arterioles. *Microvasc Res* 53, 113-120.

Haefliger JA, Krattinger N, Martin D, Pedrazzini T, Capponi A, Doring B, Plum A, Charollais A, Willecke K & Meda P. (2006). Connexin43-dependent mechanism modulates renin secretion and hypertension. *J Clin Invest* 116, 405-413.

Haefliger JA, Nicod P & Meda P. (2004). Contribution of connexins to the function of the vascular wall. *Cardiovasc Res* 62, 345-356.

Harrison DG. (1997). Cellular and molecular mechanisms of endothelial cell dysfunction. *J Clin Invest* 100, 2153-2157.

Hawkins BT & Davis TP. (2005). The blood-brain barrier/neurovascular unit in health and disease. *Pharmacol Rev* 57, 173-185.

He DS, Jiang JX, Taffet SM & Burt JM. (1999). Formation of heteromeric gap junction channels by connexins 40 and 43 in vascular smooth muscle cells. *Proc Natl Acad Sci U S A* 96, 6495-6500.

Hilgers RH, Todd J, Jr. & Webb RC. (2006). Regional heterogeneity in acetylcholine-induced relaxation in rat vascular bed: role of calcium-activated K+ channels. *Am J Physiol Heart Circ Physiol* 291, H216-222.

Hill CE, Rummery N, Hickey H & Sandow SL. (2002). Heterogeneity in the distribution of vascular gap junctions and connexins: implications for function. *Clin Exp Pharmacol Physiol* 29, 620-625.

Hirashiki A, Yamada Y, Murase Y, Suzuki Y, Kataoka H, Morimoto Y, Tajika T, Murohara T & Yokota M. (2003). Association of gene polymorphisms with coronary artery disease in low- or high-risk subjects defined by conventional risk factors. *J Am Coll Cardiol* 42, 1429-1437.

Hirst GD, Edwards FR, Gould DJ, Sandow SL & Hill CE. (1997). Electrical properties of iridial arterioles of the rat. *Am J Physiol* 273, H2465-2472.

Hirst GD & Neild TO. (1978). An analysis of excitatory junctional potentials recorded from arterioles. *J Physiol* 280, 87-104.

Horiuchi T, Dietrich HH, Hongo K & Dacey RG, Jr. (2002). Mechanism of extracellular K+-induced local and conducted responses in cerebral penetrating arterioles. *Stroke* 33, 2692-2699.

Huang A, Wu Y, Sun D, Koller A & Kaley G. (2001). Effect of estrogen on flow-induced dilation in NO deficiency: role of prostaglandins and EDHF. *J Appl Physiol* 91, 2561-2566.

Iadecola C, Yang G, Ebner TJ & Chen G. (1997). Local and propagated vascular responses evoked by focal synaptic activity in cerebellar cortex. *J Neurophysiol* 78, 651-659.

Inai T, Mancuso MR, McDonald DM, Kobayashi J, Nakamura K & Shibata Y. (2004). Shear stress-induced upregulation of connexin 43 expression in endothelial cells on upstream surfaces of rat cardiac valves. *Histochem Cell Biol* 122, 477-483.

Jackson WF. (1993). Arteriolar tone is determined by activity of ATP-sensitive potassium channels. *Am J Physiol* 265, H1797-1803.

Jackson WF. (2000). Ion channels and vascular tone. *Hypertension* 35, 173-178.

Jackson WF. (2005). Potassium channels in the peripheral microcirculation. *Microcirculation* 12, 113-127.

Jaggar JH, Wellman GC, Heppner TJ, Porter VA, Perez GJ, Gollasch M, Kleppisch T, Rubart M, Stevenson AS, Lederer WJ, Knot HJ, Bonev AD & Nelson MT. (1998). Ca2+ channels, ryanodine receptors and Ca(2+)-activated K+ channels: a functional unit for regulating arterial tone. *Acta Physiol Scand* 164, 577-587.

Jantzi MC, Brett SE, Jackson WF, Corteling R, Vigmond EJ & Welsh DG. (2006). Inward rectifying potassium channels facilitate cell-to-cell communication in hamster retractor muscle feed arteries. *Am J Physiol Heart Circ Physiol* 291, H1319-1328.

Kakoki M, Kim HS, Edgell CJ, Maeda N, Smithies O & Mattson DL. (2006). Amino acids as modulators of endothelium-derived nitric oxide. *Am J Physiol Renal Physiol* 291, F297-304.

Karagiannis J, Rand M & Li CG. (2004). Role of gap junctions in endothelium-derived hyperpolarizing factor-mediated vasodilatation in rat renal artery. *Acta Pharmacol Sin* 25, 1031-1037.

Ko EA, Han J, Jung ID & Park WS. (2008). Physiological roles of K+ channels in vascular smooth muscle cells. *J Smooth Muscle Res* 44, 65-81.

Koehler RC, Gebremedhin D & Harder DR. (2006). Role of astrocytes in cerebrovascular regulation. *J Appl Physiol* 100, 307-317.

Koehler RC, Roman RJ & Harder DR. (2009). Astrocytes and the regulation of cerebral blood flow. *Trends Neurosci* 32, 160-169.

Kohler R, Degenhardt C, Kuhn M, Runkel N, Paul M & Hoyer J. (2000). Expression and function of endothelial Ca(2+)-activated K(+) channels in human mesenteric artery: A single-cell reverse transcriptase-polymerase chain reaction and electrophysiological study in situ. *Circ Res* 87, 496-503.

Krattinger N, Capponi A, Mazzolai L, Aubert JF, Caille D, Nicod P, Waeber G, Meda P & Haefliger JA. (2007). Connexin40 regulates renin production and blood pressure. *Kidney Int* 72, 814-822.

Kruger O, Plum A, Kim JS, Winterhager E, Maxeiner S, Hallas G, Kirchhoff S, Traub O, Lamers WH & Willecke K. (2000). Defective vascular development in connexin 45-deficient mice. *Development* 127, 4179-4193.

Kwak BR, Pepper MS, Gros DB & Meda P. (2001). Inhibition of endothelial wound repair by dominant negative connexin inhibitors. *Mol Biol Cell* 12, 831-845.

Lagaud G, Karicheti V, Knot HJ, Christ GJ & Laher I. (2002). Inhibitors of gap junctions attenuate myogenic tone in cerebral arteries. *Am J Physiol Heart Circ Physiol* 283, H2177-2186.

Lang RJ & Watson MJ. (1998). Effects of nitric oxide donors, S-nitroso-L-cysteine and sodium nitroprusside, on the whole-cell and single channel currents in single myocytes of the guinea-pig proximal colon. *Br J Pharmacol* 123, 505-517.

Lee SW & Kang TM. (2001). Effects of nitric oxide on the Ca2+-activated potassium channels in smooth muscle cells of the human corpus cavernosum. *Urol Res* 29, 359-365.

Leybaert L. (2005). Neurobarrier coupling in the brain: a partner of neurovascular and neurometabolic coupling? *J Cereb Blood Flow Metab* 25, 2-16.

Li C, Huang W, Harris MB, Goolsby JM & Venema RC. (2005). Interaction of the endothelial nitric oxide synthase with the CAT-1 arginine transporter enhances NO release by a mechanism not involving arginine transport. *Biochem J* 386, 567-574.

Li X & Simard JM. (2001). Connexin45 gap junction channels in rat cerebral vascular smooth muscle cells. *Am J Physiol Heart Circ Physiol* 281, H1890-1898.

Liao Y, Day KH, Damon DN & Duling BR. (2001). Endothelial cell-specific knockout of connexin 43 causes hypotension and bradycardia in mice. *Proc Natl Acad Sci U S A* 98, 9989-9994.

Liao Y, Regan CP, Manabe I, Owens GK, Day KH, Damon DN & Duling BR. (2007). Smooth muscle-targeted knockout of connexin43 enhances neointimal formation in response to vascular injury. *Arterioscler Thromb Vasc Biol* 27, 1037-1042.

Little TL, Beyer EC & Duling BR. (1995). Connexin 43 and connexin 40 gap junctional proteins are present in arteriolar smooth muscle and endothelium in vivo. *Am J Physiol* 268, H729-739.

Little TL, Xia J & Duling BR. (1995). Dye tracers define differential endothelial and smooth muscle coupling patterns within the arteriolar wall. *Circ Res* 76, 498-504.

Locke D, Liu J & Harris AL. (2005). Lipid rafts prepared by different methods contain different connexin channels, but gap junctions are not lipid rafts. *Biochemistry* 44, 13027-13042.

Lockhart CJ, Hamilton PK, Quinn CE & McVeigh GE. (2009). End-organ dysfunction and cardiovascular outcomes: the role of the microcirculation. *Clin Sci (Lond)* 116, 175-190.

Locovei S, Wang J & Dahl G. (2006). Activation of pannexin 1 channels by ATP through P2Y receptors and by cytoplasmic calcium. *FEBS Lett* 580, 239-244.

Lohn M, Jessner W, Furstenau M, Wellner M, Sorrentino V, Haller H, Luft FC & Gollasch M. (2001). Regulation of calcium sparks and spontaneous transient outward currents by RyR3 in arterial vascular smooth muscle cells. *Circ Res* 89, 1051-1057.

London GM, Guerin AP, Pannier B, Marchais SJ & Safar ME. (1998). Large artery structure and function in hypertension and end-stage renal disease. *J Hypertens* 16, 1931-1938.

Martinez AD & Saez JC. (2000). Regulation of astrocyte gap junctions by hypoxia-reoxygenation. *Brain Res Brain Res Rev* 32, 250-258.

Mather S, Dora KA, Sandow SL, Winter P & Garland CJ. (2005). Rapid endothelial cell-selective loading of connexin 40 antibody blocks endothelium-derived hyperpolarizing factor dilation in rat small mesenteric arteries. *Circ Res* 97, 399-407.

McDonald KK, Zharikov S, Block ER & Kilberg MS. (1997). A caveolar complex between the cationic amino acid transporter 1 and endothelial nitric-oxide synthase may explain the "arginine paradox". *J Biol Chem* 272, 31213-31216.

Metea MR & Newman EA. (2006). Calcium signaling in specialized glial cells. *Glia* 54, 650-655.

Metea MR & Newman EA. (2006). Glial cells dilate and constrict blood vessels: a mechanism of neurovascular coupling. *J Neurosci* 26, 2862-2870.

Michel T & Vanhoutte PM. (2010). Cellular signaling and NO production. *Pflugers Arch* 459, 807-816.

Moncada S, Palmer RM & Higgs EA. (1991). Nitric oxide: physiology, pathophysiology, and pharmacology. *Pharmacol Rev* 43, 109-142.

Moreno AP. (2004). Biophysical properties of homomeric and heteromultimeric channels formed by cardiac connexins. *Cardiovasc Res* 62, 276-286.

Mount PF, Kemp BE & Power DA. (2007). Regulation of endothelial and myocardial NO synthesis by multi-site eNOS phosphorylation. *J Mol Cell Cardiol* 42, 271-279.

Mulligan SJ & MacVicar BA. (2004). Calcium transients in astrocyte endfeet cause cerebrovascular constrictions. *Nature* 431, 195-199.

Mulvany MJ. (1990). Structure and function of small arteries in hypertension. *J Hypertens Suppl* 8, S225-232.

Murphy ME & Brayden JE. (1995). Apamin-sensitive K+ channels mediate an endothelium-dependent hyperpolarization in rabbit mesenteric arteries. *J Physiol* 489 (Pt 3), 723-734.

Nedergaard M. (1994). Direct signaling from astrocytes to neurons in cultures of mammalian brain cells. *Science* 263, 1768-1771.

Nedergaard M, Ransom B & Goldman SA. (2003). New roles for astrocytes: redefining the functional architecture of the brain. *Trends Neurosci* 26, 523-530.

Nilius B & Droogmans G. (2001). Ion channels and their functional role in vascular endothelium. *Physiol Rev* 81, 1415-1459.

Norel X. (2007). Prostanoid receptors in the human vascular wall. *ScientificWorldJournal* 7, 1359-1374.

Nowicki PT, Flavahan S, Hassanain H, Mitra S, Holland S, Goldschmidt-Clermont PJ & Flavahan NA. (2001). Redox signaling of the arteriolar myogenic response. *Circ Res* 89, 114-116.

Okamoto T, Akiyama M, Takeda M, Gabazza EC, Hayashi T & Suzuki K. (2009). Connexin32 is expressed in vascular endothelial cells and participates in gap-junction intercellular communication. *Biochem Biophys Res Commun* 382, 264-268.

Pacicca C, Schaad O & Beny JL. (1996). Electrotonic propagation of kinin-induced, endothelium-dependent hyperpolarizations in pig coronary smooth muscles. *J Vasc Res* 33, 380-385.

Papassotiriou J, Kohler R, Prenen J, Krause H, Akbar M, Eggermont J, Paul M, Distler A, Nilius B & Hoyer J. (2000). Endothelial K(+) channel lacks the Ca(2+) sensitivity-regulating beta subunit. *Faseb J* 14, 885-894.

Polacek D, Bech F, McKinsey JF & Davies PF. (1997). Connexin43 gene expression in the rabbit arterial wall: effects of hypercholesterolemia, balloon injury and their combination. *J Vasc Res* 34, 19-30.

Quayle JM, Dart C & Standen NB. (1996). The properties and distribution of inward rectifier potassium currents in pig coronary arterial smooth muscle. *J Physiol* 494 (Pt 3), 715-726.

Rafikov R, Fonseca FV, Kumar S, Pardo D, Darragh C, Elms S, Fulton D & Black SM. (2011). eNOS activation and NO function: structural motifs responsible for the posttranslational control of endothelial nitric oxide synthase activity. *J Endocrinol* 210, 271-284.

Rath G, Dessy C & Feron O. (2009). Caveolae, caveolin and control of vascular tone: nitric oxide (NO) and endothelium derived hyperpolarizing factor (EDHF) regulation. *J Physiol Pharmacol* 60 Suppl 4, 105-109.

Retamal MA, Cortes CJ, Reuss L, Bennett MV & Saez JC. (2006). S-nitrosylation and permeation through connexin 43 hemichannels in astrocytes: induction by oxidant stress and reversal by reducing agents. *Proc Natl Acad Sci U S A* 103, 4475-4480.

Rummery NM, Hickey H, McGurk G & Hill CE. (2002). Connexin37 is the major connexin expressed in the media of caudal artery. *Arterioscler Thromb Vasc Biol* 22, 1427-1432.

Rummery NM & Hill CE. (2004). Vascular gap junctions and implications for hypertension. *Clin Exp Pharmacol Physiol* 31, 659-667.

Saez JC, Berthoud VM, Branes MC, Martinez AD & Beyer EC. (2003). Plasma membrane channels formed by connexins: their regulation and functions. *Physiol Rev* 83, 1359-1400.

Saez JC, Retamal MA, Basilio D, Bukauskas FF & Bennett MV. (2005). Connexin-based gap junction hemichannels: gating mechanisms. *Biochim Biophys Acta* 1711, 215-224.

Sandow SL, Bramich NJ, Bandi HP, Rummery NM & Hill CE. (2003). Structure, function, and endothelium-derived hyperpolarizing factor in the caudal artery of the SHR and WKY rat. *Arterioscler Thromb Vasc Biol* 23, 822-828.

Sandow SL, Looft-Wilson R, Doran B, Grayson TH, Segal SS & Hill CE. (2003). Expression of homocellular and heterocellular gap junctions in hamster arterioles and feed arteries. *Cardiovasc Res* 60, 643-653.

Schonbeck U, Sukhova GK, Graber P, Coulter S & Libby P. (1999). Augmented expression of cyclooxygenase-2 in human atherosclerotic lesions. *Am J Pathol* 155, 1281-1291.

Schubert R, Krien U, Wulfsen I, Schiemann D, Lehmann G, Ulfig N, Veh RW, Schwarz JR & Gago H. (2004). Nitric oxide donor sodium nitroprusside dilates rat small arteries by activation of inward rectifier potassium channels. *Hypertension* 43, 891-896.

Scotland RS, Madhani M, Chauhan S, Moncada S, Andresen J, Nilsson H, Hobbs AJ & Ahluwalia A. (2005). Investigation of vascular responses in endothelial nitric oxide synthase/cyclooxygenase-1 double-knockout mice: key role for endothelium-derived hyperpolarizing factor in the regulation of blood pressure in vivo. *Circulation* 111, 796-803.

Segal SS. (2000). Integration of blood flow control to skeletal muscle: key role of feed arteries. *Acta Physiol Scand* 168, 511-518.

Segal SS. (2005). Regulation of blood flow in the microcirculation. *Microcirculation* 12, 33-45.

Segal SS & Jacobs TL. (2001). Role for endothelial cell conduction in ascending vasodilatation and exercise hyperaemia in hamster skeletal muscle. *J Physiol* 536, 937-946.

Segal SS & Kurjiaka DT. (1995). Coordination of blood flow control in the resistance vasculature of skeletal muscle. *Med Sci Sports Exerc* 27, 1158-1164.

Severs NJ, Rothery S, Dupont E, Coppen SR, Yeh HI, Ko YS, Matsushita T, Kaba R & Halliday D. (2001). Immunocytochemical analysis of connexin expression in the healthy and diseased cardiovascular system. *Microsc Res Tech* 52, 301-322.

Shi Y, Liu X, Gebremedhin D, Falck JR, Harder DR & Koehler RC. (2008). Interaction of mechanisms involving epoxyeicosatrienoic acids, adenosine receptors, and metabotropic glutamate receptors in neurovascular coupling in rat whisker barrel cortex. *J Cereb Blood Flow Metab* 28, 111-125.

Shimokawa H & Morikawa K. (2005). Hydrogen peroxide is an endothelium-derived hyperpolarizing factor in animals and humans. *J Mol Cell Cardiol* 39, 725-732.

Shimokawa H, Yasutake H, Fujii K, Owada MK, Nakaike R, Fukumoto Y, Takayanagi T, Nagao T, Egashira K, Fujishima M & Takeshita A. (1996). The importance of the hyperpolarizing mechanism increases as the vessel size decreases in endothelium-dependent relaxations in rat mesenteric circulation. *J Cardiovasc Pharmacol* 28, 703-711.

Si H, Heyken WT, Wolfle SE, Tysiac M, Schubert R, Grgic I, Vilianovich L, Giebing G, Maier T, Gross V, Bader M, de Wit C, Hoyer J & Kohler R. (2006). Impaired endothelium-derived hyperpolarizing factor-mediated dilations and increased blood pressure in mice deficient of the intermediate-conductance Ca2+-activated K+ channel. *Circ Res* 99, 537-544.

Si JQ, Zhao H, Yang Y, Jiang ZG & Nuttall AL. (2002). Nitric oxide induces hyperpolarization by opening ATP-sensitive K(+) channels in guinea pig spiral modiolar artery. *Hear Res* 171, 167-176.

Simmons DL, Botting RM & Hla T. (2004). Cyclooxygenase isozymes: the biology of prostaglandin synthesis and inhibition. *Pharmacol Rev* 56, 387-437.

Simon AM & Goodenough DA. (1998). Diverse functions of vertebrate gap junctions. *Trends Cell Biol* 8, 477-483.

Smith PD, Brett SE, Luykenaar KD, Sandow SL, Marrelli SP, Vigmond EJ & Welsh DG. (2008). KIR channels function as electrical amplifiers in rat vascular smooth muscle. *J Physiol* 586, 1147-1160.

Solomonson LP, Flam BR, Pendleton LC, Goodwin BL & Eichler DC. (2003). The caveolar nitric oxide synthase/arginine regeneration system for NO production in endothelial cells. *J Exp Biol* 206, 2083-2087.

Stankevicius E, Lopez-Valverde V, Rivera L, Hughes AD, Mulvany MJ & Simonsen U. (2006). Combination of Ca2+ -activated K+ channel blockers inhibits acetylcholine-evoked nitric oxide release in rat superior mesenteric artery. *Br J Pharmacol* 149, 560-572.

Stoen R, Lossius K & Karlsson JO. (2003). Acetylcholine-induced vasodilation may depend entirely upon NO in the femoral artery of young piglets. *Br J Pharmacol* 138, 39-46.

Stout CE, Costantin JL, Naus CC & Charles AC. (2002). Intercellular calcium signaling in astrocytes via ATP release through connexin hemichannels. *J Biol Chem* 277, 10482-10488.

Straub AC, Billaud M, Johnstone SR, Best AK, Yemen S, Dwyer ST, Looft-Wilson R, Lysiak JJ, Gaston B, Palmer L & Isakson BE. (2011). Compartmentalized connexin 43 s-nitrosylation/denitrosylation regulates heterocellular communication in the vessel wall. *Arterioscler Thromb Vasc Biol* 31, 399-407.

Straub SV, Bonev AD, Wilkerson MK & Nelson MT. (2006). Dynamic inositol trisphosphate-mediated calcium signals within astrocytic endfeet underlie vasodilation of cerebral arterioles. *J Gen Physiol* 128, 659-669.

Suzuki H, Chen G, Yamamoto Y & Miwa K. (1992). Nitroarginine-sensitive and -insensitive components of the endothelium-dependent relaxation in the guinea-pig carotid artery. *Jpn J Physiol* 42, 335-347.

Takano T, Tian GF, Peng W, Lou N, Libionka W, Han X & Nedergaard M. (2006). Astrocyte-mediated control of cerebral blood flow. *Nat Neurosci* 9, 260-267.

Taylor MS, Bonev AD, Gross TP, Eckman DM, Brayden JE, Bond CT, Adelman JP & Nelson MT. (2003). Altered expression of small-conductance Ca2+-activated K+ (SK3) channels modulates arterial tone and blood pressure. *Circ Res* 93, 124-131.

Topper JN, Cai J, Falb D & Gimbrone MA, Jr. (1996). Identification of vascular endothelial genes differentially responsive to fluid mechanical stimuli: cyclooxygenase-2, manganese superoxide dismutase, and endothelial cell nitric oxide synthase are selectively up-regulated by steady laminar shear stress. *Proc Natl Acad Sci U S A* 93, 10417-10422.

van Kempen MJ & Jongsma HJ. (1999). Distribution of connexin37, connexin40 and connexin43 in the aorta and coronary artery of several mammals. *Histochem Cell Biol* 112, 479-486.

van Kempen MJ, ten Velde I, Wessels A, Oosthoek PW, Gros D, Jongsma HJ, Moorman AF & Lamers WH. (1995). Differential connexin distribution accommodates cardiac function in different species. *Microsc Res Tech* 31, 420-436.

Vanheel B & Van de Voorde J. (2000). EDHF and residual NO: different factors. *Cardiovasc Res* 46, 370-375.

Vanhoutte PM. (2004). Endothelium-dependent hyperpolarizations: the history. *Pharmacol Res* 49, 503-508.

Vanhoutte PM. (2009). COX-1 and vascular disease. *Clin Pharmacol Ther* 86, 212-215.

Vanhoutte PM, Shimokawa H, Tang EH & Feletou M. (2009). Endothelial dysfunction and vascular disease. *Acta Physiol (Oxf)* 196, 193-222.

Wagner C, de Wit C, Kurtz L, Grunberger C, Kurtz A & Schweda F. (2007). Connexin40 is essential for the pressure control of renin synthesis and secretion. *Circ Res* 100, 556-563.

Wang XL, Ye D, Peterson TE, Cao S, Shah VH, Katusic ZS, Sieck GC & Lee HC. (2005). Caveolae targeting and regulation of large conductance Ca(2+)-activated K+ channels in vascular endothelial cells. *J Biol Chem* 280, 11656-11664.

Watanabe S, Yashiro Y, Mizuno R & Ohhashi T. (2005). Involvement of NO and EDHF in flow-induced vasodilation in isolated hamster cremasteric arterioles. *J Vasc Res* 42, 137-147.

Welsh DG & Segal SS. (1998). Endothelial and smooth muscle cell conduction in arterioles controlling blood flow. *Am J Physiol* 274, H178-186.

White TW. (2003). Nonredundant gap junction functions. *News Physiol Sci* 18, 95-99.

White TW & Bruzzone R. (1996). Multiple connexin proteins in single intercellular channels: connexin compatibility and functional consequences. *J Bioenerg Biomembr* 28, 339-350.

Wolfle SE, Schmidt VJ, Hoepfl B, Gebert A, Alcolea S, Gros D & de Wit C. (2007). Connexin45 cannot replace the function of connexin40 in conducting endothelium-dependent dilations along arterioles. *Circ Res* 101, 1292-1299.

Xia J & Duling BR. (1995). Electromechanical coupling and the conducted vasomotor response. *Am J Physiol* 269, H2022-2030.

Xu HL, Mao L, Ye S, Paisansathan C, Vetri F & Pelligrino DA. (2008). Astrocytes are a key conduit for upstream signaling of vasodilation during cerebral cortical neuronal activation in vivo. *Am J Physiol Heart Circ Physiol* 294, H622-632.

Yamada Y, Ichihara S, Izawa H, Tanaka M & Yokota M. (2004). Genetic risk for coronary artery disease in individuals with or without type 2 diabetes. *Mol Genet Metab* 81, 282-290.

Yamada Y, Izawa H, Ichihara S, Takatsu F, Ishihara H, Hirayama H, Sone T, Tanaka M & Yokota M. (2002). Prediction of the risk of myocardial infarction from polymorphisms in candidate genes. *N Engl J Med* 347, 1916-1923.

Yeh HI, Lupu F, Dupont E & Severs NJ. (1997). Upregulation of connexin43 gap junctions between smooth muscle cells after balloon catheter injury in the rat carotid artery. *Arterioscler Thromb Vasc Biol* 17, 3174-3184.

Zani BG & Bohlen HG. (2005). Transport of extracellular l-arginine via cationic amino acid transporter is required during in vivo endothelial nitric oxide production. *Am J Physiol Heart Circ Physiol* 289, H1381-1390.

Zheng-Fischhofer Q, Ghanem A, Kim JS, Kibschull M, Schwarz G, Schwab JO, Nagy J, Winterhager E, Tiemann K & Willecke K. (2006). Connexin31 cannot functionally replace connexin43 during cardiac morphogenesis in mice. *J Cell Sci* 119, 693-701.

Zonta M, Angulo MC, Gobbo S, Rosengarten B, Hossmann KA, Pozzan T & Carmignoto G. (2003). Neuron-to-astrocyte signaling is central to the dynamic control of brain microcirculation. *Nat Neurosci* 6, 43-50.

Zonta M, Sebelin A, Gobbo S, Fellin T, Pozzan T & Carmignoto G. (2003). Glutamate-mediated cytosolic calcium oscillations regulate a pulsatile prostaglandin release from cultured rat astrocytes. *J Physiol* 553, 407-414.

5

Hemodynamics

Ali Nasimi
*Isfahan University of Medical Sciences,
Iran*

1. Introduction

Hemodynamics is the study of the relationship among physical factors affecting blood flow through the vessels. In this chapter these factors and their relationship were discussed.

2. Blood flow is a function of pressure difference and resistance (Darcy's law)

Blood flow (F) through a blood vessel is determined by two main factors: (1) pressure difference (ΔP) between the two ends of the vessel and (2) the resistance (R) to blood flow through the vessel (Fig. 1).

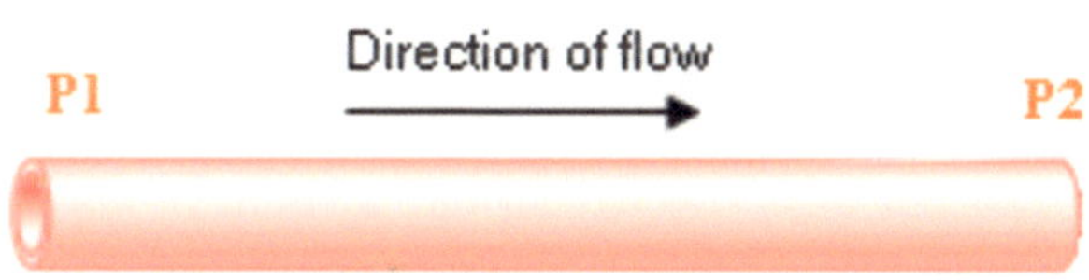

Fig. 1. Blood flow through a blood vessel.

The equation relating these parameters is:

$$F = \Delta P / R \tag{1}$$

This equation is called Darcy's law or Ohm's law.

Flow (F) is defined as the volume of blood passing each point of the vessel in one unit time. Usually, blood flow is expressed in milliliters per minute or liters per minute, but it is also expressed in milliliters per second.

Pressure which is the force that pushes the blood through the vessel is defined as the force exerted on a unit surface of the wall of the tube perpendicular to flow. Pressure is expressed as millimeters of mercury (mmHg). Since the pressure is changing over the course of the blood vessel, there is no single pressure to use; therefore the pressure parameter used is pressure difference (ΔP), also called pressure gradient, which is the difference between the pressure at the beginning of the vessel (P_1) and the pressure at the end of the vessel (P_2), i.e.

$\Delta P = P_1 - P_2$. As seen in the Darcy's law, ΔP is the cause of the flow; with no pressure difference there would be no flow. The pressure energy is produced by the ventricle and it drops throughout the vessel due to resistance. In other words, resistance is the cause of the pressure drop over the course of a vessel.

Resistance is how difficult it is for blood to flow from point 1 to point 2. Resistance impedes flow and it is a measure of interactions between flowing particles (including molecules and ions) themselves and interactions between flowing particles and the wall of the vessel. As seen Darcy's law, resistance is the impeding cause of the flow; the bigger the resistance the lesser the flow. If the resistance is ∞ (complete closure of the vessel) there will be no flow. The resistance equation is:

$$R = \frac{8}{\pi}\frac{\eta L}{r^4} \qquad (2)$$

Where η = fluid viscosity

L = vessel length

r = inside radius of the vessel

Viscosity represents the interactions between flowing particles themselves and radius represents the interactions between flowing particles and the wall of the vessel. The units of viscosity are Pa·s = Ns/m^2, or Poise (dynes·s/cm^2), with 1 Pa·s = 10 Poise.

The red blood cells, erythrocytes (RBCs), constitute 99% of the suspending particle volume of blood. Therefore viscosity of blood depends on the concentration of various constituents of plasma and volume % of red blood cells (hematocrit), as well as size, shape and deformability of RBCs. In a healthy individual all these parameters are constant, therefore blood viscosity is constant and viscosity is not a mean of control (regulation) of the resistance. In abnormal situations viscosity abnormally affects the total resistance. Low hematocrit, as in anemia, decreases viscosity of blood. Inversely, polycythemia increases viscosity and lowers blood flow. In sickle cell anemia the erythrocytes are misshapen and inflexible causing serious disturbances of regional blood flow.

In the resistance equation, L represents the vessel length. Since the length of the vessels of the body is constant, L could not be used for control of the resistance.

Resistance has an inverse relation with the 4th power of r (inside radius of the vessel); therefore radius of the vessel has the most powerful effect on the resistance, so that with small changes in radius, resistance will change dramatically. Radius is the main factor for control of the resistance by the cardiovascular system. Radius of the vessels of the body is controlled by the sympathetic system.

Resistance is mainly located in the arterioles. Assuming an aortic radius of 15 mm and an (arbitrary) length of 50 cm and an arteriole with a radius of 7.5 μm and a length of 1 mm. The ratio of the radius is 2000 and the length ratio is ~500, therefore the resistance ratio would be $(2000)^4/500$, i.e., $\sim 3 \bullet 10^{10}$. It means that the resistance of a single arteriole is $3 \bullet 10^{10}$ as large as that of a 50 cm long aorta. Since there are $3 \bullet 10^8$ parallel arterioles, their total resistance is about $3 \bullet 10^{10} / 3 \bullet 10^8 \cong 100$ times as large as the resistance of the aorta (Westerhof et al. 2010).

Even though all vessels except metarterioles and capillaries are innervated by the sympathetic system, the arterioles receive the most profound innervations and play the main role in the control of the total peripheral resistance by the sympathetic system.

The resistance of any vessel can be calculated by having ΔP and F. For systemic circulation, if mean aortic pressure (P_1) is taken to be 100 mmHg and mean right atrial pressure (P_2) is 0 mmHg, the pressure difference (ΔP) is 100 mmHg. With a cardiac output of 6 l/min (100 ml/s), the total resistance is 100/100 = 1 mmHg/ml/s. This unit is called peripheral resistance unit (PRU). Other physical units are used in the clinic and resistance is expressed in $dyn•s•cm^{-5}$ or $Pa•s/m^3$. The total peripheral resistance of the systemic circulation may change from 4 PRU in very strong constriction to 0.2 PRU in great dilation of the vessels. In the pulmonary system, the mean pulmonary arterial pressure is 16 mm Hg and the mean left atrial pressure is 2 mm Hg, giving a ΔP of 14 mm. With a cardiac output of 100 ml/sec, the total pulmonary vascular resistance is 0.14 PRU, about one seventh of that in the systemic circulation.

In the body, blood vessels arranged in series and in parallel. The arteries, arterioles, capillaries, venules and veins are arranged in series. The total resistance of a series of vessels is equal to the sum of the resistances of each vessel:

$$R_{total} = R_1 + R_2 + R_3 + \dots \quad (3)$$

Blood vessels branch extensively to form parallel circuits in all organs and tissues of the body. The total resistance of parallel vessels is calculated by:

$$\frac{1}{Rtotal} = \frac{1}{R1} + \frac{1}{R2} + \frac{1}{R3} + \dots \quad (4)$$

As a result, adding a parallel vessel to a circuit will reduce the total resistance. This is the reason that the resistance of each organ alone is far greater than the total peripheral resistance. For example in renal circulation, if blood pressure in the renal artery is taken to be 100 mmHg and that of the renal vein be 10 mmHg and renal flow is taken to be 20 ml/s (1200 ml/min), then R = 90/20 = 4.5 PRU, 4.5 times as much as the total resistance of the systemic circulation.

2.1 Poiseuille's law

In equation F= ΔP/R if we substitute R with its equation results in:

$$F = \frac{\pi \Delta P r^4}{8 \eta L} \quad (5)$$

This is called Poiseuille's law. As seen, flow is proportional to ΔP which is the main cause of flow. Flow is also proportional to the 4th power of internal radius of the vessel indicating the great importance of the radius for flow.

2.2 Physiological and clinical applications of Darcy's law

In equation F= ΔP/R if P_1 is increased, since ΔP = P_1 - P_2, ΔP will increase which results in an increase in blood flow (F) and P_2. For example, during exercise, contractility of the left ventricle increases and produces more pressure energy which results in the increase of aortic pressure (P_1), causing blood flow to various organs and capillary pressure (P_2) to increase. On the contrary, a decrease of P_1 results in a decrease of flow and capillary pressure.

An increase in P_2 results in a decrease of ΔP and blood flow. For example if the venous resistance increases or atrial pressure (P_2) increases, such as in heart failure, ΔP will be lower than that of the normal and blood flow will decrease. This subsequently results in a small increase in the arterial pressure (P_1). Therefore a change in either one of the P_1 or P_2 causes a similar change in the corresponding P which is smaller than the first one. It is smaller, since resistance always causes a pressure drop between the two points of the vessel. For example, $\uparrow P_1 \rightarrow \uparrow \Delta P$ (1st) $\rightarrow \uparrow F \rightarrow \uparrow P_2 \rightarrow \downarrow \Delta P$ (2nd), but flow is still higher, since due to resistance, the magnitude of the increase of P_2 is smaller than the increase of P_1, therefore the magnitude of the second change (decrease) of ΔP is smaller than the first change (increase) of ΔP.

Changing the resistance by adjusting the radius of the vessels is the main mechanism of controlling blood flow to each tissue and organ, called local control of blood flow. It is also one of the two major mechanisms (control of the heart and the resistance) to control arterial blood pressure.

Darcy's equation ($F = \Delta P/R$) could be rewritten as: $\Delta P = P_1 - P_2 = FR$. If R is increased by decreasing the radius, other three parameters of the equation will change. The first thing that happens is the reduction of flow, exactly as expected from the Darcy's equation. Reduction of flow then causes a pile up of flowing materials (such as blood) before resistance and a decrease in blood volume after the resistance; thus P_1 will increase and P_2 will decrease and subsequently ΔP will get bigger, exactly as expected from the 2nd form of Darcy's equation. The resultant increase in ΔP is always quantitatively smaller than the primary increase of R; therefore F is always less than before. The steps could be summarized as follows:

$$R\uparrow \Rightarrow F\downarrow = \Delta P/R\uparrow \Rightarrow P_1\uparrow \ \& \ P_2\downarrow \Rightarrow \Delta P\uparrow \Rightarrow F\downarrow = \Delta P\uparrow/R\uparrow$$

Exactly opposite will happen if R is decreased. As seen, any change in R will change both P_1 and P_2 in opposite to each other. For example when some one turns the valve of a tap clock wise, the radius of the outlet is decreased, flow decreases, output pressure (P_2) decreases and the pressure of pre-valve water (P_1) increases.

Based on Darcy's law, if the cardiovascular system is to increase blood flow, it could either increase ΔP by increasing the heart work, or decrease R by decreasing sympathetic outflow to the vessels, especially to arterioles, resulting in a decrease of resistance. Also it could do both ($\Delta P\uparrow$ and $R\downarrow$). In local control mechanism, only local resistance is adjusted to control blood flow to a tissue. High metabolism of a tissue changes the concentration of some chemical factors including oxygen. These factors make metarterioles and precapillary sphincters dilate. Based on Darcy's law, blood flow to that tissue increases so that the blood supply to that tissue will be proportional to its metabolism.

When arterial pressure is low, baroreflex stimulates the heart by increasing contractility and heart rate which results in higher P_1. Baroreflex also increases the total peripheral resistance which results in higher P_1

Resistance causes pressure drop across the vascular system (Fig. 2). In the large arteries, resistance is relatively small and pressure drop is small. The small arteries have moderate resistance to blood flow. Resistance is highest in the arterioles, which are sometimes referred to as the stopcocks of the vascular system. Therefore, the pressure drop is greatest across the terminal part of the small arteries and the arterioles (Fig. 2).

Resistance vessels make pressure drop from ~100 to 30 mmHg. Based on Darcy's law, high resistance of these vessels increases the P_1 (arterial pressure) and decreases the P_2 (capillary pressure). Both effects are absolutely necessary for survival. High arterial pressure makes it possible for blood to reach all parts of the body especially to the head which is at a higher level than the heart. The second effect, low capillary pressure, is also very useful because it prevents the capillaries from being damaged and it is necessary for stable transport between the capillaries and the interstitial fluid. High capillary pressure makes capillaries too permeable so that proteins can cross the endothelium which results in edema.

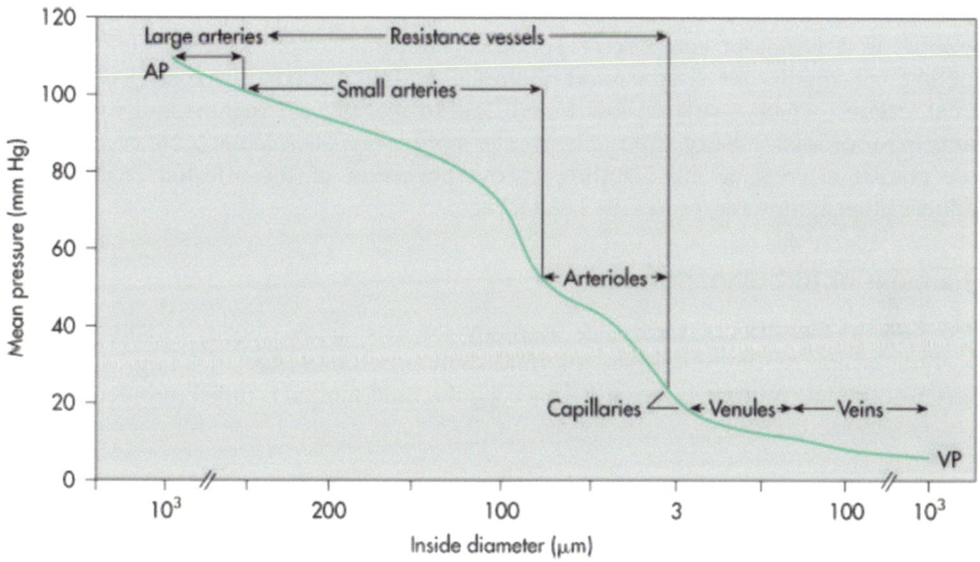

Fig. 2. Pressure drop across the vascular system in the hamster cheek pouch. AP, mean arterial pressure; VP, venous pressure (From Bern et al., Physiology, 2007, with permission).

Anaphylaxis is an allergic condition in which the cardiac output and arterial pressure often decrease drastically. It results from an antigen-antibody reaction after an antigen to which the person is sensitive enters the circulation, causing secretion of histamine by basophile and mast cells. Histamine dilates the arterioles, resulting in greatly reduced arterial pressure that could result in coma and death. Too much vasodilator drugs also could produce similar effect.

In aneurysm disease, part of an artery dilates abnormally. Based on Darcy's law, blood flow to the zone perfused by that artery is increased (F↑) which results in a higher pressure in microcirculation of that zone (P_2↑), which may produce pain and damage.

In coarctation of descending aorta, a local malformation marked by deformed aortic media, causes narrowing of the lumen. As expected from Darcy's law, blood flow to the lower parts of the body is seriously decreased (F↓). As a consequence, the arterial pressure in the lower part of the aorta decreases (P_2↓) and of the upper part of the aorta may be 40-50 per cent higher (P_1↑) than the lower aorta. Due to the low renal blood pressure, water and salt retention occurs that eventually returns the blood pressure of the lower part of the body to normal and produces hypertension in the upper part of the body.

In heart ischemic diseases, narrowing or obstruction of one or more coronary arteries, decreases or ceases blood flow to the regions supplied by the affected arteries.

In aortic stenosis, the diameter of the aortic valve opening is reduced significantly, and the aortic pulse pressure (difference between systolic and diastolic pressure) is decreased significantly because of great decrease of systolic pressure. Based on Darcy's law, due to high resistance of aortic valve, P_1 (ventricular pressure) increases and P_2 (aortic systolic pressure) decreases. This is exactly what we see in the disease. Due to high ventricular pressure, ventricle hypertrophy may occur.

Migraine, is a symptom complex of periodic headaches, often with irritability, nausea, vomiting, constipation or diarrhea and photophobia. It is preceded by constriction of some cranial arteries, which results in low blood flow to the affected regions and consequently results in prodromal sensory, especially occular symptoms. Then remarkable vasodilation of those cranial arteries occurs resulting in overperfusion of the affected regions which produces other symptoms, especially headache.

3. Laminar or turbulent flow

Blood flow in the straight vessels, is normally laminar. Blood moves in smooth parallel concentric layers. As flow increases, the fluid motion becomes wavy, leading to vortices in different seemingly random directions. This irregular fluid motion is called turbulence (Fig. 3).

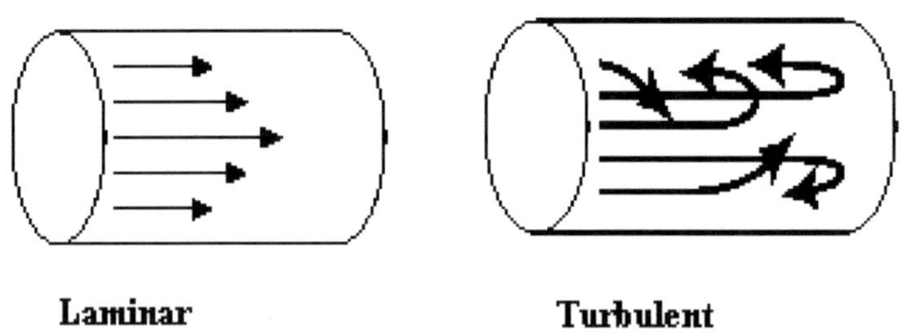

Fig. 3. Laminar and turbulent flow

In turbulent flow the resistance to flow is higher and energetically is more costly than laminar flow, since part of the mechanical energy is lost in the erratic motion between the fluid particles. The probability of turbulence is related to blood density, velocity, the diameter of the vessel and the viscosity of the blood. To judge whether a fluid flow is laminar or turbulent, the Reynolds number (Re, a dimensionless parameter: has no unit) is often used. Re is defined as:

$$Re = \rho v D / \eta \qquad (6)$$

ρ is the fluid density, v is the mean fluid velocity; D is the tube inner diameter and η is the fluid viscosity. The Reynolds number reflects the ratio of inertia and viscous effects. The critical Reynolds number is 2200. For low Reynolds numbers (<2200) the viscous effects are dominant and flow is laminar, but for high Reynolds numbers (>2200), flow is turbulent. For transitional numbers around the critical Reynolds number of 2200 flow is neither strictly laminar nor strictly turbulent (Westerhof et al. 2010, p- 22).

At normal resting conditions, arterial flows are laminar. But in heavy exercise, where flow may increase as much as five-folds, the Reynolds number may get higher than the critical value and turbulence occurs.

Laminar flow can be disturbed at the branching points of arteries resulting in turbulence which may deposit the atherosclerotic plaques.

Turbulence is delayed in accelerating flow whereas occurs faster in decelerating flows. For example turbulence occurs distal to a stenosis. Fluid particles accelerate through the narrow part of the stenosis and decelerate fast in the distal expanding part resulting in turbulence. Turbulence in severe stenosis can be initiated for Reynolds numbers as low as 50 (Westerhof et al. 2010, p- 23). This turbulence also widens the vessel after the stenotic part. Constriction of an artery likewise produces turbulence and sound beyond the constriction. This is the reason that murmurs are heard over arteries constricted by atherosclerotic plaques and the sounds of Korotkoff heard when measuring blood pressure (Barrett et al. 2010, p- 540). In severe anemia, because of low viscosity, functional cardiac murmurs are often heard.

4. Bernoulli's principle

Regarding Darcy's law alone, some aspects of hemodynamics seem puzzling. For example, mean arterial pressure of aorta is about 100 mmHg while it is 180 mmHg in the foot arteries during standing. The very high arterial pressure of the foot is due to gravitational force, as a column of blood with an altitude of ~ 130 cm produces a high pressure in the foot's arteries. Based on Darcy's law, since the pressure in the foot's arteries is higher than aorta, blood should move upward from the foot arteries to aorta, which is not the case. Also blood pressure in the venous sinuses of the brain is highly negative, while the right atrial pressure is ~0. Again based on Darcy's law, blood should move upward from right atrium to venous system of brain, which is not the case. Such problems are solved by Bernoulli's principle. Bernoulli's theory states that flow between point A and point B is dependent on the total mechanical energy difference between A and B, not on pressure difference alone. Total mechanical energy consisted of pressure energy, potential energy and kinetic energy. The pressure energy equals pressure × volume (P × V). The potential energy equals fluid mass

(m) × gravitational force (g) × height (h). Kinetic energy equals mass (m) × velocity squared (v^2) divided by 2 ($m \times v^2/2$). Thus:

$$\text{Total mechanical energy} = PV + mgh + \tfrac{1}{2} mv^2 \quad (7)$$

Based on the conditions, these pressures could easily convert to each other. For example consider the model presented in figure 4 (Burton 1972). This figure demonstrates an experiment showing some basic hydraulic points. In this experiment, flow in the tube is constant. As seen in figure 4, flow is driven by the gradient of total mechanical energy. At the first part, cross-sectional area (A) is 6 and velocity (v) is 1. Based on the equation V = F/A (V: velocity, F: flow, A: cross-sectional area), as at the middle of the tube cross-sectional area gets smaller, velocity increases with the same ratio.

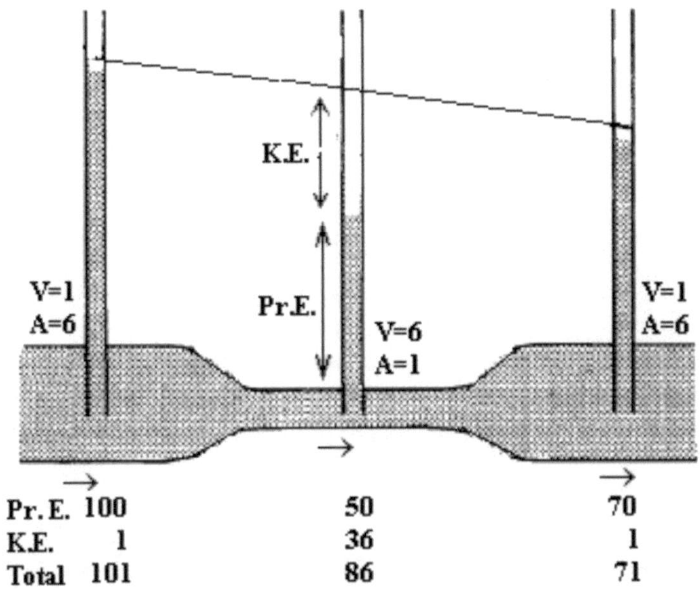

Fig. 4. Flow is driven by the total mechanical energy difference. In the middle of the tube, the cross-sectional area (A) gets smaller resulting in an increase of velocity (v). In other words, pressure energy is converted to kinetic energy. In the third part of the tube, opposite will happen. Pr.E., pressure energy; K.E., kinetic energy. (Data from Burton 1972).

It means that pressure energy is converted to kinetic energy. This is shown by the numbers at the bottom of the figure and is displayed on the middle vertical tube. Since there are both pressure and total mechanical gradients, flow from the first part to the second part of the tube is consistent with both Darcy's and Bernoulli's equations. The third part of the tube gets wider again resulting in an increase of pressure energy and a decrease of kinetic energy. Here kinetic energy is converted to pressure energy. This shows that these three mechanical energies can readily convert to each other. Flow from the middle part to the third part is not expected from Darcy's law, but is consistent with Bernoulli's principle. Another important point shown in this experiment is that due to resistance, total mechanical energy is decreasing over the course of the tube.

Now we can explain the puzzling examples mentioned above. In the upright posture, the aortic blood possesses much more gravitational potential energy than the foot arteries, so that the total mechanical energy in the aorta is higher than the foot arteries and makes blood flow from aorta to the foot.

When someone lies down, Darcy's law is sufficient for explaining blood flow, but in sitting or standing positions, the gravitational potential energy gets quite large and Bernoulli's law should be applied for more accurate explanation of the blood flow. For example in the upright posture, blood flow to the lung could not be explained well without using Bernoulli's principle. Since the pressure in the pulmonary arteries is low, the gravitational energy is comparatively large and greatly affects the pulmonary blood flow, so that during diastole, blood does not reach the apex of the lung.

5. Law of Laplace

The law of Laplace gives the relation between transmural pressure, wall tension, radius and wall thickness in a vessel (Fig. 5) as:

$$T = P \cdot r / w \tag{8}$$

Where T is the force per unit length tangential to the vessel wall called wall tension (dynes/cm), P is transmural pressure, intravascular pressure minus extravascular pressure, in dynes/cm^2 , r is radius of the vessel in cm, and w is thickness of the vessel in cm. Distending force (P·r) tends to pull apart a theoretical slit in the vessel, while the wall tension (T) will keep the parts together.

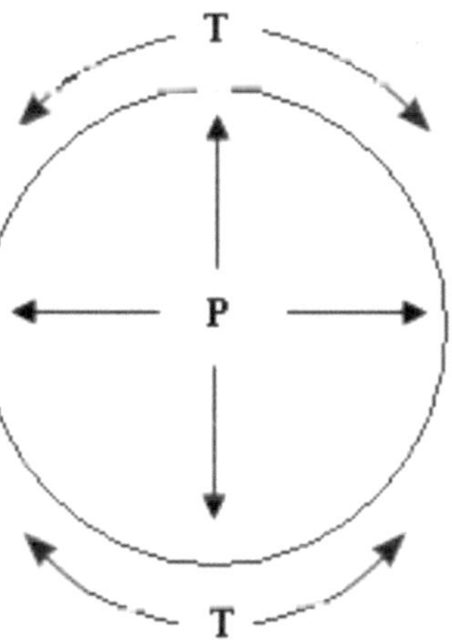

Fig. 5. Transmural pressure (P) and wall tension (T) in a vessel.

Thin-walled capillaries can withstand high internal blood pressure since even though their wall thickness is very small, their radius is also very small and their internal pressure is much smaller than that of the arteries. In aneurysm (local widening of an artery) since radius gets bigger the distending pressure gets higher and makes the vessel more prone to rupture. In eccentric hypertrophy where a ventricle dilates, due to increase in radius, distending force is higher and the ventricle must work harder to pump the normal stroke volume and it will deteriorates the already diseased ventricle.

6. Velocity is inversely related to cross-sectional area

Velocity (V) is related to flow (F) and inversely related to cross-sectional area (A) of a vessel as follows:

$$V = F/A \tag{9}$$

As blood vessels branch extensively from aorta to capillaries, cross-sectional area of each vessel decreases while the total cross-sectional area increases.

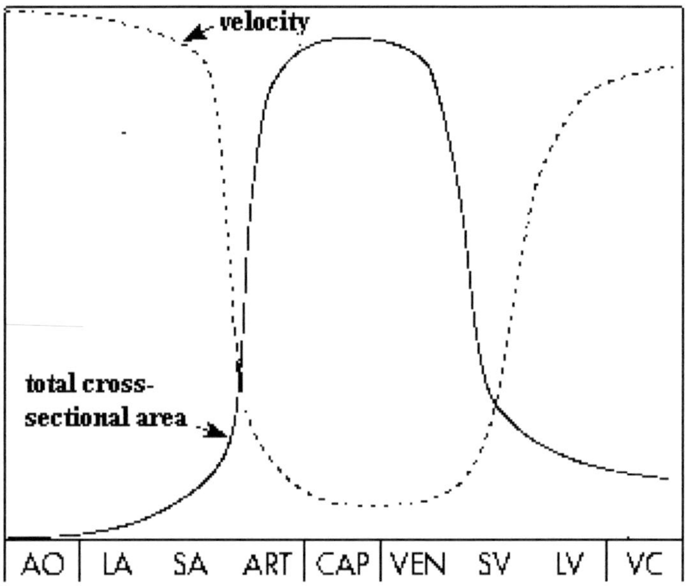

Fig. 6. Velocity and total cross-sectional area in the systemic circulation. There is the maximal cross-sectional area and minimal velocity in the capillaries. AO, Aorta; LA, large arteries; SA, small arteries; ART, arterioles; CAP, capillaries; VEN, venules; SV, small veins; LV, large veins; VC, venae cavae. (Bern et al. 2007, p-267, with permission)

As seen in figure 6, capillaries have the maximal total cross-sectional area resulting in the lowest blood velocity. This low velocity provides ample time for exchange between blood and interstitial fluid.

7. Elasticity and compliance

When a strip of material with cross-sectional area A, and length l_0, is subjected to a force (F) it will lengthen by Δl (Fig. 7). For a specimen with a larger cross-sectional area the same force will produce a smaller change of the length. Also if the starting length (l_0) is longer, the same force causes a larger length change. To have a unique characterization of the material, independent of the sample primary length and thickness, force is normalized by starting cross-sectional area, $\sigma = F/A$ called stress, and length is normalized by starting length $\varepsilon = \Delta l / l_0$ called strain. Elasticity is defined as $E = \sigma / \varepsilon$ (Westerhof et al. 2010, p-49).

The relation between stress and strain for biological material is given in the right part of the figure 7. As seen the relationship between stress and strain for biological material almost always is nonlinear. This nonlinearity implies that a biological material cannot be characterized by a single E. Therefore we should get the local slope of the stress-strain relation for the desired point. This point elasticity is called incremental elasticiy (E_{inc}). E_{inc} increases with strain, i.e., the biological materials become stiffer with increasing stress and strain.

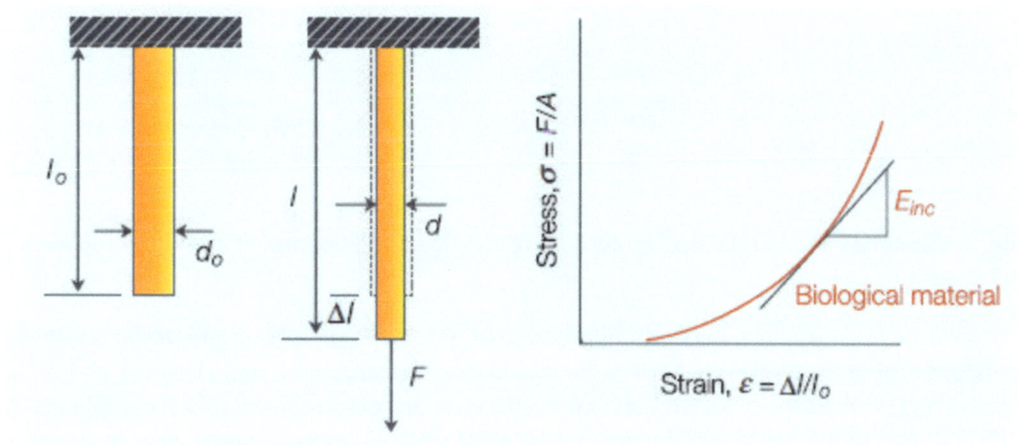

Fig. 7. Stress-strain relationship for biological materials (taken from snapshot p-49 with permission)

For a vessel or a heart, increasing its blood volume results in an increase in the internal pressure and increasing the internal pressure results in an increase in the volume. Pressure is comparable to stress and volume is comparable to strain. Therefore in cardiovascular physiology, pressure-volume relation (Fig. 8) is normally used instead of stress-strain relation. An advantage of pressure-volume relation is that it can be measured *in vivo*. It is important to note that pressure-volume relation does not characterize the material alone but includes the structure of the organ as a whole ((Westerhof et al. 2010, p-58). The change of volume per one unit change of pressure is called compliance ($C = \Delta V / \Delta P$). The change of pressure per one unit change of volume is called elastance ($E = \Delta P / \Delta V$). For biological organs like vessels and heart, the pressure-volume relation is curved toward volume axis indicating that by increasing volume or pressure stiffness increases (Fig. 8). Therefore there is not a single compliance or elastance and for a working point, the tangent of the pressure-volume curve is used. Thus, when comparing compliance or elastance the chosen working point, the pressure at which compliance or elastance was determined, should be reported.

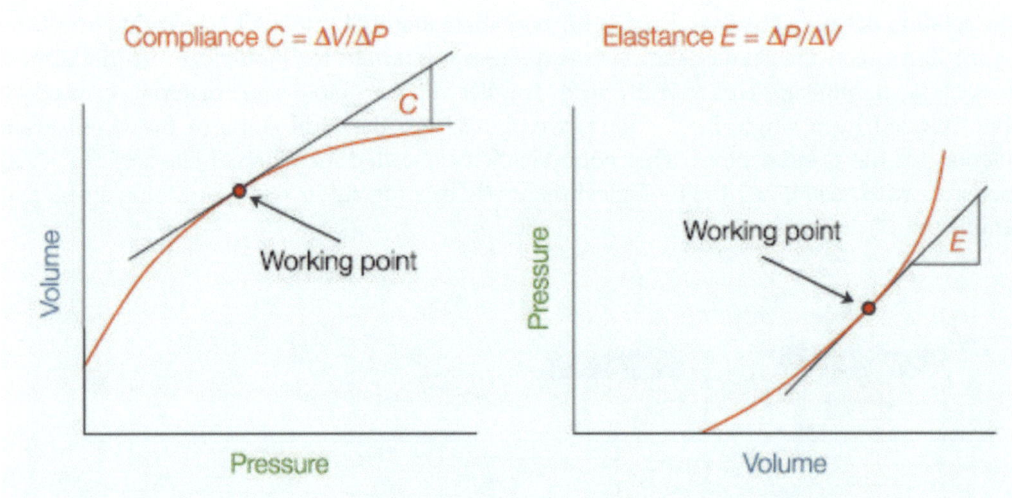

Fig. 8. Pressure-volume relationship for biological organs (Westerhof et al. 2010, p-57, with permission)

Compliance and elastance depend on the original volume (V_0) of the organ under study. To compare properties of different blood vessels, or hearts, compliance and elastance should be normalized with respect to the original volume of the organ. Normalized compliance is called distensibility [distensibility = $C/V_0 = \Delta V/(\Delta P \cdot V_0)$]. Normalized elastance is called volume elasticity [volume elasticity = $E \cdot V_0 = (\Delta P \cdot V_0)/\Delta V$].

7.1 Physiological and clinical applications

Distensibility of the veins is 8 times as much as the arteries and the original volume of the veins is 3 times as much as the arteries, thus compliance of each vein is 24 times as much as its corresponding (parallel artery and vein which have the same flow) artery. It means that perfusing a vein and its corresponding artery with the same volume of blood, increases the artery's pressure 24 times as much as the vein. Therefore veins can store large amount of blood with little increase in pressure. Veins are called capacitance vessels storing 60-70 percent of the total blood volume.

Figure 9 shows the effect of blood pressure on blood flow through an isolated vessel. As expected from Darcy's law ($F = \Delta P/R$) increasing pressure results in an increase of flow, but in fact, the effect of pressure on blood flow is greater than expected from Darcy's law (Fig. 9b), as shown by the upward curving lines in Figure 9a. This is because due to vascular distensibility, increased arterial pressure not only increases the force that pushes blood through the vessels but it also distends the elastic vessels, actually decreasing vascular resistance. Therefore elasticity makes the heart work less to pump normal cardiac output, resulting in longer survival.

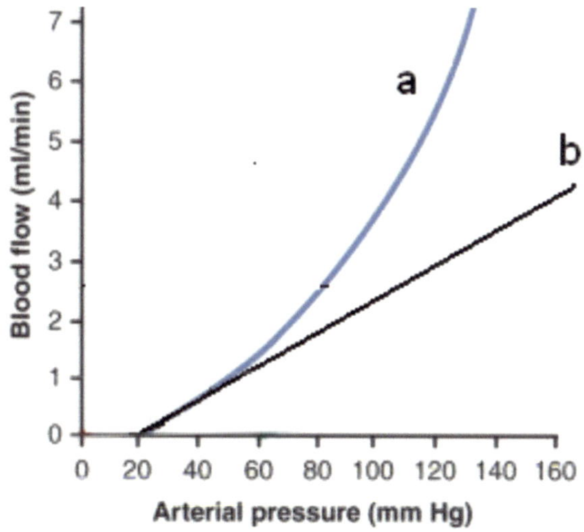

Fig. 9. Effect of blood pressure on blood flow through an isolated vessel (a), and calculated from Darcy's law (b). (Modified from Guyton and Hall, 2011, p-166, with permission).

In arteriosclerosis, blood vessels are less distensible, therefore they extend less which results in a higher resistance causing hypertension, high pulse pressure and high work load of the heart. These symptoms have serious deteriorating effects on the cardiovascular system.

During systole, due to vascular distensibility, high blood pressure distends the arteries, i.e. some pressure energy is stored in the walls of the arteries as potential energy. During diastole the wall of the arteries return to their diastolic position releasing the stored potential energy to the blood as pressure energy. This function attenuates systolic pressure and increases diastolic pressure resulting in normal pulse pressure (difference between systolic pressure and diastolic pressure) of 40 mmHg. Keeping diastolic pressure reasonably high, keeps blood flowing during diastole. In arteriosclerosis, due to stiffness of the arteries, less pressure energy is stored in the wall of the arteries causing systolic pressure to get abnormally high, resulting in a high pulse pressure which has a deteriorating effect on the arteries.

Another physiological benefit of elasticity is damping of the pulse pressure in the smaller arteries, arterioles, and capillaries. Figure 10 shows typical changes in the pulse pressure as the pulse travels into the peripheral vessels. The intensity of pulsation becomes progressively less in the smaller arteries and eventually disappears in the capillaries. In fact, only when the aortic pulsations are extremely large or the arterioles are greatly dilated can pulsations be observed in the capillaries. Lack of pulsation in the capillaries guarantees stable pressure thus stable permeability and stable transport across the capillaries' wall.

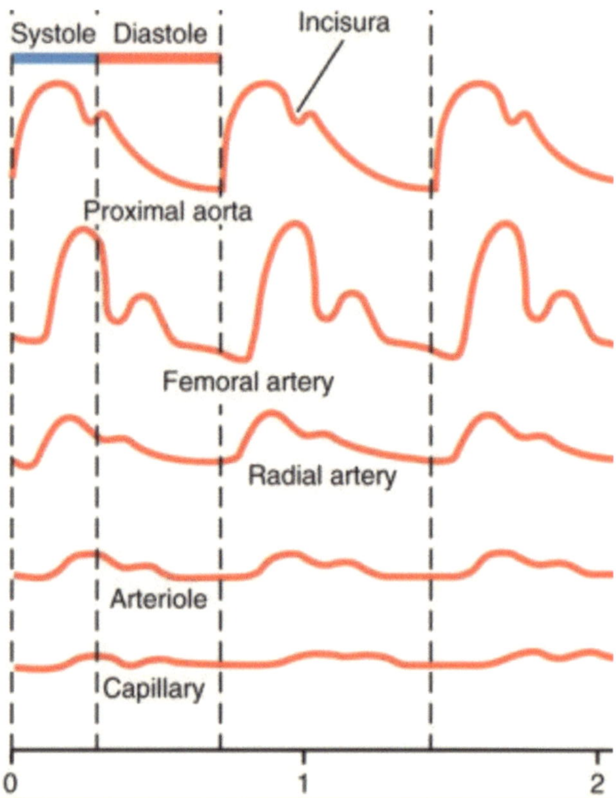

Fig. 10. Damping of the pulse pressure in the smaller arteries, arterioles, and capillaries (Guyton and Hall, 2011, p-170, with permission).

The cause of progressive diminution of the pulsations in the periphery is twofold: (1) resistance and (2) elasticity of the vessels. Resistance is the cause of pressure drop throughout of the vessels, thus decreases the pulse pressure. Elasticity continuously decreases the systole and adds to diastole pressure bringing them closer to each other.

8. References

Badeer H.S., Hemodynamics for medical students, Adv Physiol Educ, 2001, 25: 44–52.

Barrett Kim E., Boitano Scott, Barman Susan M. and Brooks Heddwen L. Ganong's Riview of Medical Physiology, 2010, The McGraw-Hill Companies, New York.

Baun J., Hemodynamics: Physical Principles in: Physical Principles of General and Vascular Sonography, 2009, ProSono publishing, San Francisco, 149-158.

Bern et al., Physiology, 2007, Elsevier ltd.

Burton A.C., physiology and biophysics of the circulation, 1972, Year Book Medical Publishers, Chicago.

Glaser R., Biophysics, 2001, Springer-Verlag Berlin Heidelberg

Guyton and Hall, Textbook of Medical Physiology, 2011, Saunders

Westerhof N., Stergiopulos N. and Noble M.I.M. Snapshots of Hemodynamics, An Aid for Clinical Research and Graduate Education, 2010, Springer, New York.

6

Adenosinergic System in the Mesenteric Vessels

Ana Leitão-Rocha, Joana Beatriz Sousa and Carmen Diniz
*REQUIMTE/FARMA, Department of Drug Science,
Laboratory of Pharmacology, Faculty of Pharmacy,
University of Porto,
Portugal*

1. Introduction

1.1 Adenosinergic pathways in the cardiovascular system

Adenine-based purines, such as adenosine, and adenosine triphosphate (ATP), are ubiquitous signalling molecules that mediate diverse biological actions and physiological processes. Adenosine is an important signalling molecule in the brain, lungs, kidneys, heart, blood vessels and immune systems (Lu et al., 2004), that exerts a potent action on many physiological processes including vasodilation, hormone and neurotransmitter release, platelet aggregation, and lipolysis (Baldwin et al., 2004; Podgorska et al., 2005). Reports of adenosine and adenosine monophosphate (AMP), effects on the heart and blood vessels (Drury & Szent-Gyorgyi, 1929), were the first in a major line of research concerning the physiological actions of purines. Since then, the list of biological processes in which extracellular purines participate has dramatically increased. Insights into the physiological roles of purines came from studies of their biological sources and the stimuli for their release.

Adenosine is composed of an adenine base, consisting of two carbon-nitrogen rings, bound to a ribose sugar group via a beta glycosidic link (Fig. 1); it is considered a nucleoside due to the absence of phosphate groups in its structure. It presents a short half-life due to its rapid conversion into inosine by adenosine deaminase, phoshorylation by adenosine kinase and rapid uptake by adenosine transporters into tissues (Thorn & Jarvis, 1996).

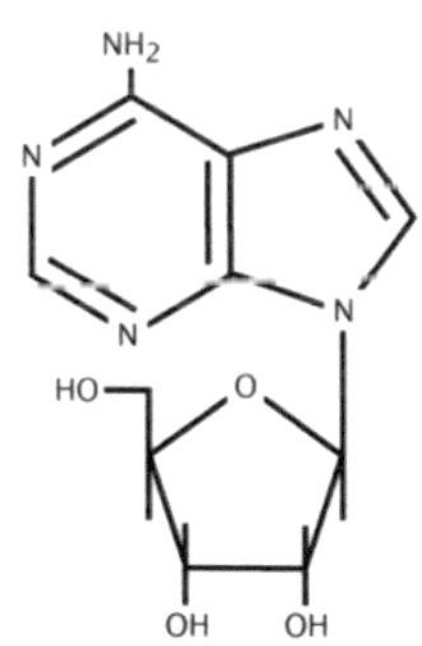

Fig. 1. Adenosine molecule.

Adenosine is a plurisystem mediator/modulator, influencing responses in various cell and tissue types, and *via* numerous receptor and cell signalling pathways. Adenosine can be generated by intracellular and extracellular enzyme pathways depending upon the specific and unique conditions, giving rise to elevated extracellular concentrations. Both equilibrative and concentrative adenosine transport proteins can move adenosine across cellular membranes, influencing extracellular adenosine concentrations (Conlon et al., 2005).

There are several pools of adenosine which arise from different sources. Firstly, there is the existing adenosine being transported in and out of cells *via* transporters. ATP present in the cytosol is dephosphorylated to AMP which can be dephosphorylated further by the action of adenosine kinase to produce adenosine. Alternatively, ATP can be released from the cell by exocytosis, which can then be acted upon by nucleotidases to form adenosine diphosphate (ADP), then AMP and finally adenosine. It can then be transported between the inside of the cell and the interstitial fluid *via* transporters. Another pool of adenosine is generated by neurons. ATP, as a neurotransmitter can be released into the interstitial fluid when carrying a nerve impulse. As before, ATP is acted on by nucleotidases to ADP which is further hydrolysed to AMP and then adenosine (Rang et al., 2007).

Under physiological conditions, adenosine is produced intracellularly (Fig. 2) by AMP dephosphorylation, and extracellularly (Fig. 2) by dephosphorylation of released adenine nucleotides (Brunton et al., 2006; Rang et al., 2007), mainly ATP (Conlon et al., 2005; Meghji et al., 1992).

1.2 Adenosine receptors

The intra and extracellular concentration of adenosine is determined, nearby their receptors, by the existence and function of the transporters. Adenosine is a potent modulator of cardiovascular function and when administered systemically, adenosine produces hypotension and bradycardia (Barraco et al., 1987; Evoniuk et al., 1987). These effects are thought to be mediated at adenosine receptors localized centrally (central nervous system) and in the periphery (heart and vasculature), through different receptor subtypes, particularly the adenosine A_1 and A_{2A} subtypes (Dhalla et al., 2003; Shryock & Belardinelli, 1997; Spyer & Thomas, 2000; Tabrizchi & Bedi, 2001). In the periphery, A_1 receptors are located primarily in the heart and mediate negative inotropic and chronotropic effects (Shryock & Belardinelli, 1997). Adenosine A_{2A} receptors are located primarily in the vasculature and mediate vasodilation (Tabrizchi & Bedi, 2001). In the central nervous system, adenosine A_1 receptors are widely distributed, while adenosine A_{2A} receptors are found in limited regions of the brain, most prominently in the striatum (Dunwiddie & Masino, 2001). However, high levels of A_{2A} receptors are also found in the cardiovascular regulation regions of the hindbrain, including the nucleus tractus solitarius and the rostral ventral lateral medulla (Thomas et al., 2000). In fact, adenosine A_{2A} receptors are thought to play a neuromodulatory role in baroreceptor reflex control (Barraco et al., 1988; Schindler et al., 2005; Thomas et al., 2000).

Adenosine receptors activation may alter vascular tonus in normotensive rats (Cox, 1979; Fresco et al., 2002; Fresco et al., 2004; Fresco et al., 2007), and its modulation differs in hypertensive rats. Thus, it is conceivable that the availability of adenosine may be altered in pathological conditions (Karoon et al., 1995), such as hypertension (Rocha-Pereira et al., 2009).

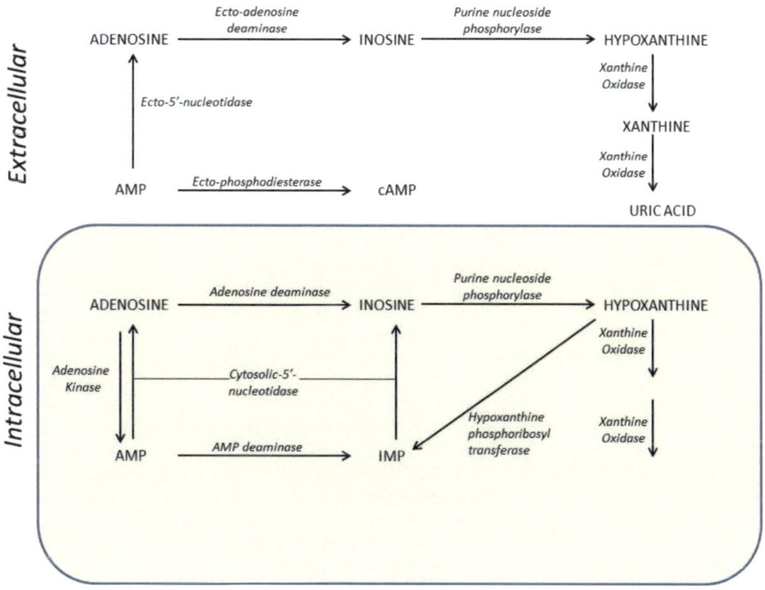

Fig. 2. Metabolism of Adenosine: extracellular. Partial schema of enzyme pathways involved in the regulation of extracellular adenosine concentrations. Cyclic adenosine monophosphate (cAMP) can be transported out of cells upon activation of adenylate cyclase. The actions of an ecto-phosphodiesterase on cAMP results in the formation of AMP. AMP can also be directly released by some cell types. AMP is acted upon by an ecto-5'-nucleotidase to form adenosine; it can then be transported into the cell, or deaminated to inosine by adenosine deaminase. Hypoxanthine is formed after removal of ribose from inosine by the actions of purine nucleoside phosphorylase. Hypoxanthine enters the xanthine oxidase pathway to sequentially form xanthine and uric acid, generating oxyradicals as a byproduct; Metabolism of Adenosine: intracellular. Partial schema of enzyme pathways involved in the regulation of intracellular adenosine concentrations. Adenosine monophosphate (AMP) can be directly deaminated to inosine monophosphate (IMP) by AMP deaminase, or acted upon by an endo-5'-nucleotidase to form adenosine; it can be rephosphorylated to AMP by adenosine kinase, or deaminated to inosine by adenosine deaminase. IMP can also be a source of inosine by the same endo-5'-nucleotidase. Hypoxanthine is formed after removal of ribose from inosine by the actions of purine nucleoside phosphorylase. Hypoxanthine can be salvaged to IMP by hypoxanthinephospho-ribosyltransferase, or by entering the xanthine oxidase pathway to sequentially form xanthine and uric acid, generating oxyradicals as a byproduct. Intracellular adenosine can be transported into and out of the cell by membrane-associated transporter proteins. Being an endogenous purine nucleoside, adenosine is constitutively present in the extracellular spaces at low concentrations. However, its levels increase dramatically in blood and interstitial fluids (extracellular level), in response to cell injury and metabolically-stressful conditions such as tissue damage, hypoxia, ischemia and inflammation. Extracellular adenosine levels have been observed to increase by dephosphorylation of ATP and so a large amount of adenosine is produced from the breakdown of adenine nucleotides by ecto-5´-nucleotidase (Fig. 2) (Cronstein, 1994; Li et al., 2009; Li et al., 2011); and then to be released through the action of specialized nucleoside transporters (Pastor-Anglada et al., 2001).

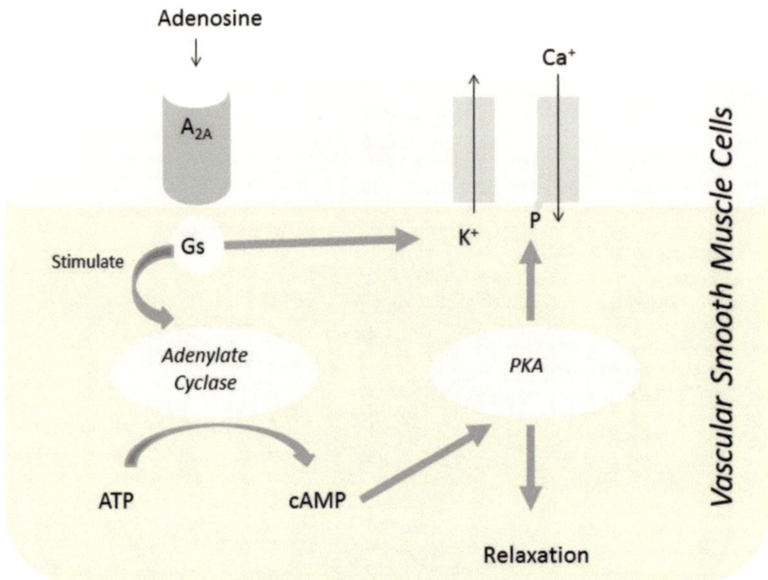

Fig. 3. Adenosine binding to purinergic receptors in smooth muscle tissue. Adenosine can bind to purinergic receptors in different cell types where it can produce diverse physiological actions. One important action is vascular smooth muscle relaxation, which leads to vasodilation. This mechanism is particularly important for matching coronary blood flow to the metabolic needs of the heart. In coronary vascular smooth muscle, adenosine binds to adenosine receptors A_{2A}, which are coupled to the Gs-protein. Activation of this G-protein stimulates adenylate cyclase, increases cAMP and causes protein kinase activation. This stimulates K_{ATP} channels, which hyperpolarize the smooth muscle, causing relaxation. Increased cAMP also causes smooth muscle relaxation by inhibiting myosin light chain kinase, which leads to decreased myosin phosphorylation and a decrease in contractile force. There is also evidence that adenosine inhibits Ca^{2+} entry into the cell through L-type Ca^{2+} channels. Since Ca^{2+} regulates smooth muscle contraction, reduced intracellular Ca^{2+} causes relaxation. In some types of blood vessels, there is evidence that adenosine produces vasodilation through increases in cGMP, which leads to inhibition of Ca^{2+} entry into the cells as well as opening of K^+ channels.

It is well established that adenosine effects occur *via* activation of specific membrane receptors, known as A_1, A_{2A}, A_{2B} and A_3 (Olsson & Pearson, 1990; Ralevic & Burnstock, 1998) that are currently accepted to be coupled to $G_{i/o}$, G_s, $G_{s/Gq}$ and $G_{i/o}/G_q$, respectively (Fredholm et al., 2001). Adenosine receptors are broadly grouped into two categories: A_1 and A_3 receptors, which couple to inhibitory G proteins, and A_{2A} and A_{2B} receptors, which couple to stimulatory G proteins. However, adenosine receptors are pleiotropic; they can couple with various G proteins and transduction systems according to their degree of activation and their particular cellular or subcellular location (Cunha, 2005).

1.2.1 Adenosine receptors and vasodilation

Adenosine receptors are present in many areas of the organism including the smooth muscle cells of blood vessels - these subtypes of receptors have been found to be distributed in different blood vessels such as the coronary artery, pulmonary artery, mesenteric artery, renal vasculature and aorta (Olah et al., 1995; Olah & Stiles, 1995).

The importance of the adenosine induced vasodilatation (Fig. 3), is known in the coronary artery of many species including rats. The vasodilatory effect appears to be mediated by A_2 receptors on vascular smooth muscle cells, thus increasing blood flow and oxygenation; also, adenosine released during preconditioning by short periods of ischemia followed by reperfusion can induce cardioprotection to subsequent sustained ischemia (Li et al., 2011). There are two pathways which can result in relaxation. The first pathway is *via* activation of A_2 receptors located on smooth muscle cells, which are linked to K_{ATP} sensitive channels, and the second is through activation of A_2 receptors located on nitric oxide associated endothelial cells. Alternatively there are blood vessels such as the pulmonary artery in which vascular control is mediated *via* both A_1 and A_2 receptor activation, with vasoconstriction occurring *via* the activation of A_1 receptors and vasodilatation mediated by the activation of A_2 receptors (Tabrizchi & Bedi, 2001). A_2 receptor agonists, including 5'-N-ethylcarboxamide-adenosine, were investigated on porcine coronary artery by King and co-workers (King et al., 1990), and their findings showed that these compounds caused vasodilation. These results support the idea that the activation of adenosine A_2 receptors on smooth muscle results in adenosine-induced relaxation. On the other hand, no evidence has been linked to A_3 receptor activation producing relaxation of blood vessels. Similar findings were obtained from a study by Hiley and co-workers (Hiley et al., 1995), which tested the effects of adenosine analogues on rat mesenteric artery which showed that adenosine analogue, 5'-N-ethylcarboxamide-adenosine acts on adenosine A_2 receptors on the mesenteric bed to produce relaxation. In addition, relaxation mediated by adenosine receptors in the mesenteric bed was sensitive to inhibition by 8-(3-chlorostyryl)caffeine, a selective adenosine A_{2A} receptor antagonist.

Signalling of the adenosine receptor occurs via a G-protein coupled mechanism, with differences between the subtypes: the A_1 subtype is thought to be coupled to G_i or G_o proteins via inhibition of adenylate cyclase or activation of phospholipase C, respectively, and conducing to the opening of K^+ channels and inhibition of Ca^{2+} channels; the A_{2A} subtype ($A_{2A}R$) interacts with the G protein G_s and the A_{2B} subtype ($A_{2B}R$) interacts with the G proteins G_s or G_q to induce adenylate cyclase activity and elevate cAMP levels and consequently, activating calcium channels; the A_3 subtype couples to the G_i or G_q proteins through activation of phospholipase C/D or inhibition of adenylate cyclase, respectively (Olah & Stiles, 1995).

It is conceivable that adenosine cardioprotective effect is mediated through the activation of adenosine receptors A_1 and A_3 in cardiomyocytes, and involves protein kinase C and mitochondrial K_{ATP} channels. However, a recent study has shown that A_{2B} receptors may also be involved since adenosine A_{2B} receptor-deficient mice are more susceptible to acute myocardial ischemia and the treatment of normal mice with an agonist of the receptor A_{2B} significantly attenuated the infarct size after ischemia (Li et al., 2011).

It has been established that adenosine receptor activation occurs via a series of signalling pathways as a result of the binding of adenosine. The affinity of these receptors for adenosine varies; thus their activation depends on the adenosine's concentration. Metabolism and transport across the plasma membrane are the main factors influencing the adenosine level (Podgorska et al., 2005).

In summary, when adenosine binds to these receptors it can cause vascular smooth muscle relaxation leading to vasodilatation of blood vessels. As mentioned above, this occurs *via* a G-protein coupled protein mechanism. On activation of the G-protein, adenylate cyclase is activated causing an increase in cAMP concentration. This then leads to protein kinase A activation which stimulates K^+ channels, hyperpolarizing smooth muscle, causing relaxation (Tawfik et al., 2005).

1.3 Nucleoside transporters

Membrane transporters are responsible for the uptake of essential nutrients, modulation of concentrations of physiologically relevant chemicals, and active release of substances such as signaling molecules (Hyde et al., 2001). Transmembrane transport is a critically important physiological process in all cells and, is likely to have evolved early to allow for controlled uptake and release of nonlipophilic compounds. Nucleoside Transporters constitute a family of membrane proteins with different pharmacological and kinetic properties (Fredholm, 2003), recently identified and characterized in humans. These transport proteins were initially purified from human blood red cells for more than two decades ago, and the lack of abundance of nucleoside transporters proteins in the membranes of mammalian cells, has hampered the analysis of the relationship between its structure and function (Endres et al., 2009; Molina-Arcas et al., 2008; Molina-Arcas et al., 2009).

As previously discussed, there are several ways in which adenosine can be produced and made available for adenosine receptors. One of such, being the transport of adenosine across the plasma membrane, through nucleoside transporters, which determine the intra and extracellular levels of nucleosides, including adenosine (Baldwin et al., 2004; Lu et al., 2004). Generally, nucleoside transporters facilitate the movement of nucleosides and nucleobases across cell membranes but their distribution is not homogeneous among tissues, and their expression can be regulated by various physiological and pathophysiological conditions (Baldwin et al., 2004; Lu et al., 2004; Molina-Arcas et al., 2008). Over the past two decades important advances in the understanding of nucleoside transporters functioning have been achieved. One of nucleoside transporters functions is to salvage extracellular nucleosides for intracellular synthesis of nucleotides; besides, they also control the extracellular concentration of adenosine in the vicinity of its cell surface receptors and regulate processes such as neurotransmission and cardiovascular activity (Anderson et al., 1999; Cass et al., 1999). Other function of nucleoside transporters is vital for the synthesis of nucleic acids in cells that lack *de novo* purine synthesis: carrier-mediated transport of this nucleoside plays an important role in modulating cell function, because the efficiency of the transport processes determines adenosine availability to its receptors or to metabolizing enzymes. Therefore, nucleoside transporters may be key elements as therapeutic targets in the cardiovascular disorders as they are, for example, in anticancer and antiviral therapy where nucleoside analogues are successfully used (Huber-Ruano & Pastor-Anglada, 2009; Lu et al., 2004; Molina-Arcas et al., 2005; Yao et al., 2002).

To date it is accepted that there are two types of transporters (Fig. 6) (Baldwin et al., 2004; Podgorska et al., 2005):

- Equilibrative Nucleoside Transporters (ENT) - equilibrative bidirectional transport processes driven by chemical gradients by facilitated diffusion. ENT are present in most, possibly all, cell types (Cass et al., 1998). They might mediate adenosine transporter in both directions, depending on the concentration gradient of adenosine across the plasma membrane. Until the present day, there are four subtypes described: ENT1, ENT2, ENT3 and ENT4 (Baldwin et al., 2004; Molina-Arcas et al., 2009; Podgorska et al., 2005).

- Concentrative Transporters (CNT) – active inwardly directed concentrative processes, driven by the Na^+ electrochemical gradient: Na^+-dependent. CNT are expressed in a tissue-specific fashion (Cass et al., 1998). Three subtypes were described: CNT1, CNT2 and CNT3 (Hyde et al., 2001; Kong et al., 2004; Molina-Arcas et al., 2009).

Identification and molecular cloning of the ENT and CNT families from mammals and protozoan parasites have provided detailed information about the structure, function, regulation, tissue and cellular localization (Baldwin et al., 2004; Molina-Arcas et al., 2008). Comparing these different types of transporters, CNT and ENT, some differences become evident. Whereas the CNT transport processes are present primarily in specialized epithelia, the ENT transport processes are found in most mammalian cell types (Cass et al., 1998).

Both types of transporters are tightly regulated, both by endocrine and growth factors and by substrate availability. They transport endogenous substrates such as adenosine, thymidine, cytidine, guanosine, uridine, inosine, and hypoxanthine (Lu et al., 2004). They are both involved in the transport of adenosine, but ENT have higher affinity for adenosine than CNT (Molina-Arcas et al., 2009), a reason why the present study focused exclusively on ENT.

ENT play an important role in the provision of nucleosides, derived from the diet or produced by tissues such as the liver, for salvage pathways of nucleotide synthesis in those cells deficient in *de novo* biosynthetic pathways. The latter include erythrocytes, leukocytes, bone marrow cells and some cells in the brain. The co-existence in many cell types of both ENT1 and ENT2, which exhibit similar nucleoside specificities, may reflect the importance of the ENT2 substrate hypoxanthine as a source of purines for salvage. Similarly, this ability to transport hypoxanthine and the higher apparent affinity of ENT2 for inosine have been suggested to reflect a role in the efflux or uptake of these adenosine metabolites during muscle exercise and recovery respectively (Baldwin et al., 2004; Endres et al., 2009). Several polymorphisms have been described in ENT proteins that could affect nucleoside homeostasis, adenosine signalling events or nucleoside-derived drug cytotoxicity or pharmacokinetics (Kong et al., 2004; Molina-Arcas et al., 2009). Although the transport of adenosine involves a simple carrier system, it is a complex process.

1.3.1 Equilibrative nucleoside transporters isoforms

The first example of the ENT family was characterized in human tissues at the molecular level only 10 years ago. Since that time, the identification of homologous proteins by functional cloning and genome analysis has revealed that the family is widely distributed in eukaryotes. The SLC29 family of integral membrane proteins, is part of a larger group of equilibrative and concentrative nucleoside and nucleobase transporters found in many eukaryotes. ENT are a unique family of proteins with no apparent sequence homology to other types of transporters, which enable facilitated diffusion of nucleosides, such as adenosine, and nucleoside analogues across cell membranes (Hyde et al., 2001). Studies performed over the past thirty years have revealed that most mammalian cells exhibit low-affinity, ENT processes, now known to be mediated by members of the SLC29 family. Some mammalian ENT have been well characterized at the molecular and pharmacological levels (Crawford et al., 1998), and currently, four isoforms are known: ENT1–4 (Hyde et al., 2001).

Human (h) and rat (r) ENT1 and ENT2 (456–457 amino acid residues) transport both purine and pyrimidine nucleosides, including ADO. They also differ in their sensitivity to vasodilator drugs (hENT1 > hENT2 > rENT1 > rENT2) and by the ability of hENT2 and rENT2 to transport nucleobases as well as nucleosides (Hyde et al., 2001).

ENT family members are predicted to possess 11 transmembrane helices, with a cytoplasmic N-terminus and an extracellular C-terminus experimentally confirmed for ENT1 (Baldwin et al., 2004). The number of molecules present of each ENT subtype depends on both the cell and the tissue type. The intra and extracellular concentration of adenosine is determined, nearby their receptors, by the existence and function of the transporters, and the four isoforms although structurally similar, show differences in their ability to regulate adenosine concentrations, which may be due to slight modifications in configuration (Baldwin et al., 2004).

Whilst the name of the family reflects the properties of its prototypical member ENT1, some family members can also transport nucleobases and some are proton-dependent, concentrative transporters. Therefore, the transporters play key roles in nucleoside and nucleobase uptake for salvage pathways of nucleotide synthesis, and are also responsible for the cellular uptake of nucleoside analogues. In addition, by regulating the concentration of adenosine available to cell surface receptors, they influence many physiological processes ranging from cardiovascular activity to neurotransmission (Baldwin et al., 2004). ENT are targets, for example, for coronary vasodilator drugs, are responsible for the cellular uptake of nucleoside analogues used in the treatment of cancers and viral diseases (Elwi et al., 2006; Young et al., 2008) and they can also act as routes for uptake of cytotoxic drugs in humans and protozoa (Hyde et al., 2001).

The best-characterized members of the family, ENT1 and ENT2, are cell surface proteins that possess similar broad substrate specificities for purine and pyrimidine nucleosides regulating, eventually, the access of adenosine to its receptors. ENT1 plays a primary role mediating adenosine transport while ENT2, in addition, efficiently transport nucleobases (Baldwin et al., 2004). More recently, the ENT3 and ENT4 isoforms have been shown to be also genuine nucleoside transporters, they are both pH sensitive, and optimally active under acidic conditions. ENT3 has a similar broad permeant selectivity for nucleosides and nucleobases and appears to function in intracellular membranes, including lysosomes. ENT4 is uniquely selective for adenosine, but yet present a low affinity to this nucleoside, and it may also transport a variety of organic cations (Baldwin et al., 2004; Kong et al., 2004).

All four isoforms are widely distributed in mammalian tissues, although their relative abundance varies. In polarised cells ENT1 and ENT2 are found in the basolateral membrane and, in tandem with CNT of the SLC28 family, may play a role in transepithelial nucleoside transport. ENT2 is known to be particularly abundant in skeletal muscle while the ENT3 isoform seems to be widely distributed and the most abundant ENT in the heart. Nevertheless, since ENT3 is a lysosomal transporter functioning in intracellular membranes, is unlikely to contribute to a direct regulation of interstitial adenosine concentrations in tissues. Finally, in what concerns the ENT4, it presents low sequence identity to the other members of the family (due to differences in its structure), is highly selective for adenosine and is also widely distributed. For instance, ENT4 is present in vascular endothelial cells and contributes to regulate the extracellular concentration of adenosine in these structures but only at acidic pH (Baldwin et al., 2004; Barnes et al., 2006).

In summary, all four members of the family share an ability to transport adenosine, but differ in their abilities to transport other nucleosides and nucleobases.

The human gene encoding the human ENT1 (hENT1) protein has been localized to region p21.1-21.2 on chromosome 6 (Baldwin et al., 2004). hENT1 protein consists of 456-residue protein and its sequence displays about 78% identity to the 457-residue rat homologue (rENT1) and 79% identical to the 460-residue mouse protein (mENT1.1) homologues. Splice variants of hENT1 have not been reported, but a 458-residue variant of the mouse homologue (mENT1.2), generated by alternative splicing at the end of exon 7, is widely distributed (Abdulla & Coe, 2007).

The two forms of mENT1 protein appear to be functionally identical, although mENT1.2 lacks the potential casein kinase II phosphorylation site. Both rENT1 and hENT1 proteins display broad substrate specificity for pyrimidine and purine nucleosides with Km values ranging from 50 mM (adenosine) to 680 mM (cytidine), but are unable to transport the pyrimidine base uracil (Yao et al., 1997). hENT1 and mENT1, which are sensitive to nitrobenzylthioinosine (NBMPR), are also inhibited by the coronary vasodilators dipyridamole, dilazep, and draflazine. In contrast, rENT1 although presenting sensitivity to NBMPR is essentially insensitive to inhibition by the coronary vasodilators dipyridamole and dilazep (Baldwin et al., 2004; Podgorska et al., 2005; Ward et al., 2000; Yao et al., 1997).

The messenger ribonucleic acid (mRNA) for hENT1 is widely distributed in different tissues, including erythrocytes, liver, heart, spleen, kidney, lung, intestine, and brain (Endres et al., 2009; Griffith & Jarvis, 1996; Lum et al., 2000, Pennycooke et al., 2001). mENT1.2 protein was shown to be commonly co-expressed with mENT1.1 (460 aminoacids) and the highest level was found in the liver, heart and testis. Moreover, studies at both the mRNA and protein levels have revealed that ENT1 is almost ubiquitously distributed in human and rodent tissues, although its abundance varies between tissues (Baldwin et al., 2005).

Human ENT2 (hENT2) protein, responsible for the *ei* type nucleoside transport, is encoded by a gene localized at position 13q on chromosome 11. hENT2 consists of 456 aminoacids and their sequence displays 88% identity to mouse (mENT2) and rat (rENT2) homologues. In humans, besides the 456-aminoacid ENT2 protein, exists at least, two shorter forms of ENT2, generated from mRNA splice variants. The 326 aminoacid protein, termed hHNP36, lacks the first three transmembrane domains and is inactive as a nucleoside transporter. Inactive is also the second splice variant, a 301-aminoacid protein named hENT2A that lacks the C-terminal domain (Crawford et al., 1998).

The ENT2 protein accepts a broad range of substrates, including purine and pyrimidine nucleosides and nucleobases. It has been postulated that hENT2 plays a role in the efflux and reuptake of inosine and hypoxanthine generated from adenosine during and after strenuous physical exercise. ENT2 (both rat and human), is much less susceptible to inhibition by NBMPR and the coronary vasodilators dipyridamole and draflazinethan ENT1 (Baldwin et al., 2004; Crawford et al., 1998; Podgorska et al., 2005; Ward et al., 2000; Yao et al., 1997, 2002).

The mRNA for ENT2 was reported to be present in several tissues including heart, kidney, brain, placenta, thymus, pancreas, intestine and prostate, but the highest expression level was found in skeletal muscle (Crawford et al., 1998; Lum et al., 2000; Pennycooke et al., 2001).

The gene encoding the human ENT3 (hENT3) protein is located at position q22.1 on chromosome 10. hENT3 is a 475-residue protein displaying 73% identity to the mouse homologue (mENT3) (Baldwin et al., 2004, 2005; Kong et al., 2004). ENT3 has a characteristic, long (51 aminoacids), hydrophilic N-terminal region preceding the first transmembrane (TM1) domain. The N-terminal region of ENT3 consists of two di-leucine motifs characteristic for endossomal, lysosomal targeting motifs. This architectural design distinguishes the ENT3 protein from other members of the equilibrative transporters family. Indeed, it was demonstrated that hENT3 protein is predominantly localized intracellularly and that mutation of the dileucine motif to alanine triggers the relocation of ENT3 protein to the cell surface (Baldwin et al., 2004, 2005).

In comparison with ENT1, the ENT3 protein is much less susceptible to inhibition by NBMPR and coronary vasodilatory drugs (dipyridamole and dilazep). hENT3 demonstrates a broad selectivity for nucleosides, but does not transport hypoxanthine. Moreover, the hENT3 protein facilitates transport of several adenosine analogues like cordycepin (3'-deoxyadenosine) (Baldwin et al., 2004; Podgorska et al., 2005). hENT3 and hENT4, which are mainly located in the intracellular organelles, are not prominent nucleoside transporters like hENT1 and hENT2 (Endo et al., 2007).

The mRNA for ENT3 has been detected in a variety of mouse and human tissues, including brain, kidney, colon, testis, liver, spleen, placenta (highest level), and in a number of neoplastic tissues (Baldwin et al., 2004, 2005; Hyde et al., 2001).

The gene encoding the human ENT4 (hENT4) protein is located on chromosome 7, at position p22.1. Interestingly, the hENT4 is more closely related to the products of the *Drosophila melanogaster* gene CG11010 (28% identity) and the *Anopheles gambiae* gene agCG56160 (30% identity), than to hENT1 (18% identity), indicating an ancient divergence from the other members of the SLC29 family (Acimovic & Coe, 2002). hENT4 is a 530-residue protein 86% identical in sequence to its 528-residue mouse homologue (mENT4) (Baldwin et al., 2004). The substrate specificity of hENT4 has not yet been established in detail, but among the ENT proteins, hENT4 has the lowest affinity for adenosine (Kong et al., 2004). The mRNA for hENT4 was detected in several human tissues. However, recent characterisation of the complementary deoxyribonucleic acids (cDNAs) encoding h/mENT4 has confirmed that these proteins are indeed nucleoside transporters, capable of low-affinity adenosine transport. Analysis of multiple tissue RNA arrays indicates that hENT4 is likely to be ubiquitously expressed in human tissues (Baldwin et al., 2005; Podgorska et al., 2005).

1.3.2 Equilibrative nucleoside transporters in the cardiovascular system

There are currently no reports implicating ENT - SLC29 transporters family, in the pathogenesis of human disease (Baldwin et al., 2004). Still, as mentioned above, adenosine transporters contribute to the intra and extracellular concentration of adenosine, modulating its concentration in the vicinity of its receptors (Li et al., 2011; Tawfik et al., 2005). It is therefore conceivable that the availability of adenosine may be altered in pathological states.

Adenosine exerts vasodilatory and cardioprotective effects, and also reduces the proliferation of vascular smooth muscle cells, inhibits platelet aggregation and attenuates the inflammatory response. Apart from adenosine receptors and ecto-5´-nucleotidase, transporter proteins can regulate adenosine function by modulating extracellular levels of adenosine. The extracellular adenosine is rapidly taken up into cells by nucleoside transporters and is, subsequently, metabolized to inosine by adenosine deaminase and phosphorylated to AMP by adenosine kinase. Nucleoside transporters are supposed to play an integral part in adenosine functions by "fine-tuning" local levels of adenosine in the vicinity of adenosine receptors (Li et al., 2011).

Recent studies have proposed the occurrence of a greater degree of adenosine release from cells that are metabolically stressed. In other words, cells with a high oxygen demand such as the vascular smooth muscle cells in the hypertensive state (Conlon et al., 2005; Tabrizchi & Bedi, 2001). Several studies have been conducted in order to further understand the role of ENT in cardiovascular diseases (Chaudary et al., 2004; Li et al., 2011; Reyes et al., 2010; Rose et al., 2010). Adenosine seems to be a cardioprotective metabolite. Hypoxia and ischemia lead to a large increase in extracellular adenosine, which is released by cardiomyocytes. Extracellular adenosine activates G-protein coupled adenosine receptors linked to various signalling pathways, which initiate compensatory responses. Intracellular and extracellular levels of adenosine fluctuate, considerably, depending on the metabolic state of the heart, the flux of adenosine (down its concentration gradient), across the cardiomyocyte cell membrane, is facilitated by the ENT. These transporters are highly expressed in the cardiovascular system but very little is known about their role in cardiomyocyte physiology (Baldwin et al., 2004; Chaudary et al., 2004; Reyes et al., 2010).

As previously mentioned, ENT are bidirectional, allowing adenosine to be released from cells (to act as an autocrine/paracrine hormone), or transported into the cell (to terminate receptor activation, or restore adenosine metabolite pools). Thus, cardiomyocyte adenosine physiology is dependent on the adenosine receptor profile, and on the presence and activity of the ENT. In the past years, ENT have been shown to be important in modulating the effects of adenosine in human epithelial cells. Moreover, a correlation was found between ENT1 and A_1 adenosine receptor distribution in the brain, suggesting potential interactions and/or feedback between receptors and transporters. Nevertheless, there is an extensive literature on adenosine and adenosine receptor physiology in the cardiovasculature, whereas very little is known about ENT (Baldwin et al., 2004; Chaudary et al., 2004).

ENT inhibitors, by virtue of their effect on extracellular adenosine concentrations, can also modulate a variety of physiological processes, potentially leading to therapeutic benefits. For example, by inhibiting nucleoside uptake into endothelial and other cells the coronary vasodilator draflazine substantially increases and prolongs the cardiovascular effects of adenosine. The latter exerts beneficial, cardioprotective effects in the ischaemic/reperfused myocardium mediated, at least in part, *via* activation of A_1 and possibly also A_3 receptors, probably involving the protein kinase C and mitochondrial K_{ATP} channels. Transport inhibitors have also potential value in the context of ischaemic neuronal injury: pre-ischaemic administration of the pro-drug NBMPR phosphate has been shown to increase brain adenosine levels and reduce ischaemia-induced loss of hippocampal neurons in the rat. In a clinical setting, pharmacological inhibition of ENT, using drugs such as dipyridamole, dilazep and draflazine, is used to promote cardiovascular health. However, despite the clinical relevance of ENT as drug targets, very little is known about them (Baldwin et al., 2004; Tabrizchi & Bedi, 2001; Takahashi et al., 2010).

Recent studies have challenged the role of ENT in purine nucleoside-dependent physiology of the cardiovascular system. Rose and co-workers (2010), investigated whether the ENT1-null mouse heart was cardioprotected in response to ischaemia. In that study, the authors observed that ENT1-null mouse hearts showed significantly less myocardial infarction compared with wild-type littermates, demonstrating that ENT1 activity may contribute to cardiac injury. A posterior study (Reyes et al., 2010), confirmed that isolated wild-type adult mouse cardiomyocytes express predominantly ENT1, which is primarily responsible for purine nucleoside uptake in these cells. However, ENT1-null cardiomyocytes exhibit severely impaired nucleoside transport and lack ENT1 transcript and protein expression. Adenosine receptor expression profiles and expression levels of ENT2, ENT3, and ENT4 were similar in cardiomyocytes isolated from ENT1-null adult mice compared with cardiomyocytes isolated from wild-type littermates. Moreover, small interfering RNA knockdown of ENT1 in the cardiomyocyte cell line, mimics findings in ENT1-null cardiomyocytes. Taken together, the data from the study conducted by Rose and co-workers (2010), demonstrated that the absence of ENT1 plays an essential role in cardioprotection, most likely due to its effects in modulating purine nucleoside-dependent signalling and that the ENT1-null mouse is a powerful model system for the study of the role of ENT in the physiology of the cardiomyocyte.

Other authors, determined that adenosine and inosine accumulate extracellularly during hypoxia/ischaemia and that both may act as neuroprotectors (Takahashi et al., 2010). In the spinal cord, there was pharmacological evidence for an extracellular adenosine levels increase during hypoxia, but no direct measurements of purine release have been done; furthermore, the efflux pathways and origin of extracellular purines are still not defined. Therefore, to characterize hypoxia-evoked purine accumulation, Takahashi and co-workers (2010), examined the effect of acute hypoxia on the extracellular levels of adenosine and inosine in isolated spinal cords from rats, and these authors found that both inhibitors of adenosine deaminase or ENT, abolished the hypoxia-evoked increase in inosine but not adenosine: extracellular level of inosine was about 10-fold higher than that of adenosine. These data suggest that hypoxia releases adenosine itself from intracellular sources, on the other hand, inosine formed intracellularly may be released through ENT (Takahashi et al., 2010).

Gestational diabetes has been associated with increased L-arginine transport and nitric oxide (NO) synthesis as well as a reduced adenosine transport in human umbilical vein endothelial cells. Adenosine increases endothelial L-arginine/NO pathway via A_2 adenosine receptors in human umbilical vein endothelial cells, in normal pregnancies (Vasquez et al., 2004; Vega et al., 2009) compared to the reduction in adenosine transport observed in veins of women with gestational diabetes. Additionally, an association between L-arginine transport and NO synthesis was also found. In fact, Vásquez and co-workers (2004), demonstrated that in gestational diabetes, stimulation of L-arginine transport and NO synthesis occurs with a reduction in adenosine transport in human umbilical vein endothelial cells.

The effect of gestational diabetes on the L-arginine/NO pathway may result from an increased extracellular adenosine level, due to low adenosine uptake as a consequence of a reduced *hENT1*mRNA expression. Accumulation of extracellular adenosine could activate A_{2A} adenosine receptors, which leads to an increased expression of cationic amino acid transporter-1 *(hCAT-1)* mRNA, and of endothelial nitric oxide synthase *(eNOS)*, mRNA or protein expression, an increased L-arginine transport activity, as well as, of the NO synthesis. The effect of gestational diabetes on adenosine and L-arginine transport involves activation of protein kinase C, and p42/44 MAPK pathways and increased the NO levels. Thus, the authors hypothesized the establishment of a functional link between adenosine transport and the L-arginine/NO pathway, governing the normal function of human fetal endothelium from gestational diabetic pregnancies (Vasquez et al., 2004; Vega et al., 2009).

These results also highlight the physiological effects of purinoceptors, particularly of adenosine receptors, in the umbilical vein endothelium, in pathologies, where alterations of blood flow from the mother to the fetus (via the umbilical vein may occur), altering the normal supply of nutrients to the developing fetus, such as in intrauterine growth restriction, fetal hypoxia or gestational diabetes. Finally, these findings also demonstrate that gestational diabetes induces alterations in the phenotype of human fetal endothelium (Vasquez et al., 2004).

It has been demonstrated that insulin inhibited elevated ENT1 expression in human umbilical arterial smooth muscle cells from pregnancies in diabetic subjects (Aguayo et al., 2001). However this is probably due to the activation of adenylate cyclase rather than the effect of insulin on glucose metabolism. The effects of oral anti-diabetic agents on nucleoside transporters are rarely reported: Li and co-workers (2011), studied the effects of different oral anti-diabetic agents such as metformin, sulfonyureas, meglitinides and thiazolidinediones on nucleoside transporters; among them, only the thiazolidinedione troglitazone showed inhibitory effects on nucleoside transporters, but unfortunately it was withdrawn because of hepatic toxicity.

To our knowledge, until the present date, only one study has been carried out to investigate the relationship between hypertension and nucleoside transporters. The binding of a ENT1 probe [^{3}H]NBMPR in membranes prepared from platelets, as well as renal, pulmonary, cardiac and brain tissues of Spontaneously Hypertensive Rats (SHR), was compared to those of age matched Wistar-Kyoto (WKY) controls (Williams et al., 1990). The number of [^{3}H]NBMPR binding sites were higher in the kidneys of SHR but lower in platelets, whereas no difference was found in the heart, lung or brain. Age-dependent decreases were also observed in the heart and platelets of SHR and WKY. The results indicated that the expression of ENT1 changed with age as well as with the pathogenesis of hypertension. Li and co-workers (2011), compared the expressions of nucleoside transporters in basilar arteries in SHR and WKY rats and they found that ENT1 and ENT2 were unaffected by hypertension. Interestingly, the mRNA expression of CNT2 was higher than that seen in WKY; nevertheless, whether the upregulation of CNT2 is a primary or secondary event in the development of hypertension is questionable. It has been speculated that the increase in the activities of ENT1 and CNT2 may reduce the availability of adenosine to its receptors, thereby weakening the vascular functions of adenosine. It may explain why patients with diabetes and hypertension suffer greater morbidity from ischemia and atherosclerosis (Li et al., 2011).

2. Mesenteric vessels

The branches of the abdominal aorta are divided into parietal and visceral parts. The visceral arteries are in turn divided into paired and unpaired branches. The mesenteric artery is an elasto-muscular resistance vessel. In adult rats, for example WKY, the mesenteric artery branches from the abdominal aorta and is composed of five to seven concentric layers of smooth muscle cells, separated by three to four medial laminae. The medium is separated from the endothelial cells of the intima by the continuous internal elastic lamina and from the adventitia, which contains a few fibroblasts and nerve terminals, by the external elastic lamina (McGuire et al., 1993; Sullivan et al., 2002).

Three major unpaired branches exist: the celiac trunk, the superior mesenteric artery and the inferior mesenteric artery. Each has several major branches supplying the abdominal organs: the superior mesenteric artery, supplies the pancreas, small intestine and the colon, whereas the inferior mesenteric artery supplies the descending colon and rectum (Fig. 4).

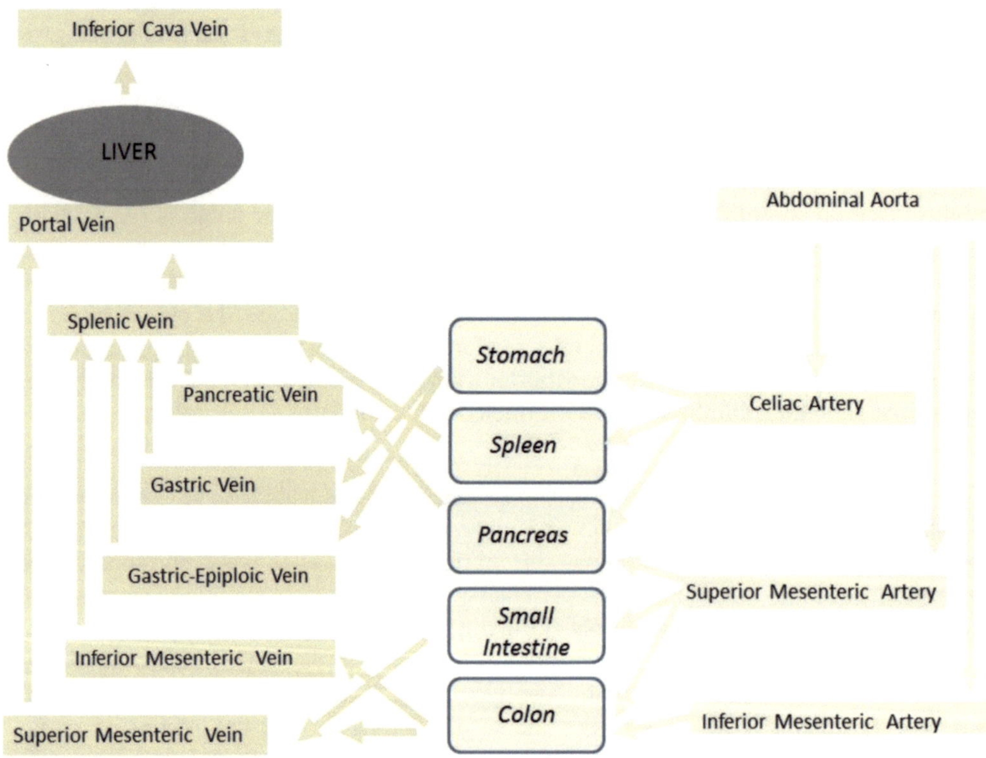

Fig. 4. Schematic representation of splanchnic circulation. Under normal resting conditions in humans, total hepatic blood flow is 1200 to 1400 mL/min (~100 mL/min/100g), which represents about 25% of cardiac output. Blood flow to the four lobes of the liver is derived from two major sources, the portal vein and the hepatic artery. The hepatic artery is a branch of the celiac axis and accounts for 25 to 30 percent of total hepatic blood flow and 45 to 50 percent of the oxygen supply. The portal vein is a valveless afferent nutrient vessel of the liver that carries blood from the entire capillary system of the stomach, spleen, pancreas, and intestine (McGuire et al., 1993).

The mesenteric circulation plays an important role in maintenance of systemic blood pressure, and regulation of tissue blood flow. Actually, the entire splanchnic circulation can receive up to 60% of cardiac output and contains about one third of the total blood volume. Mesenteric arteries and veins have significant resistance and capacitance functions in the systemic circulation, respectively. In comparison to the associated veins, the mesenteric artery has a high resting basal tone mediated in part by a thicker layer of vascular smooth muscle (Kreulen, 2003). Constriction of the mesenteric artery is thought to increase total peripheral resistance in the systemic circulation greatly. In contrast, the mesenteric vein, contains fewer layers of vascular smooth muscle cells and are more compliant vessels. The function of these low pressure vessels is to store significant quantities of blood that can be utilized to maintain the central venous pool of blood and cardiac output. As such, the degree of vascular tone in mesenteric vasculature plays a major role in the regulation of systemic blood pressure and overall body hemodynamics (Ross & Pawlina, 2006).

2.1 Vascular tonus regulation and physiology in mesenteric vessels

The tone of the mesenteric artery and resistance blood vessels are mainly regulated by sympathetic adrenergic nerves through the release of neurotransmitter noradrenaline. It is also controlled by nonadrenergic noncholinergic nerves, and possibly by parasympathetic cholinergic nerves. Noradrenaline and adrenergic cotransmitters including neuropeptide Y, and ATP, act as a vasoconstrictor neurotransmitter for sympathetic nerves. While, dopamine, calcitonin gene-related peptide and acetylcholine act as a vasodilator neurotransmitter for adrenergic, nonadrenergic noncholinergic and cholinergic nerves, respectively. In the mesenteric circulation, these nerves containing various neurotransmitters and cotransmitters interact and modulate each other *via* feedback autoregulatory mechanisms and neuromodulation of various vasoactive substance to regulate vascular resistance (Takenaga & Kawasaki, 1999). In fact, net vascular tone in the mesenteric vasculature is under the influence of several key factors. These factors include locally acting and circulating hormones, intrinsic myogenic properties of the vessel, as well as neurotransmitters released from perivascular post-ganglionic sympathetic neurons. In general, the arteries and veins of the splanchnic circulation are richly innervated with sympathetic nerves that act to constrict these vessels. Maximal activation of the sympathetic constrictor nerves can produce an 80% reduction in blood flow to the splanchnic region (Morhrman & Heller, 2006).

In vivo, sympathetic neurogenic influence of vascular tone is mediated by three neurotransmitters: neuropeptide Y, noradrenaline, and ATP make up the sympathetic triad of neurotransmitters. Perivascular neurons store the sympathetic neurotransmitters in synaptic vesicles and release these neurotransmitters from varicosities to act on postjunctional receptors on the vascular smooth muscle cells. The arrangement of the sympathetic neurons differs between arteries and veins. The nerve plexus for the mesenteric artery consists of a bundle of axons arranged in a mesh-like network with nerve fibres equally likely to run parallel or perpendicular to the longitudinal axis of the vessel. In contrast, in mesenteric vein the nerve plexus consists of single axons with a circumferential nerve fibre arrangement about the vessel. In both cases, the sympathetic neurotransmitters released cause depolarization of the nearby vascular smooth muscle cells. As a whole, activation the sympathetic postjunctional receptors mediates contraction of the vascular smooth muscle cells and, therefore, constriction of the artery or vein (Park et al., 2007).

In vitro, electrical field stimulation studies have found that upon stimulation of mesenteric perivascular nerves a measurable amount of noradrenaline is released (Bobalova & Mutafova-Yambolieva, 2001). Once released, noradrenaline can act on a variety of receptors on the vascular smooth muscle cells. Previous *in vitro* studies have found contractile responses to be mediated by activation of the α_1 adrenoceptor in mesenteric arteries and both α_1 and α_2 adrenoceptors in the mesenteric vein (Perez-Rivera et al., 2007). These adrenoceptors are G-protein linked receptors that are coupled to an intracellular increase of inositol 1,4,5-triphosphate (IP3). Contraction of the smooth muscle is mediated by IP3 acting on sarcoplasmic reticulum receptors to release intracellular Ca^{2+} stores. Additional Ca^{2+} is taken up into the vascular smooth muscle cells following depolarization via L-type voltage-gated calcium channels (Lee et al., 2001).

Like noradrenaline, a measurable amount of ATP is released from perivascular sympathetic neurons when activated by electrical field stimulation (Bobalova & Mutafova-Yambolieva, 2001). *In vivo,* ATP is thought to mediate neurogenic contractions of vascular smooth muscle by acting on various purinergic receptors present on the smooth muscle cells. The two subtypes of purinergic receptors are the P2X and P2Y receptors. The P2X receptors are ATP-gated ion channels that cause an influx of Ca^{2+} into the smooth muscle cells from the extracellular environment (Donoso et al., 2004). Though there are several P2X receptor isoforms, there is evidence that vascular smooth muscle cells primarily express the P2X1 receptors (Wang et al., 2002). P2X receptors are thought to be responsible for the excitatory junction potentials (rapid and short depolarization of vascular smooth muscle) present in mesenteric artery (Kreulen, 2003). In contrast, excitatory junction potentials are not present in mesenteric vein. This is largely thought to be the result of selective expression of only the P2Y receptor subtype in mesenteric vein (Mutafova-Yambolieva et al., 2000). The P2Y receptors mediate slower contractile responses than the P2X receptors, and are G-protein linked receptors that have similar intracellular effects as the α-adrenoceptors. The isoforms of the P2Y receptors that are thought to be expressed in vascular smooth muscle cells are the P2Y2 and the P2Y4 receptors (Galligan et al., 2001).

Noradrenaline and ATP contract the mesenteric artery and the mesenteric vein through the activation of adrenergic and purinergic vascular smooth muscle receptors respectively. The use of selective adrenoceptor agonists and antagonists suggests that the α_1 adrenoceptor is the primary adrenoceptor mediating responses to noradrenaline in these vessels. In addition, the data collected suggests that the P2X and/or the P2Y1 receptors contract the mesenteric artery, but do not mediate substantial contractile responses in rat mesenteric vein. Therefore, this data suggests that other purinergic receptors, such as the P2Y2 and the P2Y4 receptor subtypes, mediate vasoconstriction in these vessels in response to ATP. The Sympathetic Nervous System, is an important modulator of net vascular tone in mesenteric arteries and veins, and that sympathetic modulation of these vessels is an important regulator of the resistance function of mesenteric artery and the capacitance function of mesenteric vein.

Splanchnic veins and venules account for most of the active capacitance responses in the circulation and are richly innervated by the Sympathetic Nervous System. In fact, it has been estimated that innervation to the non hepatic splanchnic organs accounts for half of the total noradrenaline released in the entire body. Therefore, the recent observations in Angiotensin II salt hypertension of neurogenically mediated increases, in whole body venous tone, would best be explained by increased Sympathetic Nervous System activity to the splanchnic circulation. The splanchnic vascular resistance rises in proportion to the blood pressure, and the transvascular escape rate of plasma proteins is increased. Vascular resistance increases in the hepatosplanchnic circulation before any other bed in humans with borderline hypertension. Therefore, increased sympathetic activity to the splanchnic circulation may represent a common stage in the development of hypertension (King et al., 2007).

The various animal models of hypertension show variable results, but in general support the concept that vascular resistance changes in the splanchnic organs are similar in direction and magnitude to pressure changes. These resistance changes appear to result from increased responsiveness of the arterioles to a variety of constrictor influences, and they may result from either structural or functional changes. Hypertension appears to alter splanchnic arteriolar permeability *via* a pressure-dependent mechanism. These vessels may also undergo degenerative histological changes. In addition to the resistive and exchange alterations, the capacitance function of splanchnic veins is reduced, probably via a structural change (Nyhof et al., 1983).

Also, chronic hypertension is associated with resistance artery remodelling and mechanical alterations. A study by Briones and co-workers (2003), evaluated the role of elastin in vascular remodelling of mesenteric artery from SHR. When compared with WKY, the mesenteric artery of SHR showed: smaller lumen, decreased distensibility at low pressures, a leftward shift of the stress–strain relationship, redistribution of elastin within the internal elastic lamina leading to smaller fenestrae but no change in fenestrae number or elastin amount. Elastase incubation fragmented the structure of internal elastic lamina in a concentration-dependent fashion, abolished all the structural and mechanical differences between strains, and decreased distensibility at low pressures. Mesenteric artery remodelling and increased stiffness are accompanied by elastin restructuring within the internal elastic lamina and elastin degradation reverses structural and mechanical alterations of SHR mesenteric artery. Differences in elastin organisation are, therefore, a central element in small artery remodelling in hypertension (Briones et al., 2003).

The rat superior mesenteric vein, which drains blood from the intestine, or the splenic vein, which drains from the spleen, is a capacitance vein. The blood flow in the superior mesenteric vein is the primary source of irrigation of the rat liver and this vein plays an important role in maintaining bile flow, bile acid excretion, and bilirubin conjugation and in preventing the precipitation of bile (possibly preventing hepatolithiasis) (Adachi et al., 1991).

The splanchnic venous bed is the largest vascular bed in terms of capacitance because 50% of the intestinal blood volume is in the venules and small mesenteric veins (Dunbar et al., 2000). Also, many animal studies have shown that the splanchnic bed is very responsive to baroreceptor and sympathetic stimulation (Haase & Shoukas, 1991, 1992; Shoukas & Bohlen, 1990), pointing to this vascular bed as a primary source of blood volume changes. These studies have demonstrated that sympathetic stimulation of splanchnic veins and venules will cause them to constrict, leading to significant volume shifts out of this vascular bed. Consequently, changes in splanchnic venous capacitance can have large effects on venous filling pressure. Capacitance changes can occur through changes in both vessel compliance and unstressed vascular volume. One way to experimentally assess these changes is to examine changes in the pressure-diameter relationships of individual vessels, particularly in the splanchnic regions of the body. The mesenteric veins are also critical in modulating cardiac filling through venoconstriction.

The mesenteric circulation is regulated by multiple mechanisms and there is sufficient amount of aspects described in the literature that support the suspicion that local metabolic factors are especially important in the control of intestinal vasculature. Of these, adenosine, which is a mesenteric vasodilator, may be the messenger of the intestinal tissue to signal appropriate responses of the intestinal vessels. The evidence supporting the candidacy of this nucleoside as a local regulator of mesenteric circulation may be summarized, as follows: adenosine is present in the tissue of the gut in measurable quantities; exogenous adenosine is a powerful dilator of mesenteric resistance vessels; blockade of adenosine receptors in the mesenteric circulation interferes significantly with three autoregulatory phenomena, i.e., postprandial hyperaemia, pressure-flow autoregulation, and reactive hyperaemia (Jacobson & Pawlik, 1992).

3. Adenosinergic system and hypertension

Some lines of investigation have already used both these models to study the role of adenosine in hypertension. For example, in 1987, Jackson performed an interesting assay, where the author compared the *in vivo* role of adenosine, as a modulator of noradrenergic neurotransmission, in the SHR and WKY. In the *in situ* blood-perfused rat mesentery, vascular responses to sympathetic periarterial nerve stimulation, and to exogenous noradrenaline, were enhanced in SHR compared with WKY. In both SHR and WKY, vascular responses to periarterial nerve stimulation were more sensitive to inhibition by adenosine, than were responses to noradrenaline. At matched base-line vascular responses, compared with WKY, SHR were less sensitive to the inhibitory effects of adenosine on vascular responses to periarterial nerve stimulation, but SHR and WKY were equally sensitive with respect to adenosine-induced inhibition of responses to noradrenaline. Antagonism of adenosine receptors with 1,3-dipropyl-8-p-sulfophenylxanthine, shifted the dose-response curve to exogenous adenosine six-fold to the right, yet did not influence vascular responses to periarterial nerve stimulation or noradrenaline in either SHR or WKY. Furthermore, periarterial nerve stimulation did not alter either arterial or mesenteric venous plasma levels of adenosine in SHR or WKY, and plasma levels of adenosine in both strains were always lower than the calculated threshold level required to attenuate neurotransmission. According to these findings, the author concluded that *in vivo* exogenous adenosine interferes with noradrenergic neurotransmission in both SHR and WKY; SHR are less sensitive to the inhibitory effects of exogenous adenosine on noradrenergic neurotransmission than are WKY; endogenous adenosine does not play a role in modulating neurotransmission in either strain under the conditions of this study; and enhanced noradrenergic neurotransmission in the SHR is not due to defective modulation of neurotransmission by adenosine (Jackson, 1987).

Other studies have found differences in blood vessels when comparing SHR and WKY (Cox, 1979; Gisbert et al., 2002; Leal et al., 2008; Lee, 1987); Rocha-Pereira et al., 2009). Findings from the study by Gisbert and co-workers (2002), showed that the population of constitutively active α_{1D}-adrenoceptors is significantly increased in aorta and mesenteric artery from adult SHR when compared to WKY - these results verify that the vessels in question, from hypertensive animals, have an increased population of constitutively active receptors as well as an increased functionality of the α_{1D}-subtype, with respect to normotensive animals. Other studies (Villalobos-Molina & Ibarra, 1999; Villalobos-Molina et al., 1999; Xu et al., 1998), highlighted the importance of the α_{1D}-adrenoceptor in the pathology of hypertension, suggesting that, it appears first in the vasculature, followed by a rise in blood pressure. α_{1D}-adrenoceptors can be found on smooth muscle cells and the activation of these receptors by noradrenaline (released by sympathetic postganglionic terminals), conduce mainly to vasoconstriction. These can lead to an increase in blood pressure playing, therefore, a role in the development of hypertension observed in SHR animals. The opposite effect to the contraction of smooth muscle can occur as a result of adenosine acting on A_2 adenosine receptors, thus causing smooth muscle relaxation. The levels of extracellular adenosine, which can act on those receptors to produce this effect, can be altered by ENT. These transporters play a role in determining the levels of adenosine available extracellularly and hence the extent of vasodilation which can occur (Rang et al., 2007).

On the other hand, previous studies have shown that the vasodilatory response to adenosine and its analogues is weakened in hypertension and in other pathological conditions affecting blood vessels (Lockette et al., 1986; Luscher et al., 1987). Lüscher and co-workers (1987) investigated the effects of antihypertensive therapy on hypertensive rats and their findings demonstrated a prevention or reversal of decreased endothelium-dependent relaxations in response to agonists, suggesting that antihypertensive treatment normalizes endothelium-dependent relaxations. It was, therefore, proposed that antihypertensive treatment may be important in preventing cardiovascular complications in hypertensive individuals. A possible explanation for the attenuated vasodilatory response to adenosine in hypertension can be linked to the levels of adenosine receptors and their functionality in hypertensive models. Vasodilation of blood vessels occurs via the activation of adenosine receptors by adenosine and so an alteration in these receptors can result in a modified vasodilatory response (Rocha-Pereira et al., 2009). This hypothesis can be associated with adenosine transporters, which are partly responsible for making adenosine available to adenosine receptors. It is, therefore, legitimate to hypothesize that an increase or decrease in transporter population could indirectly alter the physiology of the adenosinergic system and, contributing indirectly to the contractility of blood vessels and conducing to an elevated blood pressure (correspondent to the pathologic situation of hypertension).

4. Nucleoside transporters as therapeutic tools – Future perspectives

Nucleoside derived drugs or nucleobase analogues are being developed and investigated for a number of different applications, in order to pursue a better and more efficient way of treating several diseases. The studies conducted in several other conditions might shed some light in this challenging pathway, as promising results have already been published, for example in cancer and infection by Human Immunodeficiency Virus (Cano-Soldado et al., 2008; Damaraju et al., 2003; Endo et al. 2007; Hyde et al., 2001; Kong et al., 2004; Molina-Arcas et al., 2005, 2009; Ritzel et al., 2001; Yao et al., 2002), chronic pain and inflammation (Eltzschig et al., 2005; Li et al., 2009, 2011; Reyes et al., 2010).

The amount of research being done in these past years is indicative of the interest and potential that the area of ENT have in many scientific fields, especially in what concerns its role in a pharmacological perspective. Hopefully, in the future, as the knowledge increases and the mechanisms involving these transporters are better understood, the application of ENT will have an impact, particularly, in cardiovascular diseases, such as hypertension.

5. References

Abdulla, P.& Coe, I.R.(2007). Characterization and functional analysis of the promoter for the human equilibrative nucleoside transporter gene, hENT1. *Nucleosides Nucleotides Nucleic Acids*, 26, 99-110.

Acimovic, Y. & Coe, I.R.(2002). Molecular evolution of the equilibrative nucleoside transporter family: identification of novel family members in prokaryotes and eukaryotes. *Mol Biol Evol*, 19, 2199-210.

Adachi, Y., Kamisako, T.& Yamamoto, T.(1991). The effects of temporary occlusion of the superior mesenteric vein or splenic vein on biliary bilirubin and bile acid excretion in rats. *J Lab Clin Med*, 118, 261-8.

Aguayo, C., Flores, C., Parodi, J., Rojas, R., Mann, G.E., Pearson, J.D.& Sobrevia, L. (2001). Modulation of adenosine transport by insulin in human umbilical artery smooth muscle cells from normal or gestational diabetic pregnancies. *J Physiol*, 534, 243-54.

Anderson, C.M., Xiong, W., Geiger, J.D., Young, J.D., Cass, C.E., Baldwin, S.A.& Parkinson, F.E. (1999). Distribution of equilibrative, nitrobenzylthioinosine-sensitive nucleoside transporters (ENT1) in brain. *J Neurochem*, 73, 867-73.

Baldwin, S.A., Beal, P.R., Yao, S.Y., King, A.E., Cass, C.E. & Young, J.D.(2004). The equilibrative nucleoside transporter family, SLC29. *Pflugers Arch*, 447, 735-43.

Baldwin, S.A., Yao, S.Y., Hyde, R.J., Ng, A.M., Foppolo, S., Barnes, K., Ritzel, M.W., Cass, C.E .& Young, J.D. (2005). Functional characterization of novel human and mouse equilibrative nucleoside transporters (hENT3 and mENT3) located in intracellular membranes. *J Biol Chem*, 280, 15880-7.

Barnes, K., Dobrzynski, H., Foppolo, S., Beal, P.R., Ismat, F., Scullion, E.R., Sun, L., Tellez, J., Ritzel, M.W., Claycomb, W.C., Cass, C.E., Young, J.D., Billeter-Clark, R., Boyett, M.R. & Baldwin, S.A.(2006). Distribution and functional characterization of equilibrative nucleoside transporter-4, a novel cardiac adenosine transporter activated at acidic pH. *Circ Res*, 99, 510-9.

Barraco, R.A., Campbell, W.R., Schoener, E.P., Shehin, S.E. & Parizon, M.(1987). Cardiovascular effects of microinjections of adenosine analogs into the fourth ventricle of rats. *Brain Res*, 424, 17-25.

Barraco, R.A., Janusz, C.J., Polasek, P.M., Parizon, M. & Roberts, P.A.(1988). Cardiovascular effects of microinjection of adenosine into the nucleus tractus solitarius. *Brain Res Bull*, 20, 129-32.

Bobalova, J. & Mutafova-Yambolieva, V.N.(2001). Co-release of endogenous ATP and noradrenaline from guinea-pig mesenteric veins exceeds co-release from mesenteric arteries. *Clin Exp Pharmacol Physiol*, 28, 397-401.

Briones, A.M., Gonzalez, J.M., Somoza, B., Giraldo, J., Daly, C.J., Vila, E., Gonzalez, M.C., McGrath, J.C. & Arribas, S.M.(2003). Role of elastin in spontaneously hypertensive rat small mesenteric artery remodelling. *J Physiol*, 552, 185-95.

Brunton L.L., Lazo J.S. & Parker K.L. (2006) Goodman & Gilman's The Pharmacological Basis of Therapeutics (11th edition), The McGraw-Hill Companies, ISBN 8577260111.

Cano-Soldado, P., Molina-Arcas, M., Alguero, B, Larrayoz, I., Lostao, M.P., Grandas, A., Casado, F.J. & Pastor-Anglada, M. (2008). Compensatory effects of the human nucleoside transporters on the response to nucleoside-derived drugs in breast cancer MCF7 cells. *Bioch Pharmacol,* 75, 639-48.

Cass, C.E., Young, J.D. & Baldwin, S.A.(1998). Recent advances in the molecular biology of nucleoside transporters of mammalian cells. *Biochem Cell Biol,* 76, 761-70.

Cass, C.E., Young, J.D., Baldwin, S.A., Cabrita, M.A., Graham, K.A., Griffiths, M., Jennings, L.L., Mackey, J.R., Ng, A.M., Ritzel, M.W., Vickers, M.F. & Yao, S.Y.(1999). Nucleoside transporters of mammalian cells. *Pharm Biotechnol,* 12, 313-52.

Chaudary, N., Naydenova, Z., Shuralyova, I. & Coe, I.R. (2004). Hypoxia regulates the adenosine transporter, mENT1, in the murine cardiomyocyte cell line, HL-1. *Cardiovasc Res,* 61, 780-8.

Conlon, B.A., Ross, J.D. & Law, W.R.(2005). Advances in understanding adenosine as a plurisystem modulator in sepsis and the systemic inflammatory response syndrome (SIRS). *Front Biosci,* 10, 2548-65.

Cox, R.H.(1979). Comparison of arterial wall mechanics in normotensive and spontaneously hypertensive rats. *Am J Physiol,* 237, H159-67.

Crawford, C.R., Cass, C.E., Young, J.D. & Belt, J.A.(1998). Stable expression of a recombinant sodium-dependent, pyrimidine-selective nucleoside transporter (CNT1) in a transport-deficient mouse leukemia cell line. *Biochem Cell Biol,* 76, 843-51.

Cronstein, B.N.(1994). Adenosine, an endogenous anti-inflammatory agent. *J Appl Physiol,* 76, 5-13.

Cunha, R.A.(2005). Neuroprotection by adenosine in the brain: From A(1) receptor activation to A (2A) receptor blockade. *Purinergic Signal,* 1, 111-34.

Damaraju, V.L., Damaraju, S., Young, J.D., Baldwin, S.A., Mackey, J., Sawyer, M.B. & Cass, C.E. (2003). Nucleoside anticancer drugs: the role of nucleoside transporters in resistance to cancer chemotherapy. *Oncog Nat,* 22, 7524-36.

Dhalla, A.K., Shryock, J.C., Shreeniwas, R. & Belardinelli, L. (2003). Pharmacology and therapeutic applications of A1 adenosine receptor ligands. *Curr Top Med Chem,* 3, 369-85.

Donoso, M.V., Miranda, R., Briones, R., Irarrazaval, M.J. & Huidobro-Toro, J.P. (2004). Release and functional role of neuropeptide Y as a sympathetic modulator in human saphenous vein biopsies. *Peptides,* 25, 53-64.

Drury, A.N.& Szent-Gyorgyi, A. (1929). The physiological activity of adenine compounds with especial reference to their action upon the mammalian heart. *J Physiol,* 68, 213-37.

Dunbar, S.L., Berkowitz, D.E., Brooks-Asplund, E.M. & Shoukas, A.A.(2000). The effects of hindlimb unweighting on the capacitance of rat small mesenteric veins. *J Appl Physiol,* 89, 2073-7.

Dunwiddie, T.V. & Masino, S.A.(2001). The role and regulation of adenosine in the central nervous system. *Annu Rev Neurosci,* 24, 31-55.

Eltzschig, H.K., Abdulla, P., Hoffman, E., Hamilton, K.E., Daniels, D., Schonfeld, C., Loffler, M., Reyes, G., Duszenko, M., Karhausen, J., Robinson, A., Westerman, K.A., Coe,

I.R. & Colgan, S.P.(2005). HIF-1-dependent repression of equilibrative nucleoside transporter (ENT) in hypoxia. *J Exp Med*, 202, 1493-505.

Elwi, A.N., Damaraju, V.L., Baldwin, S.A., Young, J.D., Sawyer, M.B. & Cass, C.E.(2006). Renal nucleoside transporters: physiological and clinical implications. *Biochem Cell Biol*, 84, 844-58.

Endo, Y., Obata, T., Murata, D., Ito, M., Sakamoto, K., Fukushima, M., Yamasaki, Y., Yamada, Y., Natsume, N. & Sasaki, T. (2007). Cellular localization and functional characterization of the equilibrative nucleoside transporters of antitumor nucleosides. *Cancer Sci*, 98, 1633-7.

Endres, C.J., Moss, A.M., Govindarajan, R., Choi, D.S. & Unadkat, J.D.(2009). The role of nucleoside transporters in the erythrocyte disposition and oral absorption of ribavirin in the wild-type and equilibrative nucleoside transporter 1-/- mice. *J Pharmacol Exp Ther*, 331, 287-96.

Evoniuk, G., von Borstel, R.W. & Wurtman, R.J.(1987). Antagonism of the cardiovascular effects of adenosine by caffeine or 8-(p-sulfophenyl)theophylline. *J Pharmacol Exp Ther*, 240, 428-32.

Fredholm, B.B., AP, I.J., Jacobson, K.A., Klotz, K.N. & Linden, J.(2001). International Union of Pharmacology. XXV. Nomenclature and classification of adenosine receptors. *Pharmacol Ver*, 53, 527-52.

Fredholm, B.B. (2003). Adenosine receptors as targets for drug development. *Drug News Perspect*, 16, 283-9.

Fresco, P., Diniz, C., Queiroz, G. & Goncalves, J.(2002). Release inhibitory receptors activation favours the A2A-adenosine receptor-mediated facilitation of noradrenaline release in isolated rat tail artery. *Br J Pharmacol*, 136, 230-6.

Fresco, P., Diniz, C. & Goncalves, J.(2004). Facilitation of noradrenaline release by activation of adenosine A(2A) receptors triggers both phospholipase C and adenylate cyclase pathways in rat tail artery. *Cardiovasc Res*, 63, 739-46.

Fresco, P., Oliveira, J.M., Kunc, F., Soares, A.S., Rocha-Pereira, C., Goncalves, J.& Diniz, C., (2007). A2A adenosine-receptor-mediated facilitation of noradrenaline release in rat tail artery involves protein kinase C activation and betagamma subunits formed after alpha2-adrenoceptor activation. *Neurochem Int*, 51, 47-56.

Galligan, J.J., Hess, M.C., Miller, S.B. & Fink, G.D.(2001). Differential localization of P2 receptor subtypes in mesenteric arteries and veins of normotensive and hypertensive rats. *J Pharmacol Exp Ther*, 296, 478-85.

Gisbert, R., Ziani, K., Miquel, R., Noguera, M.A., Ivorra, M.D., Anselmi, E. & D'Ocon, P.(2002). Pathological role of a constitutively active population of alpha(1D)-adrenoceptors in arteries of spontaneously hypertensive rats. *Br J Pharmacol* 135, 206-16.

Griffith, D.A. & Jarvis, S.M. (1996). Nucleoside and nucleobase transport systems of mammalian cells. *Biochim Biophys Acta*, 1286, 153-81.

Haase, E.B. & Shoukas, A.A.(1991). Carotid sinus baroreceptor reflex control of venular pressure-diameter relations in rat intestine. *Am J Physiol*, 260, H752-8.

Haase, E.B. & Shoukas, A.A.(1992). Blood volume changes in microcirculation of rat intestine caused by carotid sinus baroreceptor reflex. *Am J Physiol*, 263, H1939-45.

Hiley, C.R., Bottrill, F.E., Warnock, J. & Richardson, P.J.(1995). Effects of pH on responses to adenosine, CGS 21680, carbachol and nitroprusside in the isolated perfused superior mesenteric arterial bed of the rat. *Br J Pharmacol*, 116, 2641-6.

Huber-Ruano, I. & Pastor-Anglada, M. (2009). Transport of nucleoside analogs across the plasma membrane: a clue to understanding drug-induced cytotoxicity. *Curr Drug Metab*, 10, 347-58.

Hyde, R.J., Cass, C.E., Young, J.D. & Baldwin, S.A. (2001). The ENT family of eukaryote nucleoside and nucleobase transporters: recent advances in the investigation of structure/function relationships and the identification of novel isoforms. *Mol Membr Biol*, 18, 53-63.

Jackson, E.K. (1987). Role of adenosine in noradrenergic neurotransmission in spontaneously hypertensive rats. *Am J Physiol*, 253, H909-18.

Jacobson, E.D. & Pawlik, W.W.(1992). Adenosine mediation of mesenteric blood flow. *J Physiol Pharmacol*, 43, 3-19.

Karoon, P., Rubino, A. & Burnstock, G. (1995). Enhanced sympathetic neurotransmission in the tail artery of 1,3-dipropyl-8-sulphophenylxanthine (DPSPX)-treated rats. *Br J Pharmacol*, 116, 1918-22.

King, A.D., Milavec-Krizman, M. & Muller-Schweinitzer, E.(1990). Characterization of the adenosine receptor in porcine coronary arteries. *Br J Pharmacol*, 100, 483-6.

King, A.J., Osborn, J.W. & Fink, G.D. (2007). Splanchnic circulation is a critical neural target in angiotensin II salt hypertension in rats. *Hypertension*, 50, 547-56.

Kong, W., Engel, K. & Wang, J. (2004). Mammalian nucleoside transporters. *Curr Drug Metab*, 5, 63-84.

Kreulen, D.L. (2003). Properties of the venous and arterial innervation in the mesentery. *J Smooth Muscle Res*, 39, 269-79.

Leal, S., Sa, C., Goncalves, J., Fresco, P. & Diniz, C.(2008). Immunohistochemical characterization of adenosine receptors in rat aorta and tail arteries. *Microsc Res Tech*, 71, 703-9.

Lee, C.H., Poburko, D., Sahota, P., Sandhu, J., Ruehlmann, D.O. & van Breemen, C.(2001). The mechanism of phenylephrine-mediated [Ca(2+)](i) oscillations underlying tonic contraction in the rabbit inferior vena cava. *J Physiol*, 534, 641-50.

Lee, R.M., 1987. Structural alterations of blood vessels in hypertensive rats. Can J Physiol Pharmacol, 65, 1528-35.

Li, R.W., Seto, S.W., Au, A.L., Kwan, Y.W., Chan, S.W., Lee, S.M., Tse, C.M. & Leung, G.P., (2009). Inhibitory effect of nonsteroidal anti-inflammatory drugs on adenosine transport in vascular smooth muscle cells. *Eur J Pharmacol*, 612, 15-20.

Li, R.W., Yang, C., Sit, A.S., Lin, S.Y., Ho, E.Y. & Leung, G.P.(2011). Physiological and Pharmacological Roles of Vascular Nucleoside Transporters. *J Cardiovasc Pharmacol*,

Lockette, W., Otsuka, Y. & Carretero, O.(1986). The loss of endothelium-dependent vascular relaxation in hypertension. *Hypertension*, 8, 1161-6.

Lu, H., Chen, C. & Klaassen, C.(2004). Tissue distribution of concentrative and equilibrative nucleoside transporters in male and female rats and mice. *Drug Metab Dispos*, 32, 1455-61.

Lum, P.Y., Ngo, L.Y., Bakken, A.H. & Unadkat, J.D.(2000). Human intestinal es nucleoside transporter: molecular characterization and nucleoside inhibitory profiles. *Cancer Chemother Pharmacol*, 45, 273-8.

Luscher, T.F., Vanhoutte, P.M. & Raij, L.(1987). Antihypertensive treatment normalizes decreased endothelium-dependent relaxations in rats with salt-induced hypertension. *Hypertension*, 9, III193-7.

McGuire, P.G., Walker-Caprioglio, H.M., Little, S.A.& McGuffee, L.J. (1993). Isolation and culture of rat superior mesenteric artery smooth muscle cells. *In Vitro Cell Dev Biol*, 29A, 135-9.

Meghji, P., Pearson, J.D.& Slakey, L.L.(1992). Regulation of extracellular adenosine production by ectonucleotidases of adult rat ventricular myocytes. *Am J Physiol*, 263, H40-7.

Molina-Arcas, M., Marce, S., Villamor, N., Huber-Ruano, I., Casado, F.J., Bellosillo, B., Montserrat, E., Gil, J., Colomer, D. & Pastor-Anglada, M.(2005). Equilibrative nucleoside transporter-2 (hENT2) protein expression correlates with ex vivo sensitivity to fludarabine in chronic lymphocytic leukemia (CLL) cells. *Leukemia*, 19, 64-8.

Molina-Arcas, M., Trigueros-Motos, L., Casado, F.J. & Pastor-Anglada, M.(2008). Physiological and pharmacological roles of nucleoside transporter proteins. *Nucleosides Nucleotides Nucleic Acids*, 27, 769-78.

Molina-Arcas, M., Casado, F.J. & Pastor-Anglada, M.(2009). Nucleoside transporter proteins. *Curr Vasc Pharmacol*, 7, 426-34.

Morhrman D.E. & Heller L.J. (2006). *Cardiovascular Physiology* (6th edition), The McGraw-Hill Companies, ISBN 0071465618.

Mutafova-Yambolieva, V.N., Carolan, B.M., Harden, T.K. & Keef, K.D. (2000). Multiple P2Y receptors mediate contraction in guinea pig mesenteric vein. *Gen Pharmacol*, 34, 127-36.

Nyhof, R.A., Laine, G.A., Meininger, G.A. & Granger, H.J. (1983). Splanchnic circulation in hypertension. *Fed Proc*, 42, 1690-3.

Olah, M.E., Ren, H. & Stiles, G.L.(1995). Adenosine receptors: protein and gene structure. *Arch Int Pharmacodyn Ther*, 329, 135-50.

Olah, M.E. & Stiles, G.L. (1995). Adenosine receptor subtypes: characterization and therapeutic regulation. *Annu Rev Pharmacol Toxicol* 35, 581-606.

Olsson, R.A.& Pearson, J.D.(1990). Cardiovascular purinoceptors. *Physiol Ver*, 70, 761-845.

Park, J., Galligan, J.J., Fink, G.D. & Swain, G.M.(2007). Differences in sympathetic neuroeffector transmission to rat mesenteric arteries and veins as probed by in vitro continuous amperometry and video imaging. *J Physiol*, 584, 819-34.

Pastor-Anglada, M., Casado, F.J., Valdes, R., Mata, J., Garcia-Manteiga, J.& Molina, M.(2001). Complex regulation of nucleoside transporter expression in epithelial and immune system cells. *Mol Membr Biol* 18, 81-5.

Pennycooke, M., Chaudary, N., Shuralyova, I., Zhang, Y. & Coe, I.R.(2001). Differential expression of human nucleoside transporters in normal and tumor tissue. *Biochem Biophys Res Commun*, 280, 951-9.

Perez-Rivera, A.A., Hlavacova, A., Rosario-Colon, L.A., Fink, G.D. & Galligan, J.J. (2007). Differential contributions of alpha-1 and alpha-2 adrenoceptors to vasoconstriction in mesenteric arteries and veins of normal and hypertensive mice. *Vascul Pharmacol* 46, 373-82.

Podgorska, M., Kocbuch, K. & Pawelczyk, T. (2005). Recent advances in studies on biochemical and structural properties of equilibrative and concentrative nucleoside transporters. *Acta Biochim Pol*, 52, 749-58.

Ralevic, V. & Burnstock, G.(1998). Receptors for purines and pyrimidines. *Pharmacol Rev*, 50, 413-92.

Rang H.P., Dale M.M. & Ritter J.M. (2006) *Rang and Dale's Pharmacology* (6th edition),Churchill/Livingstone, ISBN 0443069115.

Reyes, G., Naydenova, Z., Abdulla, P., Chalsev, M., Villani, A., Rose, J.B., Chaudary, N., DeSouza, L., Siu, K.W. & Coe, I.R. (2010). Characterization of mammalian equilibrative nucleoside transporters (ENTs) by mass spectrometry. *Protein Expr Purif*, 73, 1-9.

Ritzel, M.W., Ng, A.M., Yao, S.Y., Graham, K., Loewen, S.K., Smith, K.M., Hyde, R.J., Karpinski, E., Cass, C.E., Baldwin, S.A. & Young, J.D.(2001). Recent molecular advances in studies of the concentrative Na+-dependent nucleoside transporter (CNT) family: identification and characterization of novel human and mouse proteins (hCNT3 and mCNT3) broadly selective for purine and pyrimidine nucleosides (system cib). *Mol Membr Biol*, 18, 65-72.

Rocha-Pereira C., Fresco P., Arribas S.M., Gonzalez M.C., Conde M.V., Goncalves J. & Diniz C. (2009) Evidence for a Less Efficient A1 Receptor-Mediated Inhibition of Noradrenaline Release in Mesenteric Arteries from Spontaneously Hypertensive Rats (SHR). Hypertension, 54, 1183-4.

Rose, J.B., Naydenova, Z., Bang, A., Eguchi, M., Sweeney, G., Choi, D.S., Hammond, J.R.& Coe, I.R.(2010). Equilibrative nucleoside transporter 1 plays an essential role in cardioprotection. *Am J Physiol Heart Circ Physiol*, 298, H771-7.

Ross M.H. & Pawlina W. (2006) *Histology: a text and atlas with correlated cell and molecularbiology* (5th edition), Lippinicott Williams & Wilkins, ISBN 0781772214.

Schindler, C.W., Karcz-Kubicha, M., Thorndike, E.B., Muller, C.E., Tella, S.R., Ferre, S.& Goldberg, S.R.(2005). Role of central and peripheral adenosine receptors in the cardiovascular responses to intraperitoneal injections of adenosine A1 and A2A subtype receptor agonists. *Br J Pharmacol*, 144, 642-50.

Shoukas, A.A. & Bohlen, H.G. (1990). Rat venular pressure-diameter relationships are regulated by sympathetic activity. *Am J Physiol*, 259, H674-80.

Shryock, J.C. & Belardinelli, L.(1997). Adenosine and adenosine receptors in the cardiovascular system: biochemistry, physiology, and pharmacology. *Am J Cardiol*, 79, 2-10.

Spyer, K.M. & Thomas, T.(2000). A role for adenosine in modulating cardio-respiratory responses: a mini-review. *Brain Res Bull*, 53, 121-4.

Sullivan, J.C., Giulumian, A.D., Pollock, D.M., Fuchs, L.C. & Pollock, J.S.(2002). Functional NOS 1 in the rat mesenteric arterial bed. *Am J Physiol Heart Circ Physiol*, 283, H658-63.

Tabrizchi, R.& Bedi, S.(2001). Pharmacology of adenosine receptors in the vasculature. *Pharmacol Ther*, 91, 133-47.

Takahashi, T., Otsuguro, K., Ohta, T. & Ito, S.(2010). Adenosine and inosine release during hypoxia in the isolated spinal cord of neonatal rats. *Br J Pharmacol*, 161, 1806-16.

Takenaga, M.& Kawasaki, H.(1999). [Neuronal control of mesenteric circulation]. *Nihon Yakurigaku Zasshi*, 113, 249-59.

Tawfik, H.E., Schnermann, J., Oldenburg, P.J. & Mustafa, S.J.(2005). Role of A1 adenosine receptors in regulation of vascular tone. *Am J Physiol Heart Circ Physiol*, 288b H1411-6.

Thomas, T., St Lambert, J.H., Dashwood, M.R. & Spyer, K.M. (2000). Localization and action of adenosine A2a receptors in regions of the brainstem important in cardiovascular control. *Neuroscience*, 95, 513-8.

Thorn, J.A. & Jarvis, S.M.(1996). Adenosine transporters. *Gen Pharmacol*, 27, 613-20.

Vasquez, G., Sanhueza, F., Vasquez, R., Gonzalez, M., San Martin, R., Casanello, P. & Sobrevia, L.(2004). Role of adenosine transport in gestational diabetes-induced L-arginine transport and nitric oxide synthesis in human umbilical vein endothelium. *J Physiol*, 560, 111-22.

Vega, J.L., Puebla, C., Vasquez, R., Farias, M., Alarcon, J., Pastor-Anglada, M., Krause, B., Casanello, P. & Sobrevia, L. (2009). TGF-beta1 inhibits expression and activity of hENT1 in a nitric oxide-dependent manner in human umbilical vein endothelium. *Cardiovasc Res*, 82, 458-67.

Villalobos-Molina, R. & Ibarra, M.(1999). Vascular alpha 1D-adrenoceptors: are they related to hypertension? *Arch Med Res*, 30, 347-52.

Villalobos-Molina, R., Lopez-Guerrero, J.J., Ibarra, M.(1999). Functional evidence of alpha1D-adrenoceptors in the vasculature of young and adult spontaneously hypertensive rats. *Br J Pharmacol*. 126, 1534-6.

Wang, L., Karlsson, L., Moses, S., Hultgardh-Nilsson, A., Andersson, M., Borna, C., Gudbjartsson, T., Jern, S. & Erlinge, D. (2002). P2 receptor expression profiles in human vascular smooth muscle and endothelial cells. *J Cardiovasc Pharmacol*, 40, 841-53.

Ward, J.L., Sherali, A., Mo, Z.P. & Tse, C.M. (2000). Kinetic and pharmacological properties of cloned human equilibrative nucleoside transporters, ENT1 and ENT2, stably expressed in nucleoside transporter-deficient PK15 cells. Ent2 exhibits a low affinity for guanosine and cytidine but a high affinity for inosine. *J Biol Chem*, 275, 8375-81.

Xu, K., Lu, Z., Wei, H., Zhang, Y. & Han, C.(1998). Alteration of alpha1-adrenoceptor subtypes in aortas of 12-month-old spontaneously hypertensive rats. *Eur J Pharmacol*, 344, 31-6.

Yao, S.Y., Ng, A.M., Muzyka, W.R., Griffiths, M., Cass, C.E., Baldwin, S.A. & Young, J.D. (1997). Molecular cloning and functional characterization of nitrobenzylthioinosine (NBMPR)-sensitive (es) and NBMPR-insensitive (ei) equilibrative nucleoside transporter proteins (rENT1 and rENT2) from rat tissues. *J Biol Chem*, 272, 28423-30.

Yao, S.Y., Ng, A.M., Vickers, M.F., Sundaram, M., Cass, C.E., Baldwin, S.A. & Young, J.D.(2002). Functional and molecular characterization of nucleobase transport by recombinant human and rat equilibrative nucleoside transporters 1 and 2. Chimeric constructs reveal a role for the ENT2 helix 5-6 region in nucleobase translocation. *J Biol Chem*, 277, 24938-48.

Young, J.D., Yao, S.Y., Sun, L., Cass, C.E. & Baldwin, S.A.(2008). Human equilibrative nucleoside transporter (ENT) family of nucleoside and nucleobase transporter proteins. *Xenobiotica*, 38, 995-1021.

7

Endothelial Nitric Oxide Synthase, Nitric Oxide and Metabolic Disturbances in the Vascular System

Grażyna Lutosławska
University of Physical Education, Warsaw, Poland

1. Introduction

It is well documented that hyperlipidemia, obesity and diabetes increase the risk for the development of atherosclerosis and subsequent cardiovascular disease (Vinik, 2005, Ritchie & Connell 2007, Stapleton et al. 2010). However, until now the precise mechanism by which the above mentioned metabolic perturbations contribute to atherosclerosis has not been fully elucidated.

Numerous studies have focused on the detrimental effects of excessive body fat stores as a possible reason for both insulin resistance and disturbed lipoprotein metabolism with special attention paid to the adverse effects of visceral fat (Sharma et al., 2002, Matsuzawa, 2005). In overweight and/or obesity, free fatty acids (FFA) are released into the circulation and their availability for lipoprotein synthesis in the liver is markedly elevated (Jensen, 2006).

Moreover, high circulating FFA negatively affects whole body insulin sensitivity and disturbs carbohydrate and lipid metabolism (Kohen-Avramoglu et al., 2006). Furthermore, body fat excess brings about increased secretion of adipokines which depress insulin sensitivity (e.g. leptin, resistin), and decreased secretion of insulin-sensing adiponectin. Additionally, IL-6 and TNF-α, derived from adipose tissue, on the one hand induce inflammation, and on the other stimulate adipose tissue lipolysis and augment FFA availability for lipid and lipoprotein synthesis (Lago et al., 2009).

In addition, both insulin resistance and adipokines affect endothelial nitric oxide synthase (eNOS) and nitric oxide (NO) production and in consequence deteriorate blood vessel contractility (Muniyappa et al., 2008). Moreover, there are data indicating an adverse effect of LDL-cholesterol and positive action of HDL cholesterol on eNOS expression and NO production (Stepp et al., 2002, Rämet et al., 2003).

All the above-mentioned metabolic disturbances have pronounced consequences for the cardiovascular system due to inflammation, atherosclerotic plaque formation and structural alterations in the endothelium and subsequently lead to its dysfunction.

Thus, in this sequence of metabolic perturbations the endothelium was recognized rather as a target of unfavorable events related to excessive body fat stores, insulin resistance and dyslipidemia, but not as an independent player contributing to dysfunction of the cardiovascular system.

2. Vascular dysfunction – Primary or secondary target

However, there were also data suggesting that endothelial dysfunction was a major mechanism involved in the development of metabolic disturbances and subsequent atherogenesis (Yang & Ming, 2006).

Recently this hypothesis has been the focus much attention mostly as a consequence of data concerning a wide spectrum of metabolic eNOS/NO action. It has been recognized that eNOS itself is indispensable for physiological insulin action and glucose disposal in the working muscle (Roberts et al., 1997, Kingwell et al., 2002, Ross et al., 2007). Moreover, *in vitro* NO markedly increases glucose transporter (GLUT 4) expression in the muscle and regulates AMP- kinase (AMPK) signaling (Lira et al., 2007). Taking into account the special role of AMPK in the regulation of substrate utilization it is clear that eNOS activity and NO production markedly affect energetic processes in the muscle (Smith A.C., et al., 2005).

In contrast, eNOS deficiency in eNOS $^{-/-}$ mice depresses oxidative processes and brings about defective mitochondrial fatty acid oxidation (Momken et al., 2002, Le Gouill et al., 2007). Recent data have shown that the ablation of eNOS in mice accelerates glucose and free fatty acid uptake by muscles and increases liver and muscle glycogenolysis (Lee-Young et al., 2010). In consequence, eNOS knockout animals exhibit hypoglycemia and limited exercise capacity during exercise.

It is well documented that in vitro NO contributes to the regulation of lipid metabolism in the liver by inhibiting acetyl-CoA carboxylase (ACC) activity and *de novo* free fatty acid synthesis (Garcia-Villafranca et al., 2003). There are also data suggesting that both *in vitro* and *in vivo* NO exerts a hypocholesterolemic effect, since stimulation of NO synthesis in rabbits decreases circulating LDL-cholesterol (Kurowska & Carrol, 1998).

At present eNOS/NO system contribution to the regulation of metabolism is far from being fully elucidated. However, it is accepted that the vascular endothelium is not exclusively a target responding to metabolic disturbances accompanying cardiovascular disease, but is an important and independent player in the complicated relationships between cardiovascular disease, obesity and diabetes.

This assumption is partially supported by research indicating that adverse changes in vasculature in response to high fat diet (inflammation, insulin resistance, reduced NO production) precede detrimental effects in muscle, liver, or adipose tissue (Kim et al., 2008).

3. Endothelial Nitric Oxide Synthase (eNOS) and Nitric Oxide (NO) system coupling and uncoupling

It should be pointed out that the endothelium is one of the largest systems in human body spread throughout the capillaries and arterioles in all tissues, forming a selectively permeable barrier between the outer vascular wall and the bloodstream. It also the tissue producing nitric oxide (NO) responsible for vasorelaxation, platelet aggregation, leukocyte-endothelium adhesion and vascular smooth muscle cell migration and proliferation (Michel & Vanhoutte, 2010).

The mechanism of endothelial eNOS regulation is not fully elucidated due to its complexity. However, there are data indicating that enzyme activity is subjected to complicated regulation by many intracellular factors including heat shock protein (HSP90), different phosphatases, kinases, but also by enzyme location in the cell and potentially motor proteins (Dudzinski & Michel, 2007).

On the other hand, it is well documented that eNOS activity is also regulated by factors generated outside the endothelium - negatively by resistin, TNF-α, and leptin and positively by estrogen ((Dai et al., 2004, Kougias et al., 2005, Valerio et al., 2006, Korda et al,. 2008, LeBlanc et al. 2009).

Nitric oxide is synthesized from L-arginine in a reaction catalyzed by the endothelial eNOS (Moncada et al., 1991) (Fig. 1). Thus, any factors decreasing eNOS activity and/or increasing NO degradation i.e. affecting the eNOS/NO system have been recognized as a potential source of disturbed endothelium function.

Under physiological conditions and optimal eNOS activity L-arginine in the presence of O_2 is converted to NO and citrulline with minor production of superoxide (Alp & Channon, 2004). In consequence, NO production is "coupled" with eNOS activity.

In contrast, inadequate L-arginine intake and deficiency of the eNOS cofactor - tetrahydropterin (BH4) brings about depressed NO synthesis, and promotes superoxide and peroxynitrite generation - a phenomenon named eNOS uncoupling (Huang, 2009).

Taking into account that L-arginine is the exclusive substrate for NO synthesis it is clear that its metabolism catalyzed by arginase has the potential to decrease eNOS activity and NO production (Wu et al., 2009).

In mammals there are two types of arginase, encoded by two genes – arginase I and II. Arginase I is expressed mostly in the liver catalyzing L-arginine conversion into urea and ornithine and in this way participating in ammonia detoxication. Arginase II is a mitochondrial enzyme of extrahepatic tissues contributing to biosynthesis of amino acids (glutamate, proline and ornithine) and polyamines, but also playing a fundamental role in the depression of endothelial NO production decreasing L-arginine availability for eNOS action. In addition, arginase II overexpression seems to induce superoxide and peroxynitrite generation – *per se* harmful for the endothelium. There are data suggesting increased arginase activity in atherosclerosis and hypertension, thus diseases characterized by endothelial dysfunction (Ryoo et al., 2011)

BH4 bioavailability within the endothelium plays a fundamental role in eNOS/NO coupling. It has been demonstrated that the inhibition of the rate-limiting enzyme responsible for *de novo* BH4 synthesis - GTP cyclohydrolase 1 - brings about eNOS/NO uncoupling and elevated superoxide production in isolated bovine or mouse aortic endothelial cells. Moreover, superoxide production was reduced by the sepiapterin – BH4 precursor (Tiefenbacher et al. ,2000, Wang et al., 2008).

However, recent data have indicated that the regulation of BH4 levels in the endothelium is even more complicated since it is oxidized to 7,8-dihydrobiopterin (BH2) which in turn is recycled into BH4 in the reaction catalyzed by dihydrofolate reductase (DHFR). Moreover, a genetic DHFR knockout or pharmacological inhibition of the enzyme suppresses BH4 synthesis and causes eNOS uncoupling (Crabtree et al., 2009) (Fig.2).

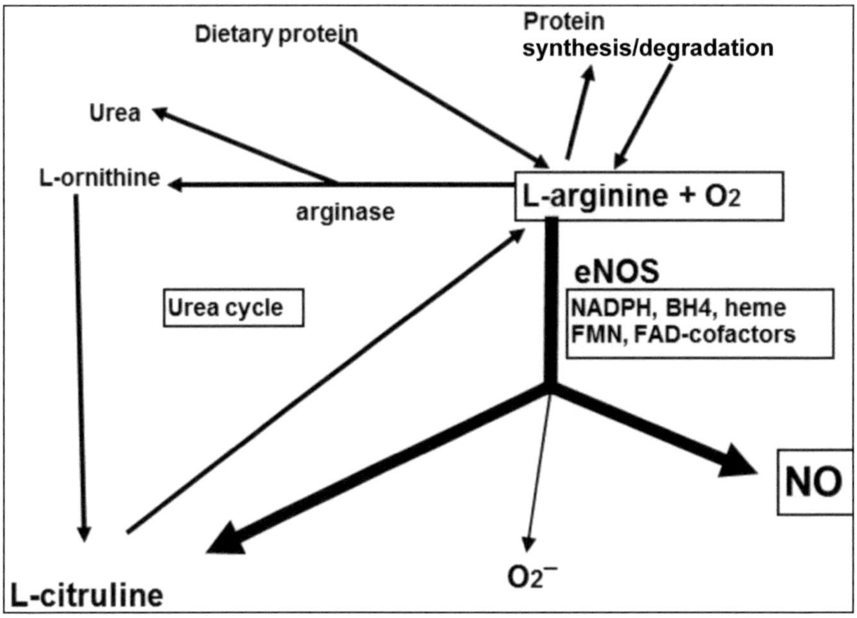

Fig. 1. L-arginine as a source of nitric oxide (NO) under physiological condition and minor superoxide production.

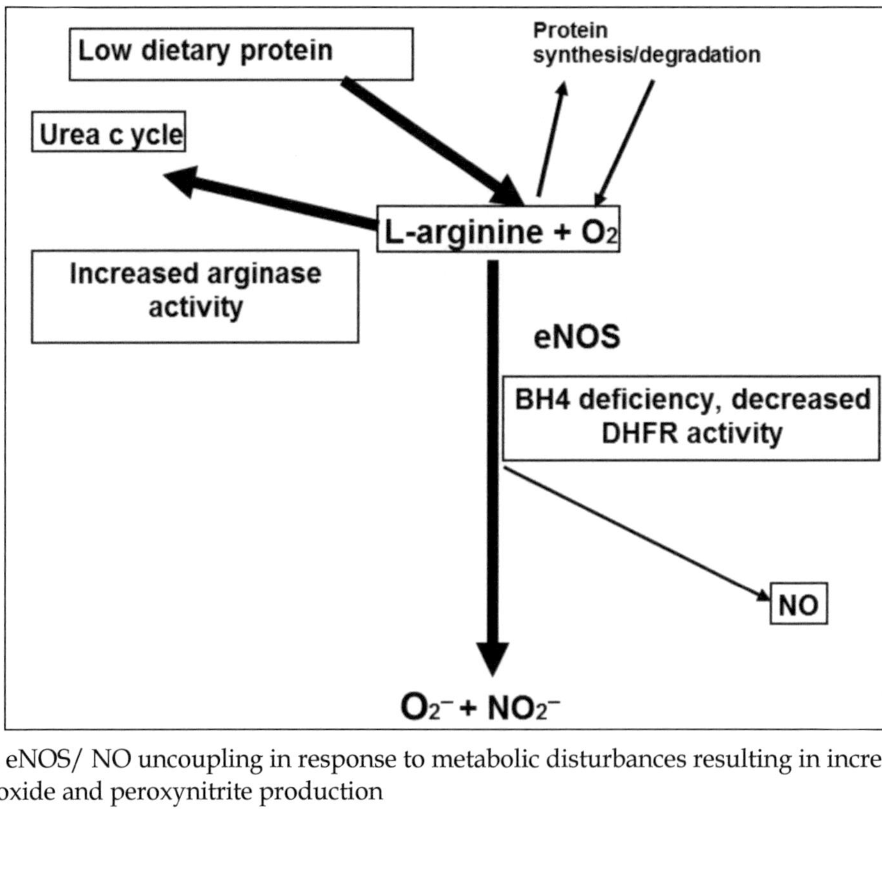

Fig. 2. eNOS/ NO uncoupling in response to metabolic disturbances resulting in increased superoxide and peroxynitrite production

It should be pointed out that regulation of cardiovascular system is not limited to eNOS action. Numerous research focus on neuronal (nNOS) and inducible (iNOS) nitric oxide synthase role in the cardiovascular system. It has been postulated that nNOS expressed outside of the vascular system might protect mice from diet-induced atherosclerosis through indirect action on hormonal and/or nervous system and blood pressure regulation. (Lowenstein, 2006). On the other hand, iNOS is expressed in a wide range of cells in response to cytokines and is overexpressed in macrophage and cardiovascular system of diabetic rats (Soskić et al.,2011). However, much more studies are needed to fully elucidate the relationship between three isoforms of NO in vascular system dysfunction.

4. Asymmetrical dimethylarginine (ADMA) and the vascular system

Recently numerous studies have focused on the role of endogenous inhibitor of eNOS activity and NO production - asymmetrical dimethylarginine (ADMA). ADMA is synthesized in many tissues, including the endothelium, by the methylation of L-arginine released from proteins which undergo regular turnover. The methylation process is catalyzed by arginine methyltransferase type I (PRMT I) and ADMA production is related to both protein turnover and enzyme activity (Pope et al., 2009) (Fig.3). However, about 90% of ADMA is metabolized to citrulline and dimethylamine by dimethylarginine dimethylaminohydrolase (DDAH), with the remainder partially excreted with urine (Tran et al., 2003). Numerous studies have indicated a substantial role for DDAH in ADMA turnover. DDAH is expressed as two isoforms (DDAH I and DDAH II) encoded by different genes (Leiper et al,. 1999). Animal studies have revealed that in mice overexpressing DDAH I plasma ADMA levels are reduced with concomitant increase in tissue NOS activity. (Dayoub et al., 2003). Moreover, in humans genetic variants of DDAH I and DDAH II genes are significantly associated with plasma ADMA levels (Abhary et al., 2010). Moreover, ADMA concentration in tissues and plasma is also affected by cationic amino acid transporter (CAT) in exchange for arginine and other cationic amino acids (Teerlink et al., 2009). Reference values of circulating ADMA in healthy subjects vary widely, even when similar analytic methods are used (Meinitzer et al., 2007). However, the risk of acute coronary events and mortality increases with elevated plasma ADMA concentrations (Valkonen et al., 2001, Zoccali et al., 2001) Moreover, it is well documented that circulating ADMA is inversely related to endothelial function in hypertensive and healthy subjects (Perticone et al., 2003, Böger et al., 2007). Furthermore, it has been established that the intima-media thickness of the carotid artery and aortic stenosis are related to circulating ADMA (Furuki et al., 2007, Ngo et al., 2007). Additionally, circulating ADMA has been recognized as an independent factor determining flow mediated dilatation in cardiac syndrome X (Haberka et al., 2010).

The mechanism of detrimental ADMA action in the vascular system is not fully established. It is still under debate whether ADMA represents a novel risk factor for the development of endothelial dysfunction or its production reflects endothelium response to other metabolic disturbances such as oxidative stress (Sydow & Münzel, 2003). This latter hypothesis could not be excluded since *in vitro* oxidative stress decreases ADMA-demethylating enzyme (DDAH) activity and causes elevated ADMA levels (Leiper et al., 2002).

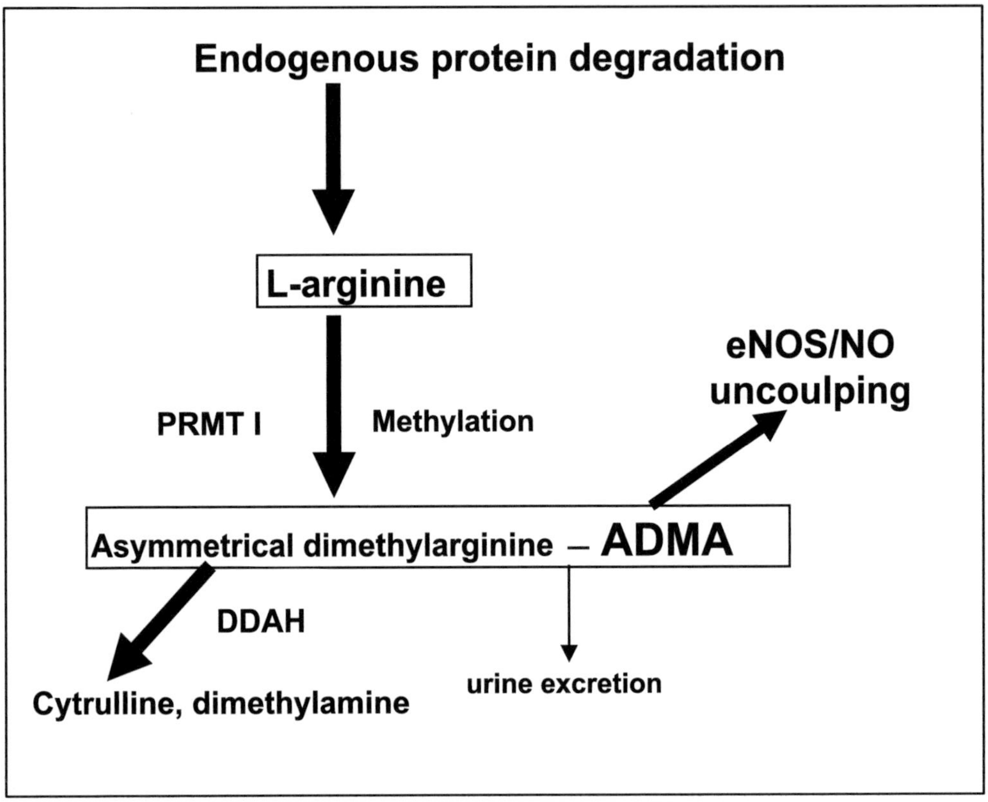

Fig. 3. Asymmertical dimethyl arginine (ADMA) synthesis and action on eNOS/NO system

On the other hand, the analysis of 131 cases with coronary heart disease (CHD) and 131 controls matched for age, sex and body mass index has revealed that plasma ADMA concentrations in patients were higher than in controls and ADMA is an independent risk factor for CHD (Schultze et al., 2006). Similarly, in 138 patients with acute myocardial infartion ADMA was recognized as a marker of cardiovascular risk independent of traditional risk factors (Korandji et al., 2007).

Despite these doubts the detrimental effects of ADMA on the endothelium are well documented. First of all ADMA is a potent inhibitor of eNOS inducing eNOS/NO uncoupling (Jin & Loscalzo, 2010). Moreover, it has been found that ADMA is an endogenous inhibitor of mobilization, differentiation and function of endothelial progenitor cells which participate in continuous endothelial renewal and neovascularization of ischemic tissues (Thum et al., 2005). Additionally, *in vitro* pathological concentrations of ADMA are sufficient to elicit marked changes in coronary artery endothelial cell gene expression of bone morphogenic protein receptor, and PRMT - the enzyme responsible for methylation of arginine to ADMA Moreover, in mice treated with high ADMA doses (2 μM) more than 50 genes in endothelium were significantly altered (Smith C.L., et al., 2005). Some data also data suggest proinflammatory ADMA action in human endothelial cells (Chen et al., 2007)

Thus, it should be pointed out that ADMA-mediated pathological processes are not exclusively due to eNOS uncoupling, however, eNOS inhibition is most likely being the dominant ADMA vascular effect (Cooke, 2004).

5. Lifestyle and vascular system

There is no doubt that lifestyle has a pronounced effect on health, decreasing body fat stores, improving insulin sensitivity, lipid and lipoprotein metabolism and positively affecting the cardiovascular system (Lamon-Fave et al., 1996, Lee et al., 2005, Takahashi et al., 2011). Numerous data have revealed that both eNOS and NO production are the target of lifestyle interventions such as dietary habits and physical activity.

5.1 Dietary habits, eNOS and NO

Dietary habits are associated with both acute and chronic effects on the vascular system. In healthy, normolipidemic young and middle-aged men a single high fat meal has been found to adversely affect endothelial function depressing the flow-mediated vasodilation of the brachial artery (Vogel et al., 1997, Marchesi et al., 2000). Moreover, a decrease in endothelial function has been observed in response to both glucose and fat load, with a more pronounced effect when high fat and glucose were combined (Ceriello et al., 2002). Thus, postprandial state has to be taken into consideration as a possible reason for diet-induced depression in vascular reactivity.

The mechanism of the effects of postprandial state on vascular function is not fully elucidated, however it seems that oxidative stress due to elevated plasma remnant lipoproteins, triglycerides, and glucose concentrations contributes to the adverse effects of a single meal on vascularity (Doi et al., 2000, Bae et al., 2001, Ceriello et al., 2004). Moreover, recent data have suggested that in addition to oxidative stress, oral fat load enhances metalloproteinase-2 and metalloproteinase-9 activity which in turn bring about unfavorable vascular remodeling (Derosa et al., 2010).

However, it should be pointed out that adverse effects of fat load on the vascular system are mostly due to saturated fat (Vogel et al., 2000, Cortěz et al,. 2006, Berry et al., 2008). In contrast, an exchange of saturated for unsaturated fat load has been found to improve postprandial vascular function probably due to the positive effect of the latter on endothelial eNOS/NO system (Armah et al., 2008, Masson & Mesink, 2011).

Numerous experimental studies have focused on chronic effects of dietary habits on endothelium function and vasoreactivity, however, their results are inconsistent. In patients with coronary artery disease a long-term (6 weeks) treatment with purified eicosapentaenoic acid (EPA) markedly improved NO-mediated forearm vasodilatation (Tagawa et al., 1999). Similarly, improved forearm microcirculation has been noted in hyperlipidemic, overweight subjects following a 6 week treatment with purified docosahexaenoic acid (DHA), but not with EPA (Mori et al., 2000). On the contrary, positive action of longer (7 weeks) EPA and DHA supplementation on systemic arterial compliance has been demonstrated in dyslipidemic elderly men (Nestel et al., 2002). Additionally, it has been noted that 32 weeks EPA and DHA-rich fish oil supplementation improve endothelial function and vascular tone in healthy middle-aged men and women (Khan et al., 2003).

Thus, it seems that duration of supplementation possibly contributes to discordant results concerning the response of the vascular system to polyunsaturated fatty acid (PUFA) treatment.

There are also data suggesting that EPA and DHA-rich fish oil exert a more pronounced effect on vascular function than other oils In rats fed a fish-oil rich diet the aortic content of eNOS protein and enzyme activity are markedly (by 70% and 102 %, respectively) higher than in rats fed corn oil (Lopez et al., 2004). Moreover, improved vascular reactivity and enhanced eNOS expression have been indicated in aortic rings of spontaneously hypertensive rats fed diet rich in pomace olive oil, but not refined olive or corn oil (Rodriguez-Rodriguez et al., 2007). Thus, the positive effect of unsaturated fat provision seems to be related to its composition.

Recent data have indicated a positive effect of conjugated linoleic acid (CLA) on vascularity in obese *fa/fa* rats due to CLA-induced elevation in adiponectin production and subsequent eNOS phosphorylation increasing enzyme activity and NO production (DeClerq et al., 2011). Therefore, it seems feasible that well-known beneficial effects of oil consumption on health are at least partially due to its action on the eNOS/NO system.

Much attention has been paid to effects of dietary protein on vascular function. It has been demonstrated that in hypertensive men there is an inverse relationship between blood pressure and protein consumption with more pronounced action of soy and fish than animal protein intake. Further studies have shown that this effect is due to various amino acids such as cysteine, glutamate, and arginine which decrease oxidative stress, improve renal function and insulin resistance (Vasdev & Stuckles, 2010). However, numerous studies have focused on L-arginine contribution to vascular system regulation since, as was mentioned earlier, L-arginine serves as a substrate for NO synthesis.

In young hypercholesterolemic adults after 4 week L-arginine supplementation (7 grams x 3/day) marked improvement in endothelium-dependent vasodilation has been noted (Clarkson et al.,1994). Similarly, it has been observed that in patients with heart failure 6 weeks L-arginine treatment (5.5 to 12.6 g/ day) positively affects vascular system (Rector, et al. 1996).

Growing evidence indicates that L-arginine supplementation brings about improved insulin sensitivity and decreases circulating free fatty acids and triglycerides in chemically induced diabetic and genetically obese rats (Kohli et al., 2004, Fu et al., 2005). Moreover, similar effects have been observed in obese and type II diabetic patients receiving oral/or intravenous L-arginine (Lucotti et al,. 2006). Furthermore, it has been documented that postprandial lipemia-induced endothelial dysfunction is neutralized by addition of proteins to the fatty meals due to increased L-arginine to ADMA ratio (Westphal et al.,2006). Moreover, in healthy volunteers addition of 2.5 g L-arginine to fatty meal prevents the lipemia-induced endothelial dysfunction (Borucki et al., 2009).

The above data suggest a possible beneficial effect of L-arginine treatment in cardiovascular dysfunction. However, it should be pointed out that some studies do not show any beneficial effect of L-arginine treatment (Chin-Dusting et al., 1996, Oomen et al., 2000). It could not be excluded that this discrepancy is due to individual variability in the response to L-arginine treatment (Evans et al., 2004). Recently it has been postulated that beneficial L-arginine action in vascular system is related to circulating ADMA with no effect in subjects with low metabolite levels (Böger, 2007).

On the other hand, it should be stressed that the acute provision of exogenous L-arginine possibly depresses NO production due to induction of arginases which metabolize L-arginine to urea and in consequence divert it from eNOS and in this way adversely affects cardiovascular system (Dioguardi, 2011).

Data concerning dietary carbohydrate effects on the eNOS/NO system are fragmentary. In obese Zucker rats a low carbohydrate diet (10 %) improves vascular function with no effect on NO production in comparison with that containing 59 % carbohydrates (Focaroli et al., 2007).

However, it is well documented that in the rat excessive fructose supply adversely affects endothelium-dependent vasodilation both *in vitro* and *in vivo* and this effect is probably due to inhibition of NO synthesis (Verma et al., 1997, Rickey et al., 1998, Kamata et al., 1999). Similarly, high glucose concentration *iv vitro* decreases eNOS protein expression and enzyme activity as a result of destroyed enzyme interaction with HSP-90 (Noyman et al,. 2002, Mohan et al., 2009).

On the other hand, many diet components have the potential to reduce detrimental effects of poor dietary habits.

Consumption of antioxidant - rich products such as fruits and vegetables in humans prevents the detrimental action of a saturated fat load due to their positive effect on the eNOS/NO system (Plotnick et al., 2003, Traber & Stevens, 2011). Similarly, low cholesterol , walnut-enriched and the Mediterranean diets are effective in improving the eNOS/NO system and vascular function (Winkler- Möbius et al., 2010).

Data concerning diet effects on ADMA - an endogenous eNOS inhibitor and risk factor are scarce. Päivä et al., (2004) have indicated that in a middle-aged population with mild hypercholesterolemia circulating ADMA is inversely related to carbohydrate consumption. Additionally, Puchau et al. (2009) have demonstrated that in healthy young men circulating ADMA is inversely related to zinc and selenium status.

In elderly subjects polyunsaturated fatty acid (PUFA) supplementation markedly elevates circulating L- arginine and in this way decreases L-arginine/ADMA ratio what might be discussed as an improvement of endothelial function (Eid et al., 2006). However, there are also data which question the fat contribution to increased ADMA level in the blood. Recently Engeli et al. (2011) have revealed that the variation in fat consumption (20% and above 40% of energy) exerts divergent effect on circulating ADMA. In obese subjects higher fat consumption slightly (by 4%) decreases ADMA level. In contrast, in lean subjects both low and high fat consumption causes 6% elevation in ADMA concentration. The authors have postulated that contradictory data concerning dietary fat intake on ADMA levels are mostly due to methodological issues concerning ADMA determination.

Thus, the effects of dietary habits on ADMA plasma levels are far from being elucidated. Moreover, in analysis of the effect of the diet on the eNOS/NO system not only diet composition but also total caloric intake has to be taken into consideration. Animal studies have demonstrated that caloric restriction for 3 or 13 months significantly improves the expression of eNOS protein in various tissues (Nisoli et al., 2005).

5.2 Physical activity and eNOS/NO system

For many years physical activity which decreases body fat stores, improves lipid and lipoprotein metabolism and insulin sensitivity and positively affects cardiovascular system has been recommended in the therapy of obesity, hypertension, type 2 diabetes and cardiovascular disease (Shephard & Balady, 1999).

Assuming the importance of the eNOS/ NO system in the regulation of many metabolic processes in recent years numerous studies have focused on the relationship between endothelial function and physical activity. This issue seems to be of special importance since animal studies have indicated that physical inactivity induces endothelial dysfunction due to decreased eNOS activity (Suvarova et al., 2004).

It is well documented that in rats both acute exercise and regular physical activity (2-4 weeks) markedly enhance eNOS activity and endothelial NO synthesis in skeletal muscle arterioles (Sun et al., 1994, Roberts et al., 1999). Similarly, in dogs following exercise elevated NO synthesis has been noted in coronary circulation being responsible for ¼ of the vasodilation response (Bernstein et al., 1996, Ishibashi et al., 1998). Moreover, in active animals eNOS phosphorylation and activity is significantly elevated after 12 weeks of training (Touati et al., 2011).

In apparently healthy young men and women acute aerobic exercise markedly counteracts detrimental effects of a high-fat meal on flow-mediated dilatation (FMD), but also improves FMD in participants consuming a low-fat meal possibly due to reduction of circulating lipids, insulin resistance and oxidative stress (Padilla et al,. 2006, Silvestre et al., 2008, Tyldum et al.,2009). Thus, it has been postulated that physical activity can attenuate adverse postprandial changes in vascular function (Johnson et al., 2011).

It should be pointed out that a positive effect of physical activity on the eNOS/NO system has also been noted in patients with stroke, chronic heart failure, and myocardial infarction (Gertz et al., 2006, Mendes-Ribeiro et a.,2009, De Waard et al., 2010).

The mechanism of exercise-induced positive changes in the eNOS/NO system is not fully elucidated. However, it is well documented that physical activity brings about hyperemia and subsequently endothelial shear stress (ESS) defined as a fractional force exerted by blood flow (Boushei et al,. 2000, Taylor et al., 2002, Boo & Jo, 2003).

It is well documented that shear stress markedly affects a myriad of intracellular events in endothelial cells including remodeling, inflammation and NO production with low ESS inducing plaque formation (Harrison, 2005, Koskinas et al., 2010).

Early studies have demonstrated that in bovine aortic endothelial cells the elevation of shear stress causes elevation in eNOS phosphorylation and expression which in turn increases enzyme activity (Corson et al., 1996, Malek et al. 1999). Furthermore, in human vessels increase in shear stress inhibits lipid peroxidation induced by high glucose and arachidonic acid in the medium (Mun et al., 2008). Thus, direct effects of physical activity on eNOS/NO system and inhibition of oxidative processes contribute to exercise - induced improvement in endothelium function. However, it is worth noting that positive action of physical activity is limited to moderate intensity, since it has been demonstrated that high intensity exercise (90 % $VO_{2}max$) enhances platelet reactivity to shear stress and induces coagulation which in turn increases the risk of thrombosis (Ikaguri et al., 2003).

Taking into account all data cited in this review it is clear that eNOS/NO system undergoes complicated regulation by both genetic and lifestyle factors (Fig. 4).

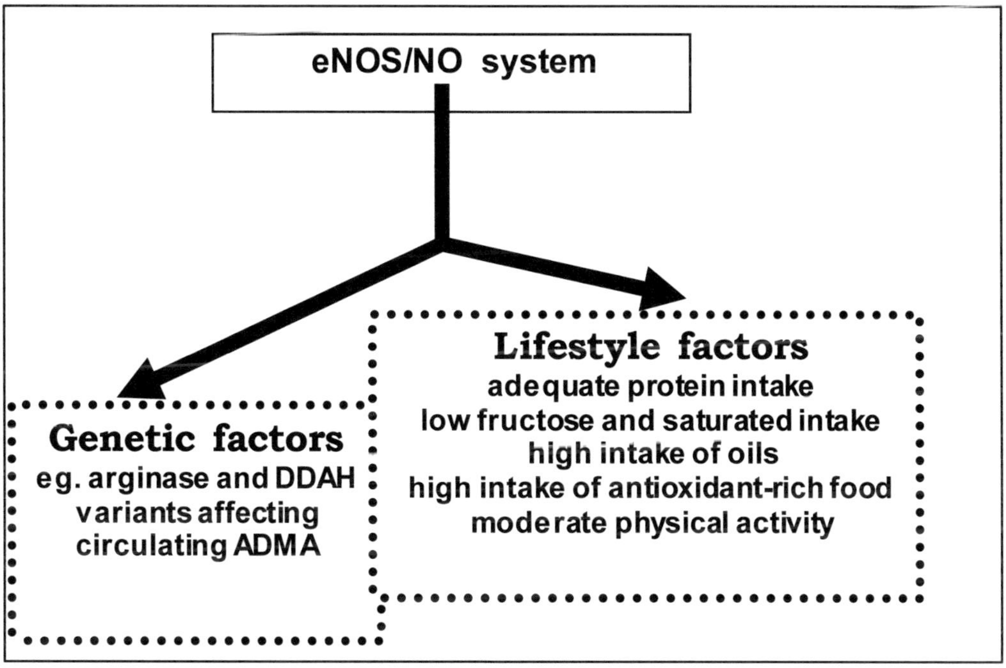

Fig. 4. Interplay between genetic and lifestyle factors affecting eNOS/NO system

6. Conclusion

Our present knowledge about eNOS and NO effects on overall metabolic processes at least partially supports the hypothesis concerning a special and possibly central role of endothelium as an active tissue, and not only the target of metabolic disturbances. Moreover, circulating ADMA seems to be a risk factor of endothelial disturbances and disturbed cardiovascular system. In consequence, further research is required on strategies improving the eNOS/NO system and decreasing ADMA synthesis, including both pharmacological and lifestyle interventions.

7. References

Abhary,S., Burdon, KP., Kuot, A. et al. (2010). Sequence variations in DDAH1 and DDAH2 genes is strongly and additively associated with serum ADMA concentrations in individuals with type 2 diabetes. *PLos one*. Vol. 5, No. 3, pp. e9462. www.plosone.org

Alp, NJ., & Channon, KM. (2004). Regulation of endothelial nitric oxide synthase by tetrahydropterin in vascular disease. *Arteriosclerosis Thrombosis and Vascular Biology*. Vol. 24, December 4, pp. 413-420.

Armah ChK., Jackson, KG., Doman, I. et al. (2008). Fish oil fatty acids improve postprandial vascular reactivity in healthy men. *Clinical Science*. Vol. 114, No. 11, June, pp. 679-686.

Bae, J-H., Bassenge, E., Kim, K-B. et al. (2001). Postprandial hypertriglyceridemia impairs endothelial function by enhanced oxidative stress. *Atherosclerosis.* Vol. 155, No. 2, April, pp. 517-523.

Bernstein, RD., Ochoa, FY., Xu, X. et al. (1996). Function and production of nitric oxide in the coronary circulation of the conscious dog during exercise. *Circulation Research.* Vol. 79, pp. 840-848.

Berry, SE., Tucker, S., Banerji, R. et al. (2008). Impaired postprandial endothelial function depends on the type of fat consumed by healthy men. *Journal of Nutrition.* Vol. 138, No. 10, October, pp. 1910-1914.

Böger, GI., Rudolph, TK., Maas, R. et al. (2007). Asymmetric dimetylarginine determines the improvement of endothelium-dependent vasodilation by simvastatin. *Journal of the American College of Cardiology.* Vol. 49, May, pp. 2274-2282.

Böger, RH. The pharmacodynamics of L-arginine. *Journal of Nutrition.* Vol. 137, (6 Suppl.2), pp. 1650S-1655S.

Boo, YCh., Jo, H. (2003). Flow-dependent regulation of endothelial nitric synthase: role of protein kinases. *American Journal of Physiology Cell Physiology.* Vol. 285, No. 3, September, pp. C499-C508.

Borucki, K., Aronica, S., Starke, I. et al. (2009). Addition of 2.5 g L-arginine in a fatty meal prevent the lipemia-induced endothelial dysfunction in healthy volunteers. *Atherosclerosis.* Vol. 205, No. 1, July, pp. 251-254.

Boushei, R., Landberg, H., Olesen, J. et al. (2000). Regional blood flow during exercise in humans measured by near-infrared spectroscopy and indocyanine green *in vivo.* *Journal of Applied Physiology.* Vol. 89, No. 5, pp. 1868-1678.

Ceriello, A., Quagliaro, L., Piconi, L. et al. (2004). Effect of postprandial hypertriglyceridemia and hyperglycemia on circulation adhesion molecules and oxidative stress generation and a possible role of simvastatin treatment. *Diabetes.* Vol. 53, No. 3, March, pp. 701-710.

Ceriello, A., Taboga, C., Tonutti, L. et al. (2002). Evidence for an independent and cumulative effect of postprandial hypertriglyceridemia and hyperglycemia on endothelial dysfunction and oxidative stress generation: effects of short-and long-term simvastatin treatment. *Circulation.* Vol. 106, August, pp. 2111-1218.

Chen M-F., Vie, X-M., Yang, Y-L. et al. (2007) Role of asymmetric dimethylarginine in inflammatory response by angiotensin II. *Journal of Vascular Research.* Vol. 44. No. 5, May, pp. 391-402.

Chin-Dusting, JPF., Kaye ,DM., Lefkovits, J. et al. (1996). Dietary supplementation with L-arginine fails to restore endothelial function in forearm resistance arteries of patients with severe heart failure. *Journal of he American College of Cardiology.* Vol. 27, No. 5, April, pp. 1207-1213.

Clarkson, P., Adams, MR., Powe, AJ. Et al. (1996). Oral L-arginine improves endothelium-dependent dilation in hypercholesterolemic young men. *Journal of Clinical Investigation.* Vol. 97, No. 8, April, pp. 1989-1994.

Cooke, JP. (2004). Asymmetrical dimethylarginine. The über marker?. *Circulation.* Vol. 109, No. 15, April, pp. 1813-1819.

Corson, MA., James, NZ., Lakka, SE. et al. (1996). Phoshorylation of endothelial nitric oxide synthase in response to fluid shear stress. *Circulation Research.* Vol. 79, No. 5, pp. 984-991.

Cortèz, B., Nũñez, I., Cofán, M. et al. (2006). Acute effects of high-fat meals enriched with walnuts or olive oil on postprandial endothelial function. *Journal of the American College of Cardiology.* Vol. 48, pp. No. 8, October, 1666-1671.

Crabtree, MJ., Tatham, A., Hale, AB. et al. (2009). Critical role for tetrahydrobiopterin recycling by dihydrofolate reductase in regulation of endothelial nitric-oxide synthase coupling. *Journal of Biological Chemistry.* Vol. 284, No. 41, October, pp. 28128-28136.

Dai, Z., Zhu, H-Q., Jiang, D-J. et al. (2004). 17β-estradiol preserves endothelial function by reducing of the endogenous nitric oxide synthase inhibitor level. *International Journal of Cardiology.* Vol. 96, No. 2, August, pp. 223-227.

Dayoub, H., Auchan, V., Adimoolam, S. et al. (2003). Dimethylarginine dimetylaminohydrolase regulates nitric oxide synthesis: genetic and physiological evidence. *Circulation.* Vol. 108, November, pp. 3042-3047.

De Waard, MC., van Heperen, R., Soulliè, T. et al. (2010. Beneficial effects of exercise training after myocardial infraction require full eNOS expression. *Journal of Molecular and Cellular Cardiology.* Vol. 48, No. 6, June, pp. 1041-12049.

DeClercq, V., Taylor, CG., Wigle, J. et al. (2011). Conjugated linoleic acid improves blood pressure by increasing adiponectin and endothelial nitric oxide synthase activity. *Journal of Nutritional Biochemistry.* In press. Available from: www.elsevier.com

Derosa, G., Ferrari, I., D'Angelo, A. et al. (2010). Effect of a standarized oral fat load on vascular remodeling markers in healthy subjects. *Microvascular Research.* Vol. 80, No. 1, July, pp. 110-115.

Dioguardi, FS. (2011). To give or not to give? Lessons from the arginine paradox. *Journal of Nutrigenetics and Nutrigenomics.* Vol. 4, No. 2, pp. 90-98. www.karger.com/jnn

Doi, H., Kugiyama, K., Ohgushi, M. et al. (1998). Remnants of chylomicrons and very low density lipoproteins impair endothelium-dependent vasorelaxation. *Atherosclerosis.* Vol. 137, No. 2, April, pp. 341-349.

Dudzinski, DM., Michel, T. (2007). Life history of eNOS: Partners and pathways. *Cardiovascular Research.* Vol. 75, No. 2., pp. 247-260.

Eid, HMA., Arnesen, H., Hjerkinn, EM. et al. (2006). Effect of diet and omega-3 fatty acid intervention on asymmetric dimethylarginine. *Nutrition & Metabolism.* Vol. 3, No. 3. www.biomedcentral.com

Engeli, S., Tsikas, D., Lehman, AC. et al. (2011). Influence of dietary fat ingestion on asymmetrical dimethylarginine in lean and obese human subjects. *Nutrition, Metabolism & Cardiovascular Diseases.* In press. www.elsevier.com/locate.nmcd

Evans, RW., Fernstrom, JD., Thompson, J. et al. (2004). Biochemical responses of healthy subjects during dietary supplementation with L-arginine. *Journal of Nutritional Biochemistry.* Vol. 15, No. 9, September, pp. 534-539.

Focaroli, M., Dick, GM., Picchi, A. et al. (2007). Restoration of coronary endothelial function in obese Zucker rats by a low carbohydrate diet. *American Journal of Physiology Heart and Circulatory Physiology.* Vol. 292, , No. 5, May, pp. H2093-H2099.

Fu, WJ., Haynes, TE., Kohli R. et al. (2005). Dietary L-arginine supplementation reduces fat mass in Zucker diabetic rats. *Journal of Nutrition.* Vol. 135, No. 4, April, pp. 714-721.

Furuki, K., Adachi, H., Matsuoka, H. et al. (2007). Plasma levels of asymmetric dimetylarginine (ADMA) are related to intima-media thickness of the carotid artery: an epidemiological study. *Atherosclerosis.* Vol. 191, No. 1, March, pp. 206-210.

Garcia-Villafranca, J., Guillen, A., & Castro, J. (2003). Involvement of nitric oxide/cyclic GMP signaling in the regulation of fatty acid metabolism in rat hepatocytes. *Biochemical Pharmacology.* Vol. 65, No.5, March, pp. 807-812.

Gertz, K., Priller, J., Kronenberg, G. et al. (2006). Physical activity improves long-term stroke outcome via endothelium nitric oxide synthase-dependent augmentation of neovascularization and cerebral blood flow. *Circulation Research.* Vol. 99, No. 10, pp. 1132-1140.

Haberka, M., Mizia-Stec, K., Gąsior, Z. et al. (2009). Serum ADMA concentration - an independent factor determining FMD impairment in cardiac syndrome X. *Uppsala Journal of Medical Sciences.* Vol. 114, No. 4, December, pp. 221-227.

Harrison, DG. (2005). The shear stress of keeping arteries clear. *Nature Medicine.* Vol. 11, No. 4, April, pp. 375-376.

Huang, PL. (2009). eNOS, metabolic syndrome and cardiovascular disease. *Trends in Endocrinology and Metabolism.* Vol. 20, No. 6, August, pp. 295-302.

Ikaguri, H., Shibata, M., Shibata, S. et al. (2003). High intensity exercise enhances platelet reactivity to shear stress and coagulation during and after exercise. *Pathophysiology of Haemostasis and Thrombosis.* Vol. 33, pp. 127-133.

Ishibashi, Y., Duncker, DJ., Zhang, J. et al. (1998). ATP-sensitive K^+ channels, adenosine and nitric oxide-mediated mechanism account for coronary vasodilation during exercise.. *Circulation Research.* Vol. 82, pp. 346-359.

Jensen, MD. (2006). Adipose tissue as an endocrine organ: implications of its distribution on free fatty acid metabolism. *European Heart Journal Supplemets.* May 8, pp. B813-B819. Jin, RC., Loscalzo, J. (2010). Vascular nitric oxide: formation and function. *Journal of Blood Medicine.* Vol. 1, No. 1, August, pp. 147-162.

Johnson, BD., Padilla, J., Harris, RA. et al. (2011). Vascular consequences of high-fat meal in physically active and inactive subjects. *Applied Physiology Nurtition and Metabolism.* Vol. 36, No. 3, June, pp. 368-375.

Kamata, K., Yamashita, K. (1999). Insulin resistance and impaired endothelium dependent vasodilatation in fructose-fed hypertensive rats. *Research Communication in Medicine Pathology and Pharmacology.* Vol. 103, No. 2, pp. 195-210.

Khan, F., Elherik, K., Bolton-Smith, C. et al. (2003). The effects of dietary fatty acid supplementation on endothelial function and vascular tone in healthy subjects. *Cardiovascular Research.* Vol. 59, No. 4, pp. 955-962.

Kim, F., Pham, M., Maloney, E. et al. (2008). Vascular inflammation, insulin resistance and reduced nitric oxide production precede the onset of peripheral insulin resistance. *Arteriosclerosis Thrombosis and Vascular Biology.* Vol. 28, September 4, pp. 1982-1988.

Kingwell, BA., Formosa, M., Muhlmann, M. et al. (2002). Nitric oxide synthase inhibition reduces glucose uptake during exercise in individuals with type 2 diabetes more than in control. *Diabetes.* Vol. 51, No. 8 ,August, pp. 2572-2580.

Kohen Avramoglu, R., Basciano, H., & Adeli, K. (2006). Lipid and lipoprotein dysregulation in insulin resistant states. *Clinica Chimica Acta,* Vol. 368, No. 1-2, June, pp. 1-19.

Kohli, R., Meininger, CJ., Haynes, TE. et al. (2004). Dietary L-arginine supplementation enhances endothelial nitric oxide synthesis in streptozotocin-induce diabetic rats. *Journal of Nutrition.* Vol. 134, No. 3, March, pp. 600-608.

Korandji, C., Zeller, M., Gulland, J-C. et al. . (2007). Asymmetric dimethylarginine (ADMA) and hyperhomocysteinemia in patients with acute myocardial infarction. *Clinical Biochemistry*. Vol. 40, No. 1-2, January, pp. 66-72.

Korda, M., Kubant, R., Patton, S. et al. (2008). Leptin-induced endothelial dysfunction in obesity. *American Journal of Physiology, Heart and Circulatory Physiology*. Vol. 295, No. 4, April, pp. H1514-H1521.

Koskinas, KC., Feldman, ChL., Chatzizisis, YS. et al. (2010). Natural history of experimental atherosclerosis and vascular remodeling in relation to endothelial shear stress.A serial, in vivo intravascular ultrasound study. *Circulation*. Vol. 121, No. 19, pp. 2092-2101.

Kougias, P., Chai, H., Lin, PH. et al. (2005). Adipocyte-derived cytokine resistin causes endothelial dysfunction of porcine coronary arteries. *Journal of Vascular Surgery*. Vol. 41, No. 4, April, pp. 691-698.

Kurowska, EM., Carrol, KK. (1998). Hypocholesterolemic properties of nitric oxide. In vivo and in vitro studies using nitric oxide donors. *Biochimica Biophysica Acta*. Vol. 1392, No. 1, May, pp. 41-50.

Lago, F., Gómez, R., Gómez-Reino, JJ. et al. (2009). Adipokines as novel modulators of lipid metabolism. *Trends in Biochemical Sciences*. Vol. 34, No.10, October, pp. 500-510.

Lamon-Fava, S., Wilson, PWF., & Schaefer,EJ. (1996). Impact of body mass index on coronary heart disease in men and women. The Framingham offspring study. *Arteriosclerosis, Thrombosis and Vascular Biology*. Vol. 16, No. 12, December, pp. 1509-1515.

Le Gouill, E. Jimenez, M., Binnert, Ch. et al. (2007). Endothelial nitric oxide synthase (eNOS) knockout mice have defective mitochondrial β-oxidation. *Diabetes*. Vol. 56, No. 11, November, pp. 2690-2696.

LeBlanc, AJ., Reyes, R., Kang, LS. et al. (2009). Estrogen replacement restores flow-induced vasodilation in coronary arterioles of aged and ovariectomized rats. *American Journal of Physiology Regulation Integrative and Comparative Physiology*. Vol. 297, No. 6, December, pp. R1713-1723.

Lee, S., Blair, SN., Kuk, JI. et al. (2005). Cardiorespiratory fitness attenuates metabolic risk independent of abdominal subcutaneous and visceral fat in men. *Diabetes Care*. Vol. 28, No. 4, April, pp. 895-901.

Lee-Young, RS., Ayala, JE., Hunley CHF. et al. (2010). Endothelial nitric oxide synthase is central to skeletal muscle metabolic regulation and enzymatic signaling during exercise in vivo. *American Journal of Physiology, Regulation, Integrative Comparative Physiology*. Vol. 298, No. 5, March, pp. R1399 R1408.

Leiper, J., Murray-Rust, J., McDonald, N. et al. (2002). S-nitrosylation of dimetylarginine dimethylaminohydrolase regulates enzyme activity: further interaction between nitric oxide synthase and dimetylarginine dimethylaminohydrolase. *Proceeding of National Academy of Science*. Vol. 99, No. 21, October, pp. 13527-13532.

Leiper, JM., Santa Maria, J., Chubb. A. et al. (1999). Identification of two human dimethylarginine dimethylhydrolases with distinct tissue distribution and homology with microbial arginine deaminases. *Biochemical Journal*. Vol. 343, October, pp. 209-214.

Lira, VA., Soltow, QA., Long, JHD. et al. (2007). Nitric oxide increases GLUT4 expression and regulates AMPK signaling in skeletal muscle. *American Journal of Physiology, Endocrinology and Metabolism*. Vol. 293, No. 4, October, pp. E1062-E1068.

López, D., Orta, X., Casós, K. et al. Upregulation of endothelial nitric oxide synthase in rat aorta after ingestion of fish oil-rich diet. *American Journal of Physiology, Heart and Circulatory Physiology*. Vol. 287, No.2, April, pp. H567-H572.

Lowenstein ChJ. (2006). Beneficial effects of neuronal nitric oxide synthase in atherosclerosis. *Arteriosclerosis Thrombosis and Vascular Biology*. Vol.25, pp. 1417.

Lucotti P., Setola, E., Monti, LD. et al. (2006). Beneficial effect of a long-term oral arginine treatment added to a hypocaloric diet and exercise training program in obese, insulin resistant type 2 diabetic patients. *American Journal of Endocrinology and Metabolism*. Vol. 291, No. 5, November, pp. E906-E912.

Malek, AM., Izumo, S., & Alper, SL. (1999). Modulation by pathophysiological stimuli of the shear stress-induced up-regulation of endothelial nitric oxide synthase expression in endothelial cells. *Neurosurgery*. Vol. 45, No. 2, August, pp. 334-344.

Marchesi, S., Lupattelli, G., Schillaci, G. et al. (2000). Impaired flow-mediated vascoactivity during post-prandial phase in young healthy men. *Atherosclerosis*. Vol. 153, No. 2, December, pp. 397-402.

Mason, CJ., Mensink, RP. (2011). Exchanging saturated fatty acids for (n-6) polyunsaturated fatty acids in a mixed meal may decrease postprandial lipemia and markers of inflammation and endothelial activity in overweight men. *Journal of Nutrition*. Vol. 141, No. 5, May, pp. 816-821.

Matsuzawa, Y. (2005). White adipose tissue and cardiovascular disease. *Best Practice & Research Clinical Endocrinology & Metabolism*. Vol. 19, No. 4, December, pp. 637-647.

Meinitzer, A.,Puchinger, M., Winklhofer-Roob, BM. et al. (2007) Reference values for plasma concentrations of assymetricalal dimethylarginine (ADMA) and other arginine metabolites in men after validation of a chromatographic method. *Clinica Chimica Acta*. Vol. 384, No.1-2, September, pp. 141-148.

Mendes-Ribeiro, AC., Mann, GE., de Meirelles, LR. et al. (2009). The role of exercise on L-arginine nitric oxide pathway in chronic heart failure. *The Open Biochemistry Journal*. Vol. 3, October 3, pp. 55-65. Available from: http://creativecommons.org

Michel, T., Vanhoutte, PM. (2010). Cellular signaling and NO production. *Pflügers Archives-European Journal of Physiology*. Vol. 459, No. 6, pp. 807-816.

Moncada, S., Palmer, RMJ., & Higgs, EE. (1991). Nitric oxide: physiology, pathophysiology and pharmacology. *Pharmacological Reviews*. Vol. 43, No. 4, June, pp. 109-142.

Mohan, S. Konopinski, R., Yan, B. et al. (2009). High-glucose induces IKK-HSP-90 interaction contributes to endothelial dysfunction. *American Journal of Physiology, Cell Physiology*. Vol. 296, No. 1, January, pp. C182-C192.

Momken, I., Fortin, D., Serrurier, B. et al. (2002). Endothelial nitric oxide synthase (eNOS) deficiency affects energy metabolism pattern in murine oxidative skeletal muscle. *Biochemical Journal*. Vol. 368, No. 15, November, pp. 341-347.

Mori, TA., Watts, GF., Burke, V. et al. (2000). Differential effects of eicosapantaeonic acid and docosahexaenoic acid on vascular reactivity of the forearm microcirculation in hyperlipidemic, overweigh men. *Circulation*. Vol. 102, pp. 1264-1269.

Mun, GI., An, SM., Park, H. et al. (2008). Laminar shear stress inhibits lipid peroxidation induced by high glucose plus arachidonic acid in endothelial cells. *American Journal of Physiology Heart and Circulatory Physiology*. Vol. 295, No. 5, November, pp. H1966-H1973.

Muniyappa, R., Iantoro, M., Quon, MJ. (2008). An integrated view of insulin resistance and endothelial dysfunction. *Endocrinology Metabolism Clinics of North America.* Vol. 37, No. 3, September, pp. 685-711.

Nestel, P., Shige, H., Pomeroy, S. et al. (2002). The n-3 fatty acids eicosapantaeonic acid and docosahexaenoic increase systemic arterial compliance in humans. *American Journal of Clinical Nutrition.* Vol. 76, No. 2, August, pp. 326-330.

Ngo, DTM., Heresztyn, T., Mishra, K. et al. (2007). Aortic stenosis is associated with elevated plasma levels of asymmetric dimethylarginine (ADMA). *Nitric Oxide.* Vol. 16, No. 2, March, pp. 197-201.

Nisoli, E., Tonello, C., Cardile, A. et al. (2005). Calorie restriction promotes mitochondrial biogenesis by inducing the expression of eNOS. *Science.* Vol.310, No. 5746, pp. 314-317.

Noyman, I., Marikovsky, M., Sasson, S. et al. (2002). Hyperglycemia reduces nitric oxide synthase and glycogen syntase activity in endothelial cells. *Nitric Oxide.* Vol. 7, No. 3, pp. 187-193.

Oomen, CM., van Erk, MJ., Feskens, EJM. et al. (2000). Arginine intake and risk of coronary heart mortality in elderly men. *Arteriosclerosis Thrombosis and Vascular Biology.* Vol. 20, No. 9, September, pp. 2134-2139.

Padilla, J., Harris, RA., Fly, AD. et al. (2006). The effect of acute exercise on endothelial function following a high-fat meal. *European Journal of Physiology.* Vol. 93, No. 3, pp. 256-262.

Päiva, H., Lehtimaki, T., Laakso, J. et al. (2004). Dietary composition as a determinant of plasma asymmetric dimethylarginine in subjects with mild hypercholesterolemia. *Metabolism.* Vol. 53, No. 8, August, pp. 1072-1075.

Perticone, F., Sciacqua, A., Maio, R. et al. (2005). Assymetric dimethyarginine, L-arginine and endothelial dysfunction in essential hypertension. *Journal of the American College of Cardiology.* Vol. 46, No 3, August, pp. 58-523.

Plotnick, GD., Corretti, MC., Vogel, RA. et al. (2003). Effect of supplemental phytonutrients on impairment of the flow-mediated brachial artery vasoactivity after a single high-fat meal. *Journal of the American College of Cardiology.* Vol. 41, No. 10, May, pp. 1744-1749.

Pope, AJ., Karuppiah, K., & Cardounel, AJ. (2009). Role of the PRMT-DDAH-ADMA axis in the regulation of endothelial nitric oxide production. *Pharmacological Research.* Vol. 60, No. 6, December, pp. 461-465.

Puchau, B., Zulet, MA., Urtiaga, G. et al. (2009). Asymmetric dimethylarginine association with antioxidants intake in healthy young adults: a role as an indicator of metabolic syndrome features. *Metabolism.* Vo. 58, NO. 10, October, pp. 1483-1488.

Rämet, ME., Rämet,, M., Lu, Q. et al. (2003). High-density lipoproteins increases the abundance of eNOS protein in human vascular endothelial cells by increasing its half-life. *Journal of the American College of Cardiology.* Vol. 41, No. 12, June, pp. 2288-2297.

Rector, TS., Bank, AJ., Mullen, KA. et al. (1996). Randomized, double-blind, placebo controlled study of supplemental oral L-arginine in patients with heart failure. *Circulation.* Vol. 93, pp. 2135-2141.

Rickey, JM., Halter, JB., & Webb, RC. (1998). Fructose perfusion in rat mesenteric arteries impairs endothelium-dependent vasodilatation. *Life Sciences.* Vol. 62, pp. No. 4, pp.55-62.

Ritchie, S., Connell JMC. (2007). The link between abdominal obesity, metabolic syndrome and cardiovascular disease. *Nutrition, Metabolism & Cardiovascular Diseases.* Vol. 17, No. 4, pp. 319-326.

Roberts, CK., Barnard. RJ., Jasman, A. et al. (1997). Exercise-stimulated glucose transport in skeletal muscle is nitric oxide dependent. *American Journal of Physiology, Endocrinology and Metabolism.* Vol. 273, No. 1, (July), pp. E220-E225.

Roberts, ChK., Barnard, RJ., Jasman, A. et al. (1999). Acute exercise increases nitric oxide synthase activity in skeletal muscle. *American Journal of Physiology Endocrinology and Metabolism. Vol.* 277, pp. E390-E394.

Rodriguez-Rodriguez, R., Herrera, MD., de Sotomayor, MA. et al. (2007). Pomace olive oil improves endothelial function in spontaneously hypertensive rats by increasing endothelial nitric oxide synthase expression. *American Journal of Hypertension.* Vol. 20, No.5, July, pp. 728-734.

Ross, RM., Wadley, GD., Clark, MG. et al. (2007). Local nitric oxide synthase inhibition reduces skeletal muscle glucose uptake but not capillary blood flow during in situ muscle contraction in rats. *Diabetes.* Vol. 56. No. 12, December, pp. 2885-2892.

Ryoo, S., Berkowitz , DE., Lim HY. (2011). Endothelial arginase and atherosclerosis. *Korean Journal of Anasthesiology.* Vol. 61, No. 1, pp. 3-11

Schulze, F., Lenzen, H., Hanefeld, Ch. et al. (2006) Asymmetric dimethylarginine is an independent risk factor for coronary heart disease: results from the multicenter Coronary Artery Risk Determination investigating the influence of ADMA concentration (CARDIA study. *American Heart Journal.* Vol. 152, No. 3,pp. e1 -e8.

Sharma, AM. (2002). Adipose tissue: a mediator of cardiovascular risk. *International Journal of Obesity and Related Metabolic Disorders.* Suppl. 4., December 26, pp. 5-7.

Shephard, RJ., Balady, GJ. (1999). Exercise as cardiovascular therapy. Circulation. Vol. 99, pp.963-972.

Silvestre, R., Kraemer, WJ., Quann, EE. et al. (2008). Effects of exercise at different times on postprandial lipemia and endothelial function. *Medicine and Science in Sport and Exercise.* Vol. 40, No. 2, pp. 264-274.

Smith, AC., Bruce, CR., & Dyck, DJ. (2005a). AMP-kinase activation with AICAR simultaneously increases fatty acid oxidation and glucose oxidation in resting rat soleus muscle. *Journal of Physiology.* Vol. 565, No. 2, June, pp. 547-553.

Smith, CL., Anthony, S., Hubank, M. et al. (2005b). Effects of ADMA upon gene expression: an insight into pathophysiological significance of raised plasma ADMA. *PloSmedicine.* Vol. 2. No. 10, pp. e264. Available from: www.plosmedicine.org

Soskić, SS. Dobutović, BD., Sudar, EM. et al. (2011). Regulation of inducible nitric oxide synthase (iNOS) and its potential role in insulin resistance, diabetes and heart failure. *The Open Cardiovascular Medicine Journal.* Vol. 5, pp. 153-163.

Stapleton, PA., Goodwill, AG., James ME. et al. (2010). Hypercholesterolemia and microvascular dysfunction: intervention strategies. *Journal of Inflammation,* Vol. 7, No.1, pp. 54-63. www.journal-inflammation.com

Stepp, DW., Ou. J., Ackerman, AW. et al. (2002). Native LDL and minimally oxidized LDL differentially regulate superoxide anion in vascular endothelium. *American Journal of Physiology, Heart and Circulatory Physiology.* Vol. 283, No. 2, August, pp. H750-H759.

Sun, D., Huang, A., Koller, A. et al. (1994). Short-term daily activity enhances endothelial NO synthesis in skeletal muscle arterioles of rats. *Journal of Applied Physiology.* Vol. 76, No. 5, May, pp. 2241-2247.

Suvarova, T., Lauer, N., & Kojda G. (2004). Physical inactivity causes endothelial dysfunction in healthy young mice. *Journal of the American College of Cardiology.* Vol. 44, No. 6, September, pp. 1320-1327.

Sydow, K., Münzel, T. (2003). ADMA and oxidative stress. *Atherosclerosis Supplements.* Vol. 4, No. 4, December, pp. 41-51

Tagawa, H., Shimokawa, H., Tatsuya, T. et al. (1999). Long-term treatment with eicosapantaenoic acid augments both nitric-mediated and non-nitric oxide-mediated endothelium dependent forearm vasodilation in patients with coronary artery disease. *Journal of Cardiovascular Pharmacology.* Vol. 33, No. 4, April, pp. 633-640.

Takahashi, M., Prado de Oliveira, E., Rochiti de Carvalho, AL. et al. (2011). Metabolic syndrome and dietary components are associated with coronary disease risk score in free-living adults: a cross-sectional study. *Diabetology & Metabolic Syndrome.* Vol.3, pp. 1-7. http://www.dmsjournal.com/content/3/1/7

Taylor, ChA., Christopher, PCh., Espinosa, LA. et al. (2002).*In vivo* quantification of blood flow and wall shear stress in the human abdominal aorta during lower limb exercise. *Annals of Biomedical Engineering.* Vol. 30, No. 3, pp.402-408.

Teerlink, T., Luo, Z., Palm, F. et al. (2009). Cellular ADMA: regulation and action. *Pharmacological Research.* Vol. 60, No. 6, December, pp. 448-460.

Thum, T., Tsilas, D., Stein, S. et al. (2005). Suppression of endothelial progenitor cells in human coronary artery disease by endogenous nitric oxide synthase inhibitor asymmetric dimethylarginine. *Journal of American College of Cardiology.* Vol. 46, No. 9, November, pp. 1693-1701.

Tiefenbacher, ChP., Bleeke, T., Vahl, Ch. et al. (2000). Endothelial dysfunction of coronary resistance arteries is improved by tetrahydrobiopterin in atherosclerosis. *Circulation.* Vol. 102, pp. 2172-2179.

Touati, S., Meziri, F., Devaux, S. et al. (2011). Exercise reverses metabolic syndrome in high-fed diet-induced obese rats. *Medicine and Science in Sport and Exercise.* Vol. 43, No. 3, pp. 398-407.

Traber, MG., Stevens, JF. (2011).Vitamins C and E: beneficial effects from a mechanistic perspective. *Free Radicals in Biology and Medicine.* In press. Available from: www.ncbi.nml.nih.gov/pubmed21664268

Tran, CT., Leiper, JM., & Vallance, P. (2003). The DDAH/ADMA/NOS pathway. *Atherosclerosis Supplements.* Vol. 4, No. 4, December, pp. 33-40.

Tyldum, GA., Shjerve, IE., TJønna, AE. et al. (2009). Endothelial dysfunction induce by post-prandial lipemia: complete protection afforded by high-intensity aerobic interval exercise. *Journal of the American College of Cardiology.* Vol.53, No. 2, January, pp. 200-206.

Valerio, A., Cardile, A., Cozzi, V. et al. (2006). TNF-α downregulates eNOS expression and mitochondrial biogenesis in fat and muscle of obese individuals. *Journal of Clinical Investigation.* Vol. 116, No. 10, pp. 2791-2798.

Valkonen, V-P., Päivä, H., Salonen JT. et al. (2001). Risk of acute coronary events and serum concentration of asymmetrical dimetylarginine. *The Lancet.* Vol. 358, No. 9299, December, pp. 2127-2128.

Vasdev, S., Stuckless, J. (2010). Antihypertensive effects of dietary protein and its mechanism. *International Journal of Angiology.* Vol. 19, No. 1, Spring, pp. e7-e20.

Verma, S., Bhaout, S. Yao, L. et al. (1997). Vascular insulin resistance in fructose-fed hypertensive rats. *European Journal of Pharmacology.* Vol. 322, No. 2-3, pp. R1-R2.

Vinik, AI. (2005). The metabolic basis of atherogenic dyslipidemia. *Clinical Cornerstone,* Vol.7, No 2/3, pp. No. 27-35.

Vogel, RA., Corretti, MC., & Plotnic, DG. (1997). Effect of a single high-fat meal on endothelial function in healthy subjects. *Amercan Journal of Cardiology.* Vol.79, No. 3, February, pp. 350-354.

Vogel, RA., Corretti, MC., & Plotnic, G. (2000). The postprandial effects of components of the Mediterranean diet on endothelial function. *Journal of the American College of Cardiology.* Vol. 36, No. 5, November, pp. 1455-1460.

Wang, S., Xu, J., Song, P. et al. (2008). Acute inhibition of guanosine triphosphate cyklohydrolase 1 uncouples endothelial nitric oxide synthase and elevates blood pressure. *Hypertension.* Vol. 52, No. 3, September, pp. 484-490.

Westphal, S., Taneva, E., Kästner, S. et al. (2006). Endothelial dysfunction induced by postprandial lipemia is neutralized by addition of proteins to the fatty meal. *Atherosclerosis.* Vol. 185, No. 2, April, pp. 313-319.

Winkler-Möbius, S.,_Linke, A., Adams, V. et al. . (2010). How to improve endothelial repair mechanism: the lifestyle approach. *Expert Reviews in Cardiovascular Therapy.* Vol. 8, No. 4, April, pp. 573-580.

Wu, G., Bazer, FW., Davis, TA. et al. (2009). Arginine metabolism and nutrition in growth, health and disease. *Amino Acids.* Vol. 37, No. 1, pp. 153-168.

Yang, Z., Ming, X-F. (2006). Recent advances in understanding endothelial dysfunction in atherosclerosis. *Clinical Medicine & Research.* Vol. 4. No. 1, June, pp. 53-65.

Zoccali, C., Bode-Böger, S., Mallamaci, F. et al. (2001). Plasma concentration of asymmetrical dimetylarginine and mortality in patients with end-stage renal disease. A prospective study. *The Lancet.* Vol. 358, No. 9299, December, pp. 2113-2117.

Section 2

Cardiovascular Diagnostics

8

The Diagnostic Performance of Cardiovascular System and Evaluation of Hemodynamic Parameters Based on Heart Cycle Phase Analysis

Mikhail Rudenko et al.*
Russian New University,
Russia

1. Introduction

The heart cycle phase analysis based on the mathematical equations by G. Poyedinstev and O. Voronova is a foundation for practically obtaining new data on normal performance of the human cardiovascular system, cardiovascular pathology, and therapy control aimed at recovery processes [1]. It provides a way to establish cause-effect relationship between the mechanism and the behavior of pathological processes.

Considering the fact that the application of this method in clinical practice has been producing further novel data and ideas, it is obvious that even the results already achieved can radically change the conventional approaches in electrophysiology. This gives us an opportunity to utilize electrocardiography in a more efficient way in solving practical problems.

This implies the following:

1. Screening to reveal risk groups.
2. Establishing diagnosis and deciding on treatment strategy.
3. On-line monitoring of therapy efficiency.
4. On-line acute and surgical monitoring.
5. Monitoring of age-related changes.
6. Evaluation of efficiency of training procedures for conditioning in sports.

For these purposes, an electrocardiogram (ECG) is recorded according to an innovative technology developed by the authors hereof in order to identify the phase pattern of a heart cycle. This technology is easier in use than the existing one and can delivers data of higher informative value.

There are certain difficulties which exist in early diagnosis of the cardiovascular diseases since it is very often the case when variations of hemodynamic parameters of a person, who

*Olga Voronova[1], Vladimir Zernov[1], Konstantin Mamberger[1], Dmitry Makedonsky[1], Sergey Rudenko[1], Yuri Fedossov[1], Alexander Duyzhikov[2], Anatoly Orlov[2] and Sergey Sobin[2]
[2]*Rostov Cardiology & Cardiovascular Surgery Center*

is absolutely healthy but who stands under exercise load, may be even far beyond the scope of pathology changes.

Many questions might come to mind of how age-related changes affect the performance of the cardiovascular system. Of great importance is an evaluation of the coronary flow.

Another subject treated by the authors in their researches is the problem of sudden cardiac death. The authors succeeded in establishing criteria for early diagnosis for the said death cases that makes possible now to forecast and avoid such potential risks by taking adequate preventive measures.

All results of the researches described herein have been clinically verified and validated. Contrary to many conventional well-known methods of diagnosis, the informative potentialities of which have been already exhausted, the method of the heart cycle phase analysis is well under way

2. Development of innovative ECG recording technology

As mentioned above, one of the key issues in the heart cycle phase analysis is an ECG recording technology. Beginning with W. Einthoven, the challenges to research was how to record electrical activity of different parts of the cardiac muscle. In more exact terms, the final goal of those investigations was to develop methods of diagnostics of the structural features and the performance of the individual heart segments (left & right ventricles and atria) by interpreting an ECG curve. Making step by step on the road to the said goal, the investigators have come to their conclusion that there is a phase mechanism in existence, which is responsible for the proper performance of our heart. Therefore, most attention has been concentrated on this subject in further research.

That has become a driving force for an increase in ECG channels, the number of which reaches one hundred. Then, computer-assisted equipment offered new opportunities in an advanced mathematical modeling. In particular, as a consequence, that gave rise to a radically new method of ECG recording. Next step in the history of electrocardography was the EASI method [1] (fig.1). Thereupon, a new trend made its appearance: to reduce the number of the recording electrodes and provide at the same time a greater volume of information.

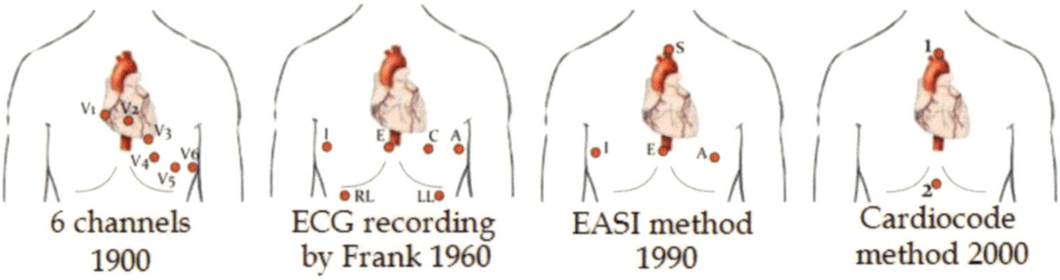

Fig. 1. Development of ECG recording methods

But all that has not assisted in the development of the heart cycle phase analysis. In the 1980s, the mode of elevated fluidity of liquid was discovered by G. Poyedintsev and O. Voronova (the so called "third" mode of flow), an innovative mathematical model of the blood flow through blood vessels and new methods how to calculate hemodynamic parameters, based on durations of the respective phases of every heart cycle were offered by the above scientists [2]. By this means the theoretical foundation was created in order to develop the phase analysis at a new level. But the only way to implement the above mathematics was an elaboration of a new reliable method of recording of the phase pattern of the heart cycle.

At that time there was no unambiguous interpretation available how to identify the heart cycle phase boundaries on an ECG curve. Different research schools gave their different descriptions of criteria of how to properly record the phases. First of all, it was applicable to key wave point S on an ECG curve. For instance, each channel in 6-lead ECG recording delivers different values of the same R-S interval.

The EASI method at its core delivers additional sources of errors in ECG processing. In order to properly record all phases, it was required to minimize the number of the channels for error reduction. At the beginning of the 2000s, medical scientists succeeded in identifying those areas on the human body where ECG recording electrodes are to be placed to obtain all fine points of electric activity of the heart [1]. It has been detected that the area delivering the most informative signals is located within the zone of the ascending aorta (Fig.1). It should be mentioned, that it is important that the second electrode is not neutral but an active one, contrary to other known methods. This electrode should be located within the area of the heart apex. As a result, using one ECG channel only, we obtain full information about electric activity within the area located between the aorta and the apex of the heart. Principally, it is essential that we deal with a signal that is not integrated because of parallel influence of conductivity of the close-located tissues, as it may be the case with other conventional methods where the second electrode is used as the neutral zone (Fig.2). In particular, it is critical for recording of interval S – T, which includes 4 periods of the phase pattern of the heart cycle.

Searching for criteria of how to record point S was successfully completed by the authors on the basis of the equations by G.Poyedintsev – O.Voronova. It follows from the equiations that the sum of diastolic phase volumes PV1 and PV2, should be equal and that of systolic phase volumes PV3 and PV4 as well as stroke volume SV that can be expressed as follows [1]:

$$PV1+PV2 = PV3 + PV4 = SV \quad (1)$$

Taking into account the fact that the above equations include several phases of the heart cycle, to make this exactly equal is possible only when all phases are recorded in the absolutely proper way. By experiment, the required criteria for the appropriate recording of every phase have been found by local extrema on the first order derivative of an ECG. It is of importance that first time a universal criterion has been established to record any phase at all.

In the course of the investigations, another thing has been revealed: the widely used conventional electronic filters are not substantiated from the scientific point of view, when selecting the proper pass bands, so that they produce signal distortions. Of special note is in this case the lower cut-off frequency of the filters. It is just the frequency that is favorably used in Cardiocode technology based on the many years' experience.

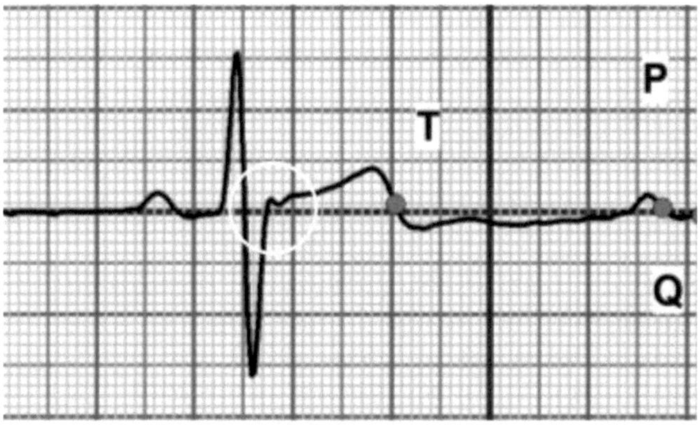

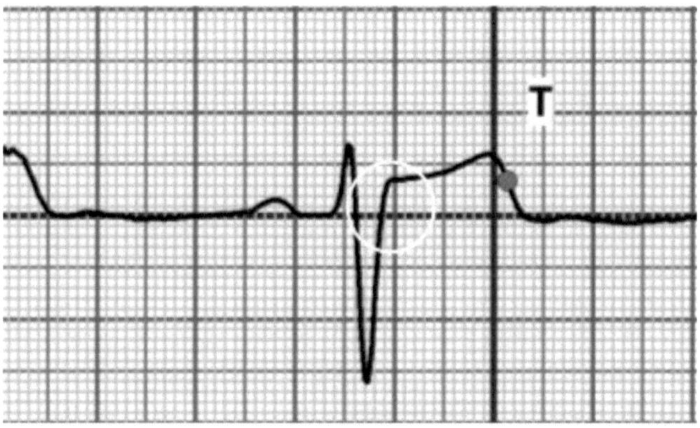

Fig. 2. A clear ECG signal according to Cardiocode single-channel method versus standard V3 lead ECG signal modified due to integration. A difference between the durations of the same R - S interval is about 25 %

Finally, according to equation (1), only the Cardiocode technology is capable of recording an ECG from the aorta with identification of every phase at local extrema of the first derivative. Any other methods or procedures are not acceptable for making heart cycle phase analysis.

But it was found that recording of an ECG curve alone is not sufficient for analysis of the performance of the cardiovascular system. Therefore, it was required to develop the so called pin-point rheography, when a rheogram is recorded from the ECG electrodes simultaneously with the ECG. Two signals of different nature that are recorded at the same time give a comprehensive idea of how the cardiovascular system performs.

3. Single-channel recording of ECG from ascending aorta, supplemented by simultaneous recording of aortic pin-point RHEOgram (Cardiocode technology)

A synchronous recording of a RHEOgram from the ECG electrodes is possible when an additional external sinusoidal high-frequency signal, supplied by a generator, passes the electrode area. This frequency is amplitude-modulated by blood circulation. The modulation shape is equivalent to changes in blood filling within the given area. By detecting a signal, we obtain a RHEO signal, the shape of which is equivalent to changes in arteric pressure. According to the Cardiocode technology, the RHEO signal is picked off the ECG electrodes, therefore the generating electrodes for RHEO recording should be placed adjacent to the ECG electrodes. A scheme of electrode arrangement is shown in Figure 3 below.

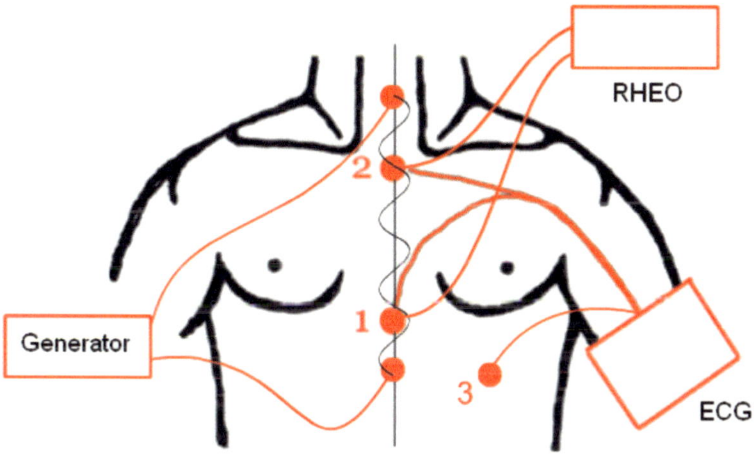

Fig. 3. Scheme of electrode arrangement for synchronous recording of ECG and RHEO from ascending aorta

An ECG and a RHEO produced in such a way contain full information of hemodynamics and the performance of the cardiovascular system. Figure 4 displays ECG and RHEO signals recorded synchronously.

The said figure consists of two parts. "A" exhibits actual ECG and RHEO curves demonstrated on the instrument display after recording. The first derivative of the ECG curve is located in between them. Local extremes on the derivative which are used for identification of the heart cycle phases are clearly marked. For instance, phase S - L is identified in such a manner. There is no other way available to detect this phase with a high accuracy. For convenience, in order to properly analyze the relations between the phases on the ECG and RHEO curves, their ideal models are presented in figure "B".

Specific criteria established for identification of the phase boundaries make it easy to identify wave point j. Little is known about this wave from the literature: it is called M. Osborn wave. Phase L - j refers to the phase of rapid ejection, and it is characterized by hemodynamic parameter PV3. The systolic pressure can be evaluated by a slope ratio of the RHEO curve in this phase.

Of particular interest is segment j - T (initiation of wave T), that is an integral part of slow ejection phase. This interval has never been identified or described in the electrophysiology literature. This period of time is required to distribute stroke volume SV throughout the space within the aorta, expanding the latter. The duration of this segment depends on elastic properties of the aorta, so that it increases with loss of its elasticity. Following this way, we can produce a criterion for evaluation of the aorta elasticity status.

The distinctive feature of our innovative technology and methodology is that it is now possible to evaluate the coronary flow qualitatively. For this purpose, wave U is analyzed. The said wave appears in premature diastole phase T (wave decay) - P (wave initiation). The authors think that the appearance of this wave is associated with the coronary flow features. But many other questions remain to be answered in this connection. At present, some preliminary conclusions can be made only. We are carrying out our further investigations in this area, and there are good grounds to believe that they will be successful.

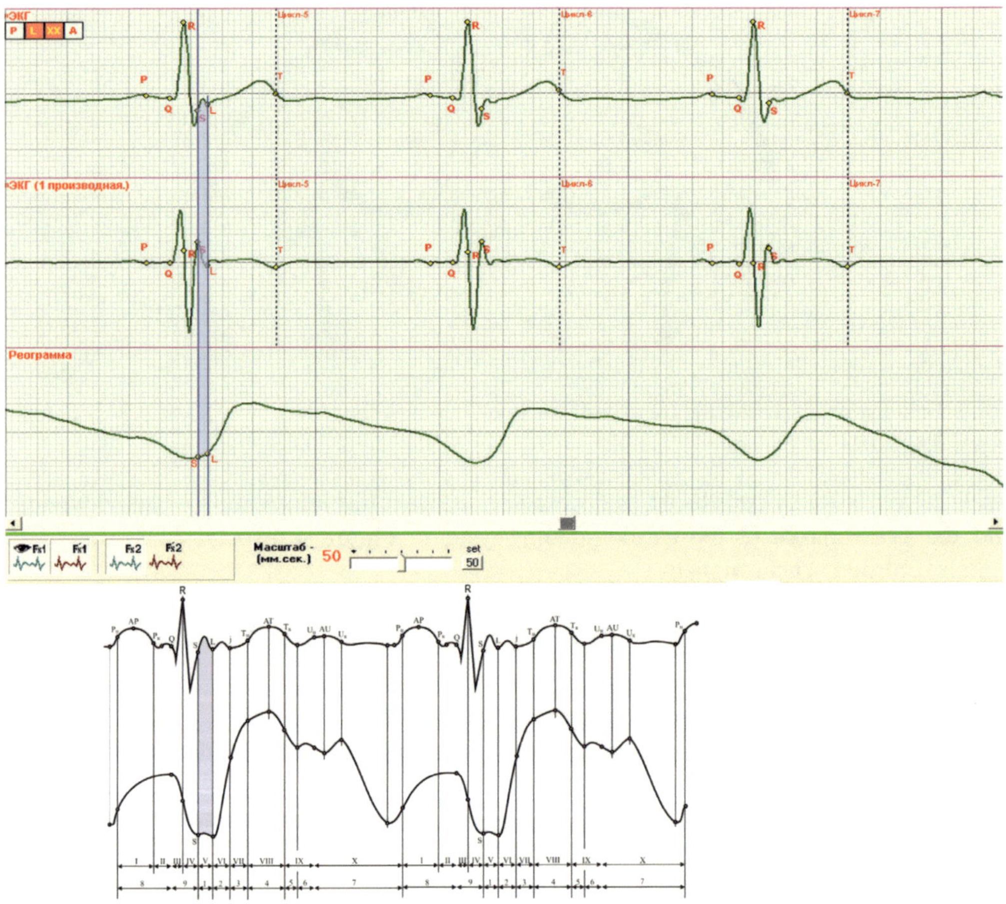

Fig. 4. A: real ECG and RHEO curves recorded from ascending aorta; B: ideal ECG and RHEO curves theoretically constructed

In order to analyze an ECG in combination with a RHEO, both curves should be synchronized. This step is of great importance. To do this, provided should be that the RHEO curve meets the isoelectric line at a point corresponding to point S on the respective ECG. In this case, it becomes possible to analyze arterial pressure development in the aorta both before and after opening of the aortic valve as shown in Figure 5 below.

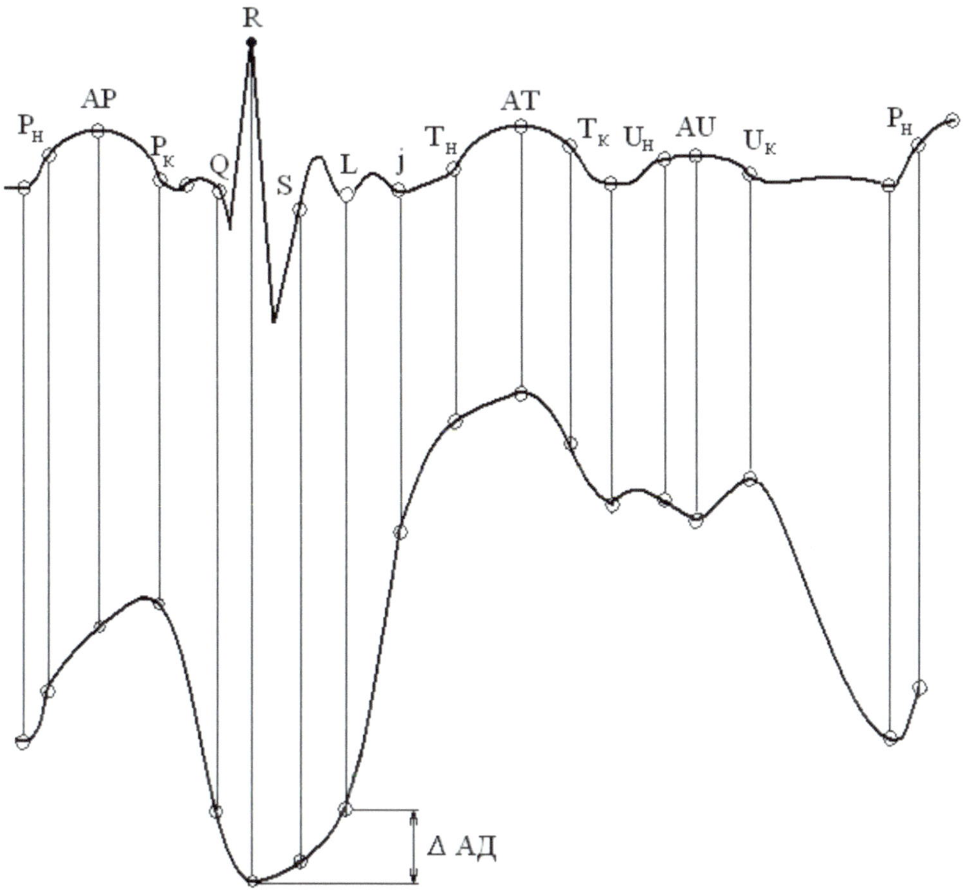

Fig. 5. Ideal ECG and RHEO curves. An interval is marked where a diastolic AP buildup can be evaluated

The RHEO isoelectric line meets point S on the ECG curve. It makes possible to evaluate an AP increase both before and after opening of aortic valve. Normally, the RHEO curve in phase S – L should be horizontal, and the AP buildup should be started at point L.

4. Classification of ECG curve shapes by reference criteria

The long-time researches of the performance of the cardiovascular system by the Cardiocode technology result in identification of such ECG and RHEO curve shapes that can be considered to be the reference curves. Figure 6 displays some recorded curves which are accepted by us as the references. Considering the fact that “a reference” is a matter of convention, such axiomatic approach, as it is often the case in practice, can solve a lot of problems in introducing the phase analysis theory.

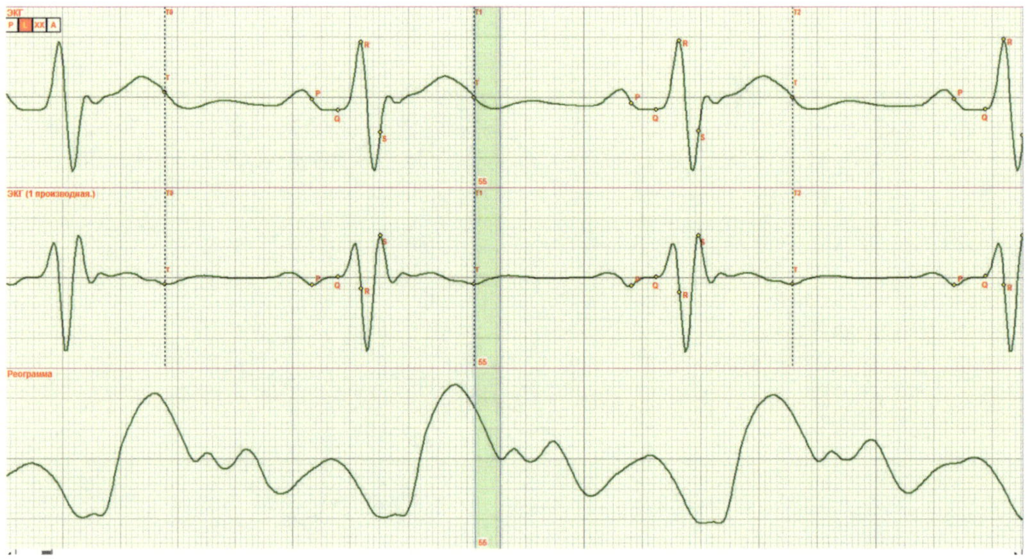

Fig. 6. ECG and RHEO reference curves applied in practice for phase analysis

The recorded curves should be classified by changes in the contraction function of the respective heart muscle area in each phase. On an ECG curve we can find the contraction function being expressed as phase amplitudes. Let us denote the respective maxima and minima on an ECG by conventional letters P; - Q; R; - S; L; j; T and U (s. Fig.7). It should be noted that it is our own legend since the same lettering is typically used for the conventional ECG waves but in our case the same letters carry other information, and, in order to avoid any confusion, they are underlined herein.

Let us denote the amplitudes of waves on the reference ECG curve as follows:

P1; - Q1; R1; - S1; L1; j1; T1; U1

If amplitudes of the waves on a real ECG differ from their reference, numerical coefficients should be other, too. For instance, if amplitude R is greater, we obtain R1,5 or R2 . With a decrease in the amplitude, we have R0,5 or R0 (for the Brugada syndrome).

Information about the performance of the cardiovascular system presented in such a way is suitable to be processed automatically. The only thing for a doctor is in this case to analyze the obtained data in the context of the actual cause-effect relations and establish the primary cause of the changes in the performance. To make it easier, the changed amplitudes may be marked only. As an example, a recorded curve indicating an increased pumping function of the aorta and a diminished function of the myocardium contraction should be presented as follows:

T2 ; - S 0,1

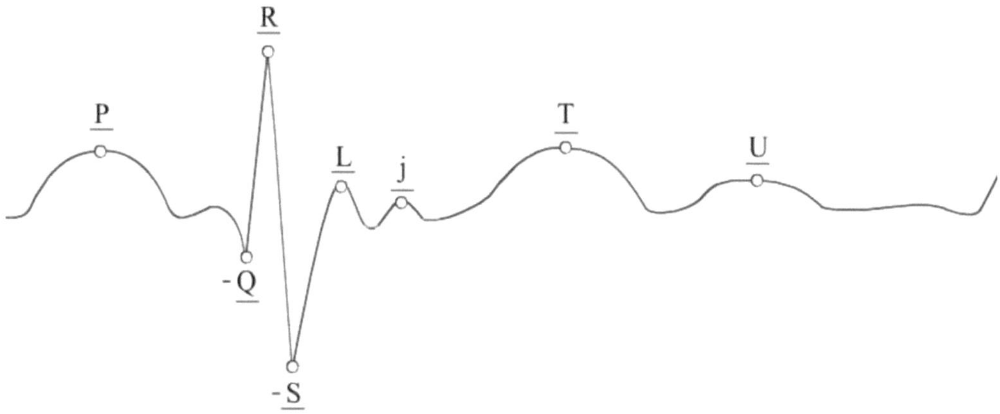

Fig. 7. Maxima and minima on ECG, which correspond to the respective heart cycle phases and characterize the contraction function of the muscle groups in the given phase. An indication is amplitude displacement of maxima or minima

The investigations carried out by us create a basis for classification of 19 most significant cases of functional changes that may occur in a staged manner and lead to some cardiovascular pathology cases. These cases are as given below:

1. Increased function of contraction of interventricular septum (IVS).
2. Diminished function of contraction of IVS.
3. Diminished function of contraction of IVS and myocardium
4. Diminished function of contraction of myocardium.
5. Reduced level of relaxation of heart in premature diastole (appearance of multiple P waves).
6. Condition of coronary flow.
7. Condition of function of regulation of diastolic AP.
8. Condition of function of regulation of systolic AP.
9. Effect of reverse contraction of IVS (at 100% passivity of myocardium).
10. Q wave dip
11. No-S-wave and P variation effect.
12. No-premature-diastole effect.
13. Regurgitation of aortic and mitral valves.
14. R-wave-bifurcation effect.
15. T-wave inversion effect.
16. No-P-wave effect.
17. P – Q phase changes
18. Respiratory arrhythmia (QRS after T wave).
19. T and P wave bifurcation.

It is impossible to present here all possible variations of the functional changes. Maybe, it should be treated separately in another book. Therefore, it is reasonable to outline general approaches to the proposed classification only and give some exemplary cases herein.

In practice, we always deal with a great variety of ECGs and RHEO curves so that no two curves are alike. It depends on individual features of the performance of the cardiovascular system of everybody. Therefore, it is expedient to consider a certain scope of functional changes and their peculiarities which may be typical for any pathology case.

The significance of the above classification is based on its practical effect. It allows for evaluating a deviation of a function from its conventional norm and detecting primary cause of the changes. Moreover, this approach makes possible early diagnostics in case of a pathology developing process well in advance so that the most favorable conditions are met to apply the most efficient ways to improve the functions.

4.1 Increased function of contraction of interventricular septum (IVS)

Table 1 illustrates one of 19 cases of the functional changes. It is a staged increase of the function of the contraction of the IVS up to its limiting critical level.

Temporal development (stage)	R	- S	L	Associated features	Symptom	Clinical aspect
				Increased Q -S width		
1	R1,5	- S0,5				
2	R2	- S2	-L2	Increased		
3	R3	- S2	-L3	Increased	Periodical short-time vertigo	Manifestation not in every heart cycle
4	R4	- S4	-L4	High probability of IVS "attenuation" in contraction	Periodical loss of consciousness	
5						Sudden cardiac death

Table 1. Increased function of contraction of IVS up to its limiting critical level

Figures 8, 9 and 10 display the recorded curves to be classified.

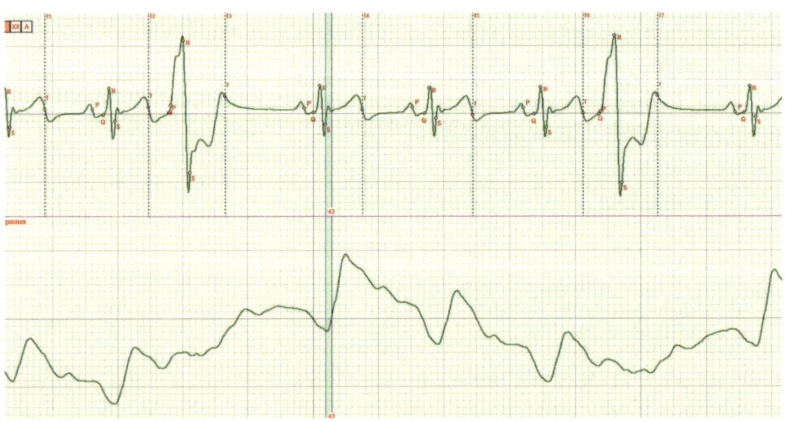

Fig. 8. Stage 2: R2; – S2; -L2

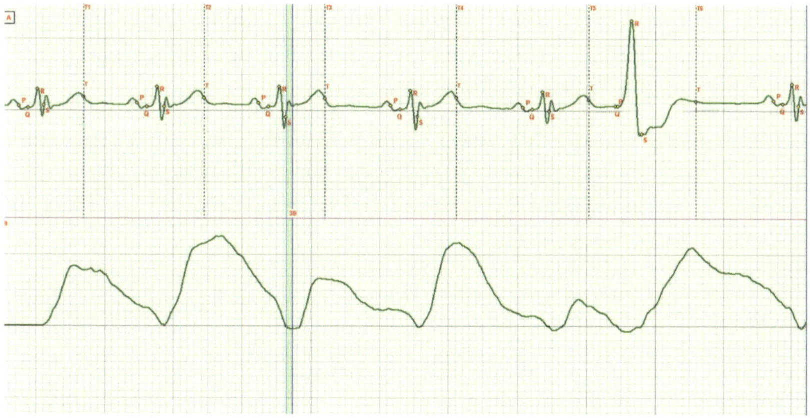

Fig. 9. Stage: R3; - S3; -L3

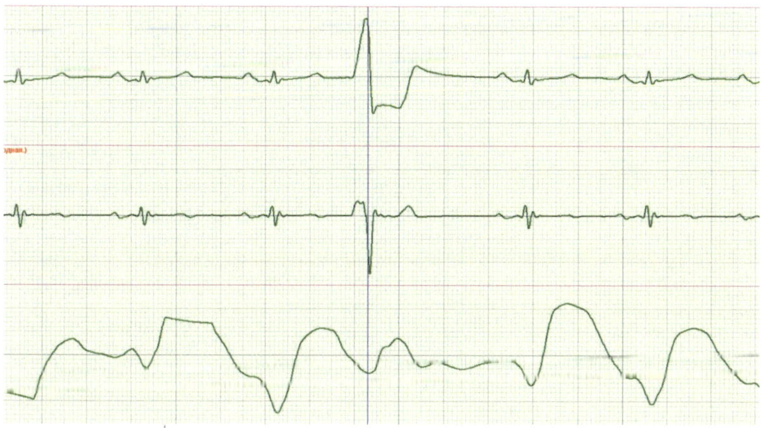

Fig. 10. Stage 4: R4; - S4; -L4

4.2 Diminished function of contraction of interventricular septum (IVS)

Item number two in the list of the significant functional changes is diminished function of contraction of the IVS (s. Table 2 below).

Energetical processes which occur in the muscle cells of the septum, the myocardium and the atria play a decisive role in the performance of the heart. The energetics depends on biochemical processes that maintain the functioning of mitochondria in tissue cells. The cell membranes and the transport elements are key factors in the said processes. Changes in mitochondria energetics are directly proportional to the function of the muscle contraction. The authors have recorded in practice a complete range of ECG changes of one patient from the extremely pathological Brugada syndrome before therapy up to the normal condition after the required treatment received. The recovery of the functions of the cardiovascular system was provided by re-establishing of functioning of mitochondria and restoring the carbon dioxide - oxygen balance in blood. Figures 11 - 16 show the ECG and RHEO curves recorded in orthostatic testing within the period of time from the beginning the therapy up to achieving the acceptable treatment results. The said figures in the above case illustrate the curves arranged in the reverse order in order to provide insight into the development of the ECG characteristics, beginning with the achieved normal status and ending with the initial extreme pathology, i.e., the Brugada syndrome.

The represented history can be described on the basis of the classification as mentioned above. The exemplary curves illustrate how the compensation mechanisms start their operation. It should be noted that the compensation mechanism takes effect at MV > 4,5 l/min.

Temporal development (stage)	R	- S	L	T	Associated features Increased R - S width	Symptom	Clinical aspect
1	R0,75		L1,5	T1,5		Increased diastolic AP	Manifestation in every heart cycle
2	R0,5		L2	T1,75	Increased	Manifestation of periodical extrasystoles. Increased systolic AP at increased diastolic AP	
3	R0,25	- S1,25	L2	T1,75	Wide	Increased systolic AP at increased diastolic AP	
4	R0,25	- S1,25	L2	T2	Wide	S-wave double contraction at normalization of its width. Instability of this process is recorded	
5	R0,25	- S1,5	L2	T2	Wide	Increased systolic AP at increased diastolic AP	
6	R0,1	- S1,5	L2,5	T2,5		High systolic AP at high diastolic AP	
7	R-wave dip						

Table 2. Diminished function of contraction of IVS

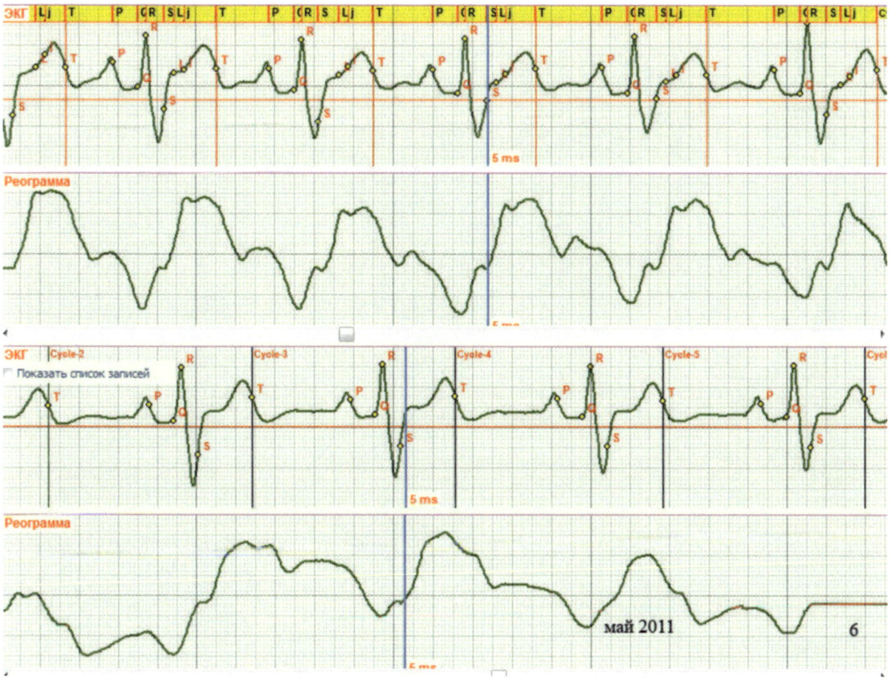

Fig. 11. Stage 1: R0,75; L1,5; T1,5

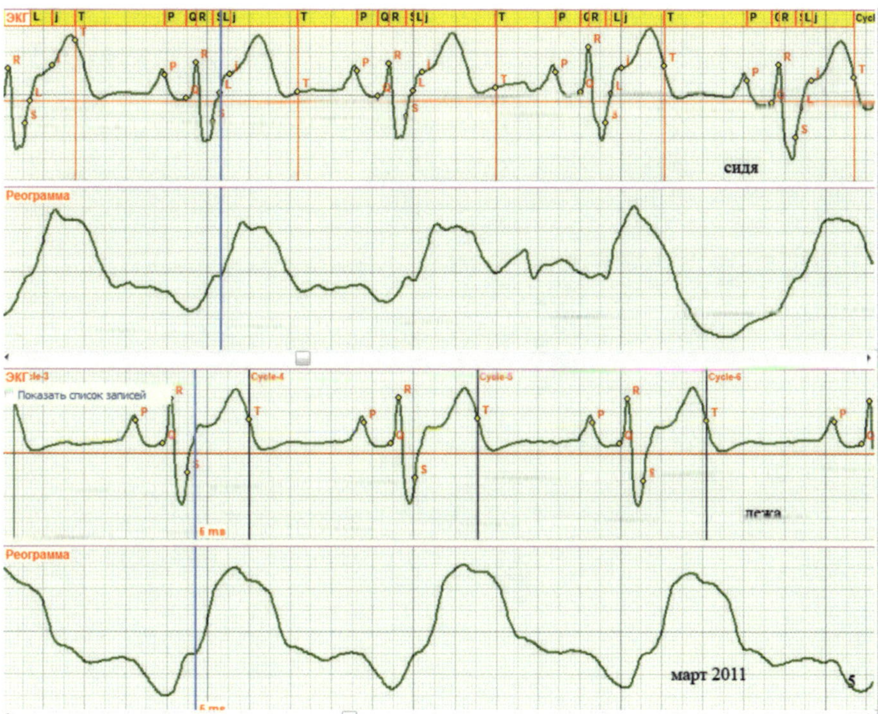

Fig. 12a. Stage 2: R0,5; L2; T1,75

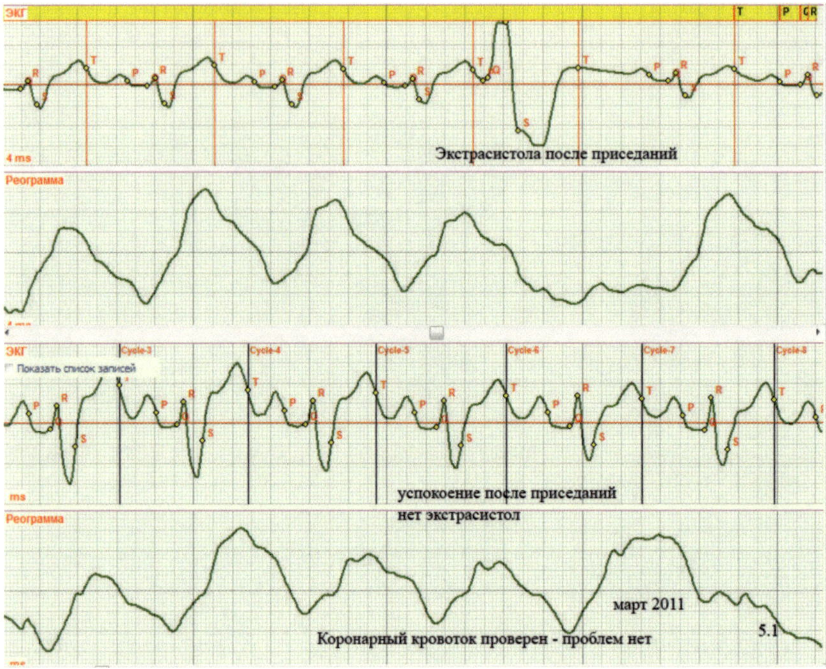

Fig. 12b. Stage 2: Appearance of extrasystoles after exercise stress or poor sleep

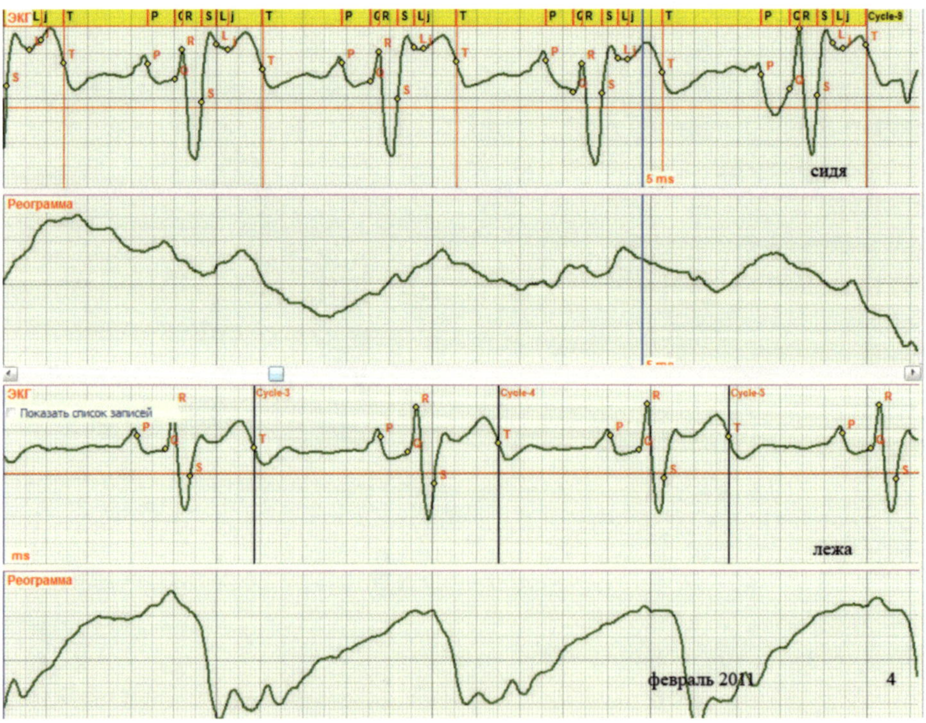

Fig. 13. Stage 3: R0,25; - S1,25; L2; T1,75

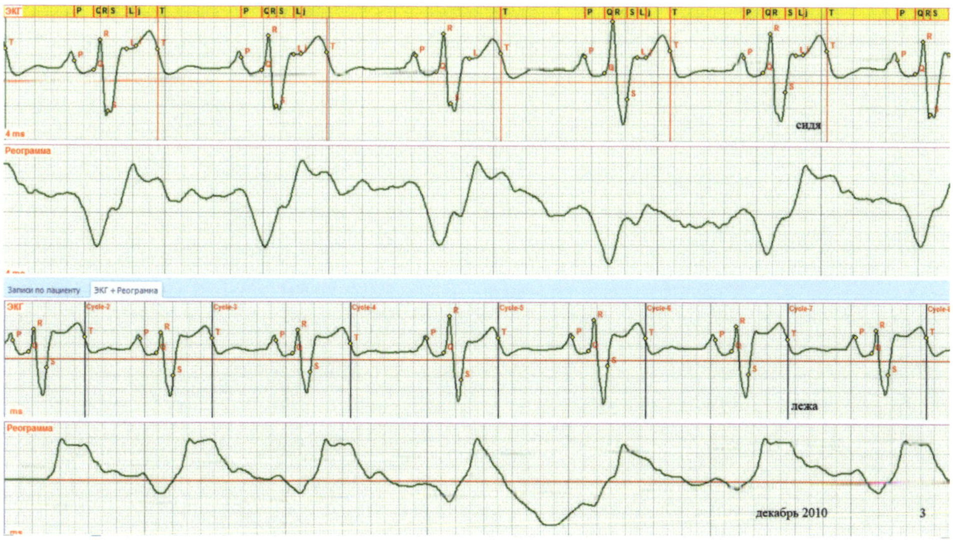

Fig. 14. Stage 4: R0,25; - S1,25; L 2; T2. S wave recovering after double contraction is observable. The record was produced in orthostatic testing

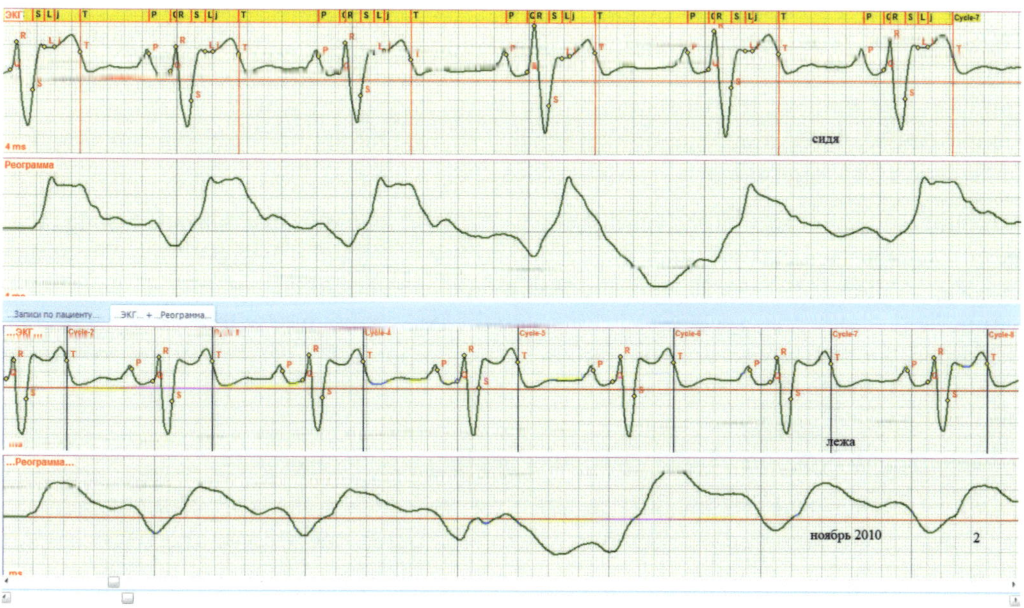

Fig. 15. Stage 5: R0,25; - S1,25; L2; T2

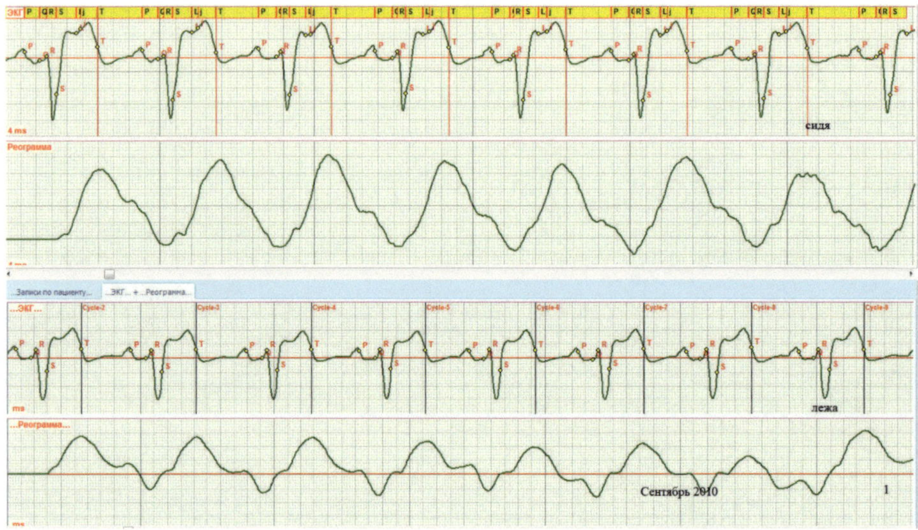

Fig. 16. Stage 6: R0,1; - S1,5; L1,25; T2,5. Brugada syndrome manifestation

Next to last stage 6 offers ECG curves where R wave is not available at all and where we observe a considerable widening of the S-wave and a significant increase in amplitude of wave S – L. This ECG curve shape is typical for the Brugada syndrome.

The suggested classification can be very effectively used in practice. Table 2 given above shows that every stage has its own risk level, considering changes in the function of contraction of the IVS. It enables to identify in the very efficient way certain risk groups among patients to be examined during either their routine periodic health examination or under emergency conditions.

It should be mentioned that the Cardiocode technology requires an orthostatic testing. That means that cardiac signals should be recorded both in lying and sitting positions. Recording in lying position lasts over 20 seconds, then the patient should change his/her position to sitting, and another 20 second-recording should be carried out within next 1 minute thereupon. It is also advisable to offer to the patient to squat 10 – 15 times, and thereupon to record the curves the third time in a session with the same patient in standing position.

4.3 Diminished function of interventricular septum and myocardium

Cases of diminished contraction function of the interventricular septum and the myocardium are observed in clinical practice (Fig. 17). In these cases, the QRS complex shows very small amplitudes. It indicates that the contraction function of the IVS and the myocardium is diminished. The relaxation of the heart in the premature diastole phase is weakened. In order to provide the proper blood filling of the heart, the contraction function of the atria increases, as evidenced by the high amplitude of the P wave. In the given case, the pressure, actually built up by the heart, is not high enough due to the diminished function of the myocardium. As a consequence, in order to reduce the resistance to the blood flow, the aorta is expanded and exceeds its normal volume that is reflected on the ECG curve in an increasing of amplitude of wave T.

According to the lettering used for the suggested classification, the ECG can be described as follows:

R0,25; - S0,25; P3; T3

Considering the fact that the reference ECG curves, as shown in Fig.6, are taken as the basis, we can obtain more precisely coefficients in automatic measuring of the actual ECG version given in Figure 17. These coefficients assist in understanding of what group is applicable to the given record. In order to qualify the primary cause of any cardiovascular pathology, it is also required to involve the respective RHEO into the phase analysis. It should be mentioned that it is not our intention to treat this issue in this Chapter.

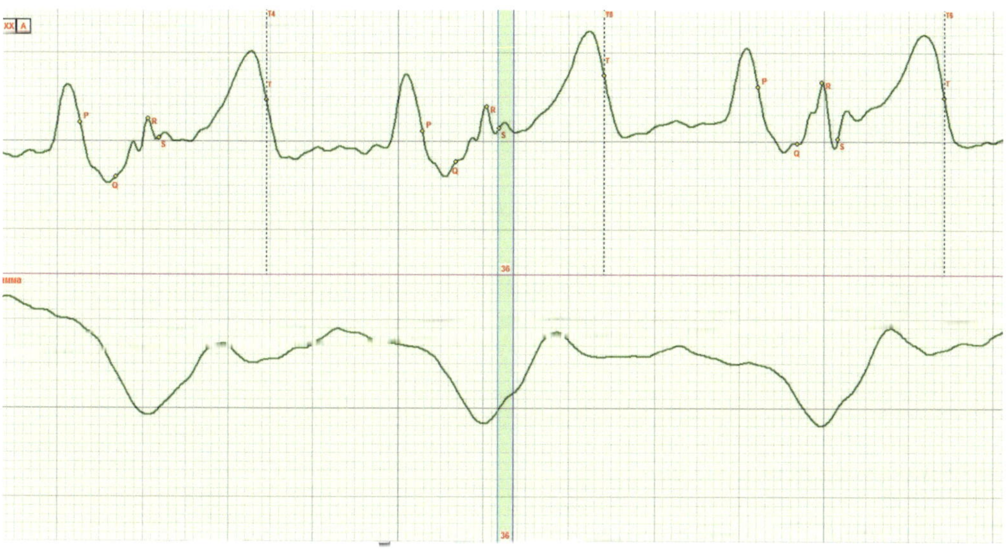

Fig. 17. Diminished contraction function of IVS and myocardium

4.4 Condition of functioning of regulation of diastolic AP (R-wave bifurcation effect)

The process of regulation of diastolic pressure, as described in Chapter 1 above, in case of pathology, is provided by different compensation mechanisms. In the instance illustrated in Figure 18, the problem with the myocardium contraction is connected with the coronary flow. The compensation mechanism manifested as R-wave bifurcation makes possible to maintain the blood flow unhindered in the ventricles and provide the blood flow with the valves closed due to additional vibration of the IVS.

The classification can be expressed as follows: (R1,5; R1,5); - S0,25.

4.5 Condition of function of regulation of diastolic AP. IVS reverse contraction effect at 100 % passivity of myocardium

Another case of the operation of the compensation mechanism, when the myocardium is passive, is an IVS reverse contraction effect (s. Fig. 19). It can be treated as an extreme case of R-wave bifurcation. But it is caused by a pathology problem other than the coronary flow. As a rule, the case history of such patients contains records of close-spaced respiratory diseases in infancy.

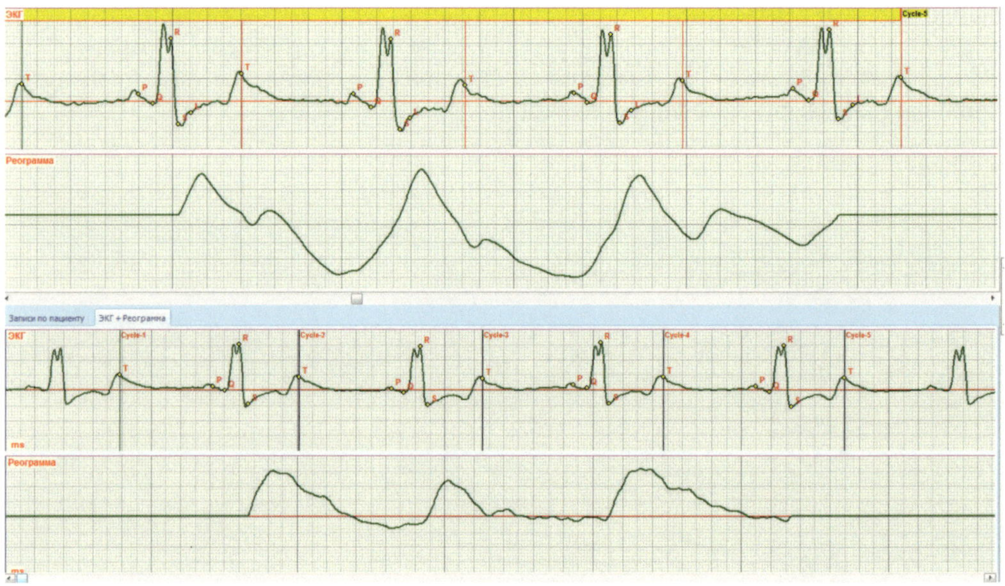

Fig. 18. Condition of function of regulation of diastolic AP (R-wave bifurcation effect)

This curve version can be classified as given below: (-R1,5; R1,5); S0,25.

One more case of the manifestation of the IVS reverse effect was recorded during the orthostatic testing of one of the patients. Figure 20a demonstrates the R wave bifurcation for horizontal position of the patient. When changing to the vertical position, appeared is permanently the said IVS reverse effect (s. Fig. 20 b). By analyzing the respective RHEO curve shape we can detect an aortic dilatation since there is no increase in the AP in the slow ejection phase for the patient's vertical position available.

4.6 No-S-wave & P-variation effect

The authors recorded and investigated the case of no-S-wave & P-variation effect (s. Fig. 21). On these conditions, the compensation mechanisms are not capable of providing the proper hemodynamics, therefore, it is the septum only which is in operation. It is evident from Figure 21 that hemodynamics is maintained due to the second P-wave periodically appearing on the ECG. Thereupon, the arterial pressure reaches its norm but in subsequent cycles it rapidly drops and remains at its low level, and the P-wave is not available. Such fluctuations are synchronized by respiratory rhythm. It is remarkable that this patient visited the doctor unaccompanied, and before visiting the doctor he had not received any treatment at hospital.

The record of this type can be classified as given below: (R3); -S0,25.

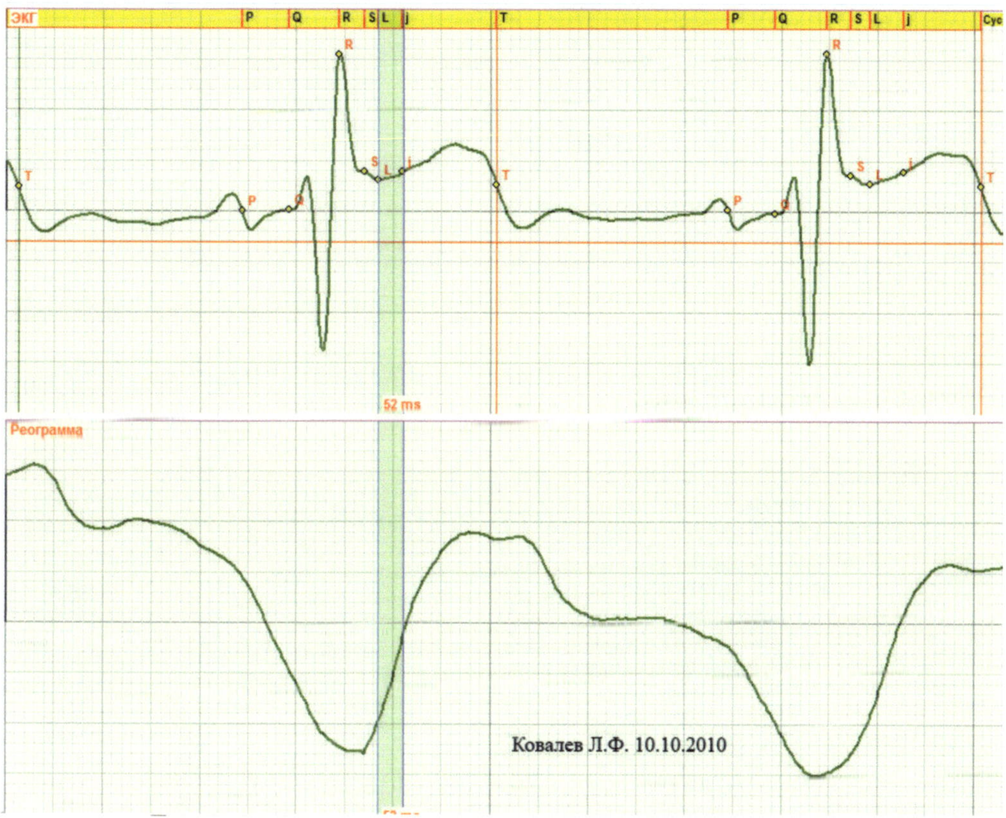

Fig. 19. IVS reverse contraction effect at 100 % passivity of myocardium. It appears at all times irrespective of the patient's position in orthostatic testing

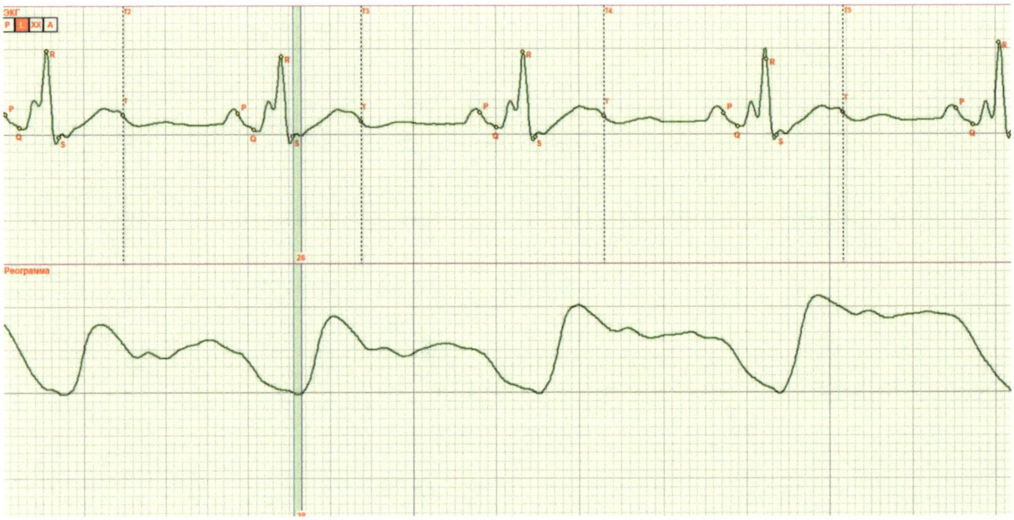

Fig. 20a. The classified curve can be presented as follows: (R1,25; R1,5); -S0,25

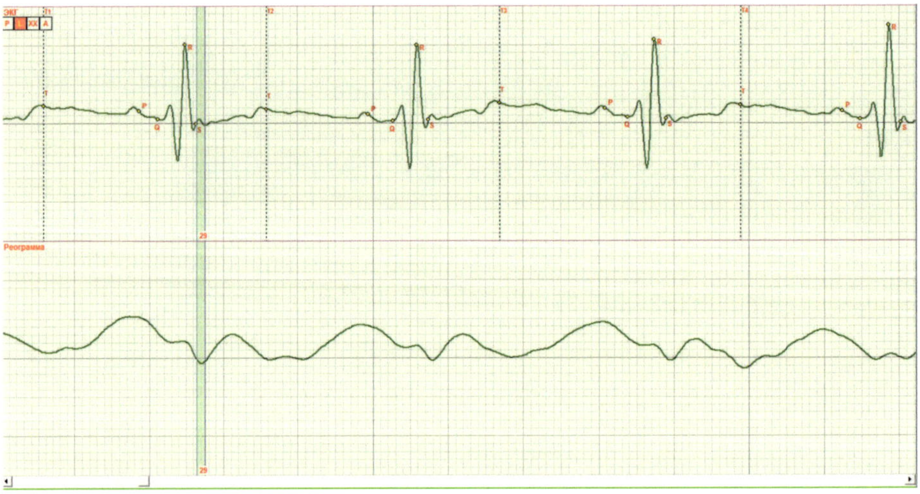

Fig. 20b. The curve can be classified as follows: (-R0,5; R1,5); -S0,25

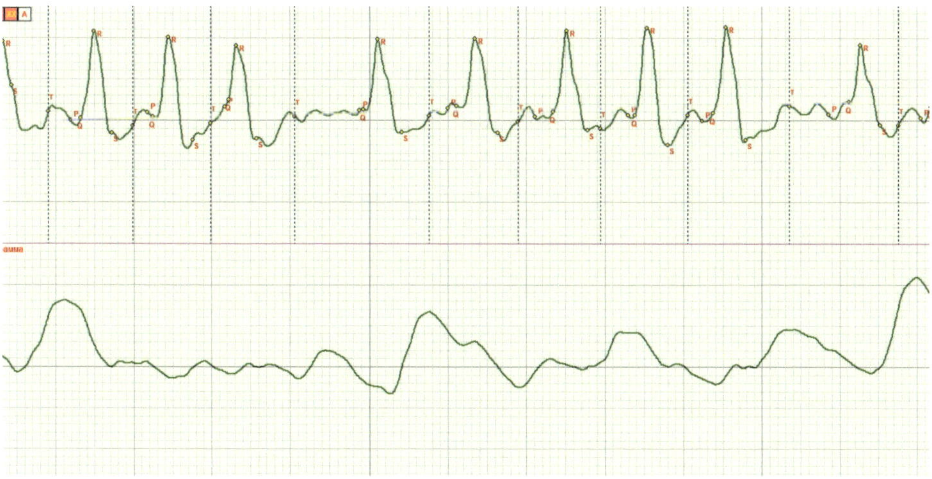

Fig. 21. No-S-wave & P-variation effect

5. Conclusion

The materials presented herein create primarily a bridge for applying theory to practice. Based on the concept of the heart cycle phase analysis, the authors have developed their own innovative diagnostics equipment Cardiocode that is now in production. All cardiac signal records contained herein were produced with this equipment. We expect that its merits like easy-in use and high informative value will be recognized by practicing physicians. But to justify the expectations is always not easy. New knowledge is finding the proper way accompanied with great difficulties. To overcome every difficulty, our team carried out a large body of research work the results of which are reflected herein.

We have focused on the basic definitions. Well-defined is also the range of problems solved by the heart cycle phase analysis theory. The way offered by the authors which is the way of systematization, unification and associated perception of new knowledge should support the medical experts in phase analysis application by them. It is commonly supposed that every innovation goes through three stages in order to be generally recognized which are as follows: it is stage one when everybody says that it is in principle impossible; then stage two comes when people say that there's something in it, and last stage three appears, when it is believed that it seems to be very simple! The authors adhere to an opinion that the heart cycle phase analysis theory is now between stage two and three from the point of view of its recognition procedure.

6. Acknowledgements

We would like to express our gratitude to all doctors who participated in the clinical testing of our methodology. We have completed a 30- year investigation cycle that includes last five years of very hard work. All opinions, comments and recommendations submitted to us by our colleagues during our researches have been considered and embodied in this Chapter.

7. References

[1] M. Rudenko, M.; Voronova, O. & Zernov. V. (2009). *Theoretical Principles of Heart Cycle Phase Analysis.* Fouqué Literaturverlag. ISBN 978-3-937909-57-8, Frankfurt a/M. München London - New York

[2] Voronova O. (1995) *Development of Models & Algorithms of Automated Transport Function of the Cardiovascular System.* Doctorate Thesis Prepared by Mrs O. K. Voronova, PhD, VGTU, Voronezh

[3] Rudenko, M.; Voronova, O. & Zernov. V. (2009) Study of Hemodynamic Parameters Using Phase Analysis of the Cardiac Cycle. *Biomedical Engineering. Springer New York.* ISSN 0006-3398 (Print) 1573-8256 (Online). Volume 43, Number 4 / July, 2009. P. 151 -155.

[4] Caro, C.; Padley, T.; Shroter, R. & Sid, W. (1981) *Blood Circulation Mechanics.* Mir. M.

[5] Eman A.A. *Biophysical principles of arterial pressure measurement.* – Л., 1983.

9

Biophysical Phenomena in Blood Flow System in the Process of Indirect Arterial Pressure Measurement

Mikhail Rudenko, Olga Voronova
and Vladimir Zernov
*Russian New University,
Russia*

1. Introduction

Diagnostic parameter "arterial pressure" known in medical practice from the earliest times is now widely used for assessment of body state. Indirect occlusive methods are the most popular measurement techniques. Although the indirect method of measurement is more than one hundred years old there is no precise understanding of biophysical processes taking place in compressed blood flow.

The idea of indirect arterial pressure measurement with the help of occlusive cuff belongs to Riva-Rocci. However, the phenomenon of noise appearing and disappearing in the blood flow distal of the brachial artery compression during the equality moments of occlusive, systolic and diastolic pressure was called Korotkov sounds. The origin of the sounds is considered from different viewpoints [1]. But it is important to mention that their identification has no valid criteria. If their appearance corresponds to the systolic pressure, their disappearance is not always characteristic for the diastolic pressure. Thus, during the Olympic Games in Mexico continuous sounds were recorded with the swimmers. But this fact didn't mean that they had zero diastolic pressure.

In case of measurement method computerization more reliably recorded biosignals in the form of oscillogram are used [1]. Nowadays Korotkov sounds are out of use in case of computerization of the arterial pressure measurement. The oscillometrical method of measurement is more reliable. But this method has no explanation from the point of view of biophysics as well.

The authors of the present research work have studied biophysics of the processes in the occlusive blood flow for a long time. The study resulted in discovery of the objective law concerning the origin of arterial pressure waves interference in occlusive blood flow. It enabled to understand the processes taking place in occlusive blood flow and find the criteria which systolic pressure and diastolic pressure correspond to.

2. Biophysical processes of origin of the arterial pressure waves interference in occlusive blood flow

Let us consider the occlusive method of the arterial pressure measurement. Big blood vessels are compressed with occlusive pressure artificially produced in the rubber cuff put as a rule on one of the patient's arms. Then the pressure is measured at the moments of its balance with the arterial pressure using the corresponding criteria. This method enables the measurement of two parameters - systolic arterial pressure and diastolic arterial pressure.

Which criteria can be used for accurate measurement?

In practice the method of Korotkov sounds and the oscillometrical method are used. In case of the measurement process computerization the sounds method is not used. It is not reliable for noise recording. Oscillometrical method seems to be more reliable. Oscillogram is the signal of pulse wave oscillations modulated by the occlusive pressure. When recorded, these oscillations are extracted from the pressure signal in the cuff as a variable component with the help of the filtering method. This process is technically simple and reliable.

To understand the biophysics of occlusive blood flow it is necessary to have at least its hypothetical model. We propose to study the model 'living body–mechanic system'. It can help to define the real biophysical processes. In this case the model is represented by the 'artery–cuff' system.

Electronic converters quite accurately register the processes taking place in the system. However different existing theories of biophysical processes give ambiguous characteristic of the criteria of arterial and occlusive pressure balance [3]. This prevents the provision of electronic arterial pressure measuring instruments with the corresponding metrology. Practically metrology of the indirect method of arterial pressure measurement does not exist.

Although the problem is quite serious we will try to study it. Let us consider the biophysical phenomena in the system of the proposed 'artery–cuff' hypothetical model in the process of indirect arterial pressure measurement [4].

Figure 1 shows the simplified version of this model. For convenience only a half of the cuff is shown, it is conventionally in contact with the artery. Pulsating blood flow contacting with the cuff influences it which is recorded in the form of the corresponding signals.

a. beginning of phase 1;
b. end of phase 1, beginning of phase 2;
c. transitory moment of phase 2;
d. end of phase 2, beginning of phase 3;
e. the first inflection moment in phase 3;
f. the second inflection moment in phase 3.

→ travel direction of the arterial pressure wave;

- - → changed travel direction of the arterial pressure wave influenced by the occlusive pressure.

Figure 2 shows the synchronous record of decompression occlusive pressure. The oscillogram (Fig.2, b) is received by means of filtration in the frequency band and increase of the oscillations which exist against the background of occlusive pressure as pulsations with

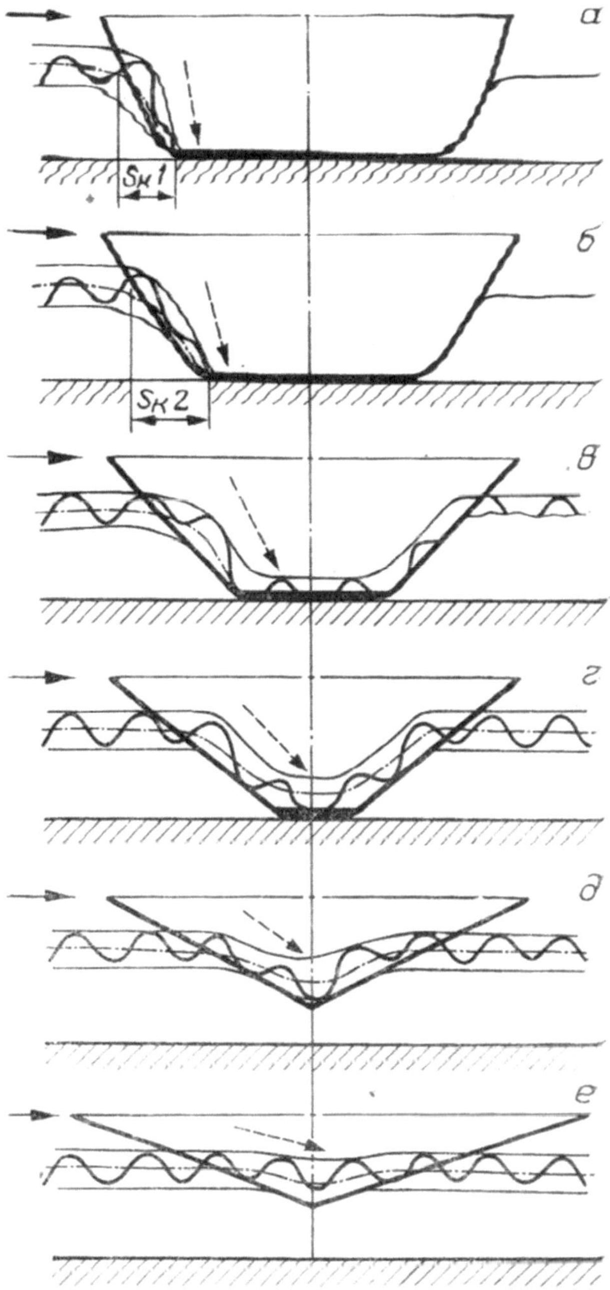

Fig. 1. Changes in the 'artery–cuff' contact profile during different phases of arterial pressure measurement.

small amplitudes (Fig.2, a). Several heart cycles of the oscillogram and its derivatives can be more closely seen in Fig.3. The extreme values of one cardiac cycle and the corresponding derivatives are marked by points *1*, *2* and *3*.

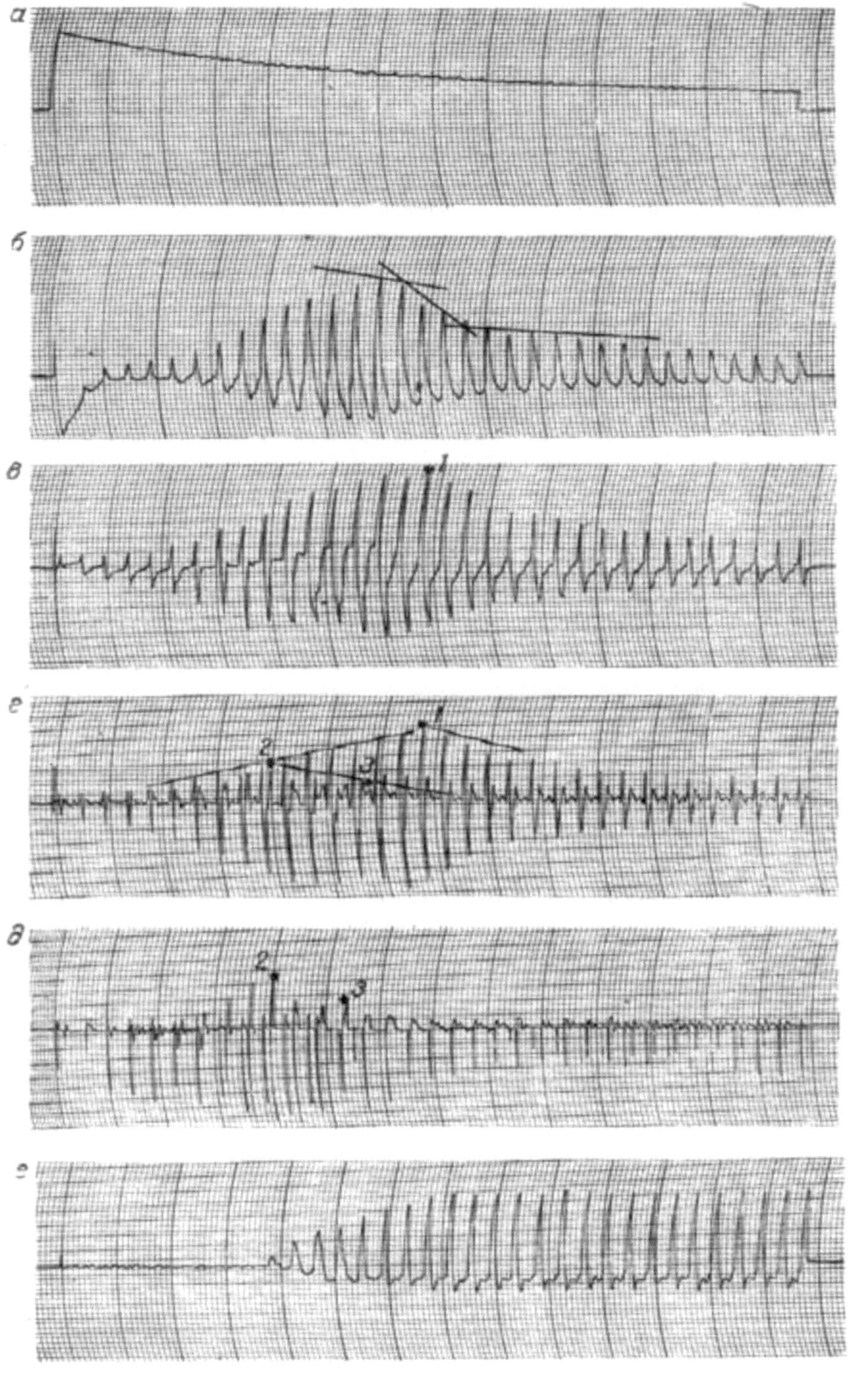

Fig. 2. Synchronous record of decompression occlusive blood pressure (*a*); oscillogram of first-order derivative (*b*); oscillogram of second-order derivative (*c*); oscillogram of the part of the second derivative (*d*); oscillogram of the plethysmogram (*e*). The explanation is to be found in the text.

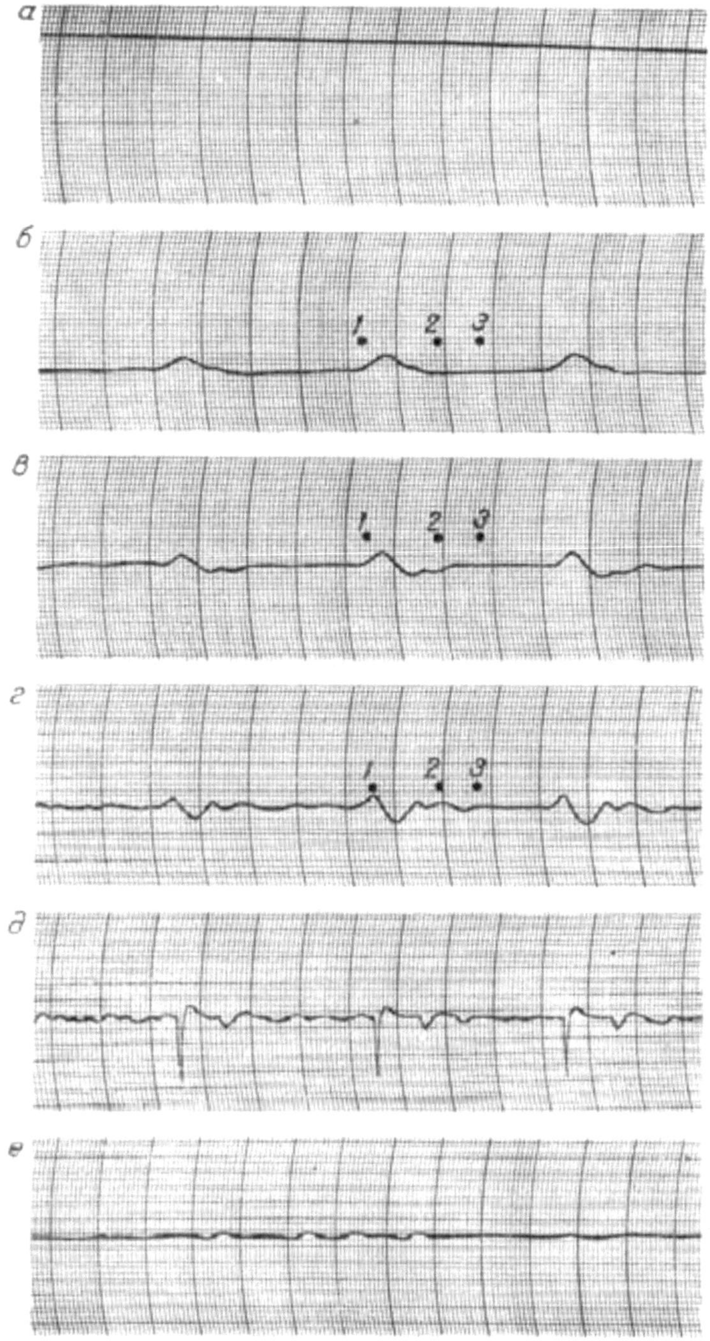

Fig. 3. Synchronous record of several cardiac cycles in the first phase of occlusive pressure (*a*); oscillogram (*b*); first-order derivative (*c*); second derivative (*d*); part of the second derivative (*e*) and photoplethysmogram (*f*). *1, 2, 3* are extreme values of one cardiac cycle and their corresponding derivatives.

In the process of modulation of blood flow by occlusive pressure additional characteristic vessel impedance is needed. Its value is calculated in compliance with the formula:

$$Z = \frac{\rho \cdot c}{S}$$

where:

ρ – blood density; c – arterial pressure wave velocity; S – vessel area.

Increase of the additional characteristic vessel impedance causes the appearance of standing wave proximal the occlusive place. Designed in such a manner interference pattern is registered by the cuff against the background of the occlusive blood pressure (see Fig. 2, a).

We should mention that reflected waves emergence in physiological blood flow is considered from a perspective of characteristic impedance disagreement in vessel branching and curving points [2]. In scientific literature this approach is based on research in rigid pipes imitating blood vessels. The received results are not proved by the experiments over the living bodies [3]. Theoretic calculations of the arterial wave reflection level in case of vessel branching for physiological blood flow can be found in [2]. It is marked that even in case of 10% mismatch of the vessel impedances which significantly exceeds the real one, the reflected waves are imperceptible and can not considerably influence the falling pressure wave. Scientific literature does not provide the investigation of the process in case of local increase of the characteristic vessel impedance which cuff occlusion under condition of arterial pressure measurement is. Thus, the study of the phenomena in case of maximum impedance change range arouses interest.

Deviation in extreme points amplitude by the falling wave is characteristic for interference [5]. This phenomenon is presented on the second derivative (see Fig. 2,d; 3,d).

For convenience we shall divide the process of arterial pressure measurement into three phases (see Fig. 1).

During the first phase (see Fig.1, a, b) the occlusive pressure exceeds the systolic pressure and the characteristic impedance is maximum. In case of decompression in one phase it remains constant. Increase of the 'cuff-artery' contact area leads to cuff elasticity growth (see Fig. 1, a, b). As a result the amplitudes of the recorded oscillations on the oscillogram rise (see Fig. 2, b). Herewith the deviations of the extreme points remain maximum. This fact is proved by the first and second derivatives character (see Fig. 2, c, d). Distal of the occlusion place the arterial pressure oscillations are not to be found (see Fig. 2, f).

The second measurement phase starts from the moment of occlusive and systolic pressure balance when the oscillating part of the arterial pressure wave begins to recover distal of the occlusion place (see Fig., b, c; Fig.2, f) and finishes at the moment of occlusive and systolic pressure balance (see Fig.1, d; Fig.2, b, d).

There exist two characteristic features of this phase. Firstly, the elasticity and area of the 'artery–cuff' contact continue to increase when the occlusive pressure falls. As a result condition for continuous oscillation amplitudes growth on the oscillogram is created.

Secondly, characteristic impedance remains maximum for the arterial pressure values that are lower than those of the occlusive pressure. For the values that exceed the occlusive pressure ones the impedance is proportional to difference of the current occlusive and systolic pressure values. This fact is related to the alteration of the straight-line travel direction of arterial pressure wave influenced by the occlusion (see Fig.1). The reflected wave amplitude will decrease proportionately with the decrease of the vessel characteristic impedance for the arterial pressure wave layers the values of which exceed the occlusive pressure. This will lead to decrease of the corresponding layers amplitude offset against the overall interference background. As a result offset of the indicated extreme points will proportionally decrease.

For the described process of layer-by-layer vessel characteristic impedance alteration for the arterial pressure falling waves the corner of triangle (marked with *2* in Fig.2, d, e) with a definite error can serve as a criterion for systolic pressure measurement. In Fig. 2 ,e a part of the second derivative shown in Fig.2 ,d can be seen. Point *2* characterizes the amplitude offset of the dicrotic oscillogram part in case of interference of falling and reflected arterial pressure waves during the occlusion. Figure 3 shows that point *2* being extreme corresponds with the dicrotic oscillogram part.

Along the same line consideration of the extreme values of the oscillogram and its derivatives indicated with *1* and *3* in Fig. 3 enables to mark similar triangles with the corresponding corners (see Fig.2, d).

The triangle corner indicated with point *1* corresponds to the moment of diastolic pressure and occlusive pressure balance (see Fig.1, d and Fig.2, d). At this moment the oscillating blood flow part is fully recovering distal of the occlusion (Fig. 2,f). On the oscillogram the oscillation with maximum amplitude and maximum leading edge steepness which corresponds to the maximum of the first derivative conforms to the described process (see Fig 2, c)

The considered model of biophysical processes enables the pressure measurement of different arterial wave layers according to characteristic maximums of oscillogram derivatives, in particular, systolic and diastolic pressure.

The beginning of the third measurement phase is the moment of diastolic and occlusive pressure balance (see Fig.1, d). This phase is characterized by the two inflections of enveloping oscillogram, defined by the alteration of the cuff shape and elasticity as a result of occlusive pressure fall (see Fig.1, e, Fig.2, b).

For the oscillating part of arterial pressure characteristic impedance is defined only by the alteration of the arterial wave travel direction influenced by the occlusive pressure. At the moment of enveloping oscillogram inflection (see Fig.2, b) the cuff loses its shape rigidness (see Fig.1, *d*). At the same time characteristic impedance changes rapidly. During the period preceding the second inflection (see Fig.1, f) the cuff takes almost the same shape as it would have without the creation of the occlusive pressure. After the second inflection the cuff perceives the arterial pressure oscillations at the expense of the occlusive pressure. Herewith the cuff elasticity does not change.

The described biophysical phenomena allow concluding that indirect method can be used to measure systolic and diastolic pressure with a definite error in the process of the oscillogram and its derivatives recording. To accomplish this it is necessary to search and record the first oscillogram derivative maximum (see Fig.2,b) and a part of the second oscillogram derivative maximum (see Fig.2, e).

The described process of falling and reflected arterial pressure waves interference is accompanied by turbulence distal of the occlusion place. Let us consider the equation of continuity:

$$\upsilon_1 \bullet S_1 = \upsilon_2 \bullet S_2 = \upsilon_3 \bullet S_3$$

where:

υ_1 stands for velocity proximal of the occlusion place; υ_2 is velocity at the place of occlusion; υ_3 is velocity distal of the occlusion place; $S_{1,2,3}$ - artery cross-section area at the corresponding places.

Considering the equation of continuity it is possible to state that if S_2 at the place of occlusion tends to zero velocity υ_2 should tend to infinity. Velocity υ_2 in Reynolds number equation defining the interrelation of inertial and viscous forces in the blood flow is found in numerator:

$$\mathrm{Re} = \frac{\upsilon . d}{v}$$

where:

υ - velocity; d - vessel diameter; v - kinematic viscosity coefficient.

As velocity $\upsilon 2$ is found in the numerator of the above equation then during the systolic time interval Reynolds number will exceed the value of 2500 which corresponds to turbulence emersion. Turbulence promotes the acoustic noise called Korotkov sounds.

Synchronous record of occlusive decompression pressure is shown in Figure 4. According to considered above criteria of occlusive and arterial pressure balance Korotkov sounds appearance corresponds to the moment of systolic pressure measurement. The peak amplitude of the sounds corresponds to the moment of diastolic pressure measurement and the disappearance of sounds occurs during the second presented inflection of the enveloping oscillogram. The connection of Korotkov sounds disappearance with the moment of their maximum amplitude and the diastolic pressure measurement criterion is possible using the 'cuff–artery' contact measurement. To achieve this, the cuff should not bear against the patient's arm. As a result the second inflection almost matches the peak amplitude and a drastic decrease of the enveloping oscillation and the sounds is registered.

3. Measurement criteria of systolic and diastolic arterial pressure based on recording by the oscillogram derivative extreme point

3.1 The peculiarities of oscillogram recording

In the first part of this chapter the biophysical processes forming the oscillogram were considered. It was proved that the oscillogram is a reflection of arterial pressure waves interference process in the place of artery occlusion. The process of falling and reflected

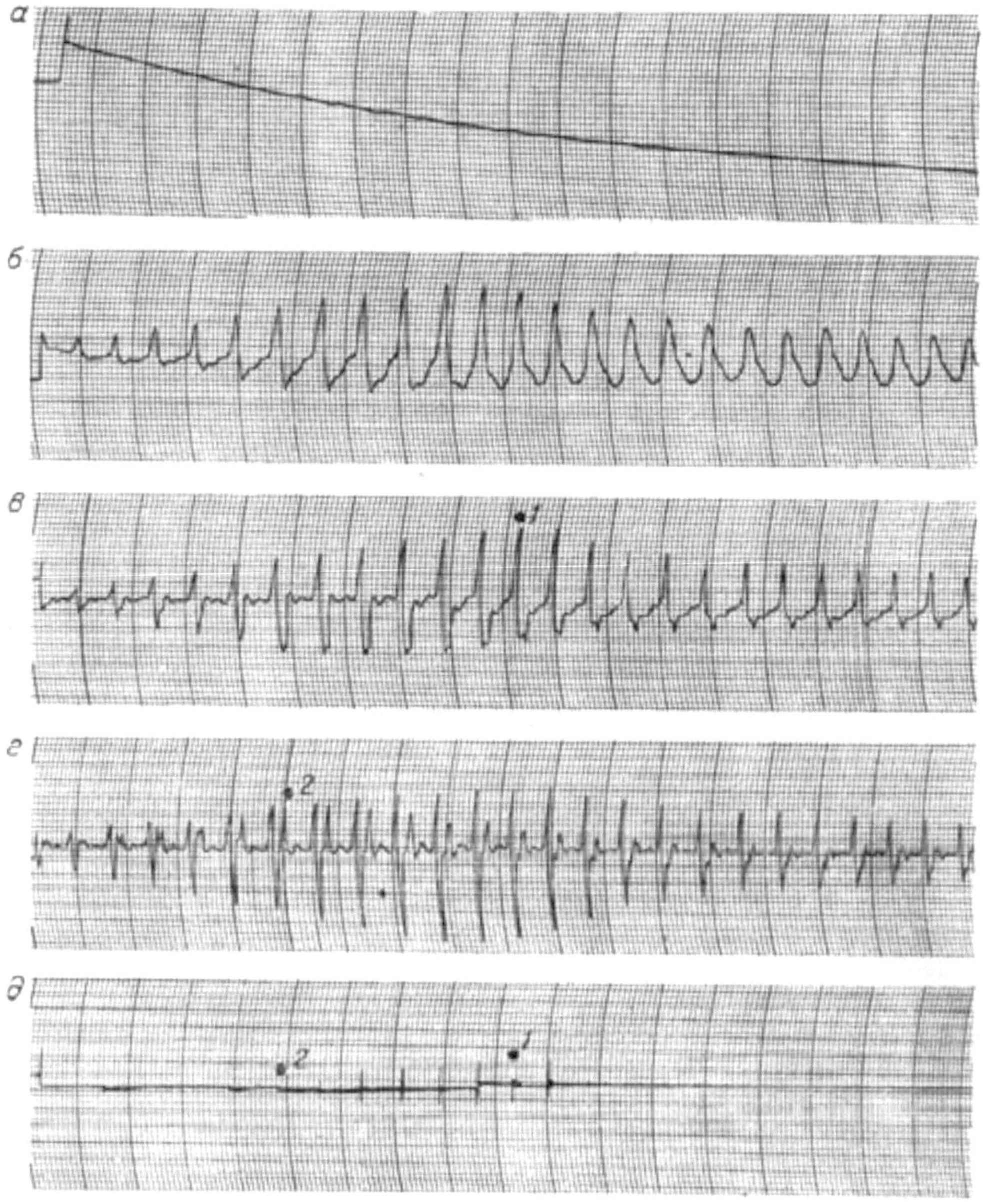

Fig. 4. Synchronous record of decompression occlusive pressure (a); oscillogram (b); the first derivative (c); the second derivative (d) and Korotkov sounds (e).

waves interference modulated by external pressure can be investigated only with the help of mathematical derivatives. In this case we used the first-order and second-order derivatives. We should notice that the first derivative reflects the process of the object alteration. The extreme points of the first derivative always indicate the moment of transformation of an object's state or its function to a different state or function. The second derivative is a result of interaction of the object or its functions with ambient environment. Here the extreme points are also informative. But their amplitude indicates the end result i.e. the fact of interaction and its result.

In the process of investigation the authors faced an interesting problem. We would name it "take something - not known what". The fact is that both the engineers and the doctors worked on the development of ECG and other bioelectric signals recording. The engineers tried to provide the doctors with the instruments that show "a fine signal". They were unaware of the degree of distortion during the filtration process and its difference from the real processes. Our research showed that these distortions are significant and reach 25% [5]. This situation could be improved but the received distorted ECG have for a long time served for creation of cardiological standards in diagnostics. Moreover, the theory which was formed had many "blank spaces".

That is why here we shall reveal a secret. It is essential that the lower cut-off band in the filter should be equal:

$$F_H = 0{,}35 \text{ Hz}.$$

The signal upper this value is differentiated, the signal lower the value is integrated. If the frequencies differ from the indicated ones it would be very difficult to understand what happens in the occlusive blood flow. The same could be said about rheography.

For the engineers we should note that for the filtration process the rate of signal increase is important as well. Different ECG phases have different amplitudes. In case of incorrect choice of filtration band *R* deflection can be integrated increasing the *RS* phase to a considerable extent. This process is influenced by the upper cut-off band. Inserting this phase time in G.Poedintsev–O.Voronova hemodynamics equation we shall obtain "fantastic" results which will be different from the real results.

3.2 Criteria of systolic and diastolic arterial pressure measurement

The considered above criteria of systolic and diastolic arterial pressure measurement using the oscillometric method and Korotkov sounds method allow to obtain identical values. But these methods have considerable discrepancies concerning diastolic pressure measurement. When the oscillometric method is used diastolic pressure is measured by the maximum of the first oscillogram derivative. When Korotkov sounds method is used diastolic pressure is measured by the sounds disappearance. Figure 5,c shows these discrepancies in points 2 and 3.

The study showed that the difference approximately accounts for 15 mm.Hg (Fig.5, points 2 and 3). How do the engineers solve this problem when developing commercial arterial pressure measuring instruments?

1. The oscillogram is recorded (Fig.5, b). At the beginning of its amplitude's increase comparator threshold is selected. Thus, systolic pressure is recorded.
2. Diastolic pressure is recorded when the oscillogram amplitude decreases below the comparator threshold.
3. In automatic devices the oscillogram resembles the first derivative. It occurs due to minimization of transient phenomena influence in the process of pumping pressure into cuff.

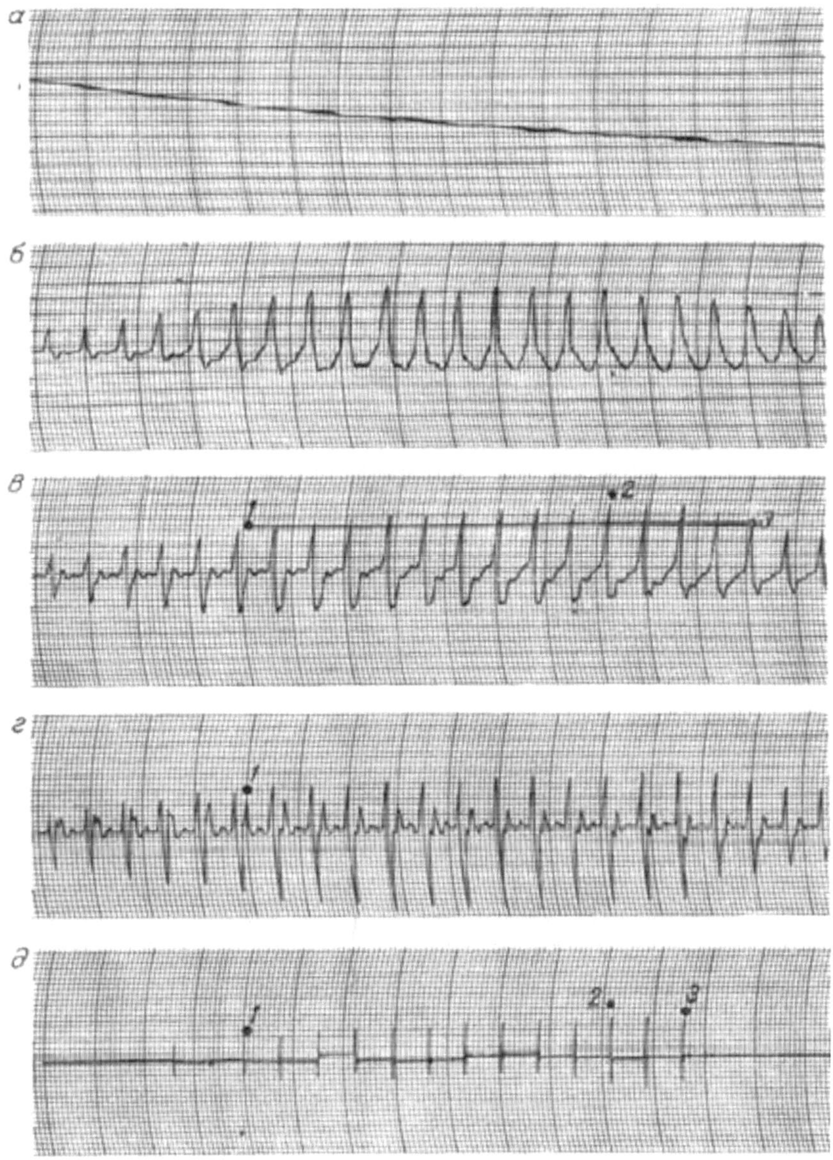

Fig. 5. Diastolic pressure measurement using the moment of Korotkov sounds disappearance: a - occlusive pressure; b - oscillogram; c -first-order derivative; d - second derivative; e Korotkov sounds.

Thus, all automatic machines with comparator threshold of signal amplitude do not measure diastolic pressure accurately. The measuring instrument developed by the authors of the present research work makes it possible to solve the problem in the following way. Figure 6 shows the signal records received from the commercially produced instrument. These signals are used to record systolic and diastolic pressure by derivatives maximum. After the measurement 15 mm.Hg. are deducted from diastolic pressure value.

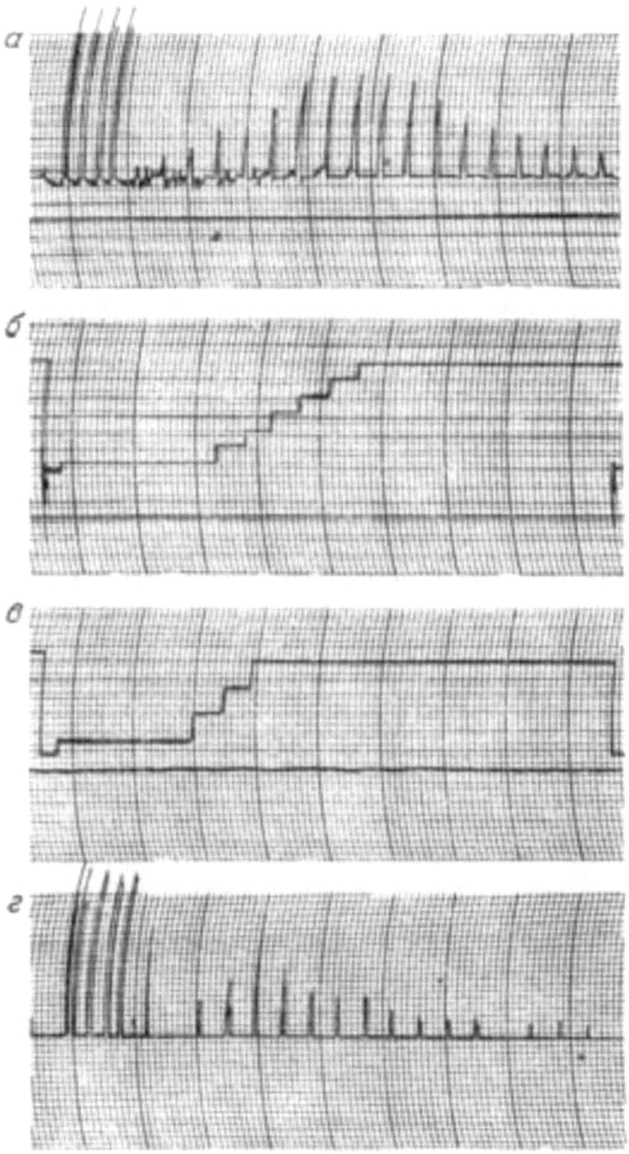

Fig. 6. Synchronous record of processed oscillogram derivatives and signals of amplitudes relation analyses unit. The amplitudes were extracted from the commercially produced measuring instrument based on arterial pressure waves interference. a –first-order derivative; b – search of diastolic pressure measurement criterion; c - search of systolic pressure measurement criterion; d –second-order derivative.

The end result will correlate with Korotkov sounds method and will not leave the doctors asking questions. Thus, the measuring instrument provides two variants of the measurement results presentation: 1) systolic pressure and average pressure (average pressure conforms to the time of maximum of the first derivative and maximum sounds amplitude i.e. true diastolic pressure (point 2 on Fig.5,b); 2) systolic pressure and diastolic pressure (diastolic pressure conforms to the second inflection of the enveloping oscillogram or the moment of Korotkov sounds disappearance (point 3 on Fig. 5,b). It is close to the value of comparator threshold in the measuring instruments produced by different firms.

4. Conclusion

1. The conditions of local increase of vessel characteristic impedance leading to interference of falling and reflected arterial pressure waves are considered. Criteria of systolic and diastolic pressure measurement compared with the used in practice Korotkov sounds are revealed.
2. The described method enables to measure systolic and diastolic arterial pressure accurately.
3. Commercially produced automatic arterial pressure measuring instruments using comparator functioning as criteria for diastolic arterial pressure measurement during oscillogram amplitude decrease do not measure diastolic pressure accurately; they rather show the value which is 15 mm.Hg lower than the true value.

5. Acknowledgement

The problem of arterial pressure measurement is given much attention in the world scientific literature. Specialized magazines are published. Scientific subpanels formed at symposiums study the results of research in this scientific field. Having studied in Radio-technical institute the authors of the present research work took interest in the popular at that time idea of computerization of arterial pressure measurement process. In the 1970s the

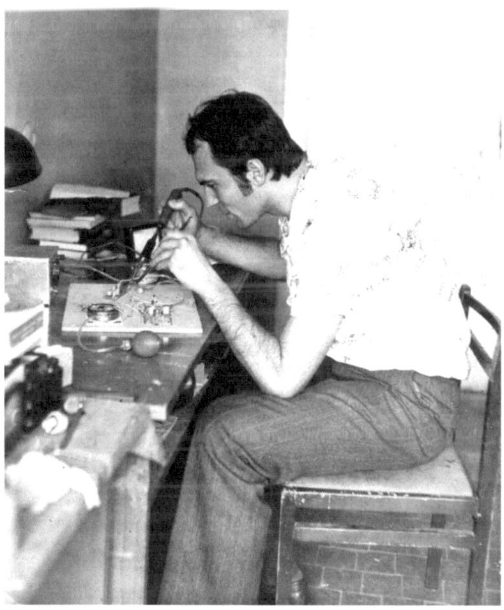

Fig. 7. M. Rudenko is in the hostel soldering the pressure-voltage transformation junction. The strain indicator is glued to the shoe cream box. Thus, the Big Science started (1978).

problem of pressure measurement in the place of brachial artery and temporal artery was set. Their magnitude relation should be equal to two. This coefficient was supposed to indicate good physical fitness of the sportsmen. The young authors started to work enthusiastically. We could not know then that the study of this problem would become a foundation for considerable scientific research the authors would devote their life to. A group of professionals would carry on research and develop medical instruments. Many of the researchers would found their schools of thought and achieve good results in business. Thirty years later the authors would receive a diploma for scientific discovery "Objective laws of arterial pressure waves propagation in blood-vessels in the areas of their impedance local increase".

An outstanding school of thought with distinguished scientists was formed. Over the past twenty years more than 150,000 copies of books were published. There emerged a need in system research of human biophysics. All of the research works found practical use.

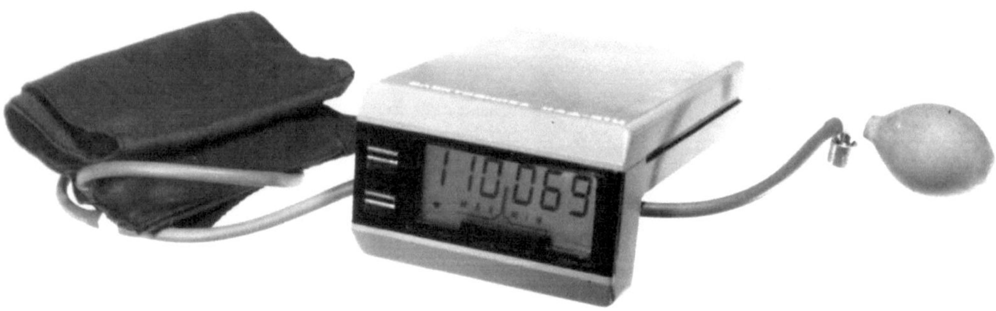

Fig. 8. The first in the world commercial instrument for indirect arterial pressure measurement based on artery pressure waves interference (1986).

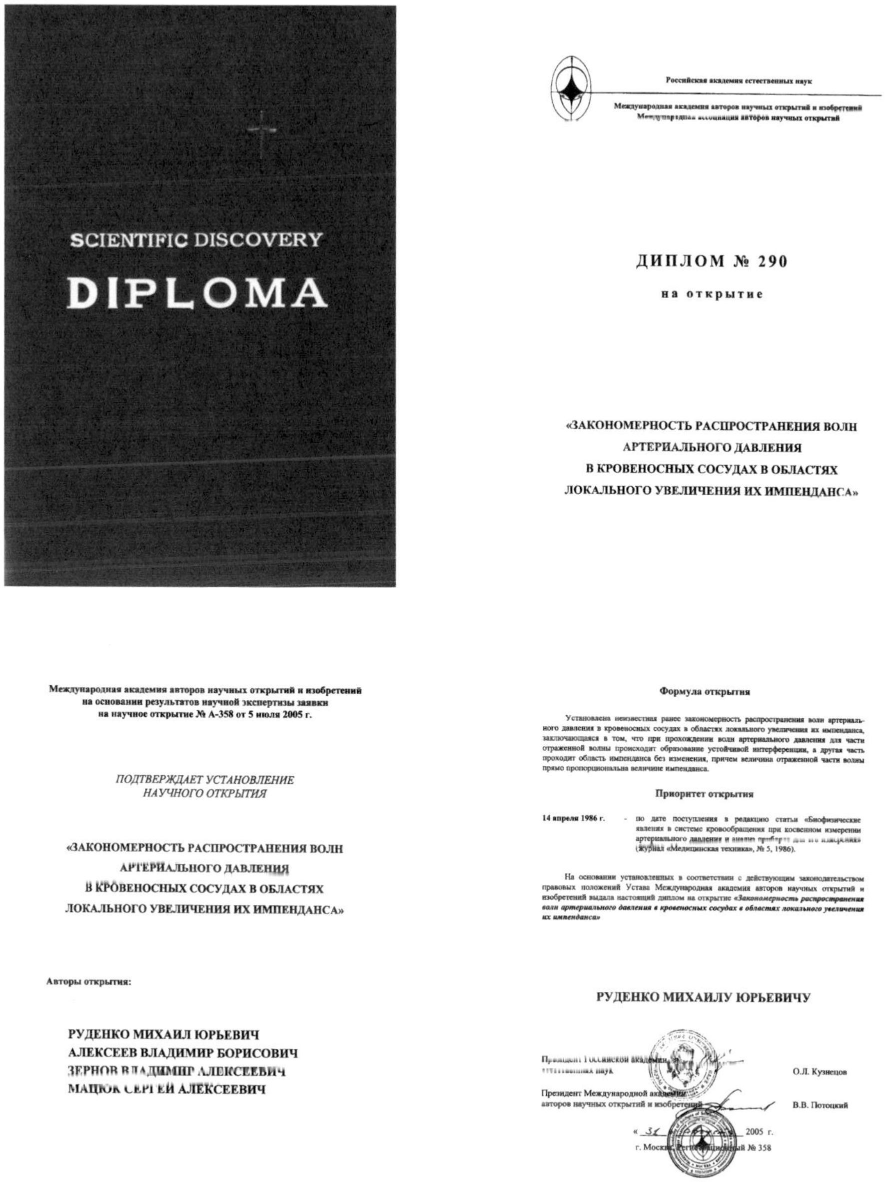

SCIENTIFIC DISCOVERY

DIPLOMA

Российская академия естественных наук

Международная академия авторов научных открытий и изобретений
Международная ассоциация авторов научных открытий

ДИПЛОМ № 290

на открытие

«ЗАКОНОМЕРНОСТЬ РАСПРОСТРАНЕНИЯ ВОЛН
АРТЕРИАЛЬНОГО ДАВЛЕНИЯ
В КРОВЕНОСНЫХ СОСУДАХ В ОБЛАСТЯХ
ЛОКАЛЬНОГО УВЕЛИЧЕНИЯ ИХ ИМПЕНДАНСА»

Международная академия авторов научных открытий и изобретений
на основании результатов научной экспертизы заявки
на научное открытие № А-358 от 5 июля 2005 г.

ПОДТВЕРЖДАЕТ УСТАНОВЛЕНИЕ
НАУЧНОГО ОТКРЫТИЯ

«ЗАКОНОМЕРНОСТЬ РАСПРОСТРАНЕНИЯ ВОЛН
АРТЕРИАЛЬНОГО ДАВЛЕНИЯ
В КРОВЕНОСНЫХ СОСУДАХ В ОБЛАСТЯХ
ЛОКАЛЬНОГО УВЕЛИЧЕНИЯ ИХ ИМПЕНДАНСА»

Авторы открытия:

РУДЕНКО МИХАИЛ ЮРЬЕВИЧ
АЛЕКСЕЕВ ВЛАДИМИР БОРИСОВИЧ
ЗЕРНОВ ВЛАДИМИР АЛЕКСЕЕВИЧ
МАЦЮК СЕРГЕЙ АЛЕКСЕЕВИЧ

Формула открытия

Установлена неизвестная ранее закономерность распространения волн артериального давления в кровеносных сосудах в областях локального увеличения их импенданса, заключающаяся в том, что при прохождении волн артериального давления для части отраженной волны происходит образование устойчивой интерференции, а другая часть проходит область импенданса без изменения, причем величина отраженной части волны прямо пропорциональна величине импенданса.

Приоритет открытия

14 апреля 1986 г. - по дате поступления в редакцию статьи «Биофизические явления в системе кровообращения при косвенном измерении артериального давления и анализ приборов для его измерения» (журнал «Медицинская техника», № 5, 1986).

На основании установленных в соответствии с действующим законодательством правовых положений Устава Международная академия авторов научных открытий и изобретений выдала настоящий диплом на открытие *«Закономерность распространения волн артериального давления в кровеносных сосудах в областях локального увеличения их импенданса»*

РУДЕНКО МИХАИЛУ ЮРЬЕВИЧУ

Президент Российской академии естественных наук — О.Л. Кузнецов

Президент Международной академии авторов научных открытий и изобретений — В.В. Потоцкий

« 31 » ... 2005 г.
г. Москва. Регистрационный № 358

Fig. 9. The documents of the official registration of scientific discovery "Objective laws of arterial pressure waves propagation in blood-vessels in the areas of their impedance local increase" (2005).

6. References

[1] *Savitsky N.N.* Biophysical principles of circulation and clinical methods of hemodynamic study. - 3-d ed. – Л., 1974.

[2] *Caro, C.; Padley, T.; Shroter, R.& Sid,W.* (1981). Blood Circulation Mechanics. - Mir. M.

[3] *Eman A.A.* Biophysical principles of arterial pressure measurement. – Л., 1983.

[4] *Rudenko, M.; Voronova, O.; & Zernov, V.* (2009). Study of Hemodynamic Parameters Using Phase analyses of the Cardiac Cycle. Biometrical Engineering. *Springer New York*. ISSN 0006-3398 (Print) 1573-8256 (Online). Volume 43, Number 4 / July 2009. P. 151-155.

[5] *Rudenko, M.; Voronova, O.; & Zernov, V.* (2009). Theoretical Principles of Heart Cycle Phase Analyses. Fouqué Literaturverlag. ISBN 978-3-937909-57-8, Frankfurt a/M. München - London - New York.

10

Interrelation Between the Changes of Phase Functions of Cardiac Muscle Contraction and Biochemical Processes as an Algorithm for Identifying Local Pathologies in Cardiovascular System

Yury Fedosov, Stanislav Zhigalov, Mikhail Rudenko, Vladimir Zernov and Olga Voronova
New Russian University, Russia

1. Introduction

Investigations of cardiovascular system based on mathematical models of hemodynamics developed by the authors allowed studying in details the cardiac cycle functions of different parts of the heart during different phases of the cardiac cycle. The proposed fundamentally novel diagnostic method based on phase analysis of cardiac cycle made it possible to track any functional and hemodynamic changes in the cardiovascular system. However, treatment of patients was always an issue after the diagnosis was established.

The existing understanding of the interrelations between the shape of the ECG an clinical meaning of the pathology were often in conflict with the insights gained from the phase analysis of cardiac cycle. New knowledge was needed about the processes occurring in the normal and pathological cardiovascular systems at the cellular level. The unique method of cardiac cycle phase analysis allowed verifying all the theoretical concepts based on the biochemical processes underlying development of the pathology, affecting functions of each segment of the cardiovascular system. Moreover, it proved possible to establish a number of recurring patterns of the influence of biochemical processes in the heart cells upon the observed shape of ECG and RHEOgrams.

In this chapter the authors outline their vision of the main biochemical processes determining the clinical meaning of the pathology diagnosed with the aid of the cardiac cycle analysis method. Selection of the therapeutic agents aimed at normalization of the diagnosed functional deviations taking into account the biochemical processes underlying these functions resulted in the recovery of the functions.

2. Interrelation between the contraction functions of myocardial muscles and biochemical processes in the cardiovascular system

2.1 Cardiac muscle contraction function and cell energy balance

Investigations with the aid of cardiac cycle phase analysis have revealed a compensatory mechanism for maintaining normal hemodynamics [1]. The essence of the mechanism is that a decrease of the contraction phase function of one segment of the heart entails an increase of the contraction phase function in an adjacent segment. E. g., decrease of amplitude of contraction of the ventricular septum causes the amplitude of contraction of ventricles to increase. E. g., decrease of amplitude of contraction of the ventricular septum causes the amplitude of contraction of ventricles to increase. Such transformations of cardiovascular system can only be diagnosed with the aid of cardiac cycle phase analysis.

Without knowing the compensatory mechanisms, neither a precise localization of the pathology nor its controlled treatment is possible. Phase analysis taking into account the compensatory mechanisms and cause-and-effect relation logics also allows identifying the origin of the pathology. Elimination of the original cause of the disease results in normalization of functions of other segments that used to perform compensatory functions for the affected segment.

In this manner, the authors attempted to control the process of influencing local pathological zones. Assessment of the recovery of the affected segments revealed that the cause of the change of function was not in the degradation of conductivity of the cardiac electrical system, but in the biochemical processes taking place within the myocardial cells.

According to publications of other authors, there is a number of various factors affecting the effectiveness of myocardial cell recovery in terms of their energy supply functions and further normalization of the muscle contraction function. [2] I. Leontieva and V. Sukhorukov have introduced a new term - mitochondrial cardiomyopathy.

Mitochondria are the major consumers of oxygen in the body. Hypoxia resulting from insufficient saturation of blood with oxygen is causing tissue damage up to necrosis. The primary symptom of hypoxia is swelling of mitochondria. The mitochondria of heart muscles have anatomic specificities. These are associated with the increased intensity of oxidation processes occurring in the cardiovascular system. The main function of mitochondria is ATP synthesis based on the uptake of fatty acids, pyruvate, glucose and amino acids from cell cytoplasm and their oxidative cleavage with generation of H2O и CO2. Fatty acids can only be delivered to mitochondria upon interaction with carnitine. Importantly, the quantative content of carnitine depends on the amount of secreted endorphins, thus regulating ATP synthesis. Besides that, carnitine regulates the exchange of phospholipids, essential substances required for normal function of the peripheral and central neural system. Its active form, L-carnitine is used for treating anorexia, extreme exhaustion.

It is due to effective functioning of mitochondria that muscle contraction occurs. They are, however, the weakest link in the cell functioning. Hypoxia substantially alters their energy budget. Oxidative phosphorylation is inhibited, transferring the mitochondria into free operation mode. Normally, oxidation in mitochondria takes place aerobically. In case of ischemia, this process becomes anaerobic. Anaerobic processes also start to become predominant at the heart rates above 150 beats per minute.

2.2 Stress and functional phase changes

In order to elucidate the influence of stress upon the work of heart and associated changes, normal energy supply to cardiac myocytes should be considered.

Contractility is the main function of cardiomyocytes. This is an energy dependent process requiring sufficient amount of ATP and Ca^{2+}. Energy supply to heart cells is a complex of sequential processes, such as binding by carnitine and transportation into mitochondria of the oxidation products, ATP generation, its transportation and consumption in various energy-dependent reactions.

Following are the main specific features of the cardiomyocyte metabolism:

1. The metabolism is predominantly aerobic. The main route of energy generation is oxidative phosphorilation.
2. The main substrates of oxidation are fatty acids.
3. High rate of energy-dependent processes in the myocard.
4. Minimal inventory of high-energy compounds.

Metabolism of cardiomyocytes is predominantly aerobic. Thus, they receive most of the energy through electron transfer from organic substrates to molecular oxygen. Therefore, contraction function of the cardiac muscle is a linear function of the oxygen uptake rate [3,4]. Synthesis of molecular ATP occurs in the process of oxidative phosphorylation in mitochondria. The amount of ATP generated depends on the amount of acetyl-CoA (EC 6.4.1.2), which gets oxidized in the tricarbonic acid cycle. When myocard is normally supplied with oxygen, 60 to 80% of the acetyl-CoA is generated due to β-oxidation of fatty acids, and 20-30 % - in the course of aerobic glycolysis. As a result of one loop of tricarbonic acid cycle, one molecule of acetyl-CoA gets decomposed to CO_2 and H_2O, 38 molecules of ATP being formed. Protons enter the mitochondrial respiratory chain in the form of reduced nicotineamides (NAD+ and NADF+). The main sources of reducing agents and their interrelation with mitochondrial respiratory chain are illustrated in figure 1.

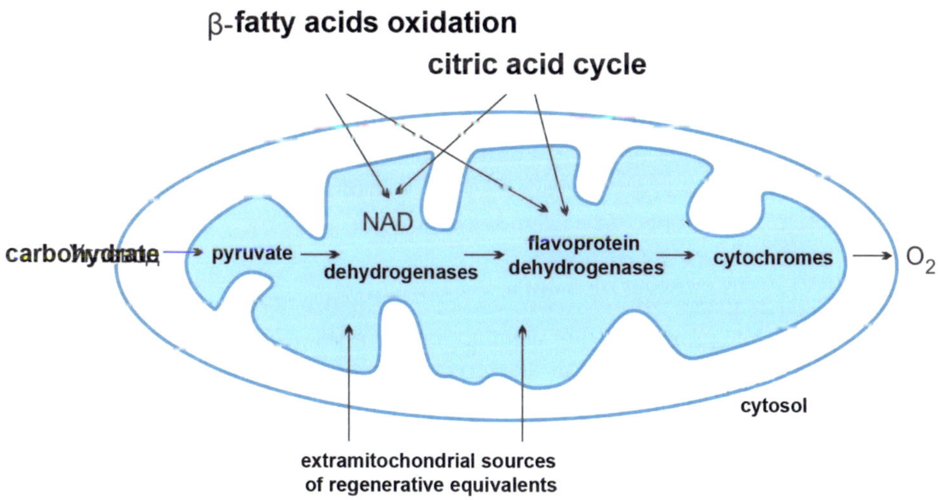

Fig. 1. The main sources of reducing agents and their interrelation with mitochondrial respiratory chain (NAD – nicotineamides).

The main transporter of ATP in cardiomyocytes is creatine phosphate. ATP-ADP translocase transports ATP to the outer side of the inner mitochondrial membrane, where creatine is phosphorylated under the action of creatine kinase (EC 2.7.3.2). Thus, creatinine phosphate and ADP are generated. Thereafter, ADP is transported inside the mitochondrial membrane.

The most energy-consuming process in the cardiomyocyte is contraction of myofibrils. Translocation of counter-lateral actin filaments against myosin filaments towards the center of sarcomeres and formation of actin-myosin bridges in the myofibrils occurs when sufficient amount of ATP is present.

Having considered the energy balance of cardiomyocytes, let us move to the metabolic processes occurring under the conditions of local stress.

From the standpoint of heart muscle, stress primarily results in hypoxia. Lack of oxygen affects all the stages of the cell energy supply (synthesis, transportation and consumption of ATP). In order to compensate for this, cardiomyocyte mobilizes energy from the intracellular inventories and reduces energy consumption. The inventories of the energy-rich substances - creatine phosphate, glucose and triglycerides are insignificant, and the cell soon starts to experience energy shortages. Anaerobic glycolysis is then activated to overcome the energy shortage.

Changes to fatty acid metabolism during hypoxia is characterized by disruption of β-oxidation of fatty acids, which is associated with the decrease of L-carnitine level caused by stress. Intracellular accumulation of fatty acids, acyl-carnitine and acyl-CoA (EC 6.2.1.3) occurs. The increase of acyl-CoA concentrations suppresses transportation of adenine nucleotides in mitochondria.

Development of hypoxia decreases the share of aerobic glycolysis to 5%. Thus, under conditions of stress caused by lack of oxygen energy, energy supply in cardiomyocytes is reduced by 65-95% of its normal value. Anaerobic glycolysis is then activated to compensate for the energy deficiency. Generation of ATP is reduced to 2 molecules per a molecule of glucose (as compared to 38 molecules under normal conditions). Increase of the share of the anaerobic glycolysis covers about 60-70% of the energy consumption. However, if this compensation occurs for an extensive period, it becomes dangerous.

In the course of anaerobic glycolysis, lactate builds up causing lactic acidosis. Against this background, accumulation of ATP hydrolysis products, and free fatty acids causes intracellular acidosis. This is accompanied by the loss of integrity of lysosomal membranes, release of lysosomal ferments, which, under conditions of energy deficiency, results in the damage of mitochondria ultra structure.

The energy deficiency also contributes to loss of ion balance. Reduced concentration of ATP inhibits the Na^+/K^+ pump of the cellular membranes. Consequentially, sodium and potassium ion concentration gradients start to decrease. Accumulation of sodium ions in the cardiomyocytes along with the increase of concentration of potassium ions in the extracellular solution result in the decrease of the resting potential and reduced duration of the action potential. Such deviations from the normal concentrations of ions in the intracellular and extracellular solutions cause hyperosmia, i.e. cell swelling, disrupting calcium homeostasis in the cardiomyocytes. Permittivity and contractility of certain sections of the cardiac muscle degrade, whereas neighboring parts of the cardiac muscle take additional load in a compensatory manner. These processes are clearly reflected in the cardiac cycle phases on the ECG. Relevant examples are given in the end of the chapter.

These abnormalities can be tracked with the aid of detecting functional phase contractions of the heart muscle.

2.3 Neural pulse – Interaction with cells

The influence of neural pulse on cardiac cells is associated primarily with initiation of sequential interrelated processes supporting cardiac muscle contraction.

Normal rhythmic contractions of cells occur as a result of spontaneous activity opf the pacemaker cells located in the sinoatrial node (SA node). Time interval between the heart contractions is determined by the time needed by the membranes of the pacemaker cells to reach the threshold level due to depolarization. Autonomous frequency of heart contractions is about 100 beats per minute without external impacts. An external impact is needed in order to increase or decrease this heart rate.

Vegetative neural system produces two most significant impacts on the heart beat rate. The fibers of both sympathetic and parasympathetic parts of the vegetative neural system terminate on the cells of the SA node and affect the heart rate beat. The impact is caused by a change of the process of spontaneous (autonomous) depolarization of the resting potential in the pacemaker cells of the sinoatrial node.

Acetylcholine released by parasympathetic neural fibers going to the heart as a part of branches of vagus nerve increases permeability of the membranes at rest to K^+ and decreases diastolic permeability for Na^+. These changes of permeability have two effects on the resting potential of the pacemaker cells. Firstly, they cause initial hyperpolarization of the membrane resting potential, making it closer to the potassium equilibrium potential. Secondly, they decrease the rate of spontaneous depolarization of the membrane at rest. Both these effects tend to increase the lag between heart contractions due to increased period of depolarization of the resting membrane to the threshold value.

Sympathetic neural fibers release noradrenalin. The most essential effect of noradrenalin is the increase of the Na^+ and Ca^{2+} intake by the cell during the diastole. These changes increase heart beat rate due to increased rate of diastolic depolarization.

Besides the influence on the heart beat rate, vegetative neural fibers affect the rate of conduction of action potentials through heart tissues. Enhanced sympathetic influence increases the conduction rate, whereas the enhanced parasympathetic influence decreases the conduction rate of action potentials.

Cardiomyocyte contraction is initiated by the action potential signal to the intracellular organelles, resulting in increased tension and contraction of the cell. This process is known as excitation-contraction coupling. The key element of these processes is an abrupt increase of intracellular concentration of free Ca^{2+}. Concentration of Ca^{2+} changes from less than 0.1 mkm at rest to 100 mkm during maximal activation of the contraction machinery.

If we now recall the influence of local stress on cardiomyocytes and mechanisms of occurrence of this influence, the reasons behind and abnormalities in conduction and contraction of heart muscle become clear.

When the energy transformation processes in the mitochondria become abnormal, parts of the respiratory chain are inhibited by specific therapeutic agents, chemical reagents or antibiotics, decrease of the amplitude of cardiomyocyte contraction due to lack of ATP is the first consequence to be observed. Thereafter, due to accumulation of free fatty acids, hydrolysis products, and lactate, due to development of internal acidosis and loss of ion balance of cell, conductance of action potential starts degrading, resulting not only in degraded conductivity of heart muscle and disturbance of the regulatory influence of the neural system on the work of heart as a whole.

2.4 Endorphin stimulation as a natural way of enhancing stress resistance

Having considered the specifics of biochemical processes taking place in stressed cardiac muscle, we can touch upon another important question: "How does the body fight stress?".

It is a common knowledge that when stress factors appear, all the systems of the body are activate. These processes are aimed at maintaining integrity, normal operability and survival of an organism. Regulation of the cascades of biochemical reactions occurring in response to stress factors is mediated by interactions of neural and endocrinal systems.

As shown in figure 2, as a result of stress the central neural system activates the following pathway of endocrinal regulation: hypothalamus - corticoliberin - pituitary gland - adrenocorticotropic (AcTH) hormone - suprarenal gland - cortisol. Besides the adrenocorticotropic (AcTH) hormone, β-lipotropic hormone (LPH) is generated from the C-terminal part of the protein. LPH proteolysis results in generation of either γ-LPH and β-endorphin, or β-melanotropin and γ-endorphin. Beside that, LPH can decompose to α-endorphin and met-enkephalin. Simultaneous production of all these hormones causes the following effects:

- Enhancement of carbohydrate metabolism (glucocorticoids)
- Enhancement of lipid metabolism (lipotropins)
- Reduced pain sensibility and euphoric sensation (endorphins and enkephalines)
- Stimulation of immune system (melanotropin).

Thus, there is a system of multiple regulatory signals initiated by a single stimulus regulating simultaneously a number of metabolic processes and receptor systems.

2.5 Example of application of phase analysis of cardiac cycle for controlling recovery of the function of cardiovascular system in the course of treatment

Based on our understanding of biophysical processes and having a tool for investigating phase processes of the heart function, we attempted to influence in an integrated manner the metabolic processes occurring in the myocardium and track the associated changes of the phase functions of heart contraction.

In order to influence the metabolism in an integrated manner, we performed normalization of the acid-base balance. L-carnitine and octolipen were used to affect lipid metabolism. Transcranial electrostimulation method was used in order to increase production of the pituitary gland hormones (adrenocorticotropic (AcTH) hormone, LPH, melanotropin, endorphins and enkephalines).

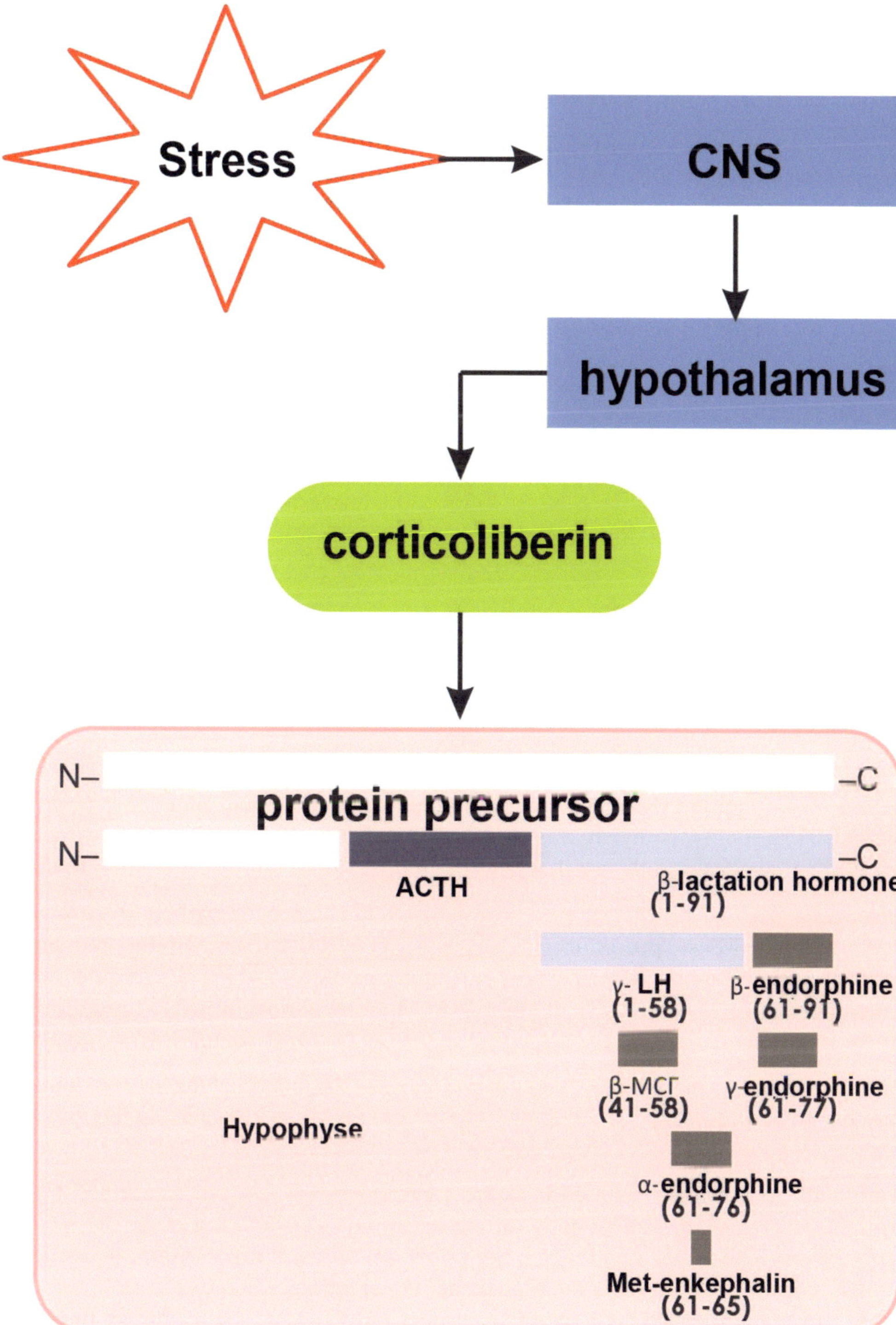

Fig. 2. Stimulation of the neuroendocrine regulation mechanism by stress

During this study, we tracked not only changes of the cardiac phase functions, but also the phase hemodynamics parameters.

The results presented below were obtained in the course of integrated impact on the patient organisms.

The figure 3 illustrates the initial results. These are ECG and RHEO records of the ascending aorta and the table of the phase hemodynamics parameters. ECG and RHEO records correspond to the same cardiac cycle. For the sake of convenience, only one cardiac cycle is represented on the figure. The table summarizes results for 18 cardiac cycles. The number of cycles is not fixed during the recording. The duration of the record is about 20 seconds. This period is sufficient to obtain information for assessing hemodynamics parameters of several cardiac cycles.

The shape of ECG corresponds to Brugada syndrome. Interventricular septum lost its contraction function. This is evidenced by minimal amplitude of the R deflection. Expansion of the S deflection is a compensatory function. Having assumed increased contraction load, myocardial muscle increased its volume. Raise of SL wave on the ECG is indicative of increased arterial pressure. In this case, there is a continuous stress of myocardium since the amplitude of the SL phase is above the isoline in each cardiac cycle

The identified factors allow making conclusions and selecting the treatment strategy. The original cause is the issue with the interventricular septum, and it is this problem that has to be addressed. Widening of the S deflection and high amplitude of the SL phase are secondary factors caused by the compensatory mechanism of substitution of its lost function. In case of successful recovery of the function of the interventricular septum, other function are to normalize on their own.

There was an assumption that the problem of the loss of contractility function is based on mitochondrial cardiomyopathy. It was therefore decided that the patient should take L-carnitine simultaneously with octolipen. In addition to that, daily use of the breathing exerciser was prescribed in order to normalize the balance of carbon dioxide and oxygen in blood. These procedures were performed domiciliary. In the outpatient conditions, he was undergoing electrical treatment, excitation of specific cranial zones with small current pulses in order to stimulate release of endorphins. No limitations in diet were imposed.

According to the table on the figure 3, in the beginning of the treatment the average value of the cardiac output (minute blood volume) of the patient ws MV = 9.71 liters. In the course of treatment, MV variations from 7.63 to 10.93 liters were recorded.

In two months, the results presented in figure 4 were recorded. The record corresponds to the upright position of the patient body during orthostatic test. Splitting of the deflection S is clearly visible. This is not a pathology, but rather a reaction of myocardium to overload. When the patient was in horizontal position, no splitting/vibrations were observed. However, already in the next cycle the ECG assumes fairly normal shape, though the shape is not yet stable. This is also evidenced both by the parameters of hemodynamics, namely the minute volume MV.

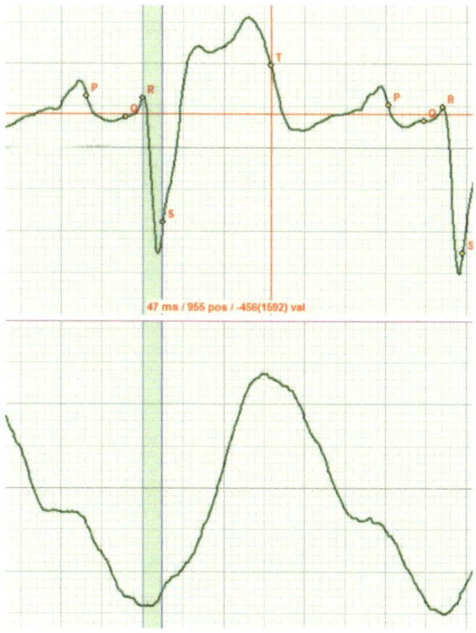

PHASE ANALYSIS RESULTS								
	HEMODYNAMIC PARAMETERS							
	SV(ml)	MV(l)	PV1(ml)	PV2(ml)	PV3(ml)	PV4(ml)	PV5(ml)	HEART RATE
AVERAGE	140.01	9.71	83.25	56.76	83.23	56.78	14.98	69.39
CYCLE №	SV(ml)	MV(l)	PV1(ml)	PV2(ml)	PV3(ml)	PV4(ml)	PV5(ml)	HEART RATE
1	148.01	10.55	85.34	62.68	87.99	60.02	15.64	71.25
2	135.47	0.40	79.68	55.79	80.53	54.94	14.59	69.85
3	135.47	9.37	81.64	53.83	80.53	54.94	14.59	69.17
4	135.47	9.70	78.64	56.83	80.53	54.94	14.59	71.61
5	135.47	10.05	73.75	61.71	80.53	54.94	14.59	74.22
6	145.76	10.87	80.17	65.59	86.67	59.10	15.11	74.61
7	145.76	10.93	79.63	66.13	86.67	59.10	15.11	75.00
8	146.89	10.68	83.19	63.70	87.33	59.56	15.38	72.70
9	135.47	9.15	82.39	53.07	80.53	54.94	14.59	67.54
10	136.45	8.27	89.77	46.68	81.11	55.35	14.84	60.64
11	137.69	7.63	95.00	42.70	81.84	55.85	15.11	55.45
12	136.45	8.38	89.18	47.28	81.11	55.35	14.84	61.42
13	136.45	9.13	84.47	51.98	81.11	55.35	14.84	66.90
14	148.01	10.49	85.89	62.12	87.99	60.02	15.64	70.90
15	148.01	10.82	82.78	65.23	87.99	60.02	15.64	73.08
16	136.45	9.97	75.35	61.10	81.11	55.35	14.84	73.08
17	135.47	9.90	75.45	60.02	80.53	54.94	14.59	73.08
18	135.47	10.11	73.17	62.30	80.53	54.94	14.59	74.61

Fig. 3. September 2010

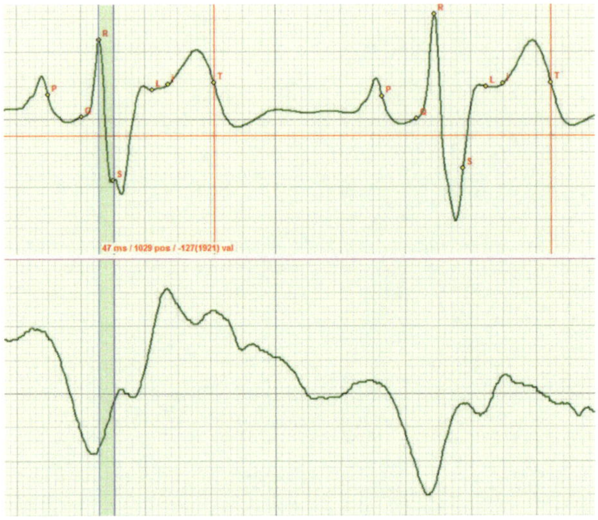

PHASE ANALYSIS RESULTS

	HEMODYNAMIC PARAMETERS							
	SV(ml)	MV(l)	PV1(ml)	PV2(ml)	PV3(ml)	PV4(ml)	PV5(ml)	HEART RATE
AVERAGE	67.09	4.14	42.51	24.58	39.80	27.29	9.98	61.66

CYCLE №	SV(ml)	MV(l)	PV1(ml)	PV2(ml)	PV3(ml)	PV4(ml)	PV5(ml)	HEART RATE
1	48.74	3.23	29.03	19.71	28.90	19.84	8.09	66.30
2	48.74	2.94	31.43	17.31	28.90	19.84	8.09	60.34
3	48.53	2.85	31.92	16.61	28.78	19.75	8.01	58.67
4	152.74	9.18	98.66	54.08	90.80	61.94	16.28	60.10
5	56.42	3.67	34.32	22.11	33.47	22.96	8.88	65.13
6	56.70	3.71	34.20	22.50	33.63	23.07	8.98	65.42
7	48.53	3.11	30.02	18.51	28.78	19.75	8.01	64.00
8	48.53	2.94	30.99	17.54	28.78	19.75	8.01	60.59
9	150.55	8.90	97.86	52.69	89.51	61.04	15.77	59.14
10	48.33	2.93	31.22	17.11	28.66	19.67	7.93	60.59
11	48.53	2.82	31.82	16.71	28.78	19.75	8.01	58.20
12	56.42	3.18	37.94	18.48	33.47	22.96	8.88	56.43
13	56.97	3.24	37.62	19.35	33.79	23.18	9.08	56.86
14	149.44	9.28	94.17	55.27	88.85	60.59	15.51	62.12
15	48.13	3.16	29.29	18.85	28.54	19.59	7.85	65.71
16	48.33	3.23	28.39	19.93	28.66	19.67	7.93	66.90

Fig. 4. November 2010

Another month later ECG remained unstable, but the average value of MV decreased to 9.06 liters.

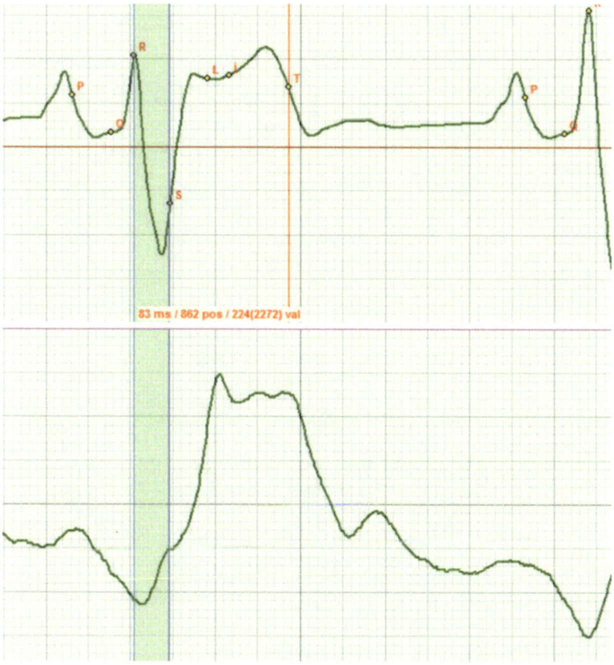

PHASE ANALYSIS RESULTS								
	HEMODYNAMIC PARAMETERS							
	SV(ml)	MV(l)	PV1(ml)	PV2(ml)	PV3(ml)	PV4(ml)	PV5(ml)	HEART RATE
AVERAGE	144.47	9.06	93.81	50.66	85.86	58.60	15.89	62.74

CYCLE №	SV(ml)	MV(l)	PV1(ml)	PV2(ml)	PV3(ml)	PV4(ml)	PV5(ml)	HEART RATE
1	153.83	10.48	93.72	60.11	91.44	62.39	16.54	68.12
2	143.42	9.22	90.88	52.54	85.23	58.18	15.98	64.27
3	129.47	7.62	87.08	42.38	76.94	52.53	14.46	58.89
4	152.81	9.18	101.82	50.99	90.84	61.97	16.29	60.09
5	152.81	9.49	99.65	53.16	90.84	61.97	16.29	62.11
6	153.83	9.47	101.72	52.11	91.44	62.39	16.54	61.59
7	143.42	8.76	94.32	49.10	85.23	58.18	15.98	61.08
8	129.47	8.18	83.24	46.22	76.94	52.53	14.46	63.17
9	142.34	9.19	90.20	52.15	84.60	57.74	15.73	64.55
10	154.89	9.87	100.00	54.89	92.07	62.82	16.80	63.71
11	153.83	9.72	99.95	53.88	91.44	62.39	16.54	63.17
12	131.22	8.15	85.82	45.40	77.87	53.24	14.91	62.11
13	143.42	9.51	89.66	53.76	85.23	58.18	15.98	66.28
14	153.83	10.06	97.17	56.66	91.44	62.39	16.54	65.40
15	143.42	8.91	93.25	50.17	85.23	58.10	15.98	62.11
16	132.29	7.82	89.90	42.39	78.60	53.68	15.16	59.12

Fig. 5. December 2010

In two months, hemodynamics parameters grew somewhat. The patient continued to receive the treatment, having only excluded the octolipen.

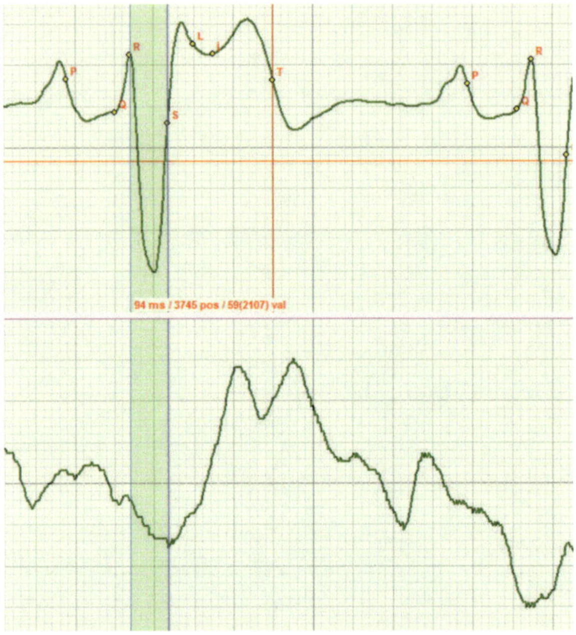

PHASE ANALYSIS RESULTS								
	HEMODYNAMIC PARAMETERS							
	SV(ml)	MV(l)	PV1(ml)	PV2(ml)	PV3(ml)	PV4(ml)	PV5(ml)	HEART RATE
AVERAGE	153.56	9.83	93.57	59.99	91.28	62.28	16.53	63.99

CYCLE №	SV(ml)	MV(l)	PV1(ml)	PV2(ml)	PV3(ml)	PV4(ml)	PV5(ml)	HEART RATE
1	154.27	10.95	80.99	73.28	91.70	62.57	16.59	70.96
2	154.27	10.35	90.02	64.25	91.70	62.57	16.59	67.09
3	141.89	8.99	86.18	55.71	84.33	57.55	15.54	63.35
4	163.53	10.59	99.38	64.15	97.23	66.29	16.83	64.74
5	156.36	10.44	92.07	64.29	92.93	63.42	17.10	66.79
6	153.25	10.62	85.26	67.99	91.10	62.15	16.34	69.30
7	165.96	10.89	98.73	67.23	98.67	67.29	17.39	65.60
8	142.76	8.97	87.05	55.71	84.85	57.91	15.77	62.81
9	153.25	10.19	89.55	63.70	91.10	62.15	16.34	66.49
10	155.34	10.66	89.07	66.27	92.33	63.00	16.85	68.65
11	154.27	10.17	91.76	62.51	91.70	62.57	16.59	65.89
12	145.65	8.46	94.29	51.36	86.55	59.10	16.49	58.11
13	142.76	8.23	94.47	48.29	84.85	57.91	15.77	57.66
14	154.27	9.77	96.32	57.94	91.70	62.57	16.59	63.35
15	175.61	11.37	106.29	69.32	104.43	71.17	17.62	64.74
16	153.25	9.46	96.84	56.41	91.10	62.15	16.34	61.76

Fig. 6. February 2011

In another month the patient stated that he had gone through a medical exam in the regional clinics, where he was offered surgery to narrow the interventricular septum. The patient rejected the surgery. Coronary angiography was also performed, having indicated that the coronary arteries were clear. The patient was concerned with premature beats (extra systole). The figure 6 illustrates the original record made during investigation of phase parameters.

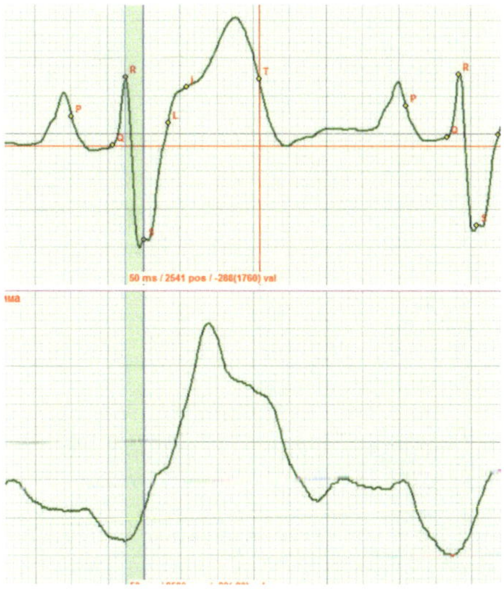

PHASE ANALYSIS RESULTS								
	HEMODYNAMIC PARAMETERS							
	SV(ml)	MV(l)	PV1(ml)	PV2(ml)	PV3(ml)	PV4(ml)	PV5(ml)	HEART RATE
AVERAGE	56.32	3.86	33.18	23.14	33.40	22.92	9.09	68.46

CYCLE №	SV(ml)	MV(l)	PV1(ml)	PV2(ml)	PV3(ml)	PV4(ml)	PV5(ml)	HEART RATE
1	65.80	4.57	37.86	27.95	39.03	26.77	10.08	69.44
2	66.13	4.59	38.46	27.67	39.23	26.90	10.19	69.44
3	41.15	2.82	23.94	17.21	24.40	16.76	7.29	68.48
4	56.92	4.07	31.21	25.72	33.76	23.16	9.07	71.45
5	48.92	3.46	27.45	21.47	29.01	19.91	8.21	70.77
6	65.80	4.55	39.22	26.58	39.03	26.77	10.08	69.12
7	57.18	3.88	34.32	22.86	33.91	23.27	9.16	67.85
8	66.45	4.39	40.63	25.83	39.42	27.04	10.30	66.03
9	48.92	3.17	29.85	19.07	29.01	19.91	8.21	64.87
10	49.16	3.29	29.74	19.41	29.15	20.01	8.30	08.93
11	65.80	4.49	39.25	26.56	39.03	26.77	10.08	68.16
12	66.45	4.47	39.83	26.62	39.42	27.04	10.30	67.23
13	48.92	3.30	29.47	19.45	29.01	19.91	8.21	67.54
14	48.69	3.33	28.78	19.91	28.87	19.82	8.08	68.48
15	48.92	3.41	28.41	20.51	29.01	19.91	8.21	09.77
16	57.65	3.95	33.85	23.80	34.19	23.46	9.34	68.48
17	57.42	3.97	33.03	24.39	34.05	23.37	9.25	69.12
18	75.60	5.23	45.30	30.30	44.85	30.75	11.24	69.12

Fig. 7. March 2011

After a series of sit-ups, extra systole was detected (see Fig. 8). Minute volume MV increased to 13.66 liters.

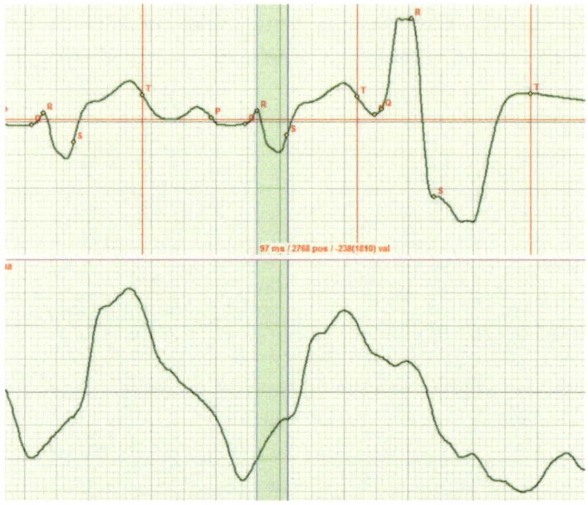

PHASE ANALYSIS RESULTS								
	HEMODYNAMIC PARAMETERS							
	SV(ml)	MV(l)	PV1(ml)	PV2(ml)	PV3(ml)	PV4(ml)	PV5(ml)	HEART RATE
AVERAGE	144.84	13.66	44.79	100.05	86.18	58.67	13.57	94.34

CYCLE №	SV(ml)	MV(l)	PV1(ml)	PV2(ml)	PV3(ml)	PV4(ml)	PV5(ml)	HEART RATE
1	146.86	14.29	35.56	111.30	87.39	59.47	13.35	97.31
2	145.44	14.25	35.22	110.22	86.55	58.89	13.06	97.95
3	128.32	12.41	35.49	92.83	76.33	52.00	12.49	96.67
4	137.00	13.16	40.04	96.95	81.51	55.49	12.81	96.04
5	157.02	14.89	42.67	114.35	93.46	63.57	13.89	94.81
6	146.86	14.10	40.62	106.24	87.39	59.47	13.35	96.04
7	148.34	14.16	44.11	104.23	88.27	60.08	13.64	95.42
8	157.02	14.98	43.43	113.59	93.46	63.57	13.89	95.42
9	155.43	14.74	44.67	110.75	92.51	62.92	13.58	94.81
10	148.34	13.80	52.30	96.05	88.27	60.08	13.64	93.02
11	155.43	14.28	57.56	97.87	92.51	62.92	13.58	91.87
12	129.46	11.75	50.68	78.78	77.00	52.46	12.74	90.74
13	148.34	13.38	58.08	90.27	88.27	60.08	13.64	90.19
14	148.34	13.54	57.40	90.94	88.27	60.08	13.64	91.30
15	146.86	13.75	49.14	97.72	87.39	59.47	13.35	93.61
16	148.34	13.89	47.64	100.71	88.27	60.08	13.64	93.61
17	148.34	13.80	49.61	98.74	88.27	60.08	13.64	93.02
18	114.25	13.20	346.18	-231.93	67.85	46.41	14.42	115.55
19	129.46	9.97	76.18	53.29	77.00	52.46	12.74	77.04
20	130.74	11.94	48.42	82.32	77.75	52.98	13.01	91.30
21	149.67	14.19	41.37	108.29	89.05	60.62	13.92	94.81
22	148.34	14.34	35.92	112.42	88.27	60.08	13.64	96.67
23	157.02	15.28	35.05	121.97	93.46	63.57	13.89	97.31
24	146.86	14.39	36.28	110.57	87.39	59.47	13.35	97.95
25	131.94	12.59	37.20	94.75	78.47	53.48	13.27	95.42
26	140.70	13.34	35.93	104.77	83.69	57.01	13.61	94.81
27	148.34	14.06	40.33	108.01	88.27	60.08	13.64	94.81

Fig. 8. March 2011, after sit-ups having caused extra systole.

After relaxation of the patient, the extra systoles disappeared. MV = 13.32.

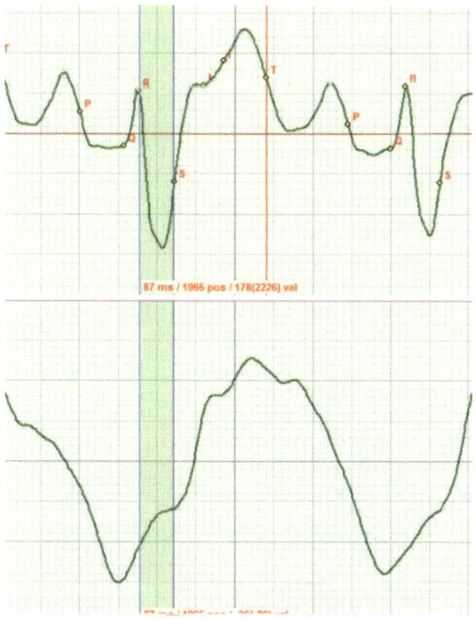

PHASE ANALYSIS RESULTS								
	HEMODYNAMIC PARAMETERS							
	SV(ml)	MV(l)	PV1(ml)	PV2(ml)	PV3(ml)	PV4(ml)	PV5(ml)	HEART RATE
AVERAGE	147.45	13.32	48.56	98.89	87.71	59.75	14.34	90.30
CYCLE №	SV(ml)	MV(l)	PV1(ml)	PV2(ml)	PV3(ml)	PV4(ml)	PV5(ml)	HEART RATE
1	149.91	14.20	38.36	111.55	89.20	60.72	13.95	94.74
2	161.90	14.95	43.35	118.55	96.34	65.56	14.83	92.37
3	164.84	15.32	42.90	121.93	98.07	66.77	15.43	92.95
4	152.67	14.37	36.39	116.28	90.82	61.85	14.52	94.13
5	143.54	13.26	41.32	102.22	85.37	58.17	14.18	92.37
6	125.82	11.34	39.19	86.63	74.79	51.03	13.56	90.11
7	134.36	12.26	42.51	91.85	79.89	54.47	13.79	91.23
8	161.90	14.59	55.40	106.50	96.34	65.56	14.83	90.11
9	161.90	14.77	54.18	107.73	96.34	65.56	14.83	91.23
10	161.90	14.77	51.23	110.68	96.34	65.56	14.83	91.23
11	153.99	13.88	47.96	106.02	91.60	62.39	14.80	90.11
12	144.92	13.14	45.85	99.07	86.18	58.73	14.46	90.67
13	135.34	12.20	42.15	93.18	80.47	54.87	14.03	90.11
14	149.91	13.76	46.72	103.19	89.20	60.72	13.05	91.79
15	160.37	14.45	56.75	103.62	95.43	64.94	14.52	90.11
16	161.90	14.68	53.35	108.55	96.34	65.56	14.83	90.67
17	143.54	12.93	49.09	94.45	85.37	58.17	14.18	90.11
18	143.54	12.78	54.76	88.78	85.37	58.17	14.18	89.03
19	119.96	10.88	44.45	75.50	71.33	48.62	12.16	90.67
20	134.36	11.54	54.93	79.43	79.89	54.47	13.79	85.92
21	161.90	14.24	60.00	101.91	96.34	65.56	14.83	87.97
22	164.84	14.50	60.10	104.05	98.07	66.77	15.43	87.97
23	153.99	13.88	50.74	103.24	91.60	62.39	14.80	90.11
24	136.42	12.00	45.29	91.13	81.10	55.31	14.28	87.97
25	123.85	11.09	41.12	82.74	73.63	50.22	13.09	89.57

Fig. 9. March 2011, Relaxation after extra systole.

The treatment course was continued. In two months, ECG was almost normal. No extra systoles were detected. MV = 7.72 liters.

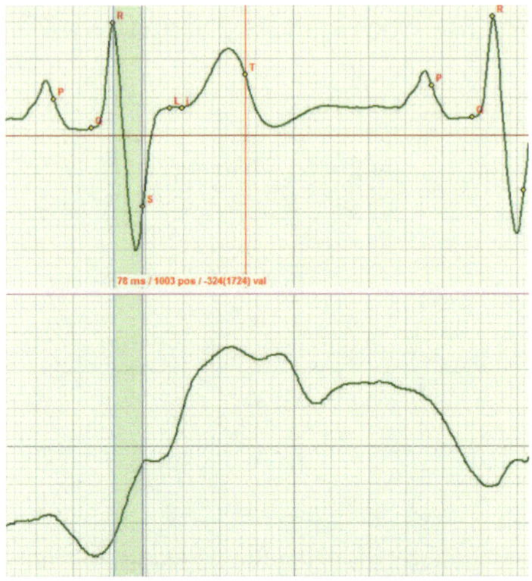

PHASE ANALYSIS RESULTS								
	HEMODYNAMIC PARAMETERS							
	SV(ml)	MV(l)	PV1(ml)	PV2(ml)	PV3(ml)	PV4(ml)	PV5(ml)	HEART RATE
AVERAGE	131.64	7.72	85.23	46.42	78.22	53.42	15.14	58.68

CYCLE №	SV(ml)	MV(l)	PV1(ml)	PV2(ml)	PV3(ml)	PV4(ml)	PV5(ml)	HEART RATE
1	121.42	6.68	80.55	40.88	72.13	49.29	14.55	54.99
2	131.13	7.85	84.32	46.81	77.91	53.21	15.02	59.86
3	141.07	8.62	89.38	51.70	83.84	57.23	15.59	61.09

Fig. 10. May 2011

3. Conclusion

Cardiac cycle phase analysis method allows tracking any changes of hemodynamics and functions of the cardiovascular system. It can be used to identify the original cause of pathologies and to efficiently monitor the treatment progress.

4. References

[1] Rudenko, M.; Voronova, O. & Zernov. V. Innovation in cardiology. A new diagnostic standard establishing criteria of quantitative & qualitative evaluation of main parameters of the cardiac & cardiovascular system according to ECG and RHEO based on cardiac cycle phase analysis (for concurrent single-channel recording of cardiac signals from ascending aorta). http://precedings.nature.com/documents/3667/version/1/html

[2] Leontieva I. & Sukhorukov V. The implications of metabolic disorders in the genesis of cardiac myopathia and possible use of L-carnitine for therapeutic correction. . Saint Petersburg. Manuscript -2006.

[3] Vasilenko V. Kh., Feldman S. B., Khotrov N.N., Miocardyodistrophia. - Moscow. Medicine. - 1989. -272.

[4] Kushakovsky M.S. Metabolic cardiac diseases. Saint Petersburg. Manuscript -2000. 128.

11

Application of Computational Intelligence Techniques for Cardiovascular Diagnostics

C. Nataraj, A. Jalali and P. Ghorbanian
Department of Mechanical Engineering, Villanova University, Villanova, Pennsylvania, USA

1. Introduction

Cardiovascular disease, including heart disease and stroke, remains the leading cause of death around the world. Yet, most heart attacks and strokes could be prevented if it were possible to provide an easy and reliable method of monitoring and diagnostics. In particular, the early detection of abnormalities in the function of the heart, called arrhythmias, could be valuable for clinicians.

Hemodynamic instability is most commonly associated with abnormal or unstable blood pressure (BP), especially hypotension, or more broadly associated with inadequate global or regional perfusion. Inadequate perfusion may compromise important organs, such as heart and brain, due to limits on coronary and cerebral auto regulation and cause life-threatening illnesses, or even death. Therefore, it is crucial to identify patients who are likely to become hemodynamically unstable to enable early detection and treatment of these life-threatening conditions (Cao, Eshelman et al. 2008). Modern intensive care units (ICU) employ continuous hemodynamic monitoring (e.g., heart rate (HR) and invasive arterial BP measurements) to track the state of health of the patients. However, clinicians in a busy ICU would be too overwhelmed with the effort required to assimilate and interpret the tremendous volumes of data in order to arrive at working hypotheses. Consequently, it is important to seek to have automated algorithms that can accurately process and classify the large amount of data gathered and to identify patients who are on the verge of becoming unstable (Cao, Eshelman et al. 2008).

Modern ICUs are equipped with a large array of alarmed monitors and devices which are used to try to detect clinical changes at the earliest possible moment so as to prevent any further deterioration in a patient's condition. The effectiveness of these systems depends on the sensitivity and specificity of the alarms, as well as on the response of the ICU staff to the alarms. However, when large numbers of alarms are either technically false, or true, but clinically irrelevant, response efficiency can be decreased, reducing the quality of patient care and increased patient (and family) anxiety (Laramee, Lesperance et al. 2006).

It is patently obvious that physiological time series such as hemodynamic and electrophysiological data represent the physiological state of subjects in a medical environment. These time series are collected over long periods of time and are usually a source of a large number of interesting behaviors or features which have the potential to be used in identifying and predicting a subject's current and future state of health. However, the high dimensionalities and complexity of the measured physiological signals make the interpretation and analysis difficult, if not impossible. Hence, although they clearly contain useful information, these signals cannot be used directly. Extraction of such hidden information can be addressed using the concept of *feature extraction*. Essentially, feature extraction is focused on dimensionality reduction and on revealing information from the different time scales that underlie physical phenomena. Also of importance is the concept of *classification*, where the features are employed in an intelligent algorithm to classify the patient, for example, as healthy or sick. Clearly, this is a broad area with an increasingly diverse set of applications. In order to illustrate the power and utility of these methods, and given the limited space, we limit ourselves to two examples both of which illustrate feature extraction and classification approaches.

The first application discussed in this chapter is the detection of cardiac arrhythmia detection. In this application, we apply continuous wavelet transform (Daubechies 2006) and principal component analysis (Jolliffe 2002) as feature extraction tools and artificial neural network algorithm as a classifier (Caudill 1989).

The second application discussed concerns the identification of ICU patients. In this example, we apply some novel feature extraction techniques to highlight the differences between healthy and patient subjects. Then we apply fuzzy decision theory (Zadeh 1968) as a final classifier.

2. An improved procedure for detection of heart arrhythmias

The electrocardiogram (ECG) plays an important role in the process of monitoring and preventing heart attacks. The typical ECG, shown in Figure 1, consists of three basic waves: P, QRS, and T. These waves correspond to the far field induced by specific electrical phenomena on the cardiac surface, namely, the atrial depolarization, P, the ventricular depolarization, QRS complex, and the ventricular repolarization, T. It should be noted however that the ECG signal does not look the same in all the leads of the standard 12-lead system used in clinical practice.

There is increasing recognition that computer-based analysis and classification of diseases could be very helpful in diagnostics and several algorithms have been reported in the literature for detection and classification of ECG beats using artificial neural networks (ANN). It has indeed been shown that neural networks are particularly able to recognize and classify ECG signals more accurately than other classification methods (Ozbay and Karlýk 2001).

The techniques, developed for automated detection of changes in electrocardiographic signals, work by transforming the mostly qualitative diagnostic criteria into a more objective quantitative signal feature classification problem. This transformation of the ECG signals has been carried out in the past using techniques such as autocorrelation function, time frequency analysis, and wavelet transforms (WT) (Maglaveras, Stamkopoulos et al. 1998; Addison, Watson et al. 2000; Kundu, Nasipuri et al. 2000; Dokur and Olmez 2001; Saxena, Kumar et al. 2002). Results of these and other studies in the literature have demonstrated that WT is the most promising method to extract features that characterize the behavior of ECG signals in an effective manner.

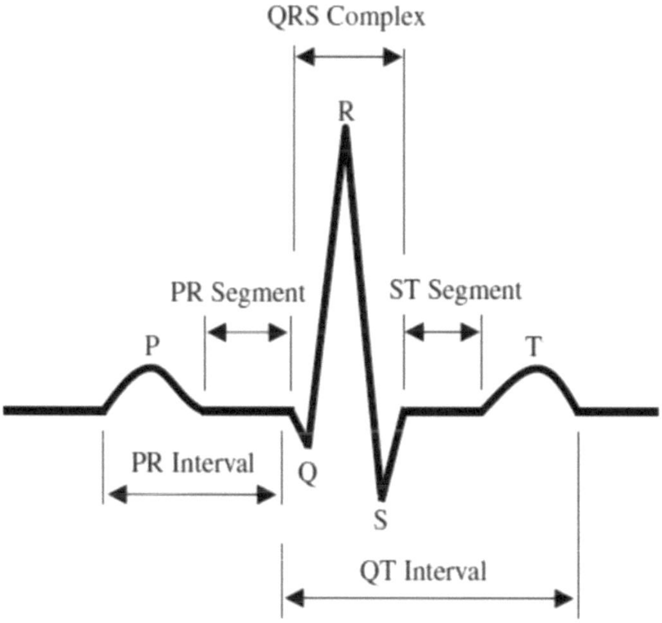

Fig. 1. The components of the ECG signal.

A study of the nonlinear dynamics of electrocardiogram signals for arrhythmia characterization was presented by Owis (Owis, Abou-Zied et al. 2002). They selected the correlation dimension and the largest Lyapunov exponent as two features for characterizing five different classes of ECG signals. The statistical analysis of the calculated features indicated that they differ significantly between the normal heart rhythm and the different arrhythmia types and, hence, can be somewhat useful in ECG arrhythmia detection. However, their study is limited by the fact that the discrimination between different arrhythmia types is difficult using those features. Application of the wavelet transform, principal component analysis (PCA) and several types of artificial neural network structures to detect and classify different kinds of heart arrhythmias have also been reported (Silipo and Marchesi 1998); this study compared results of different neural network structures in order to find the best one for the classification of specific types of arrhythmias. A neural network classifier was used by (Christov and Bortolan 2004) to recognize premature ventricular contraction arrhythmia beats in an ECG signal database. A combination of neural network and discrete wavelet transform (DWT) has also been applied for detecting four types of heart arrhythmias (Guler and Ubeyli 2005). Another application of a combination of wavelet transform and ANN in arrhythmia detection is proposed in the study by Vikas (Vikas and Sahambi 2004). In the first step, a set of discrete wavelet transform coefficients which contain the maximum information about the arrhythmia is selected from the wavelet decomposition. Then, these coefficients, in addition to the information about the RR interval, QRS duration, and amplitude of the R-peak, are fed into a multi-layer perceptron algorithm. They reach an overall accuracy of 98% in the classification of 47 patient records.

Papaloukas, et al. (Papaloukas, Fotiadis et al. 2002) used a neural network classifier to detect and classify ischemic arrhythmia episodes in the ECG signal. They also used PCA to select and extract features from the ECG signal. Lee (Lee, Park et al. 2005) applied linear discriminant analysis to 17 input features, which were based on wavelet coefficients, to reduce the feature dimension from 17 to 4, for arrhythmia detection. Then, a multi-layer perceptron classifier was applied to detect 6 types of arrhythmia beats from a 4-dimensional input feature. Foo (Foo, Stuart et al. 2002) compared and evaluated different types of multilayer neural network structures as the ECG pattern classifiers and finally settled on a two-layer feed-forward neural network. However, their work is limited to detecting only two types of patterns including normal beats and premature ventricular contractions (PVC). Acharya, et al. (Acharya, Bhat et al. 2003) proposed an algorithm based on a neural network classifier and fuzzy cluster to analyze ECG signals. They compared these two classifiers and reported the fuzzy cluster as a better classifier in comparison with the neural one. They classified 4 types of ECG signals including ischemic cardiomyopathy beat, complete heart block beat, atrial fibrillation beat, and normal beat. Also, Ozbay (Ozbay, Ceylan et al. 2006) proposed a comparative study of the classification accuracy of ECG signals using a well-known neural network architecture, a multi-layered perceptron (MLP) structure, and a new fuzzy clustering neural network architecture (FCNN) for early diagnosis; They used these two classifiers to classify 10 types of ECG signals. Based on their test results they suggested that a new proposed FCNN architecture can generalize better than ordinary MLP architecture and could also learn better and faster. The advantage of their proposed structure was a result of reduction in the number of segments by grouping similar segments in training data with fuzzy C-means clustering.

Zhang (Zhang and Zhang 2005) developed an algorithm for recognizing and classifying four types of ECG signal beats including normal beat, left bundle branch block beat, right bundle branch block beat and premature ventricular contraction PVC beat. They extracted the principal characteristics of the signals by means of the PCA technique and they showed that out of 100 principal components, the first 30 principal components have most of the total energy of the data set and hence used it as the input vector for the classifier. Among different types of classifiers, they used the support vector machine (SVM), which has exhibited very good success compared to other classification methods in complicated problems. A comparison between different classifiers is also presented in their research. A comparison between different structures for heart arrhythmia detection algorithms based on neural network, fuzzy cluster, wavelet transform and principal component analysis, was carried out by Ceylan (Ceylan and Ozbay 2007). Kutlu (Kutlu, Kuntalp et al. 2008) applied a K-nearest neighborhood algorithm for the purpose of classification. They extracted features from the electrocardiograph signals by using higher order statistics. They achieved an accuracy of 97.3% in classifying 5 types of heart arrhythmias. Cvikl (Cvikl and Zemva 2010) designed a field-programmable gate array-based (FPGA) system for ECG signal processing. Their system performs QRS complex detection and beat classification into either normal or PVC. They reached a sensitivity of 92.4% for PVC detection.

The most difficult problem faced by today's automatic ECG analysis is the large variation in the morphologies of ECG waveforms, not only of different patients or patient groups but also within the same patient. The ECG waveforms may differ for the same patient to such an extent that they could be unlike each other, and at the same time, alike for different types of beats. This is the main reason that the beat classifiers, which were reviewed in this study, perform well on the training data, while generalizing poorly when presented with the ECG waveforms of different patients (Ozbay, Ceylan et al. 2006). We address this problem of beat classifier performance by using a combination of continuous wavelet transform (CWT) and principal component analysis in order to prepare a more effective input data for the artificial neural network classifier. Since this would lead to a better input vector structure for the neural network classifier, we expect to obtain a better and more accurate performance of the classifier. Moreover, we propose to use a signal filtering method in order to remove ECG signal baseline wandering which can be further expected to improve classification.

This section is not focused on improving the processing techniques such as CWT and PCA or on improving the neural network structure. It is instead focused on designing an innovative algorithm which is a combination of these techniques in order to achieve reasonably accurate classification results in the field of heart arrhythmia detection. Although we address a better classification performance in the field of heart arrhythmia detection, another interesting achievement of this study is that the classifier in this study detects 6 types of ECG signals including the normal signal and 5 types of arrhythmia beats. This quantity of ECG signal types studied here is a much larger number in comparison with other studies in this field. The structure proposed in this section is composed of three sub stages: (a) continuous wavelet transform, which provides feature extraction; (b) principal component analysis, which performs elimination of inconsiderable features; and finally, (c) multilayer perceptron neural network, working as a final classifier.

The outline of this section is as follows; a basic definition of CWT is presented in Section 2.1. In Section 2.2 the procedure of computing principal components of a data set is provided. In Section 2.3, the designed algorithm of our study is presented with a detailed explanation. Finally, in Section 2.4, the results of our study are presented.

2.1 Continuous wavelet transform

The wavelet transform (WT) provides very general techniques, which can be applied to many tasks in signal processing. Wavelet transform can be thought of as an extension of the classic Fourier transform; the difference is that, instead of working on a single scale (time or frequency), it works on a multi-scale basis and describes the signal's frequency content at given times. This multi-scale feature of the WT allows the decomposition of a signal into a number of scales, each scale representing a particular coarseness of the signal under study.

Continuous wavelet transform (CWT) is a time-frequency analysis method which differs from the more traditional short time Fourier transform (STFT) by having a variable window width, which is related to the scale of observation. Another important distinction from the STFT is that the CWT is not limited to using sinusoidal analyzing functions (Osowski and Linh 2001); a large selection of localized waveforms can be employed as the analyzing function. The wavelet transform of a continuous time signal, $x(t)$, is defined as

$$T(a,b) = \frac{1}{\sqrt{a}} \int_{-\infty}^{+\infty} x(t) \psi^* \left(\frac{t-b}{a}\right) dt$$

where $\psi^*(t)$ is the complex conjugate of the analyzing wavelet function $\psi(t)$, a is the dilation parameter of the wavelet, which is called 'scale', and b is the location parameter of the wavelet (Osowski and Linh 2001).

2.2 Principal component analysis

Principal component analysis (PCA) has become a well-established technique for feature extraction and dimensionality reduction. An assumption made for feature extraction and dimensionality reduction by PCA is that most of the information of the observation vectors, with the dimension p, is contained in the subspace spanned by the first m principal axes, where $m<p$. Therefore, each original data vector can be represented by its principal component vector with dimensionality m (Ceylan and Ozbay 2007). This procedure decreases the data dimensionality without significant loss of information (Addison 2005). Principal components analysis has been used in a wide range of biomedical problems, including the analysis of ECG data (Silipo and Marchesi 1998; Wang and Paliwal 2003; Addison 2005; Ceylan and Ozbay 2007).

In order to apply PCA on a data set, X, the following five steps are required (Zhang and Zhang 2005; Ceylan and Ozbay 2007):

1. Subtract the mean value, μ, from each of the data dimensions.
2. Calculate the covariance matrix, S.

$$S = \frac{1}{N}\sum_{i=1}^{N}(x_i - \mu)^T (x_i - \mu)$$

where, $x_i \in X$, μ is the sample mean, and N is the number of samples.

3. Calculate the eigenvectors and eigenvalues of the covariance matrix.
4. Choose the components and form a feature vector.

In general, once the eigenvectors are found from the covariance matrix, the next step is to order them by decreasing order of the magnitude of the eigenvalue. Then the feature vector is constructed by taking the corresponding eigenvectors.

Feature Vector = (eig 1 eig 2 eig 3 … eig n)

5. Derive the new data set.

Once the components (or eigenvectors) have been chosen and the feature vector is constructed, the final data is constructed by pre-multiplying by the transpose of the feature vector as shown below.

Final Data = Row Feature Vector x Row Data Adjust

where, *'Row Feature Vector'* is the transpose of the matrix with the eigenvectors in the columns, *'Row Data Adjust'* is the transpose of the mean-adjusted data matrix, and *'Final Data'* is the final data set, with data items in columns.

2.3 Methodology

A schematic of the designed algorithm in this study is shown in Figure 2. This algorithm consists of three stages: pre-processing, main process and finally, classification of the ECG beats. The data of ECG signals used in this study are taken from the MIT-BIH ECG signal database, including normal beats and five types of different arrhythmia beats. MIT-BIH ECG signal database is a well-known standard database which has been used in many research projects reported in the literature (Silipo and Marchesi 1998; Owis, Abou-Zied et al. 2002; Zhang and Zhang 2005; Ceylan and Ozbay 2007; Cvikl and Zemva 2010). For this study, the selected types of arrhythmias are atrial premature beats (A), right bundle branch block beats (R), left bundle branch block beats (L), paced beats (P), and premature ventricular contraction beats (PVC or V).

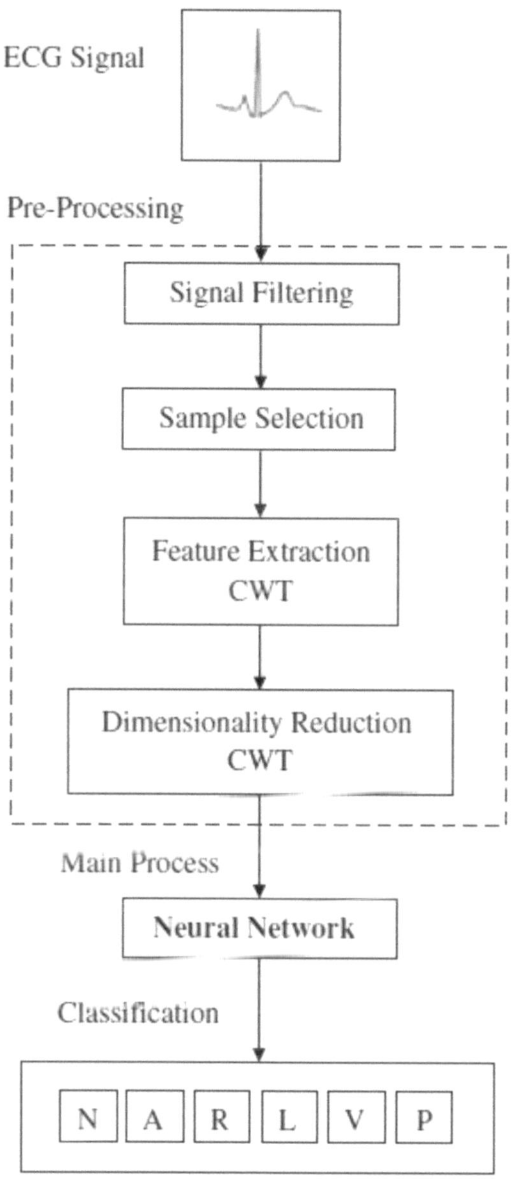

Fig. 2. Schematic of the designed algorithm

2.3.1 Pre-processing

This stage includes four levels of data processing: signal filtering, sample selection, feature extraction, and dimensionality reduction.

In the stage of signal filtering, a mathematical method presented by Ghaffari (Ghaffari, SadAbadi et al. 2006) is employed to remove baseline wandering of the ECG signal. Figures 3.a and 3.b show raw ECG signal of records 232 and 208 from the MIT-BIH database, each of which clearly exhibit baseline wandering. Figures 3.c and 3.d show the same ECG signals after applying the filtering method. It is clear that the baseline wandering has been removed, leading to a better performance of the neural classifier.

For the stage of sample selection, the suitable range of samples from the raw ECG signal was found experimentally to be 150 samples after the R wave for all types of signals, which together comprise what we call a segment. These segments are found to be an appropriate range of ECG signals which represent morphological differences between different types of ECG beats and include sufficient amount of data needed for classification of heart arrhythmias. For three types of ECG signals under study, the morphologies of ECG beats are shown in Figures 4.a - 6.a; Figures 4.b - 6.b show the selected segments of these beats.

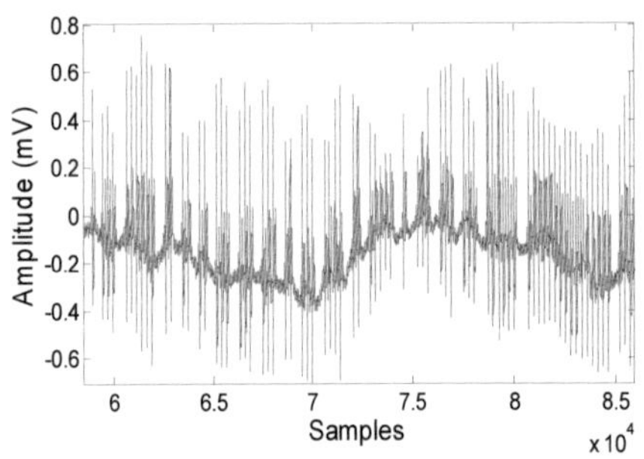

Fig. 3a. Raw ECG signal from record 232

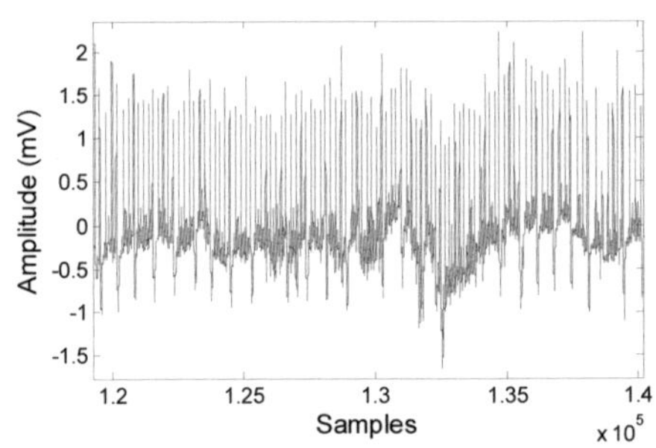

Fig. 3b. Raw ECG signal from record 208

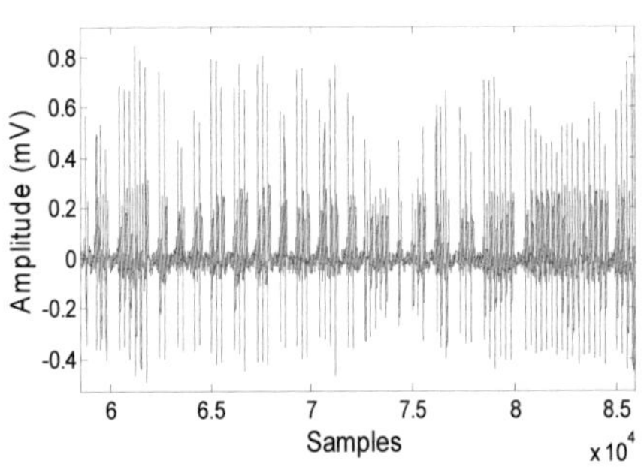

Fig. 3c. Filtered ECG signal from record 232

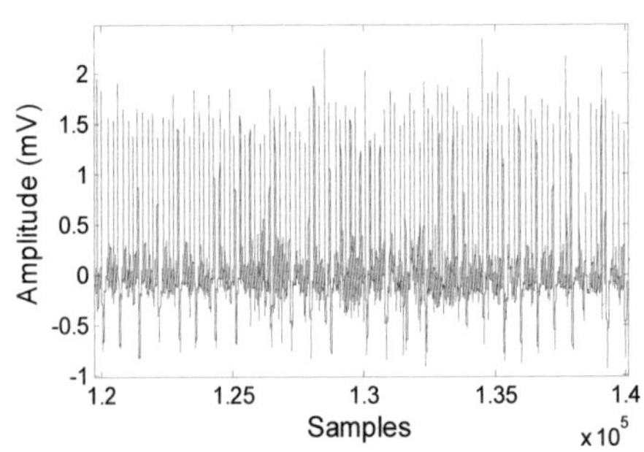

Fig. 3d. Filtered ECG signal from record 208

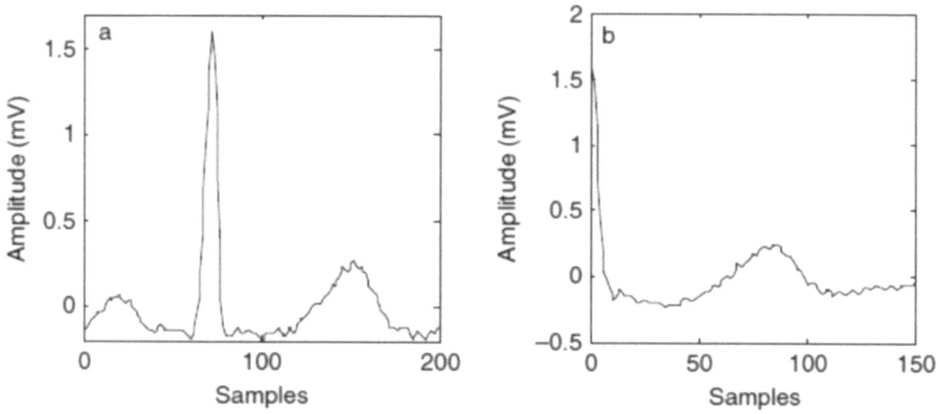

Fig. 4. (a) Normal beat, (b) selected segment for Normal beat.

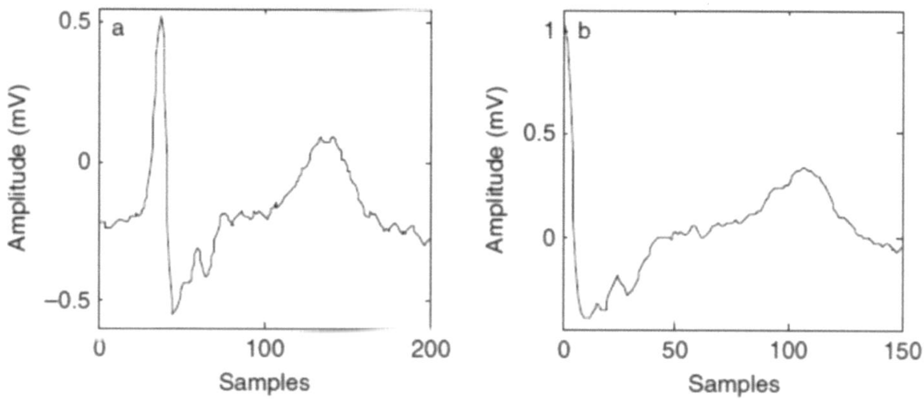

Fig. 5. (a) Atrial beat, (b) selected segment for Atrial beat.

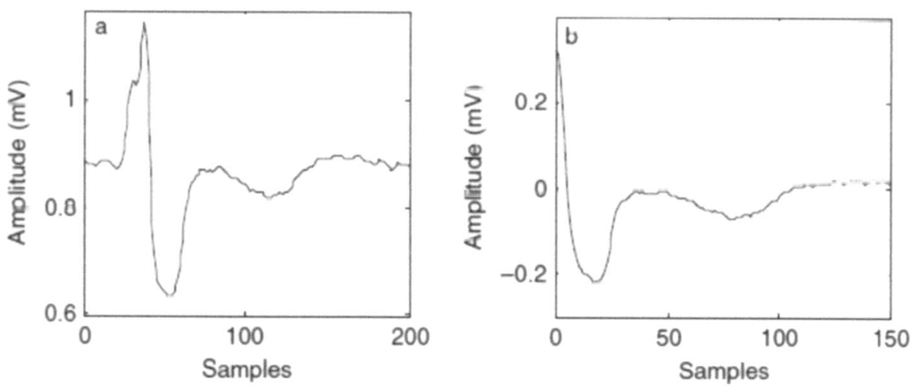

Fig. 6. (a) Right Bundle beat, (b) selected segment for Right Bundle beat.

The choice of the analyzing function in wavelet transform, which is called the mother wavelet, has a significant effect on the result of analysis and should be selected carefully based on the nature of the signal (Addison 2005). Several mother wavelets, such as Morlet and Mexican-hat, have been used in ECG signal analysis for component detection and disease diagnosis (Stamkopoulos, Diamantaras et al. 1998). Because of the harmonic nature of Morlet and Mexican-hat, they are often used for analysis of harmonic signals. These mother wavelets are not likely to be suitable options in the case of ECG signal classification. In fact, the simplicity of the computed CWT coefficients can be used as a convenient criterion to help in the selection of the mother wavelet as shown below.

Figure 7 shows a normal signal and its CWT with different mother wavelets in the scale a=10. Figure 7.a shows a normal signal beat, which has three picks. Figure 7.b shows CWT of the same signal beat with 'Haar' mother wavelet. This figure is very simple and the effects of the raw signal picks are obvious and observable. These effects can be analyzed easily and the extracted features would be suitable and appropriate for the data classification. Also, these computed coefficients can represent morphological differences very well. Figure 7.c shows CWT of the signal with 'Mexican-hat' mother wavelet. The effect of raw signal picks is not obvious in this figure and cannot be analyzed easily. Although this figure is not complicated, the extracted features do not seem to be useful for classification of the data since they are similar to each other. Figure 7.d, 7.e, and 7.f show CWT of the signal with 'Morlet', 'Daubechies8 (db8)' and 'Symlet6 (sym6)' mother wavelets, respectively. It is obvious in these figures that the computed CWT coefficients are similar to each other. Moreover, these figures are quite complicated, and the effects of raw signal picks are not obvious and cannot be analyzed easily. Therefore, the computed CWT coefficients are not suitable features for data classification, since they are similar to each other and cannot represent morphological differences very well. Hence, in this study, 'Haar' mother wavelet has been selected for feature extraction.

To compute the CWT of signals, it is not necessary to use scales in the range of 1 through 100. In view of the fact that computing CWT of signals in this range of scales will lead to a huge volume of data as extracted features, it is not advisable to use it. Instead, a specific range of scales, which is suitable and appropriate for feature extraction, is needed. The following is an analysis to determine the appropriate range of scales for the current study.

Figure 8 shows 200 samples of a raw normal signal from record 208 from MIT-BIH database and its CWT in different scales, with the 'Haar' mother wavelet. In Figure 8.a, the raw normal signal beat is shown. This signal has 3 picks, which are numbered on the figure; these picks are related to P, R, and T waves. Figure 8.b shows CWT of the signal in scale a=5. In this figure, the noise of the signal has been highlighted; however, the extent of noise is not so large as to interfere with the performance of the neural classifier, and as a result, it is possible to analyze the effect of noise of the raw signal. Moreover, the effect of picks number 1 and 3 can be analyzed to some extent. Figure 8.c shows CWT of the signal in scale a=10. In this figure the effect of the three picks is fully observable and can be analyzed completely; note that there is little noise in the figure. Figure 8.d, which shows CWT of the signal in scale a=20, has no noise and only the effect of three picks can be analyzed according to it. Figures 8.e, 8.f, and 8.g show CWT of signal in scales a=50, 80 and 100, respectively. These figures are similar to each other and neither the noise of the raw signal nor the effect of its picks can be analyzed from these figures; therefore, these figures are not useful for the analysis. It is obvious that morphological differences, which are useful and necessary for neural classifier performance, have been eliminated in these figures. Hence, these extracted features are not appropriate for the neural classifier.

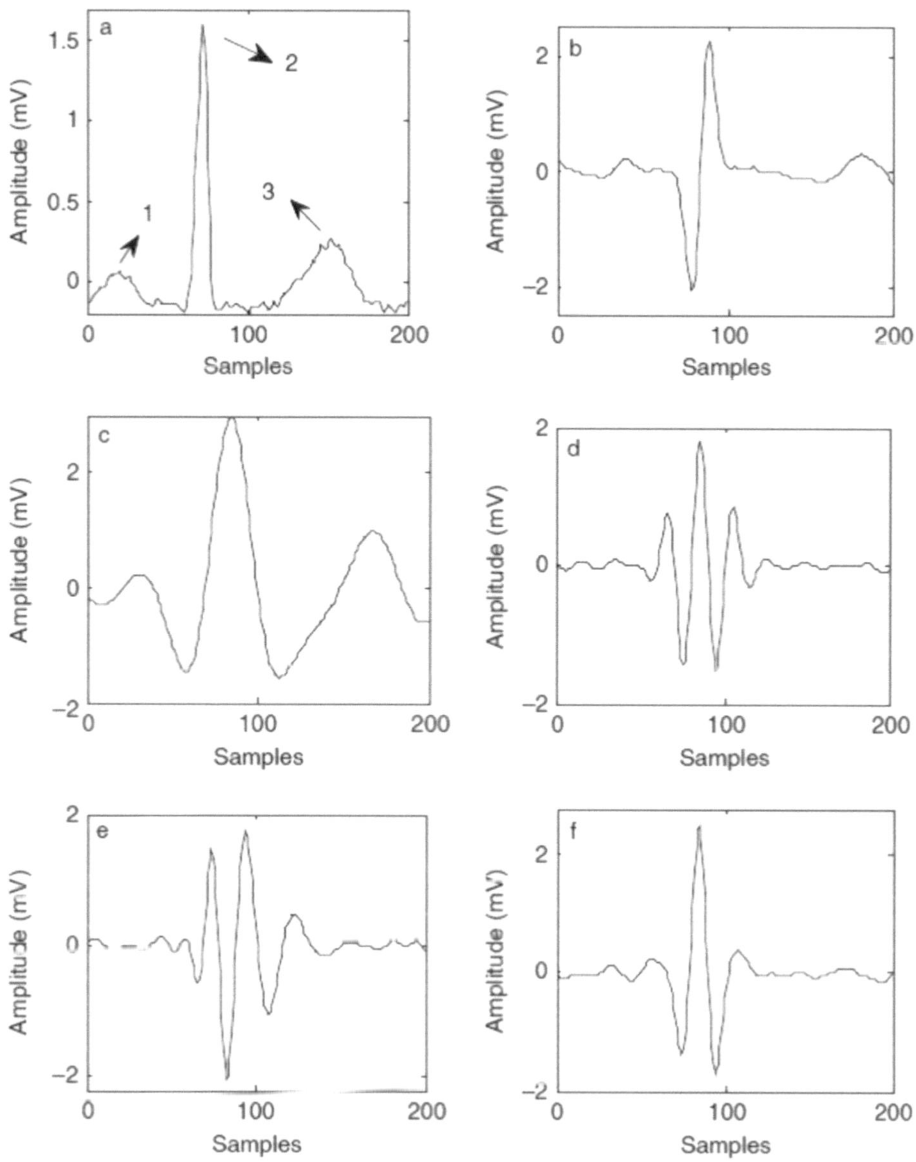

Fig. 7. (a) Normal signal beat, (b) CWT of signal with 'Haar' mother wavelet, (c) CWT of signal with 'Mexican hat' mother wavelet, (d) CWT of signal with 'Morlet' mother wavelet, (e) CWT of signal with 'db8' mother wavelet, (f) CWT of signal with 'sym6' mother wavelet.

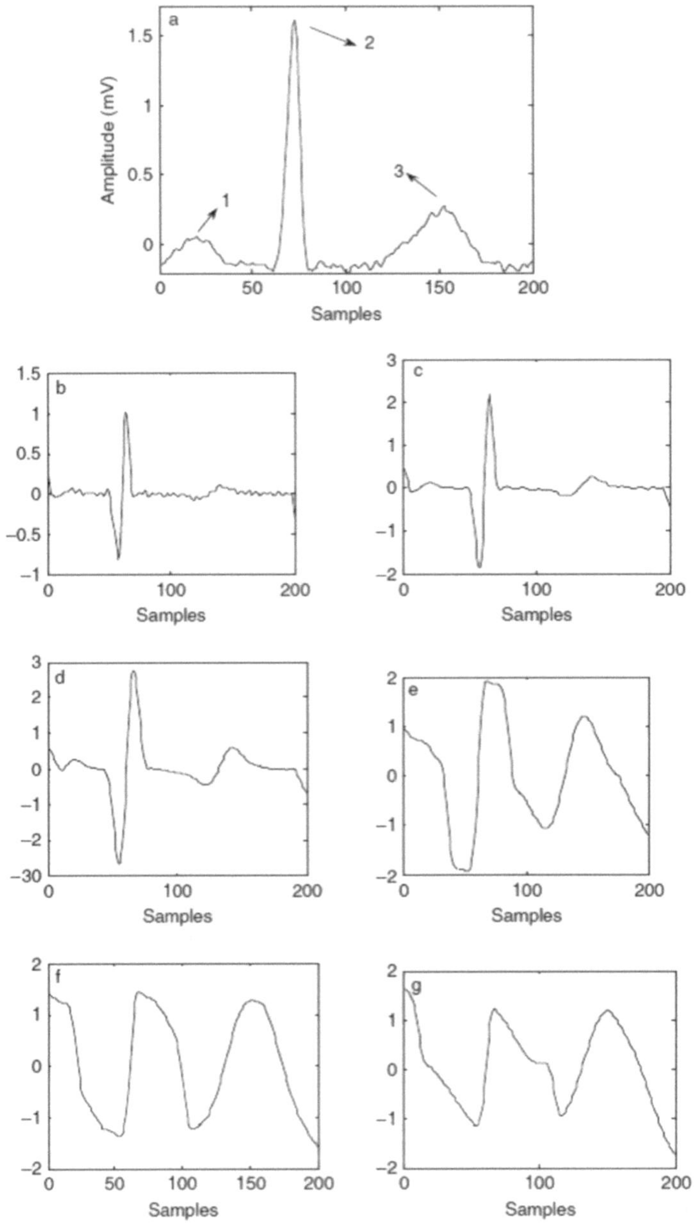

Fig. 8. (a) Raw normal signal beat, (b) CWT of signal in scale a=5, (c) CWT of signal in scale a=10, (d) CWT of signal in scale a=20, (e) CWT of signal in scale a=50, (f) CWT of signal in scale a=80, (g) CWT of signal in scale a=100.

From the above analysis, it is clear that computing CWT of the signals in the range of scales from a=5 to 20 can lead to a complete and useful analysis. Since both noise of signals and the effect of morphological differences can be analyzed in this range, the extracted features would be useful for classification of the signals under study.

In this study and for the stage of feature extraction, scales in the range of a = 6 through 15 are used that lead to matrices with 10 X 150 dimension for each segment, where each row includes the CWT coefficients in each scale. Using this range of scales has two advantages. First, by computing CWT in the range of a = 6 through 9, the ECG signal can be analyzed in detail. Second, by using the range of a = 10 through 15, the general morphology of the signal and its differences with other types of ECG signals can be highlighted.

It should be noted that computing CWT of signals in ten scales can represent morphological differences between several types of ECG signals better than computing CWT of signals in one scale only because of the fact that the differences are analyzed 10 times. This would hence be expected to result in a better performance of the neural classifier.

It would not be efficient to use a huge amount of data to perform a pattern recognition process. Hence, in the final level of pre-processing of our algorithm, PCA is applied on the computed matrices of wavelet coefficients, where each of them is a 10x150 matrixes, resulting in 10 principal component (PC) vectors.

In this study and for the stage of dimensionality reduction, the first three PC vectors have been selected and arranged as the neural network classifier input vector. This number of PC vectors was chosen according to the results which are presented in Table 1. In this table the accuracy of the neural network classifier with respect to the selected number of PC vectors is shown. According to Table 1, the accuracy of the neural network classifier increases as the number of selected PC vectors increases from 1 to 5, since, by increasing the size of data in this level and this range, the classifier will have a more appropriate set of data for classification. The accuracy of the neural network classifier decreases as the number of selected PC vectors increases from 5 to 10, since at this level, the size of the data is too much for the classifier to have a good performance. Since the difference between classification accuracy in the case of 3 PC vectors and 5 PC vectors is not that significant, we chose 3 PC vectors in order to have a reasonable accuracy, while reducing the computational effort. As a result, by selecting only three PC vectors, dimensionality reduction without significant loss of data information is achieved, leading to a better performance of the neural classifier. These results, which are based on a trial and error method, are not necessarily identical for all kinds of data and all types of algorithm structures. For any change in the algorithm, this analysis should be carried out again in order to find the appropriate number of PC vectors as a classifier input.

The prepared vectors, which are the principal components, are used as the neural network classifier input vector. The analysis for providing the input vector structure is the same for both the training and testing database.

Number of Selected PC Vectors	Classification Accuracy (%)
1	98.41 %
2	98.83 %
3	99.17 %
5	99.28 %
8	98.53 %
10	98.94 %

Table 1. Variation of classification accuracy with respect to the number of selected PC vectors

2.3.2 Main process

After finishing the pre-processing stages, data is ready as the input vector for the neural network classifier. In this study, a classical multi-layer perceptron neural network (MLPNN) structure (Silipo and Marchesi 1998; Guler and Ubeyli 2005) is used as the neural network classifier structure. This MLPNN is trained with the back propagation method of error. Selection of the neural network inputs is the most important component of designing the neural network based pattern classification since even the best classifier will perform poorly if the inputs are not selected well (Guler and Ubeyli 2005). The inputs of neural network in this study are constructed in the way which was described in previous section.

In our algorithm, we used a classical MLPNN structure with 2 hidden layers and with 60 nodes in the first hidden layer and 15 nodes in the second hidden layer for 160 iterations. The structure of this MLPNN classifier with input, hidden, and output layers is shown in Figure 9. For this structure, the training error was selected to be 0.01 in order to have precise neural network training. From all 6 types of ECG beats under study and for neural network training data, two segments have been selected and processed in the way that was described in previous section.

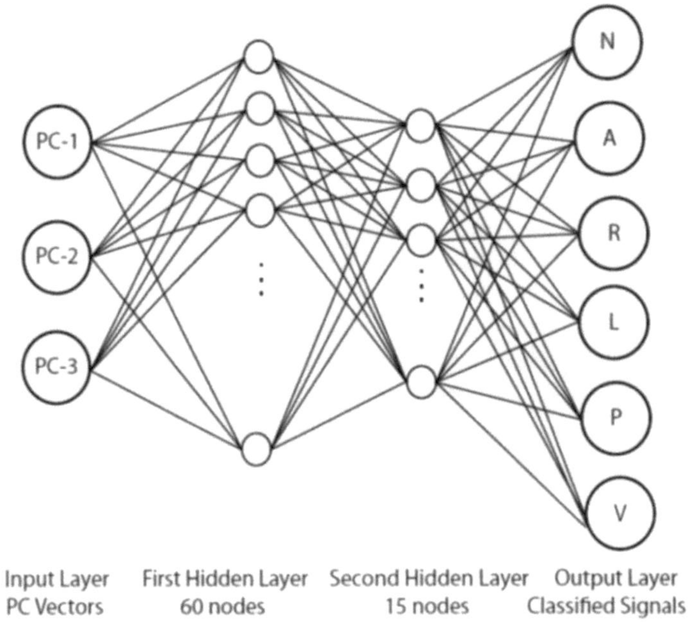

Fig. 9. MLPNN structure used as the neural classifier

2.3.3 Classification

When the neural network has been trained, it is ready as a classifier to detect and classify different types of ECG signals into one of six ECG beat groups under study. The classifier has been tested by 100 segments from each group of ECG signals. These testing segments are processed and prepared exactly like the input vector of the neural network; this means that all four levels of pre-processing stage have been applied to each segment in order to prepare it as a testing segment. These segments are used to test and evaluate the trained neural network classifier.

2.4 Results

As stated earlier, the MIT-BIH arrhythmia database is used to evaluate the proposed algorithm. To assess the accuracy of the classifier, sensitivity, positive predictive accuracy and total accuracy have been calculated. These are defined as follows:

$$Se = \frac{TP}{(TP + FN)}$$

$$PPA = \frac{TP}{(TP + FP)}$$

$$TA = \frac{TP}{(TP + FN + FP)}$$

Here, *TP* is the number of true positive detections, *FN* stands for the number of false negative detections, and *FP* stands for the number of false positive misdetections.

Table 2 shows the result of classification by the neural network. It can be seen from this table that from the whole testing data base, the classification fails only in 5 cases. According to this table, the algorithm achieves a good performance with 99.5 % *Se*, 99.66% *PPA* and 99.17% *TA*.

	Normal	Atrial premature beats	Right bundle branch block	Left bundle branch block	Paced	Premature ventricular contraction	Sum
All	100	100	100	100	100	100	600
TP	100	99	99	98	100	99	595
FN	0	0	0	2	0	1	3
FP	0	1	1	0	0	0	2
Se (%)	100	100	100	98	100	99	99.5
PPA (%)	100	99	99	100	100	100	99.66
TA (%)	100	99	99	98	100	99	99.17

Table 2. Results of the algorithm on MIT- BIH database

A comprehensive comparison between results from different studies in the field of specified ECG beat classification is very difficult since the database, signals under study, the number of arrhythmias in classification, the algorithm structure, and the data processing methods are not the same in the various studies. However, in order to present an estimate of the performance of our algorithm and our classifier we show the results of this study versus the reported results of other well-known studies in the area of selected heart arrhythmias detection in Table 3. As seen from this table, the algorithm in the present study shows reasonably accurate results, and compare favorably with other studies. The goal of this study, which was classification of ECG beats and detection of heart arrhythmias, has clearly been achieved.

	TA (%)	PPA (%)	Se (%)
Silipo et al. 1998		85 %	77 %
Papaloukas et al. 2002		89 %	90%
Foo et al. 2002	92 %	-	-
Vikas et al. 2004	-	-	98.02 %
Christov et al. 2004	-	-	99.3 %
Guler et al. 2005	96.94 %	-	96.37 %
Lee et al. 2005	-	-	98.59 %
Kutlu et al. 2008	97.3 %	-	-
Cvikl et al. 2010	-	-	92.36 %
This Study	99.17 %	99.66 %	99.5 %

Table 3. Comparison of several classifier performances on MIT-BIH database (Blank boxes have not been reported

3. A Novel technique for identifying patients with ICU needs using hemodynamic features

Modern ICUs are equipped with a large array of alarmed monitors and devices which are used in an attempt to detect clinical changes at the earliest possible moment, so as to prevent any further deterioration in a patient's condition. The effectiveness of these systems depends on the sensitivity and specificity of the alarms, as well as on the responses of the ICU staff to the alarms. However, when large numbers of alarms are either technically false, or true, but clinically irrelevant, response efficiency can be decreased, reducing the quality of patient care and increased patient (and family) anxiety (Laramee, Lesperance et al. 2006).

Medical and technical progress has extended the therapeutic possibilities of ICUs tremendously. A multitude of devices is available for monitoring and treatment in an individual assembly according to the requirements of the situation (Friesdorf, Buss et al. 1999). Due to limited physiological monitoring and a patient's individual pathophysiology, intensive care medicine has to cope with a high amount of uncertainty. Unusual circumstances caused by patients, clinicians and technology occur frequently and must be controlled and managed adequately to prevent a bad outcome and to achieve system reliability (Friesdorf, Buss et al. 1999).

Cao et al. (Cao, Eshelman et al. 2008) have used ICU minute-by-minute heart rate (HR) and invasive arterial blood pressure (BP) monitoring trend data collected from the MIMIC II database to predict hemodynamic instability at least two hours before a major clinical intervention. They derived additional physiological parameters of shock index, rate pressure product, heart rate variability, and two measures of trending based on HR and BP and they applied multi-variable logistic regression modeling to carry out classification and implemented validation via bootstrapping, resulting in 75% sensitivity and 80% specificity. Eshelman et al. (Eshelman, Lee et al. 2008) have developed an algorithm for identifying ICU patients who are likely to become hemodynamically unstable. Their algorithm consists of a set of rules that trigger alerts and uses data from multiple sources; it is often able to identify unstable patients earlier and with more accuracy than alerts based on a single threshold. The rules were generated using the machine learning techniques of support vector machines and neural network, and were tested on retrospective data in the MIMIC II ICU database, yielding a specificity of approximately 90% and a sensitivity of 60%.

Several investigations have been reported in the literature in the area of cardiovascular fault diagnosis using hemodynamic features. Javorka et al. (Javorka, Lazarova et al. 2011) compared heart rate and blood pressure variability among young patients with type I diabetes mellitus (DM) and control subjects by using Poincare plots, which are the standard tools of nonlinear dynamic analysis. They found significant reduction of all HRV Poincare plot measure in patients with type I diabetes mellitus, indicating heart rate dysregulation. The study carried out by Pagani et al. (Pagani, Somers et al. 1988) concerned patients suffering from hypertension. They showed that baroreflex gain decreases with the presence of hypertension. Blasi et al. (Blasi, Jo et al. 2003) studied the effects of arousal from sleep on cardiovascular variability. They performed time-varying spectral analyses of heart rate variability (HRV) and blood pressure variability (BPV) records during acoustically induced arousals from sleep. They found that arousal-induced changes in parasympathetic activity are strongly coupled to respiratory patterns, and that the sympathoexcitatory cardiovascular effects of arousal are relatively long lasting and may accumulate if repetitive arousals occur in close succession.

Advances in knowledge-based systems have also enhanced the functionality of intelligent alarm systems and ICU needed patient detection. Using the knowledge of a domain expert to formulate rules or an expertly classified data set to train an adaptive algorithm has proven useful for intelligent processing of clinical alarms (Laramee, Lesperance et al. 2006). Expert systems such as neural network (Westenskow, Orr et al. 1992), knowledge based decision trees (Muller, Hasman et al. 1997; Tsien, Kohane et al. 2000) and neuro-fuzzy systems (Becker, Thull et al. 1997) that encode the decisions of an expert clinician all show significant statistical improvement in the classification of alarms and ICU needed patients. Singh et al. (Singh and Guttag 2011) proposed a classification algorithm based on a decision tree method for cardiovascular risk stratification. They have shown that the decision tree method can improve performance of the classification algorithm. They have reported that the decision tree models outperform the radial basis function (RBF) kernel-based support vector machine (SVM) classifiers. Timms et al. (Timms, Gregory et al. 2011) have used a Mock circulation loop for hemodynamic modeling of the cardiovascular system in order to test cardiovascular devices, which are used in the ICU and can provide a better indication of patient's condition for nursing staff. Also, Laramee et al. (Laramee, Lesperance et al. 2006) have described an integrated systems methodology to extract clinically relevant information from physiological data. Such a method would aid significantly in the reduction of false alarms and provide nursing staff with a more reliable indicator of patient condition.

Several studies have focused on an effort to find a suitable classifier structure. Ghorbanian et al. (Ghorbanian, Jalali et al. 2011) proposed an algorithm based on a neural network classifier for heart arrhythmias detection. Their results show that the multi-layer perceptron neural network (MLPNN) structure is a strong and precise classifier. However, they used several pre-processing techniques in their algorithm to improve the performance of the NN classifier. Acharya et al. (Acharya, Bhat et al. 2003) proposed an algorithm based on a neural network classifier and fuzzy cluster for classification of heart arrhythmias. They compared these two classifiers and they reported that the fuzzy cluster is a better classifier in comparison with the neural one. Also, Ozbay et al. (Ozbay, Ceylan et al. 2006) proposed a comparative study of the classification accuracy cardiovascular diseases using a well-known neural network architecture, MLP structure, and a new FCNN for early diagnosis. Based on their test results they suggested that a new proposed FCNN architecture can generalize better than ordinary MLP architecture and also learn better and faster.

The method for classification of subjects into two categories of normal and abnormal subjects, as described in this paper, is based on the hypothesis that there should be differences between the hemodynamic data collected from normal subjects and abnormal patients. This hypothesis is constructed on the same foundation as all developed scoring methods for ICU patients. The idea behind all patient scoring methods in ICU is that critically ill patients in ICU are typically characterized by disturbance of the body's homeostasis. These disturbances can be estimated by measuring to what extent one or many physiologic variables differ from the normal range (Lacroix and Cotting 2005).

3.1 Methodology

While the proposed method in this paper shares some fundamental ideas with traditional scoring methods, it differs from them in two key areas. The first difference comes from fact that the patient scoring methods are based on the wide variety of data ranging from cardiovascular and respiratory systems to neurologic and renal systems variables. However, in our method we use a small subset of hemodynamic data, namely, HR and systolic blood pressure (SBP). The principal objection to this could be that such a small amount of data could be insufficient for identifying the patient state; the answer to this objection leads us to the second major difference of the proposed method with the scoring methods. Scoring methods just look at the data as they are being collected in the ICU, and ignore information hidden in the different time scales. In our proposed method on the other hand, this hidden information is extracted which can be expected to give us better insight into the patient's physiological condition.

The data used in this study is collected from the Physionet database. Data are collected from two databases: MIT-BIH Polysmonographic and MIMIC II databases within Physionet archive. Twenty five subjects from these databases were collected for training. For each subject, ECG signal and blood pressure waveform, in a five-hour range of the total data were collected. For the first part of the study, the HR and SBP series for each subject are derived from ECG and arterial pressure waveforms respectively.

The algorithm of the developed method of this study is shown in Figure (10). According to the proposed algorithm, in the first step and after collecting the data, four features which highlight the differences between normal subjects and patients, are extracted from data. We then define four criteria based on the extracted features. These four criteria which form the basis of our classification algorithm are: circle criterion, estimation error criterion, Poincare care plot deviation, and autonomic response delay criterion. In the next step and for the task of classification, we define three groups; namely, healthy, high risk and patient. Then we design three fuzzy membership functions for each criterion to find the subject degree of membership to each group. Finally, a scoring method is developed based on the degree of membership of each case, and subjects are classified based on this scoring method.

In the following sections, we provide a step by step description of our method, beginning with the definition of the proposed criteria.

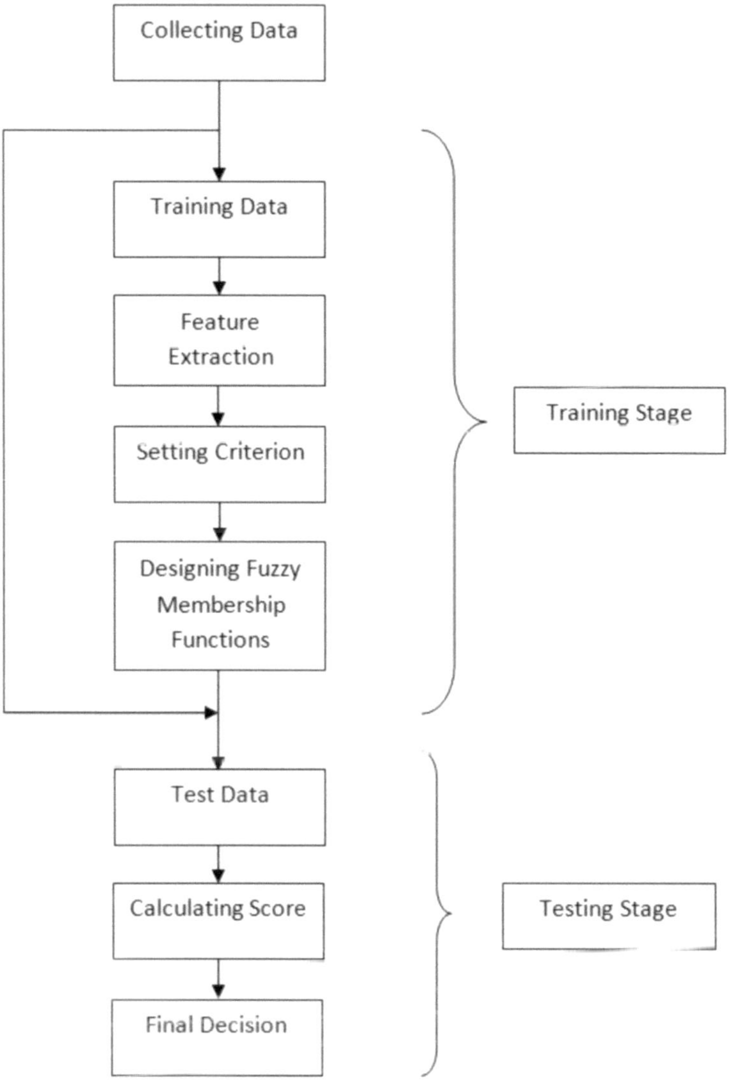

Fig. 10. Schematic of the proposed algorithm. The proposed algorithm consists of two stages: training and testing. In the training stage 25 subjects' data are used to extract features to classify patients from healthy subjects. In the test stage subjects will be divided into three predefined groups of healthy, high risk and patient, based on their assigned score.

3.1.1 Circle criterion

To evaluate the differences between healthy and patients, the SBP against HR diagram for each subject is plotted. Figure 11 shows these plots for healthy and patient cases. Clearly, the plots show a significant difference between normal subjects and abnormal patients: the data for normal subjects are concentrated, while those of the patients are scattered.

The mean value of SBP and HR for each normal subject and abnormal patient is then calculated and plotted in one diagram. Figure 12 shows the mean values for all the subjects in one diagram. The principal difference between the two groups is quite clear. This

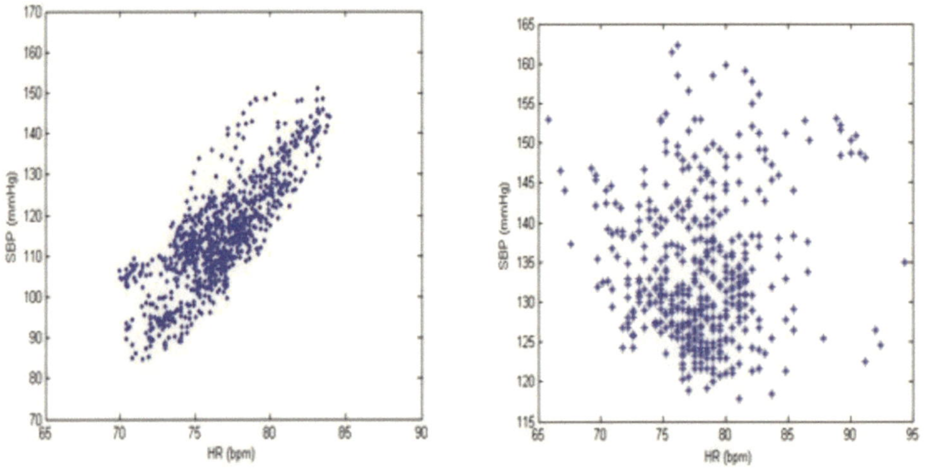

Fig. 11. SBP against HR for a healthy (left) and an abnormal (right) case

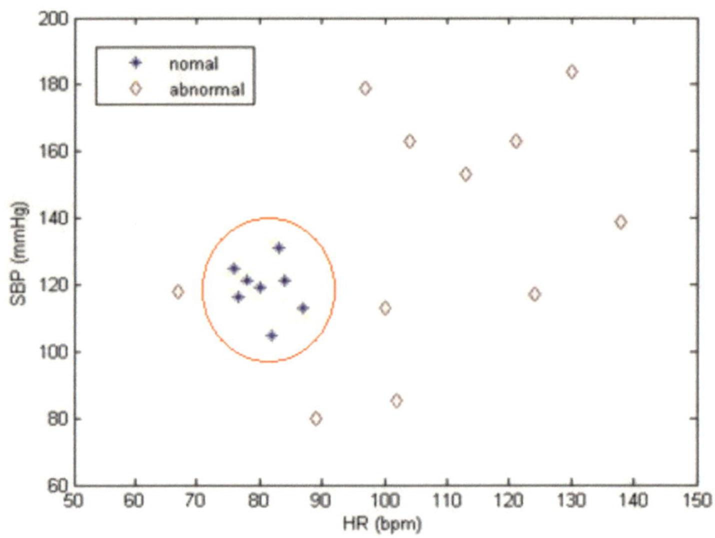

Fig. 12. Mean values of SBP versus HR for all subjects

diagram reveals the fact that there are differences between the HR and SBP data in normal subjects and abnormal ones. The plot shows that the data for the normal subjects is clustered and limited in a specific area, while those of the patients are spread out through the whole plot. The first criterion is named the "circle criterion". The center of the circle is located at point "O" where its coordinates are the mean values of HR and SBP of normal patients and, in this case, is (83, 120). The radius of this circle is calculated based on Euclidian distance between the center and the outer limit of the circle.

A given subject would be considered to be a patient if its corresponding means (HR, SBP) point is out of the healthy subject's circle (the limited area).

3.1.2 Estimation error criterion

As the second feature, a system identification method is used for the prediction of the next HR based on the current and previous HR and SBP data. A Nonlinear ARX or NARX model is employed to estimate HR series (Jalali, Ghaffari et al. 2011). NARX models in general are represented by the following equation:

$$y(t) = F\big(y(t-1), y(t-2), \dots, y(t-n_a), u(t-n_k), \dots, u(t-n_k-n_b+1)\big)$$

where, y(t) and u(t) are the output and input of the system, respectively. In Eq. (1) the matrix $[n_a \quad n_b \quad n_k]$ is the same as the order of the model. Model order is selected by use of the A-Information Criterion (AIC) method. This is the traditional method for model order selection in cardiovascular system identification research. Model order for data in this research has been calculated to be [9 6 3].

In this criterion, Artificial Neuro Fuzzy Inference System (ANFIS) structure is employed for the identification. The model has 15 inputs and one output. Membership functions for inputs are designed based on physiological facts. Since the nervous system consists of sympathetic and parasympathetic nerves, for each input, two generalized bell-shaped membership functions are assigned to designate the sympathetic and parasympathetic functions.

The system identification results are described in Table 4. The results in this table show that differences exist in the normalized root mean square error (NRMSE) with respect to the estimation of the HR for the two groups under study. In particular, the results indicate that NRMSE is smaller for normal subjects than for patients. These differences are due to the fact that the model is designed for normal subjects; thus, the output of the model for patients have higher errors than for normal subjects.

Group	Mean	Max	Min
Normal	0.193	0.238	0.119
abnormal	0.367	0.473	0.263

Table 4. Error estimation for identification of HR baroreflex

Based on these results and noting that the maximum error for healthy subject is 0.238, while the minimum error for patient is 0.263, we define a second criterion called "estimation error criterion". According to this criterion, the subject would be flagged as abnormal if the calculated error in HR estimation raise is more than 0.25.

3.1.3 Poincare plot deviation

A Poincare plot, named after Henri Poincare, is used to quantify self-similarity in processes which are usually characterized by periodic functions. This plot is commonly used in heart rate variability (HRV) analysis. The Poincare plot is a graph in which each heart rate episode is plotted as a function of previous HR, and then the line y = x is fitted to the data. In (Javorka, Lazarova et al. 2011) this method is also applied to classify patients with type I DM from healthy subjects. Drawing the Poincare plot for healthy and abnormal subjects, it is found that the deviation from the mentioned line in healthy subjects is less than in abnormal subjects. These plots are shown in Figure 13.

The deviation from the line y=x in the Poincare plot for the two groups under study is shown in Table 5. Therefore, we define the third criterion using this deviation to characterize abnormality. Based on this criterion, subjects would be called abnormal If deviation from line y=x is more than 15%.

Group	Mean	Max
Healthy	8%	13%
Patient	19%	24%

Table 5. Deviation from line y=x in Poincare plot

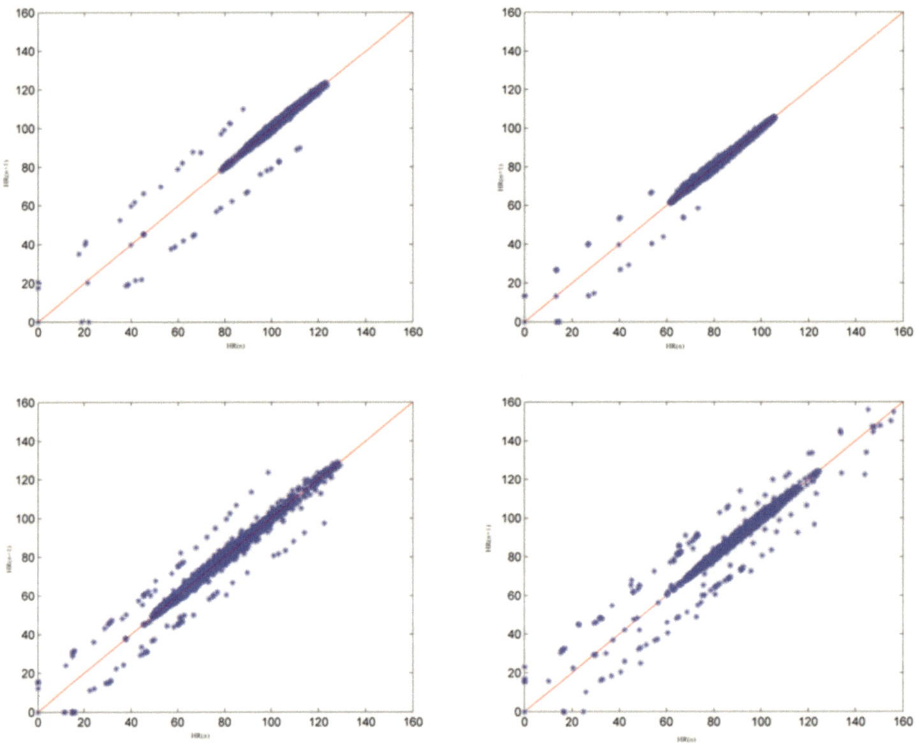

Fig. 13. Poincare plots of HR for two healthy (up) and two abnormal (down) cases. The Poincare plot is a plot of HR(n+1) vs. HR(n). Line y=x is illustrated in all pictures.

3.1.4 Autonomic response delay criterion

The normally occurring delay in the autonomic response to a stimulus has its origins in the parasympathetic nervous system. Calculating the delay for healthy subjects and patients we can infer that response delays in abnormal subjects are remarkably higher than healthy subjects. The results of calculating the delay in the autonomic response are shown in Figure 14. Fifteen abnormal patients and ten healthy subjects were involved in the training group.

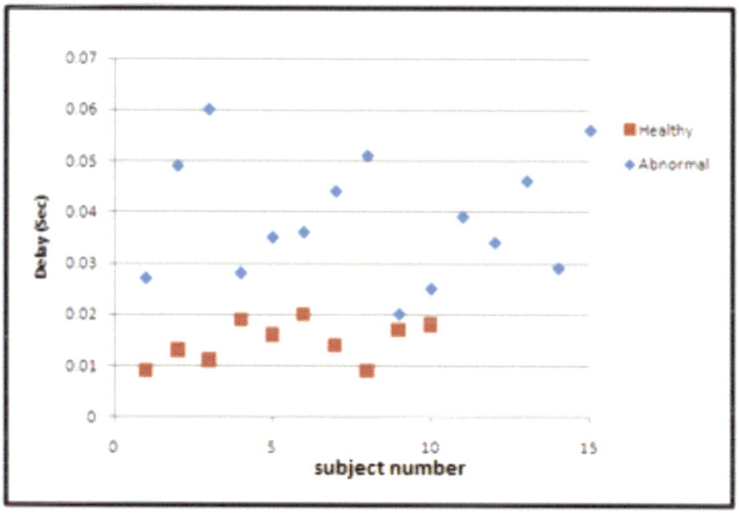

Fig. 14. Delay in autonomic response

The results of the delay calculations in the autonomic response are also represented in Table 6. Based on the above results, we define the fourth criterion where the subject is characterized as abnormal if the calculated delay in the autonomic response increases to more than 0.021 second.

Group	Mean Delay (sec)	Max Delay (sec)
Healthy	0.015	0.02
Patient	0.038	0.06

Table 6. delay in autonomic response for two groups

After deriving the four criteria discussed above, an algorithm is designed to classify healthy subjects from patients. In the following section we describe the proposed algorithm.

3.2 Scoring method and classification algorithm

Based on the evaluated criteria from training data, an algorithm is developed to automatically distinguish patients from healthy subjects. The algorithm is based on a fuzzy decision making method. First, for each criterion, three Gaussian bell membership functions are designed as an indicator of three major groups: healthy, high risk and patient. Since this algorithm is designed for clinical use and since there exists a high degree of uncertainty in clinical applications, we added the high risk groups to our predefined healthy and patient groups to account the cases that do not completely belong to the healthy or patient groups. For the training part we first made a general guess for the shape of the membership functions. The membership functions during the training round then adapt their shape parameters to the incoming data for best classification performance. Now the classifier is designed and ready for the testing stage. Figure 15 represents the adapted membership functions for each criterion based on the training data.

To test the developed algorithm, in the first step for each subject, all the mentioned features that form the basis of four criteria are extracted and used as an input for the four abnormality criteria. Then, for each criterion, the subject's degree of membership to all groups is evaluated. In this step, for each subject, we have 12 degrees of membership to the designed three groups, meaning four degrees of membership for each group. After evaluating the degree of memberships, the cumulative sum of the four degrees of membership of each group will be calculated. In this stage we have three numbers indicating subject's degree of membership to each group. We call these numbers the subject's "score" for each group. A given subject will belong to the group whose score is the largest.

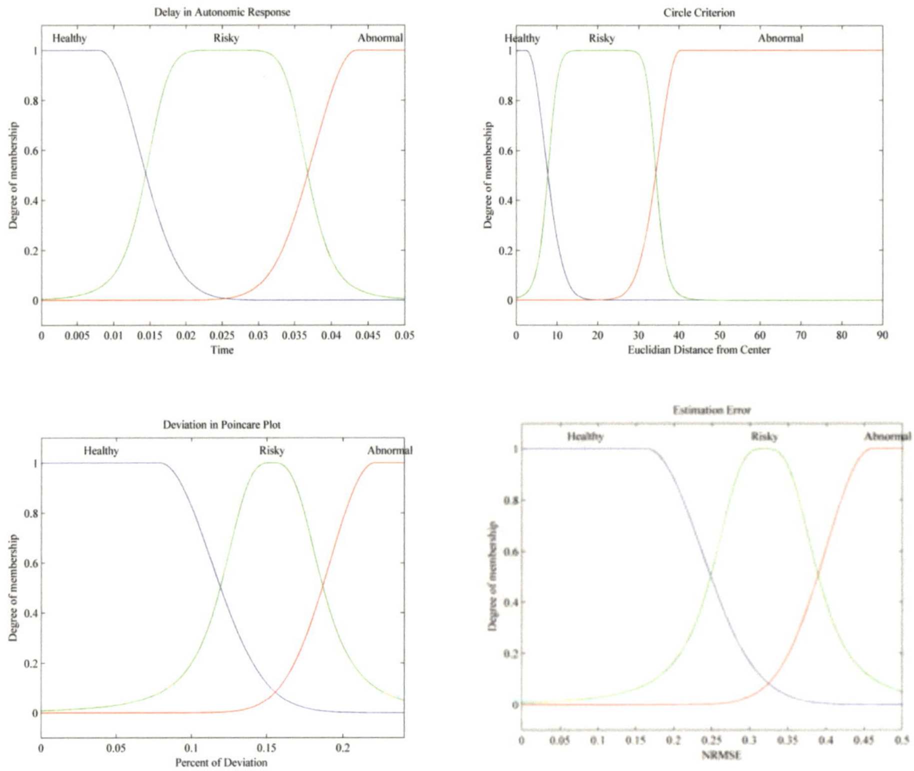

Fig. 15. The designed membership functions for each criterion

3.3 Results

From a total of seventy subject data which were collected from MIMIC II database, the algorithm was first trained with twenty five subjects including ten healthy and fifteen patients. The training data was selected randomly to avoid bias toward a specific disease. Then, three groups of subjects were tested, each group with four healthy individuals and eleven patients.

The proposed method was applied to 45 cases from Physionet database, containing 12 healthy subjects and 33 patients. From all cases, 37 cases were accurately detected, while there was one false detection. Furthermore, in five cases, a patient subject was classified as high risk and, in two cases, a healthy subject was classified as high risk.

Here, TP is the number of true positive detections, FN stands for the number of false negative detections, and FP stands for the number of false positive misdetections. Table (7) shows the overall result of the classification for all 45 cases of the 3 groups. The FP is the healthy subject who is misclassified as a high risk subject and FN is the patient who is misclassified as a high risk subject. According to this table, the scoring method of the proposed algorithm results in 86% sensitivity, 94.8% positive predictive accuracy and 82.2% total accuracy.

Group	I	II	III	All
All	15	15	15	45
TP	12	13	12	37
FN	3	1	2	6
FP	0	1	1	2
Se (%)	80	92.8	85.7	86
PPA (%)	100	92.8	92..3	94.8
TA (%)	80	86	80	82.2

Table 7. Results of testing the algorithm on Physionet database

A comprehensive comparison between the results of different studies in the field of identifying ICU needed patients by the use of hemodynamic features is very difficult since the database, signals under study, the algorithm structure, and the data processing methods are not the same in the various studies. However, in order to present an estimate of the performance of our algorithm and our classifier we show the results of this study versus the reported results of two other well-known studies in the area of ICU needed patients identifying in Table 8. As seen from this table, the algorithm in the present study shows reasonably accurate results, and compares favorably with other studies. The goal of this study, which was identifying patients with ICU needs by use of the hemodynamic features, has clearly been achieved.

Study	Se (%)
Cao et al. [1]	75
Eshelman et al. [4]	60
This study	86

Table 8. Comparison of several classifier performances on MIMIC II ICU database (Blank boxes have not been reported)

4. Conclusion

Physiological time series, including hemodynamic and electrophysiological data clearly represent the physiological state of subjects in a medical environment. Automatic detection of heart arrhythmias could be very important in clinical usage and lead to early detection of a fairly common malady and could help contribute to reduced mortality as cardiovascular disease remains the leading cause of death around the world. Hemodynamic instability is most commonly associated with abnormal or unstable blood pressure (BP), especially hypotension, or is more broadly associated with inadequate global or regional perfusion. Inadequate perfusion may compromise important organs, such as heart and brain, due to limits on coronary and cerebral autoregulation and cause life-threatening illnesses or even death. Therefore, it is crucial to identify patients who are likely to become hemodynamically unstable for an early detection and treatment of these life-threatening conditions.

In the first example of this study, the use of neural networks for classification of the ECG beats is presented. Several stages of pre-processing have been used in order to prepare the most appropriate input vector for the neural classifier. ECG signal baseline wandering is one of the most critical problems for neural classifiers, since it causes virtual morphological differences between same types of ECG beats. In this example, this wandering is removed by application of a signal filtering method which leads to better results. As the performance of the computerized ECG classification algorithms depends on the selection of the ECG features, continuous wavelet transform, which performs better than other methods, is used to extract appropriate features. Also, data dimensionality reduction is one of the most important ways of improving neural classification, since large volume of data causes problems for neural network classifier performance, and reduction in the data size is necessary for better performance of the classifier. Therefore, principal component analysis is used to achieve dimensionality reduction. Results show that PCA is more effective than other reported methods. The performance of the proposed algorithm has been shown to be reasonably acceptable and ECG beat detection and classification has been achieved. Compared to other reported work in this field, the presented algorithm shows reasonably accurate results in the field of heart arrhythmia detection.

The main advantage of this example is that, by using ten scales in computing CWT of signals, the morphological differences between several types of ECG signal are highlighted and the extracted features show the differences more clearly. Another advantage of this example is that the reduction of the dimension of data by applying PCA led to the most appropriate input vector for neural network classifier which improved the performance of the neural network classifier significantly. The main achievement of this algorithm is that the classifier in this example detects 6 types of ECG signals which include normal beats and 5 types of arrhythmia beats. Even though the number of ECG signal types considered in this example is much larger than the typical number of ECG signal types in other studies in this field, the classification results lead to a reasonably good performance.

In the second example of this study, a scoring method based on fuzzy logic and feature extraction is proposed to distinguish patients from healthy subjects. The method is based on the same principle that the ICU scoring methods follow: that of finding differences between hemodynamic data of healthy subjects and patients. Four different criteria are proposed to detect and identify patients from a group of subjects. For each criterion a fuzzy classifier is designed such that the individuals are classified into the healthy, high risk and patient fuzzy groups. In other words, a given person may have a membership grade in all three classes. A score is assigned to the subject for that group which is defined as the sum of degree of memberships to one group for different criteria. The algorithm calculates a combined criterion based on the results of the four criteria to arrive at a classification decision for each individual.

It is shown that the algorithm is highly reliable and has been able to detect correctly all members of the first group. It is also been able to detect all eleven patients in each of the next two groups correctly. Only one of the healthy members in the second and third was classified as high risk. In this example, four different criteria were proposed and used in the proposed algorithm in order to detect the abnormalities in testing subjects. From each testing subject, various features were extracted and used as input for the criteria, and based on the results of all four criteria, a decision was made about the type of subject, as to whether he/she is normal, high risk or a patient. The proposed algorithm gave reliable results in detecting the ICU needed patients but still needs to be improved. The difference between the proposed method in this example and other similar research in this field of study is that by using the presented algorithm in this example, existence of any abnormality in a patient will be found, while in most similar studies in this area, a specific abnormality is found in a patient or among a database of subjects. Therefore, our results are more general and more useful from the point of view of clinical applications. This method tends to be more detective rather than predictive, and this could be one drawback of the algorithm. Further investigations need to be carried out to render the algorithm more predictive.

5. References

Acharya, U. R., P. S. Bhat, S. S. Iyengar, A. Rao and S. Dua (2003). Classification of heart rate data using artificial neural network and fuzzy equivalence relation. *Pattern Recognition* Vol.36, No.1, (Jan 2003), pp. 61-68

Addison, P. S. (2005). Wavelet transforms and the ECG: a review. *Physiological Measurement* Vol.26, No.5, (Oct 2005), pp. R155-R199

Addison, P. S., J. N. Watson, G. R. Clegg, M. Holzer, F. Sterz and C. E. Robertson (2000). Evaluating arrhythmias in ECG signals using wavelet transforms. *IEEE Eng Med Biol Mag* Vol.19, No.5, (Sep-Oct 2000), pp. 104-109

Becker, K., B. Thull, H. KasmacherLeidinger, J. Stemmer, G. Rau, G. Kalff and H. J. Zimmermann (1997). Design and validation of an intelligent patient monitoring and alarm system based on a fuzzy logic process model. *Artificial Intelligence in Medicine* Vol.11, No.1, (Sep 1997), pp. 33-53

Blasi, A., J. Jo, E. Valladares, B. J. Morgan, J. B. Skatrud and M. C. Khoo (2003). Cardiovascular variability after arousal from sleep: time-varying spectral analysis. *J Appl Physiol* Vol.95, No.4, (Oct 2003), pp. 1394-1404

Cao, H., L. Eshelman, N. Chbat, L. Nielsen, B. Gross and M. Saeed (2008). Predicting ICU hemodynamic instability using continuous multiparameter trends, *Conf Proc IEEE Eng Med Biol Soc*, pp. 3803-3806, Vancouver, Canada, August 21-23, 2008

Caudill, M. (1989). *Neural Networks Primer*, Miller Freeman Publications, San Francisco, USA

Ceylan, R. and Y. Ozbay (2007). Comparison of FCM, PCA and WT techniques for classification ECG arrhythmias using artificial neural network. *Expert Systems with Applications* Vol.33, No.2, (Aug 2007), pp. 286-295

Christov, I. and G. Bortolan (2004). Ranking of pattern recognition parameters for premature ventricular contractions classification by neural networks. *Physiological Measurement* Vol.25, No.5, (Oct 2004), pp. 1281-1290

Cvikl, M. and A. Zemva (2010). FPGA-oriented HW/SW implementation of ECG beat detection and classification algorithm. *Digital Signal Processing* Vol.20, No.1, (Jan 2010), pp. 238-248

Daubechies, I. (2006). *Ten Lectures on Wavelet*, SIAM, Philadelphia

Dokur, Z. and T. Olmez (2001). ECG beat classification by a novel hybrid neural network. *Comput Methods Programs Biomed* Vol.66, No.2-3, (Sep 2001), pp. 167-181

Eshelman, L. J., K. P. Lee, J. J. Frassica, W. Zong, L. Nielsen and M. Saeed (2008). Development and evaluation of predictive alerts for hemodynamic instability in ICU patients. *AMIA Annu Symp Proc*2008), pp. 379-383

Foo, S. Y., G. Stuart, B. Harvey and A. Meyer-Baese (2002). Neural network-based ECG pattern recognition. *Engineering Applications of Artificial Intelligence* Vol.15, 2002), pp. 253-260

Friesdorf, W., B. Buss and M. Gobel (1999). Monitoring alarms--the key to patient's safety in the ICU? *Intensive Care Med* Vol.25, No.12, (Dec 1999), pp. 1350-1352

Ghaffari, A., H. SadAbadi and M. Ghasemi (2006). A Mathematical algorithm for ECG Signals Denoising Using Window Analysis. *Biomed Papers* Vol.151, No.73-78, 2006),

Ghorbanian, P., A. Jalali, A. Ghaffari and C. Nataraj (2011). An improved procedure for detection of heart arrhythmias with novel pre-processing techniques. *Expert Systems*2011),

Guler, I. and E. D. Ubeyli (2005). Adaptive neuro-fuzzy inference system for classification of EEG signals using wavelet coefficients. *J Neurosci Methods* Vol.148, No.2, (Oct 30 2005), pp. 113-121

Guler, I. and E. D. Ubeyli (2005). ECG beat classifier designed by combined neural network model. *Pattern Recognition* Vol.38, No.2, (Feb 2005), pp. 199-208

Jalali, A., A. Ghaffari, P. Ghorbanian and C. Nataraj (2011). Identification of sympathetic and parasympathetic nerves function in cardiovascular regulation using ANFIS approximation. *Artif Intell Med* Vol.52, No.1, (May 2011), pp. 27-32

Javorka, M., Z. Lazarova, I. Tonhajzerova, Z. Turianikova, N. Honzikova, B. Fiser, K. Javorka and M. Baumert (2011). Baroreflex analysis in diabetes mellitus: linear and nonlinear approaches. *Med Biol Eng Comput* Vol.49, No.3, (Mar 2011), pp. 279-288

Jolliffe, I. T. (2002). *Principal Component Analysis*, Springer, New York

Kundu, M., M. Nasipuri and D. K. Basu (2000). Knowledge-based ECG interpretation: a critical review. *Pattern Recognition* Vol.33, No.3, (Mar 2000), pp. 351-373

Kutlu, Y., D. Kuntalp and M. Kuntalp (2008). Arrhythmia classification using higher order statistics. *IEEE Signal Processing, Communication and Applications Conference*. Turkey: 1-4.

Lacroix, J. and J. Cotting (2005). Severity of illness and organ dysfunction scoring in children. *Pediatr Crit Care Med* Vol.6, No.3 Suppl, (May 2005), pp. S126-134

Laramee, C. B., L. Lesperance, D. Gause and K. McLeod (2006). Intelligent alarm processing into clinical knowledge. *Conf Proc IEEE Eng Med Biol Soc* Vol.Suppl, 2006), pp. 6657-6659

Lee, J., K. Park, M. Song and K. Lee (2005). Arrhythmia classification with reduced features by linear discriminant analysis. *Conf Proc IEEE Eng Med Biol Soc* Vol.2, 2005), pp. 1142-1144

Maglaveras, N., T. Stamkopoulos, K. Diamantaras, C. Pappas and M. Strintzis (1998). ECG pattern recognition and classification using non-linear transformations and neural networks: a review. *Int J Med Inform* Vol.52, No.1-3, (Oct-Dec 1998), pp. 191-208

Muller, B., A. Hasman and J. A. Blom (1997). Evaluation of automatically learned intelligent alarm systems. *Computer Methods and Programs in Biomedicine* Vol.54, No.3, (Nov 1997), pp. 209-226

Osowski, S. and T. H. Linh (2001). ECG beat recognition using fuzzy hybrid neural network. *IEEE Trans Biomed Eng* Vol.48, No.11, (Nov 2001), pp. 1265-1271

Owis, M. I., A. H. Abou-Zied, A. B. Youssef and Y. M. Kadah (2002). Study of features based on nonlinear dynamical modeling in ECG arrhythmia detection and classification. *IEEE Trans Biomed Eng* Vol.49, No.7, (Jul 2002), pp. 733-736

Ozbay, B. and B. Karlýk (2001). A recognition of ECG arrhythmias using artificial neural network, *Annual Conference of IEEE EMBS*, pp. 1680-1683, Istanbul, Turkey, 2001

Ozbay, Y., R. Ceylan and B. Karlik (2006). A fuzzy clustering neural network architecture for classification of ECG arrhythmias. *Computers in Biology and Medicine* Vol.36, No.4, (Apr 2006), pp. 376-388

Pagani, M., V. Somers, R. Furlan, S. Dell'Orto, J. Conway, G. Baselli, S. Cerutti, P. Sleight and A. Malliani (1988). Changes in autonomic regulation induced by physical training in mild hypertension. *Hypertension* Vol.12, No.6, (Dec 1988), pp. 600-610

Papaloukas, C., D. I. Fotiadis, A. Likas and L. K. Michalis (2002). An ischemia detection method based on artificial neural networks. *Artif Intell Med* Vol.24, No.2, (Feb 2002), pp. 167-178

Saxena, S. C., V. Kumar and S. T. Hamde (2002). Feature extraction from ECG signals using wavelet transforms for disease diagnostics. *International Journal of Systems Science* Vol.33, No.13, (Oct 20 2002), pp. 1073-1085

Silipo, R. and C. Marchesi (1998). Artificial neural networks for automatic ECG analysis. *Ieee Transactions on Signal Processing* Vol.46, No.5, (May 1998), pp. 1417-1425

Singh, A. and J. V. Guttag (2011). A Comparison of Non-symmetric Entropy-based Classification trees and Support Vector Machine for Cardiovascular Risk Stratification, *Annual Conference of the IEEE EMBS*, pp. 79-82, Boston, MA USA, 2011

Stamkopoulos, T., K. Diamantaras, N. Maglaveras and M. Strintzis (1998). ECG analysis using nonlinear PCA neural networks for ischemia detection. *Ieee Transactions on Signal Processing* Vol.46, No.11, (Nov 1998), pp. 3058-3067

Timms, D. L., S. D. Gregory, M. C. Stevens and J. F. Fraser (2011). Hemodynamic Modeling of Cardiovascular System Using Mock Circulation Loops to Test Cardiovascular Devices, *Annual Conference of the IEEE EMBS*, pp. 4301-4304, Boston, MA USA, 2011

Tsien, C. L., I. S. Kohane and N. McIntosh (2000). Multiple signal integration by decision tree induction to detect artifacts in the neonatal intensive care unit. *Artificial Intelligence in Medicine* Vol.19, No.3, (Jul 2000), pp. 189-202

Vikas, J. and J. S. Sahambi (2004). Neural network and wavelets in arrhythmia classification. *Asian Applied Computing* Vol.32, 2004), pp. 92-99

Wang, X. C. and K. K. Paliwal (2003). Feature extraction and dimensionality reduction algorithms and their applications in vowel recognition. *Pattern Recognition* Vol.36, No.10, (Oct 2003), pp. 2429-2439

Westenskow, D. R., J. A. Orr, F. H. Simon, H. J. Bender and H. Frankenberger (1992). Intelligent alarms reduce anesthesiologist's response time to critical faults. *Anesthesiology* Vol.77, No.6, (Dec 1992), pp. 1074-1079

Zadeh, L. A. (1968). Fuzzy Algorithms. *Information and Control* Vol.12, No.2, 1968), pp. 94-102

Zhang, H. and L. Q. Zhang (2005). ECG analysis based on PCA and Support Vector Machines, *IEEE International Conference on Neural Networks and Brain*, pp. 743-747, Beijing, China, 2005

12

Analysis of Time Course Changes in the Cardiovascular Response to Head-Up Tilt in Fighter Pilots

David G. Newman[1] and Robin Callister[2]
[1]*Aviation Discipline, Faculty of Engineering and Industrial Sciences, Swinburne University, Melbourne,*
[2]*Human Performance Laboratory, Faculty of Health, University of Newcastle, Australia*

1. Introduction

Fighter pilots are exposed to significant levels of +Gz acceleration on a frequent occupational basis (Newman & Callister, 1999). There is an emerging body of experimental research that suggests that they physiologically adapt to this frequent +Gz exposure (Convertino, 1998; Newman & Callister, 2008, 2009; Newman et al, 1998, 2000). Our previous work has shown that fighter pilots are able to maintain their cardiovascular function to a much greater extent than non-pilots when exposed to an orthostatic stimulus such as head-up tilt (Newman & Callister, 2008, 2009; Newman et al, 1998, 2000).

To further examine the mechanisms underlying these differences in cardiovascular response to +Gz, a beat-to-beat analysis of the time course of dynamic cardiovascular responses to head-up tilt (HUT) was conducted. The hypothesis was that the time course of acute changes in mean arterial pressure (MAP), heart rate (HR), stroke volume (SV) and total peripheral resistance (TPR) in +Gz-adapted fighter pilots would be different from that of non-pilots. Such differences would provide further evidence of cardiovascular adaptation to repetitive high +Gz exposure, and help to further our understanding of how this adaptation is mediated.

2. Methods

The subjects were 20 male volunteers drawn from personnel of Royal Australian Air Force (RAAF) Base Williamtown. No female subjects were recruited as the RAAF did not have any female fighter pilots at the time of the study. The control group consisted of 12 non-pilots (NP). The second group consisted of 8 current operational jet fighter pilots (FP) from RAAF Base Williamtown.

The two groups were closely matched in terms of age, height, weight, aerobic fitness level, resting blood pressure and heart rate (Newman et al, 1998, 2000). All subjects gave their written informed consent before being tested. The study was approved by both the Australian Defence Medical Ethics Committee and the Human Research Ethics Committee of the University of Newcastle. All subjects were asked to refrain from eating for 2 hours and from drinking caffeinated beverages for 4 hours prior to the test for standardisation purposes. Subjects were assigned an alpha-numeric code to maintain confidentiality.

Each subject was non-invasively instrumented for the beat-to-beat measurement of stroke volume via impedance cardiography. Four impedance cardiograph metallic band electrodes were applied to the thorax of the subject in the manner described previously (Newman et al, 1998, 2000). The leads were then attached to the impedance cardiography unit (Instrumentation for Medicine, Model 400, Greenwich, CT). Heart rate was determined via an electrocardiogram (ECG) signal generated by the impedance cardiography unit.

Data from the impedance cardiograph and other recording instruments were stored on video tape via a digital video cassette recorder (Vetter, Model 4000A, Rebersburg, PA). The video tape data were analysed using a MacLab/8s 8-channel digital chart recorder and analysis system (ADInstruments, Model ML 780, Castle Hill, Australia). MacLab Chart software (ADInstruments, Version 3.5.2/s, Castle Hill, Australia) was used to capture and analyse the digital video data.

Four cardiovascular parameters were examined in this analysis: MAP, HR, SV and TPR. MAP was calculated according to the formula MAP = DP + 1/3 (SP-DP). SV was determined using the Kubicek equation (Newman et al, 1998, 2000). TPR was calculated as MAP/(HR x SV).

The data were divided into Control (C), Anticipation (A) and Tilt (T) periods. C consisted of data from the beginning of recording until the start of A, which was defined as the 5 heart beats immediately prior to the tilting event. T consisted of the 30 heart beats from the onset of tilt. For the purposes of tracking changes across time, and for ease of description, the T period data were divided into 6 phases (I-VI) consisting of 5 heart beats each. The transition from the supine to the full $+75^0$ head-up tilt position occurred during Phase I.

Analysis of the data was performed using a statistical software package (SuperANOVA, Abacus Concepts, Inc., v1.1). Repeated measures analysis of variance with one within factor (time) and one between factor (group) was used as the test of statistical significance. An alpha level of $p<0.05$ was considered significant at the 95% confidence interval for all effects.

3. Results

Figure 1 shows the mean T period values (+ SEM) on a beat-to-beat basis for each of the four variables for both experimental groups. The mean values (+ SEM) for each group's C and A periods are shown as the first two data points. The data are divided into phases for ease of reference during description.

3.1 Responses to tilt

The NP data show an early rise (Phase I) in MAP, which then decreases to values significantly below control levels in Phase III. MAP then progressively rises to levels slightly above but not significantly different from C during the late part of the tilt (Phases IV to VI). In the FP group, MAP also rose initially during Phase I and decreases towards C values in

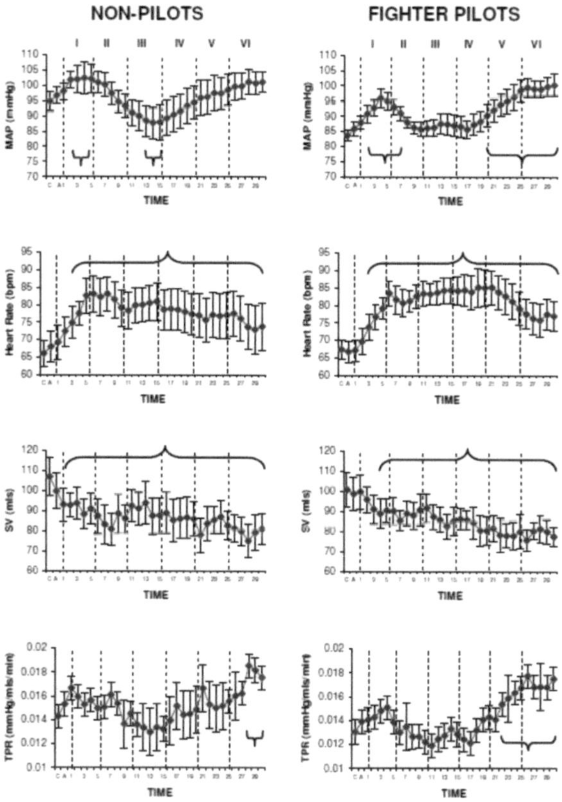

Fig. 1. Comparison of the time course of the non pilot (left columns) and fighter pilot responses to 75^{0} HUT across time. The first two data points on each plot are C and A values. The bracketed areas on each curve represent areas of significant difference ($p<0.05$) from C.

Phase II. Phase III of the FP MAP response is clearly different from that of the NP group, with MAP plateauing and never falling below the C level. Early in Phase IV, MAP rises progressively, reaching values in Phases V and VI significantly greater than the C level.

HR is elevated significantly above C in both groups within four heartbeats of tilt. In NP, HR rises immediately during Phase I, is sustained at this level during Phase II and then progressively decreases slowly towards C levels in Phases III to VI. HR is significantly different from C for most of the tilt period. In FP, HR also increases in Phase I, begins to decrease in the early part of Phase II but then increases again by the end of Phase II, and remains significantly elevated throughout Phases III and IV, reaching maximum elevation at the junction of Phases IV and V, then begins to decrease back towards C values.

In NP, SV falls precipitously at the onset of tilt, then increases slightly during the later part of Phase II and the early part of Phase III. SV then progressively decreases again, although at a slower rate in Phases III to VI. SV in the FP group falls in Phase I, but not as immediately or to the same extent as the NP group. It recovers a little in Phase II, then progressively decreases in later phases. Like the NP group, this late-phase decrease occurs at a slower rate than in Phase I.

In NP, TPR increases initially during Phase I, then decreases to levels below C values by the middle of Phase III. Phases IV to VI are marked by progressive increases in TPR to values significantly above C values by Phase VI. In FP, TPR rises during Phase I, then decreases below C values during Phase II. Phase III is marked by a small recovery in TPR, which is not evident in the same phase in the NP group. TPR increases throughout Phases IV to VI, becoming significantly different from C values earlier than in the NP group.

3.2 Group comparison

Figure 2 plots the T deviation from C values for each of the four cardiovascular variables, again divided into the same 6 phases. The analysis was performed on individual data points, although these and the error bars have been removed from the figure, purely for ease of visualising the comparison between the groups across time. This series of curves demonstrates the relative contribution of these variables to the observed time-based changes in cardiovascular dynamics.

The MAP curves show a similar overall pattern of response to tilt, although a significantly greater response is seen in the FP group to the same gravitational stimulus ($p<0.05$). The FP group maintains MAP above C values at all times, and in the second half of tilt MAP values are significantly higher than those of the NP group.

The HR curves are similar for each group, although in the later phases the group responses tend to diverge, with the FP group demonstrating a more sustained elevation. In this group, HR is maintained at its peak level until the early part of Phase V, when it begins to decrease. In the NP group HR begins to decrease in Phase II, although it remains elevated above control levels throughout tilt.

There is no statistically significant difference in the SV response to tilt of the two groups, although the initial rate and magnitude of decrease in SV appears less in the FP group.

The TPR curves show similar patterns, rising initially, then decreasing and rising again in Phase V in both groups. The FP group shows a more marked late-phase rise in TPR, which is of greater magnitude than that in the NP group, and coincides with the FP's fall in HR during Phase V. This rise in TPR becomes significantly different ($p<0.05$) from C values earlier in the FP group.

4. Discussion

The results of this analysis show similar overall patterns of response between the two groups. There are some key differences, however, in terms of the timing and magnitude of the responses. These are just sufficiently different that they produce statistically significant and physiologically meaningful differences in the MAP response between the two groups.

The NP response to HUT is the normal, well-documented human response to upright posture. On assuming the upright position, there is an initial, transient HR- and TPR-mediated rise in MAP, then both MAP and venous return fall in accordance with the applied hydrostatic force. The fall in these parameters activates the baroreceptors, both the high-pressure arterial baroreceptors and the low-pressure cardiopulmonary baroreceptors. This leads to activation of these negative feedback regulating systems and a subsequent restoration of MAP and venous return towards normal levels (Mancia & Mark, 1983).

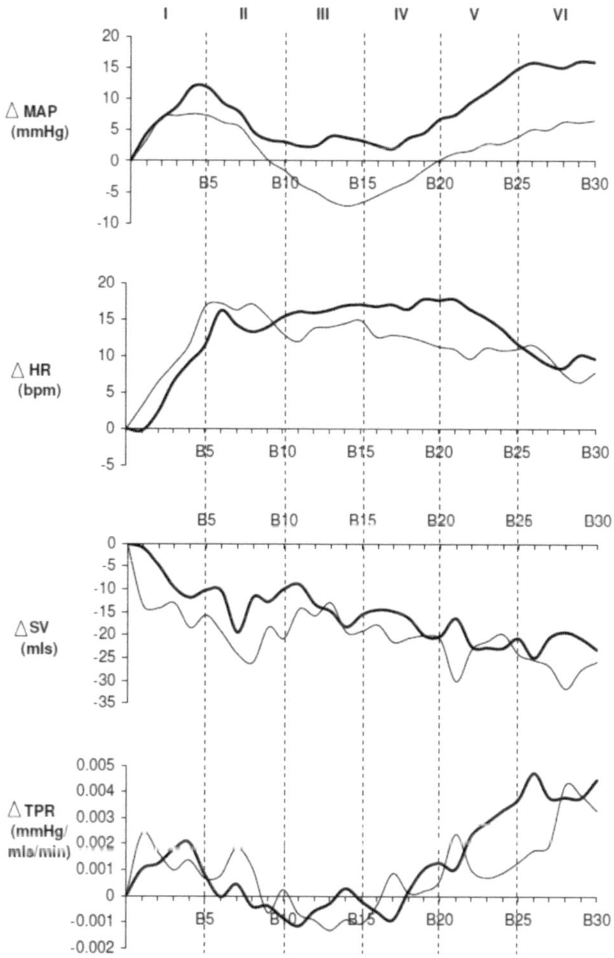

Fig. 2. Comparison of the change from control values across time of the non-pilots (thin line) and fighter pilots (thick line) in response to 75⁰ HUT. Data are mean values. SEM bars have not been drawn. The time course has been divided into 6 phases of 5 beats each, labelled I to VI (details in text).

The FP response is an adapted or modified version of the NP response. Analysis of the different phases of the groups' responses to tilt provides important information as to the mechanisms that are active during the sequence of events. The focus of this discussion will be on the integration of cardiovascular control inputs.

4.1 Cardiovascular regulation

There are four possible inputs used in the regulation of the cardiovascular system under conditions of orthostatic stress such as HUT. Firstly, there may well be some cognitive or psychological input to the autonomic nervous system at the onset of a rapid tilt or postural change, and in anticipation of this impending event. This heightened sense of arousal or alerting reaction would produce an increase in HR, vasodilation in some vascular beds (e.g., skeletal muscle) and vasoconstriction in others (e.g., gastrointestinal tract and kidneys). The rapid, almost immediate increase in HR (due to parasympathetic withdrawal) will shorten cardiac ejection time, which will in turn contribute to a fall in SV. These changes reflect an overall shift in the autonomic balance in favour of the sympathetic system. The net effect is an increase in arterial pressure (Mancia & Mark, 1983).

The arterial baroreceptors also have a well established influence on the cardiovascular system under orthostatic stress (Mancia & Mark, 1983). The overall effect is also a shift in the autonomic balance, with the sympathetic system becoming more dominant. HR increases due to parasympathetic withdrawal, while cardiac contractility and total peripheral resistance both increase due to greater sympathetic drive. A more forceful, rapid ejection of blood with higher vascular resistance results in an overall boost in mean arterial pressure. The time taken for cardiac contractility and vascular resistance to increase is much longer than that for HR, due to these sympathetically-innervated tissues taking longer to respond to neural command signals.

During HUT the aortic and carotid baroreceptors will be stimulated to different extents, based on their respective distances from the heart. In this experiment, arterial pressure was recorded effectively at aortic level, and as such does not reflect the changes occurring at the level of the carotid baroreceptors. HUT to $+75^0$ would lead to a decrease in carotid distending pressure providing a stimulus for cardiovascular compensation to drive up mean arterial pressure.

The third input source is from the cardiopulmonary baroreceptors, on the low-pressure side of the circulation. Changes in hydrostatic force will affect not only the arterial baroreflexes but also the cardiopulmonary reflexes. On standing (i.e., on exposure to the +Gz axis) central venous pressure, venous return, stroke volume and cardiac output all decrease. The drop in central venous pressure and venous return leads to activation of the cardiopulmonary baroreflexes, and subsequent reflex increases in HR and TPR. Again, HR changes will be rapid (within 1 to 2 seconds) while vascular resistance changes will take several seconds to become evident after the stimulus.

Fourthly, the vestibular system may also be involved in regulation of the cardiovascular system via the vestibulosympathetic reflex (Doba & Reis, 1974; Essandoh & Duprez, 1998; Ray et al, 1997; Shortt & Ray, 1997; Yates, 1992; Yates & Miller, 1998). The vestibular system will signal the dynamic postural change taking place, which may be supplemented by ocular inputs (the vestibulo-ocular reflex). The state of the cardiovascular system may then be altered by the action of the VSR, which may provide feed-forward adjustment of arterial pressure during dynamic postural change.

The efferent output of the vestibulosympathetic reflex will be reflected in changes in vascular resistance, based on experimental findings in animals and humans (Doba & Reis, 1974; Essandoh & Duprez, 1998; Ray et al, 1997; Shortt & Ray, 1997; Yates, 1992; Yates & Miller, 1998). The time course of changes in vascular resistance will be in the order of several seconds. A change in HR is not likely, given that this has not been reported as a feature of VSR activity.

4.2 Experimental findings

The phases seen in Figures 1 and 2 are in 5-beat intervals, which amount to approximately 4 to 6 seconds. Due to the inherent time lags in the tissue response to efferent signals of the neural control mechanisms responsible for cardiovascular regulation, the effect in a particular phase is generally a response to a stimulus that occurred in the previous one to two phases.

4.2.1 Anticipation period

During the 5-beat anticipation period, there may be changes occurring in the cardiovascular system due to an alerting response to the impending postural challenge. These changes will result in an increase in HR and changes in regional vascular resistance. While the HR change will occur rapidly, the changes in vascular resistance will take longer to develop. As such, changes in TPR due to arousal prior to tilt are likely to be seen in the tilt period phases rather than within the anticipation period itself.

4.2.2 Phase I

Phase I coincides with the dynamic phase of tilt, in which the postural change is made from 0^0 to $+75^0$. During this phase MAP rises almost immediately in both groups, and reaches a maximum at the conclusion of this phase. This rise in MAP is due to observed increases in both HR and TPR, since SV falls immediately in both groups during this phase.

Which of the four control inputs discussed above is responsible for driving the increase in HR during Phase I? An increase in arousal at the onset of HUT could account for this observed increase in HR, given that the temporal characteristics of this increase closely mirror the time taken to achieve the full HUT position (approximately 4 seconds). The HR changes seen in this early phase of HUT may be due to these arousal effects alone, and mediated by withdrawal of parasympathetic control. The fact that the FP group experienced a smaller increase in HR during Phase I could reflect a lower level of psychological arousal than in the NP group, due to the former's frequent exposure to a dynamic motion environment. This is supported by the FP group having little anticipatory rise in HR compared with the NP group, whose HR increased in anticipation of impending tilt.

The change in HR could be due to the action of the arterial or cardiopulmonary baroreflexes. However, these reflex arcs must be stimulated first, and as such some postural change must take place before baroreflex-mediated increases in HR occur. There is not likely to be a stimulus to the high- or low-pressure receptors until at least midway through this phase. Baroreflex-mediated HR increases are thus unlikely to be seen until the end of Phase I. HR increases immediately in both groups, well before the full head-up tilt position is reached, which suggests that other inputs such as arousal are responsible for the early Phase I HR increases.

Since there is no established connection between vestibular control of the cardiovascular system and HR changes, the action of the VSR is not likely to be responsible for the increase in HR.

The increase in TPR in this phase is interesting, given that changes in vascular resistance take time to occur after the initiating stimulus. The stimulus for this increase must be something that occurred prior to tilt, such as the alerting response to impending postural change.

This increase in TPR in both groups during Phase I is important, as it combines with the HR increase to boost MAP. There are several speculative explanations for this phenomenon. The first reflects the changes in vascular resistance effected by the increase in arousal during the anticipation period. Since these changes take time to develop, they may not be evident until Phase I. Vasoconstriction of some regional vascular beds (such as renal and splanchnic regions) occurs as a consequence of increased arousal. Due to the low level of skeletal muscle vasoconstrictor drive in the horizontal resting position of the anticipation period, there is likely to be little additional vasodilation occurring in these vascular beds as a result of arousal. The net result of these changes would be an increase in TPR due to the anticipatory stimulus, which is seen in Phase I.

The second explanation involves the vestibular system and its influence on the cardiovascular response to HUT. The activation of a vestibulosympathetic reflex due to the dynamic postural changes as HUT proceeds may facilitate the observed increases in TPR during Phase I. The vestibular system is in effect responding in a dynamic fashion to the postural change stimulus. The time course of this phenomenon is in accord with experimental findings that vestibular stimulation can evoke sympathetic discharges within 100 milliseconds (Yates, 1992). However, the response of vascular smooth muscle will take longer to occur, and changes in resistance values will take longer again (in the order of several seconds). The vestibular system could initiate vascular resistance changes, but these would probably not occur until late in Phase I at the earliest.

The third possible explanation may be a mechanical feature of the blood vessels themselves. As HUT proceeds, the hydrostatic force will progressively dump more blood into the dependent lower limb vessels. This sudden increase in vascular volume as HUT occurs may initiate a smooth muscle reflex in the blood vessels, in keeping with the length-tension relationship of muscle. Such a short-lived response may lead to the transient increase in TPR seen during Phase I.

The postural changes in Phase I will eventually lead to stimulation of the arterial and cardiopulmonary baroreceptors, particularly late in Phase I when the full HUT position is reached. However, the time interval involved during Phase I is too short for arterial and cardiopulmonary baroreceptor activity to have much effect in this phase. Efferent output from these baroreflexes will be seen in later phases.

What is responsible for the precipitous fall in SV during Phase I? In the NP group, SV falls in the anticipation period, reflecting a shortened ejection time as a consequence of increased HR. HR continues to increase throughout Phase I, which will exacerbate the fall in SV. As the tilt progresses, more hydrostatic force is generated. This is unlikely to be a significant input to the cardiovascular system until the second half of Phase I, and it is only at the end of the phase that it becomes maximal, once the full HUT position is achieved. The dramatic falls in SV observed in Phase I are thus due to the combination of HR changes due to the arousal effects from the anticipation period (early in Phase I) and progressive increases in hydrostatic force reducing venous return.

SV falls less in the FP group during Phase I than it does in the NP group. As a result, MAP reaches a higher peak value for the same effective increase in TPR as the NP group, while the increase in HR is slightly slower. What could account for this better SV performance in the FP group? There are two possibilities. The FP group did not have a significant fall in SV or a rise in HR during the anticipation period. As a group they begin Phase I in a better cardiovascular state. This would help defend SV against further falls due to a developing hydrostatic force. Another explanation may be an expanded circulating blood volume in the FP group. An expanded blood volume would also help to preserve SV in the face of an orthostatic challenge. There is emerging evidence that such blood volume expansion does occur in +Gz-trained individuals (Convertino, 1998). In the FP group, the important effect of even slightly improved SV performance is a greater value of MAP during this early dynamic postural change.

Therefore, it appears that the changes in HR and TPR seen in Phase I are due to the effects of a prior alerting reaction in anticipation of an impending postural change. Although the FP group has less HR rise during this phase, it is able to generate a higher level of MAP due to enhanced SV performance.

4.2.3 Phases II and III

Phase II begins with the full HUT position having been achieved. Phases II and III are marked by the progressive effects of the hydrostatic force on the cardiovascular system, and the system's attempts to compensate for these effects.

MAP falls in both groups from the peak value in Phase I towards C values. In the NP group it falls well below the C value, reaching a minimum in the late part of Phase III. In contrast, the FP response to tilt in these phases is clearly different from that of the NP group. MAP plateaus, and remains at or slightly above C levels during both phases. The difference in MAP response in Phase III is the most striking and fundamental difference between the responses of the two groups. During Phases II and III, the two groups' MAP responses diverge considerably from each other, whereas in Phase I they tracked relatively closely.

What is driving MAP down during these two phases? Heart rates in both groups during Phase II are similar, remaining at the elevated levels achieved in Phase I for most of Phase II. HR then tends to decrease during Phase III in the NP group, but increases slightly in the FP group during this phase. If the Phase I rise in HR was due to the autonomic effect of increased psychological arousal, the fact that HR tends to remain at the same elevated level during Phase II in both groups suggests that the arousal effect cannot increase HR any further. This is especially true given that arousal levels tend to be higher in the upright position compared with the supine or prone positions. HR presumably decreases towards C values in the NP group due to arousal no longer being the dominant stimulus to the cardiovascular system. The FP group, however, goes on to a further sustained HR increase during Phase III. What is responsible for this rise, which is quite different from the NP response? Further increases in HR may be due to the developing action of the arterial and cardiopulmonary baroreflexes, as a result of the ongoing effect of hydrostatic pressure. The fact that this occurs in the FP group and not in the NP group may well reflect a difference in the operating characteristics of the baroreflex in the FP group. This would suggest an enhanced level of baroreflex activity on modulation of HR.

SV continues to decrease in both groups during Phases II and III, despite a transient recovery in SV which occurs at a similar point in both groups, around the junction of Phases II and III. This temporary increase in SV may well reflect an increase in cardiac contractility, as a countermeasure against the orthostatic challenge of HUT. There is little difference in either the time course or magnitude of this contractility change between groups. This increase in contractility is mediated by the baroreflexes (arterial and cardiopulmonary). Assuming that the stimulus for this is the consequence of the full HUT position, the time course for this contractility increase would fit with the operating characteristics of cardiac tissue. Eventually, of course, this increase in contractility is unable to effectively counteract the ongoing deterioration in VR due to the upright position, and SV continues to fall.

TPR falls in both groups back to C values during Phase II after peaking in Phase I. It then effectively plateaus during Phase III. This is likely to be a reflection of the changes occurring due to the alerting reaction developed in the anticipation period. The lack of significant vasoconstrictor drive generated by the alerting reaction in the supine position is now being realised in Phases II and III. Although there may be a small contribution from vasodilation of skeletal muscle beds to this fall in TPR, it is the time lag in developing adequate vasoconstriction that is more likely to be responsible for this overall reduction in TPR. As vasoconstriction develops in Phase III, further decline in TPR is arrested. This considerable time lag between afferent input and efferent output is consistent with the operating characteristics of vascular resistance changes. The effect of arousal-induced changes in regional vascular resistance is the most likely explanation for the observed decline in TPR.

While the arterial and cardiopulmonary baroreceptors would clearly be stimulated by the decreases in MAP and VR, especially in the NP group, their ability to effect a change in vascular resistance is not evident for some time due to their inherent inertia and latency of operation. The baroreflexes are likely to contribute towards arresting further decline in both MAP and TPR and driving them up again by the very end of Phase III, but will exert their efferent effects predominantly in subsequent phases of tilt.

In both groups, the fall in MAP appears to be due to a decrease in TPR, despite the sustained increase in HR. TPR plateaus in both groups presumably due to the developing action of the baroreflexes that were initiated in Phase I. In the FP group, the fall in MAP that occurs during Phase II is arrested during Phase III by the combination of a sustained increase in HR and an increase in cardiac contractility. These increases compensate for any vasodilation-induced decrease in TPR and the ongoing deterioration in SV. Phase III demonstrates that the FP group is much better able to defend MAP against the fall in VR and SV caused by sudden exposure to an orthostatic challenge than the NP group.

4.2.4 Phases IV to VI

Phases IV to VI, the late stages of HUT, show a progressively stabilised picture, with no dynamic postural changes occurring. Hydrostatic force is constant, and the efferent outputs of all the stimulated control mechanisms are now operative. MAP rises in both groups throughout these three phases, largely due to increases in TPR. In the NP group, it is not until the end of Phase IV that MAP is restored to C levels, mediated largely by increases in TPR. In the FP group, MAP is boosted in mid-Phase IV via a combination of HR and TPR increases. HR reaches its maximum value in FP during Phase IV, but as these last three phases progress, HR decreases. TPR increases significantly and as such assumes the dominant role in maintaining MAP.

The rise in TPR is almost certainly due to the activity of the arterial and cardiopulmonary baroreflexes. These reflexes were initiated during Phase I, with the onset of the dynamic postural change. Another reflex that will have been stimulated is the vestibulosympathetic reflex. The VSR is likely to respond to the dynamic inputs of postural change, as these may have cardiovascular consequences that the VSR is presumably designed to modulate and counter.

Clearly it has taken a long time for the vascular resistance changes to occur following this initial stimulation. This is consistent with what is known about the operating characteristics of the sympathetically-mediated vascular resistance changes. The FP group's rise in TPR occurs basically at the same time as that of the NP group. This suggests that any adaptation to +Gz does not extend to shortening the time lag involved in effecting a change in vascular resistance. This may reflect a mechanical limitation in the system. Indeed, this fact helps explain why fighter pilots continue to rely on the anti-G suit, which will boost peripheral resistance almost immediately after the onset of +Gz acceleration. The FP group's TPR rise is, however, steeper than the NP group, and reaches a maximum value earlier. This reflects an increased gain.

Another contributing factor to the increase in TPR may be the putative feed-forward function of the VSR. After detecting a postural change, the vestibular system may send an excitatory signal to the medullary vasomotor centre to effect a change in vascular resistance before the efferent arm of the arterial baroreflexes becomes fully active. Such a feed-forward mechanism would clearly be an advantage to the pilot operating in the high +Gz environment. A point worthy of note is that although the vestibular input has changed from the dynamic input of Phase I to a stable static input in the full HUT position, it is likely that this static input continues to act as a command signal for the vestibulosympathetic neural link.

While both groups in this experiment presumably had some vestibulosympathetic input, it is possible that the VSR in the FP group could adapt to the demands of the high +Gz environment (and its cardiovascular effects) leading to enhancement of this feed-forward mechanism. This phenomenon would better protect the pilot from circulatory compromise due to high +Gz, and may contribute to the gain increase in vascular resistance changes observed in the FP group.

The HR and TPR changes in the FP group are very closely related. The sustained elevation in HR is effectively switched off only when TPR begins to increase substantially. This effect is not seen in the NP group, with HR progressively decreasing well before TPR rises to any great extent. It seems reasonable to suggest that this pattern of response in the FP group indicates an adaptation strategy. The +Gz-adapted baroreflexes are able to increase HR and sustain it at higher levels until such time as the increase in TPR is sufficiently established for it to assume the dominant position. Knowing that TPR increases will take a finite amount of time, the only other protective option is to keep HR up. Only when the vascular resistance changes are safely underway will the increased HR be allowed to switch off. This effect is not seen in the NP group. As such, it is highly suggestive of enhanced baroreflex function as a result of adaptation to repetitive +Gz acceleration.

4.3 Significance of the findings

Previous studies have demonstrated the existence of a difference in the cardiovascular response to an applied +Gz load in the FP group compared with the NP group (Newman et al, 1998, 2000). MAP, SP and DP all increased significantly, with PP being maintained in the FP group, whereas in the NP group MAP and SP were unchanged, DP increased and PP fell dramatically. HR, SV and TPR all demonstrated some degree of enhanced performance in the FP group relative to the NP group. These findings suggested that the FP group had more effective activation of their baroreflexes in response to a given accelerative stimulus. The FP group appeared to have enhanced baroreflex function due to their frequent and repetitive exposure to high +Gz loads.

The findings in this time course analysis support these earlier results. Indeed, from this analysis it is apparent that in fact the time course of changes in the cardiovascular response to dynamic postural change is similar between the groups, but that adaptation to +Gz appears to lead to a greater magnitude of response. The +Gz-adapted pilot demonstrates increased sensitivity of the arterial and cardiopulmonary baroreflex arcs, which in turn reflects an increase in the gain of these reflexes. This enhanced function is demonstrated by a sustained increase in HR and a more marked increase in TPR relative to the NP group.

It is likely that both arterial and cardiopulmonary baroreflexes contribute to the rise in HR and TPR seen in both groups, and that their enhanced function in the FP group acts to drive HR up (and to sustain it for longer) and to increase TPR to a greater extent over a similar time course.

Both the arterial and cardiopulmonary baroreflexes have been shown to be capable of a certain degree of functional plasticity and altered function. The central fluid shifts accompanying long-duration spaceflight have been shown to cause attenuation of both cardiopulmonary and arterial baroreflexes (Billman et al, 1981; Bungo & Johnson, 1983; Fritsch-Yelle et al, 1994; Thompson et al, 1990). Significantly, changes in cardiovascular parameters with resultant orthostatic intolerance have been observed after only 5 hours exposure to the microgravity environment. Microgravity analogue experiments, such as 60 head-down bedrest studies, have produced similar results. These studies confirm that removal of the normal gravitational gradient results in impaired baroreflex function, with these important mechanisms becoming less sensitive and as such less effective in dealing with transient changes in arterial pressure (Convertino et al, 1990).

In contrast, the research reported in this paper involving increased levels of +Gz suggests an opposite effect, with the baroreflexes becoming more effective at reacting to transient changes in cardiovascular dynamics. Other researchers have also shown enhanced baroreflex function in different settings (Krieger, 1970). It seems logical to argue that if a) both low- and high-pressure baroreflexes can develop attenuated function, and b) high-pressure baroreflexes can develop enhanced function, then the low-pressure cardiopulmonary baroreflexes must also be capable of enhanced function. The findings in this analysis would tend to support this.

These results confirm the findings in previous studies that the cardiovascular response of fighter pilots to a mild accelerative stimulus is different from that of a group of non-pilots (Newman et al, 1998, 2000). Furthermore, this analysis shows that this difference is mediated by differences in the magnitude-time course balance of the dynamic cardiovascular response to applied +Gz, specifically in terms of HR and TPR. These results provide some additional insight into the mechanisms involved in postural baroreflex adaptation to high +Gz in fighter pilots. In addition, this adaptation may not be limited to the arterial baroreflexes alone; the cardiopulmonary baroreflexes may similarly adapt to the same stimulus. Indeed, it seems likely that all reflex arcs involved in the regulation of arterial pressure undergo some form of adaptation to repetitive +Gz exposure.

The roles of the vestibular system in cardiovascular control in general and in adaptation to +Gz in particular have also been highlighted in this analysis. It is quite possible that the vestibular system also adapts to frequent exposure to high +Gz, by enhancing its normal feed-forward vestibulosympathetic action. The enhanced function of the baroreflexes may well be aided by earlier signals of changing hydrostatic force being sent via the vestibular system as a means of early alerting and correction of potentially deleterious postural changes. This certainly warrants further research attention.

5. Conclusion

The findings in this analysis support the results of previous studies, in that repetitive occupational exposure to the high +Gz environment is capable of inducing a degree of physiological adaptation. This adaptation appears to be due in part to enhanced arterial and cardiopulmonary baroreflex sensitivity, which in this analysis is illustrated by sustained rises in HR and more marked elevations in TPR. The effect of this magnitude-time course balance shift is to produce a more marked elevation in MAP in the +Gz-adapted pilot. The analysis also suggests that an increase in effective circulating blood volume may also make a contribution to the adaptation process. In addition, the results point indirectly to the possibility of a vestibulosympathetic input into the regulation of arterial pressure during an orthostatic challenge.

6. References

Billman GE, Dickey DT, Teoh KK, Stone HL. (1981). Effects of central venous blood volume shifts on arterial baroreflex control of heart rate. *Am J Physiol*, Vol. 241 (Heart Circ. Physiol. 10): pp. H571-H575.

Bungo MW, Johnson PJ. (1983). Cardiovascular examinations and observations of deconditioning during space shuttle orbital flight test program. *Aviat Space Environ Med*, Vol. 54, pp. 1001-4.

Convertino VA, Doerr DF, Eckberg DL, Fritch JM, Vernikos -Danellis J. (1990). Head-down bed rest impairs vagal baroreflex responses and provokes orthostatic hypotension. *J Appl Physiol*, Vol. 68, pp. 1458-64.

Convertino VA. (1998). High sustained +Gz acceleration: physiological adaptation to high-G tolerance. *J Grav Physiol*, Vol. 5, No. 1, pp. P51-4.

Doba N, Reis DJ. (1974). Role of the cerebellum and the vestibular apparatus in regulation of orthostatic reflexes in the cat. *Circ Res*, Vol. 34, pp. 9-18.

Essandoh LK, Duprez DA, Shepherd JT. (1998). Reflex constriction of human resistance vessels to head-down neck flexion. *J Appl Physiol*, Vol. 64, pp. 767-70.

Fritsch-Yelle JM, Charles JB, Jones MM, Beightol LA, Eckberg DL. (1994). Spaceflight alters autonomic regulation of arterial pressure in humans. *J Appl Physiol*, Vol. 77, pp. 1776-83.

Krieger, EM. (1970). Time course of baroreceptor resetting in acute hypertension. *Am J Physiol*, Vol. 218, p. 486.

Mancia G, Mark AL. (1983). Arterial baroreflexes in humans. In: *Handbook of Physiology. The Cardiovascular System*, Sect. 2, Vol III, Ch. 20, pp. 755-793, American Physiological Society, Bethesda, MD.

Newman DG, Callister R. (1999). Analysis of the +Gz environment during air combat manouevring in the F/A-18 fighter aircraft. *Aviat Space Environ Med*, Vol. 70, pp. 310-15.

Newman DG, Callister R. (2008). Cardiovascular training effects in fighter pilots induced by occupational high G exposure. *Aviat Space Environ Med*, Vol. 79, pp. 774-778.

Newman DG, Callister R. (2009). Flying experience and cardiovascular response to rapid head-up tilt in fighter pilots. *Aviat Space Environ Med*, Vol. 80, pp. 723-726.

Newman DG, White SW, Callister R. (1998). Evidence of baroreflex adaptation to repetitive +Gz in fighter pilots. *Aviat Space Environ Med*, Vol. 69, pp. 446-51.

Newman DG, White SW, Callister R. (2000). The effect of baroreflex adaptation on the dynamic cardiovascular response to head-up tilt. *Aviat Space Environ Med*, Vol. 71, pp. 255-259.

Ray CA, Hume KM, Shortt TL. (1997). Skin sympathetic outflow during head-down neck flexion in humans. *Am J Physiol*, Vol. 273 (Regulatory Integrative Comp. Physiol. 42), pp. 1142-46.

Shortt TL, Ray CA. (1997). Sympathetic and vascular responses to head-down neck flexion in humans. *Am J Physiol*, Vol. 272 (Heart Circ. Physiol. 41), pp. H1780-1784.

Thompson CA, Tatro DL, Ludwig DA, Convertino VA. (1990). Baroreflex responses to acute changes in blood volume in humans. *Am J Physiol*, Vol. 259 (Regulatory Integrative Comp. Physiol. 28), pp. R792-R798.

Yates BJ. (1992). Vestibular influences on the sympathetic nervous system. *Brain Res Rev*, Vol. 17, pp. 51-9.

Yates BJ, Miller AD. (1998). Physiological evidence that the vestibular system participates in autonomic and respiratory control. *J Vestibular Res*, Vol. 8, pp. 17-25.

Zoller RP, Mark AL, Abboud FM, Schmid PG, Heistad DD. (1972). The role of low pressure baroreceptors in reflex vasoconstrictor responses in man. *J Clin Invest*, Vol. 51, pp. 2967-2972.

Section 3

Clinical Impact of Cardiovascular Physiology and Pathophysiology

13

Physical Activity and Cardiovascular Health

Raul A. Martins
University of Coimbra,
Faculty of Sport Science and Physical Education,
Portugal

1. Introduction

The approach of this chapter makes the assumption that relationships between levels of physical activity and cardiovascular health are complex. The theoretical framework considers that physical activity can influence cardiovascular health by itself but can also influence health-related fitness, which in turn may be able to influence cardiovascular health and the level of habitual physical activity. To add more complexity, all these relationships are thought to occur in a reciprocal manner.

Cardiovascular disease corresponds to a group of disorders occurring in the heart and in the blood vessels. The various manifestations of the disease include sudden death, myocardial infarction, angina pectoris, stroke (ischemic or hemorrhagic), or peripheral vascular disease. The risk factors for the cardiovascular diseases are classified usually considering the positive or negative association with the disease and the modifiable or non-modifiable nature. On the other hand, the definition of criterions to some risk factors could be dependent of the context of prevention - primordial, primary, secondary, tertiary or even quaternary. Additionally, it is necessary the plausibility theoretic and biological, and the reversibility of the effect by the reduction or suspension of the risk factor. Modifiable risk factors like dyslipidemia, hypertension, diabetes, excess of adipose tissue, pro coagulant state, pro-inflammatory state, ignorance, sedentariness or low fitness play alone or, more frequently, in conjunction with each others, augmenting exponentially the risk of disease.

White Paper on Sport (CEC, 2007) was released by the European Union (EU) to give strategic orientation on the role of sport in Europe. The document use the definition of "sport" established by the Council of Europe: "all forms of physical activity which, through casual or organized participation, aim at expressing or improving physical fitness and mental well-being, forming social relationships or obtaining results in competition at all levels." With the ratification of the Lisbon Treaty in late 2009, sport was assumed as contributing to the EU strategic objectives of solidarity and prosperity. This follows the Olympic ideal, born in Europe, of developing sport to promote peace and understanding among nations and cultures as well as the education of young people. Member States are encouraged to implement evidence-based policies in order to improve their provision of sporting facilities and opportunities. This means that for the first time the EU is actively aiming to promote sport and physical activity at the policy level - not only with a view to improving physical wellbeing and health across the EU, which is the main focus of this chapter, but also to enhance the role of sport in boosting social cohesion and its educational value. This chapter will explore the relationship of cardiovascular health with sport, as the European understanding, or physical activity in the North American understanding. Physical activity concept, physical activity epidemiology and cardiovascular health, physical activity guidelines, prevalence of sedentariness in Europe and USA, physical activity and life expectancy, and pro-inflammatory state and physical activity are topics explored in this chapter.

2. Physical activity

Physical activity comprises any body movement produced by the skeletal muscles that results in a substantial increase over the resting energy expenditure (Bouchard & Shephard, 1994). Included in this large umbrella is considered the leisure-time physical activity (LTPA), daily physical activities, intentionally practiced exercise (frequency, intensity, type, time) and sport, or occupational work, together with other physical expressions that modify the total energy expenditure. Within the concept of physical activity, physical exercise is a narrow concept, usually defined as planned and repeated movements intending to maintain or to improve one or more components of the health-related fitness or of the performance-related fitness. Physical activity has been understood as a behavior that could also change health-related or performance-related fitness. However, it is also taken in account as a determinant behavior to health and functionality. When one is talking about the potential benefits on health, obviously, all determinants of human energy expenditure should be under careful consideration. Contrarily, sedentariness refers that people remain sitting much of the labor and leisure times.

There are a lot of methods to characterize and measure the behavior *physical activity* including calorimetry (direct and indirect), physiologic markers (heart rate or maximal oxygen uptake) mechanical and electronic devices (pedometers and accelerometers), the observation of behaviors, or the caloric intake (Welk, 2002). Independently of the selected method, the investigator should consider the complex nature of the behavior physical activity and the errors derived from the method usually used with largest number of participants - the self-reported questionnaires. The use of questionnaires imply low costs but sometimes introduces considerable error because, for instance, could exist social tendency to associate physical activity to sport participation. It means that it is desirable to use direct methods as pedometers or accelerometers. Pedometers count the number of steps but are not able to distinguish different levels of activity. This limitation is overcome by the accelerometry, and the last National Health and Nutrition Examination Survey (NHANES) realized in 2003-2004 evaluated physical activity of around 4867 American citizens with accelerometry (Troiano et al., 2008).

3. Prevalence of sedentariness

A national representative study of Portuguese people has measured directly physical activity by accelerometry (Baptista et al., 2011). Volunteered to participate 5231 adolescents (10-17 years-old; 1456 males; 1755 females), adults (18-64 years-old; 441 males; 803 females), and older adults (65+ years-old; 303 males; 473 females). All participants were measured during four days (two week days and two weekend days). The cut-off points for moderate intensity were 3-5,9 METs (adults and older adults) and 4-6,9 METs (adolescents), and for vigorous intensity were 6+ METs (adults and older adults) and 7+ METs (adolescents). Adolescents with less than 60 minutes/day of moderate/vigorous physical activity on 5 days/week, and adults or older adults with less than 30 minutes/day on 5 days/week were classified as 'insufficiently active'.

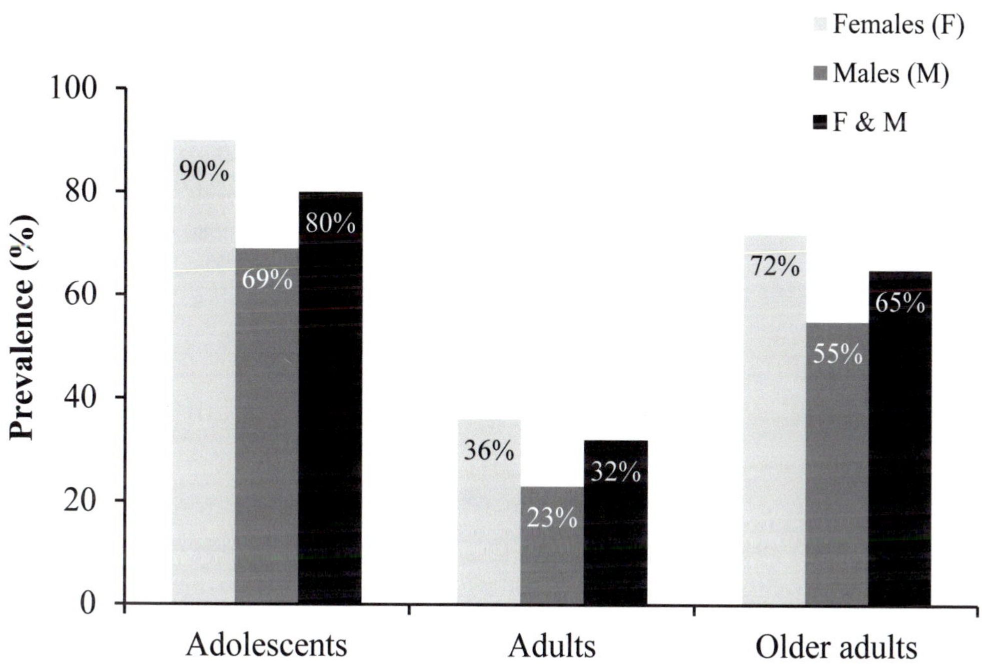

Source: Baptista et al., 2011.

Fig. 1. Prevalence of 'insufficiently active' Portuguese people measured by accelerometry.

As illustrated by Figure 1, the prevalence of insufficiently active people was particularly high in the adolescents (80%) but also in the older adults (65%). The adult people (18-64 years old) attained only 32%, which represents the group with higher volume of moderate/vigorous weekly physical activity. The prevalence of insufficiently active in all the people evaluated was 67%. Males are more active than females, in each one of the three groups, with higher difference (21%) among adolescents and lower difference among adults (13%). One can speculate that the indirect methods like self-reported questionnaires tend to overestimate physical activity when compared with a direct measure (accelerometry), as seems to result when one compares these overall data (67%) with data provided from Eurobarometer 2003 (30%) and Eurobarometer 2010 (52%) on Figure 2. However, the high prevalence of insufficiently active, particularly in adolescents and older adults, claim for the adoption of specific strategies to change these sedentary behaviors.

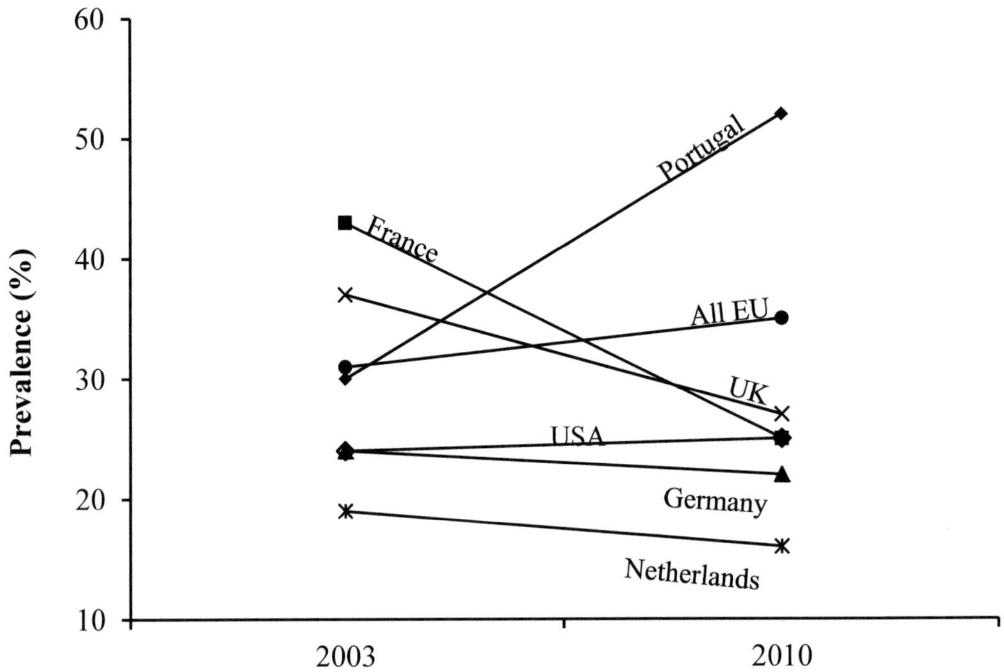

USA data is No Leisure-Time Physical Activity in 2003, and 2008.

http://www.cdc.gov/nccdphp/dnpa/physical/stats/leisure_time.htm. Extracted on 24/Oct/2011.

Fig. 2. Prevalence of the sedentariness in some EU Member States measured by self-reported questionnaires.

Data from the 2003 Eurobarometer (EC, 2003) are presented in Figure 2. Sedentary people are those not meeting the threshold for low activity. Cut-off points for low physical activity participation were 30 minutes of walking or moderate-intensity activity on at least 5 days/week, or 20 minutes of vigorous-intensity activity on at least 3 days/week. Participated people from each one of the EU Member States with 15+ years-old (N=16230), randomly sampling with probability proportional to population size (for a total coverage of the country) and to population density (metropolitan, urban, and rural areas). It was used the International Physical Activity Questionnaire (IPAQ) to characterize physical activity in a face-to-face interview in people's home and in the appropriate national language. Frequency of 5+ days/week of moderate intensity physical activity was not achieved by 72% of EU Member States citizens (equal for women and men) while 74% did not achieve 3+ days/week of vigorous intensity physical activity (81% on women, and 68% on men). Prevalence of people who do not practiced 3+ days/week of vigorous intensity increases with age from 66% (15-25 years) to 69% (26-44 years), to 76% (45-64 years), and to 89% (65+ years). Prevalence of people not engaged on 5+ days/week of moderate intensity also increases with age: 70% (15-25 years), 70% (26-44 years), 72% (45-64 years), and 79% (65+ years).

The 2010 Eurobarometer (EC, 2010) analyzed people with 15+ years-old of 27 EU Member States (N=26788), with a different self-reported questionnaire than IPAQ, and revealed a prevalence of 27% for people saying they engage in physical activity regularly at least 5 times/week, while 38% answered that exercising with some regularity (1-4 times/week) (Figure 2). The other 35% EU citizens never engage in any physical activity or engage below the desirable level (1-3 times/month). By analyzing data from some EU Member States it is possible to observe clear discrepancies in the values from 2003 to 2010. These discrepancies maybe is reflecting partially the utilization of different instruments with different self-reported answers. Sedentariness was considered in Eurobarometer 2010 to the people that engage only 1-2 times/month or even less in physical activities. With these cut-off points, sedentariness was respectively in 2003 and 2010: Portugal - 30% and 52%; France - 43% and 25%; Germany - 24% and 22%; UK - 37% and 27%; Netherlands - 19% and 16%; All EU - 31% and 35%.

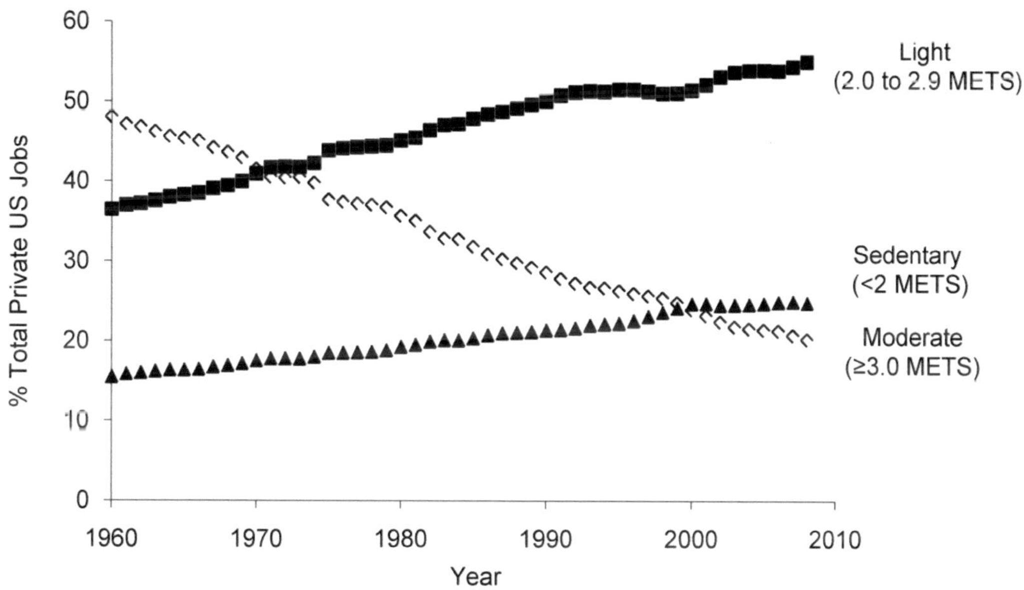

Source: Church et al., 2011.

Fig. 3. Trends in the prevalence of sedentary, light and moderate intensity occupations from 1960 to 2008.

Troiano and colleagues (2008) have described physical activity levels of children (6-11 years old), adolescents (12-19 years old), and adults (20+ years old), using objective data obtained with accelerometers from a representative sample of the U.S. population. The results were attained from the 2003-2004 National Health and Nutritional Examination Survey (NHANES), a cross-sectional study of a complex, multistage probability sample of the civilian, noninstitutionalized population. Data are described from 6329 participants who provided at least 1 day of accelerometer data and from 4867 participants who provided 4+ days of accelerometer data. Males were more physically active than females. Authors observed that physical activity declines dramatically across age groups between childhood (42% obtained the recommended 60 minutes/day) and adolescence (8% achieve 60 minutes/day) and continues to decline in adults (less than 5% attained 30 minutes/day). Objective and subjective measures of physical activity gave qualitatively similar results regarding gender and age patterns of activity. However, adherence to physical activity recommendations according to accelerometer-measured activity is substantially lower than according to self-reported questionnaire. Occupational work is also an important expression of physical activity contributing to energy expenditure and to the energy balance.

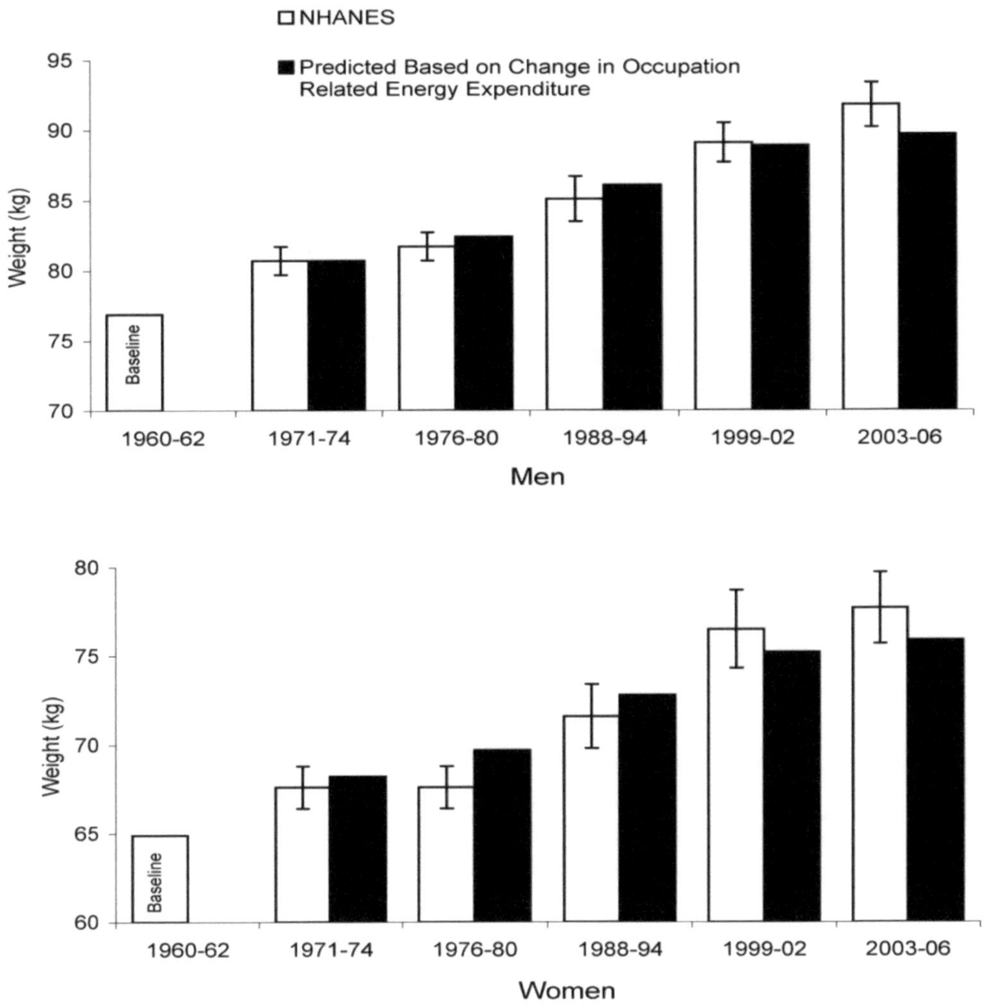

Source: Church et al., 2011.

Fig. 4. Predicted mean U.S. body weight based on change in occupation related daily energy expenditure since 1960 compared to mean U.S. weight gain based on the NHANES examination periods for 40–50 year old.

Trends in occupational physical activity during the past 5 decades (Figure 3), and the concurrent changes in body weight in the U.S. were explored by Church and colleagues (2011). Authors observed that in 1960 almost half the jobs (48%) in private industry in the

U.S. required at least moderate intensity physical activity whereas in 2008 less than 20% demand this level of energy expenditure. While there has been a steady increase in the prevalence of sedentary and light intensity physical activity occupations since 1960, the prevalence of moderate intensity physical activity occupations has decreased. At the same period (1960-2008) there was a drop in occupation-related daily energy expenditure of about 142 calories for men and 124 calories for women. Authors estimate that the decrease of 142 calories in men would result in an increase in mean weight from 76.9 kg (1960-62) to 89.7 kg (2003-06), with the results having similar pattern for women (Figure 4).

Over the last 50 years the prevalence of Americans in the labor force has increased approximately 40% to 50%, with women assuming a growing prevalence in the work force from 43% in 1970 to 60% in 2007. This fact helps to explain the decrease in the pattern of occupation-related energy expenditure (Lee & Mather, 2008). Given this, it is unlikely a return to occupations demanding moderate levels of physical activity, which addresses further strong evidence of the public health importance of promoting physically active lifestyles outside of the work day. The reduction of 124 (women) and 142 calories (men) per day in occupation-related energy expenditure over the last 50 years would have been adequately compensated for by meeting the 2008 Physical Activity Guidelines of 150 minutes/week of moderate intensity activity or 75 minutes/week of vigorous intensity activity (USDHHS, 2011). While it is often noted that the prevalence of Americans who achieve this recommendation has been constant over recent decades, the fact remains that based on self-report data only 25% adults achieve this level (CDC, 2008), but when physical activity is assessed with accelerometers the number of adult people achieving the recommendations drops dramatically to less than 5% (Troiano et al., 2008). Therefore, since energy expenditure of the labor activities has largely been removed, the relative importance of LTPA has increased and should be considered as a major focus of public health interventions and research.

Brownson and colleagues (2005) developed a revision to describe current patterns and long-term trends (up to 50 years when possible) related to (i) physical activity, (ii) employment and occupation, (iii) travel behavior, (iv) land use, and (v) related behaviors (e.g., television watching). Available data allows the following trends: relatively stable or slightly increasing levels of LTPA, declining work-related activity, declining transportation activity, declining activity in the home, and increasing sedentary activity. These reflect an overall trend of declining total physical activity, with large differences noted in the rates of walking for transportation across metropolitan areas, and a strong linear increase in vehicle miles traveled per person, coupled with a strong and consistent trend toward people living in suburbs. Authors concluded that although difficult to quantify, it appears that a combination of changes to the built environment and increases in the proportion of the population engaging in sedentary activities put the majority of the population at high risk of physical inactivity.

4. Physical activity guidelines

Vigorous activity was centrally considered to health promotion until 1995 when recommendations of the Center for Disease Control (CDC) and the American College of Sports Medicine (ACSM) pointed out for adults to accumulate at least 30 minutes of moderate-intensity physical activity on most days of the week (Pate et al., 1995). These recommendations were described in the 1996 U.S. Surgeon General's Report on Physical Activity and Health (USDHHS, 1996), and served as cornerstone for the Healthy People 2010 (HP 2010) goals on physical activity (USDHHS, 2000), inspiring public policies and programs over the next years. The HP 2010 objectives stated that adults should engage in vigorous LTPA (60-84%VO_{2Res} or %HR_{Res}; 77-93%HR_{max}; >60%VO_{2max}; >6 METs) for at least 20 minutes, at least 3 times/week, or moderate LTPA (40-59%VO_{2Res} or %HR_{Res}; 64-76%HR_{max}; 40-60%VO_{2max}; 3-6 METs) for at least 30 minutes, at least 5 times/week.

For the purposes of HP 2010, lesser amounts of vigorous and moderate activities could not be combined. In 2007, the CDC/ACSM recommendations published in 1995 were updated and clarified, emphasizing the potential health benefits of combinations of moderate and vigorous-intensity activities and of strengthening activities (Haskell et al., 2007). Meantime, the Healthy People 2020 (HP 2020) goals on physical activity were released (USDHHS, 2010) introducing some modifications, and establishing and encouraging to increase the prevalence of "sufficiently active" adults engaging in moderate-intensity aerobic physical activity of at least 150 minutes/week or vigorous-intensity aerobic activity of at least 75 minutes/week or an equivalent combination. The HP 2020 also pursue to increase the prevalence of "highly active" adults engaging in aerobic physical activity of at least moderate intensity for more than 300 minutes/week or more than 150 minutes/week of vigorous intensity or an equivalent combination. And, finally, to increase the prevalence of adults who perform muscle-strengthening activities on 2 or more days/week of 7 large muscle groups.

5. Physical activity and life expectancy

Mortality differentials by level and intensity of physical activity have been documented, with Lollgen and colleagues (2009) obtaining significant association of lower all-cause mortality for active individuals comparing with sedentary persons. Highly active men had a 22% lower risk of all-cause mortality (RR=0.78; 95% CI: 0.72 to 0.84), and women had 31% (RR=0.69; 95% CI: 0.53 to 0.90) comparing to mildly active men and women, respectively. The authors also found a similar and significant association of activity to all-cause mortality in older participants.

Schoenborn and Stommel (2011) studying the benefits of accomplish the 2008 Physical Activity Guidelines for Adults (USDHHS, 2011), which are similar to the HP 2020 goals, achieved 27% lower risk of all-cause mortality among people without existing chronic comorbidities, and by almost half among people with chronic comorbidities (such as heart disease, stroke, diabetes, cancer, respiratory conditions, or any functional limitation), regardless of age and obesity levels. Assuming several limitations present on causal interpretations, when examining for interactions of physical activity with smoking and alcohol consumption, data suggest that relative survival benefits associated with physical activity are largest among current smokers and light-moderate drinkers.

Figure 5 shows the survival curves associated with four types of adherence to the 2008 Guidelines for all adults: meeting both the aerobic and muscle-strengthening guidelines, the aerobic only, the muscle-strengthening only, and neither of the minimum recommendations. This figure suggests that meeting the 2008 Guidelines is associated with survival benefits, with stronger benefits for both the aerobic and muscle-strengthening exercises; also suggests that aerobic activity alone promotes stronger benefits than muscle strengthening alone.

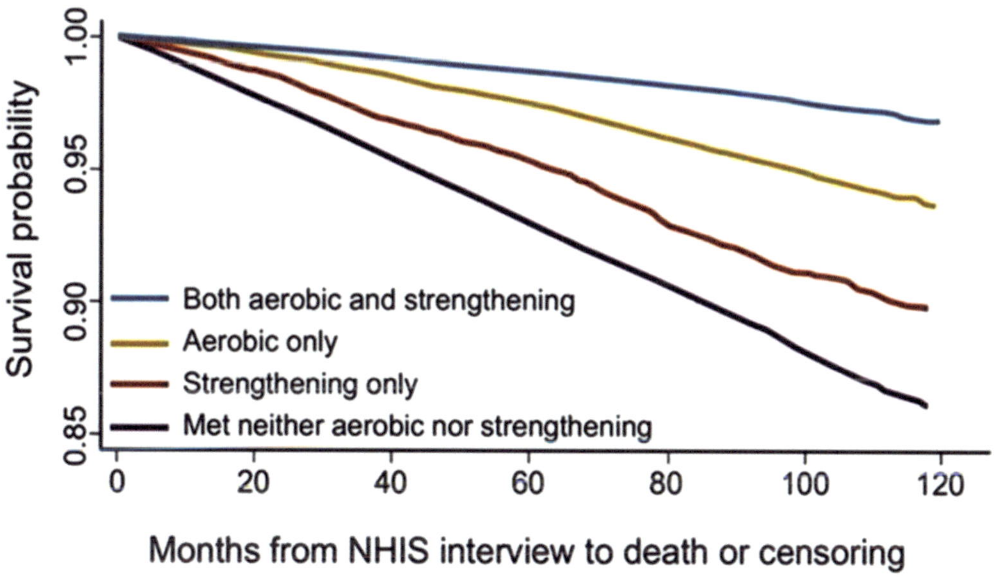

Note: U.S. adults aged ≥ 18 years (weighted); respondents not linked to death records were considered "censored", meaning they were presumed to be alive as of December 31, 2006. NHIS, National Health Interviews Survey, 1997-2004.

Adapted from Schoenborn and Stommel (2011)

Fig. 5. Survival probabilities by levels of adherence to 2008 Physical Activity Guidelines

Figure 6 illustrates that higher volumes of aerobic exercise are associated with higher increase in survival probabilities. Those who engage in none aerobic leisure-time activity attained lower survival probability while people that engaged in more than 300 minutes/week have the higher survival probability. In other words, it means that additional survival benefits can be achieved with higher levels of aerobic leisure-time activity

6. Epidemiology of physical activity and cardiovascular health

Epidemiology has been defined as "the study of the distribution and determinants of health-related states or events in specified populations, and the application of this study to the prevention and control of health problems" (Last, 2001). When this definition considers 'health-related states or events' instead of the former 'disease frequency' is having in account the contemporary definition of health that considers positive health states, as a good quality of life, or well succeeded aging, and not only the absence of disease. The word 'epidemiology' is derived from the Greek words: *epi* "upon", *demos* "people", and *logos* "study". In fact, epidemiology origin based on Hippocrates observation, made more than 2000 years ago, that environmental factors could be determinant for the occurrence of a disease. However, it was only in second half of the XIX century when the first truly epidemiologic investigations appeared (Bonita et al., 2006).

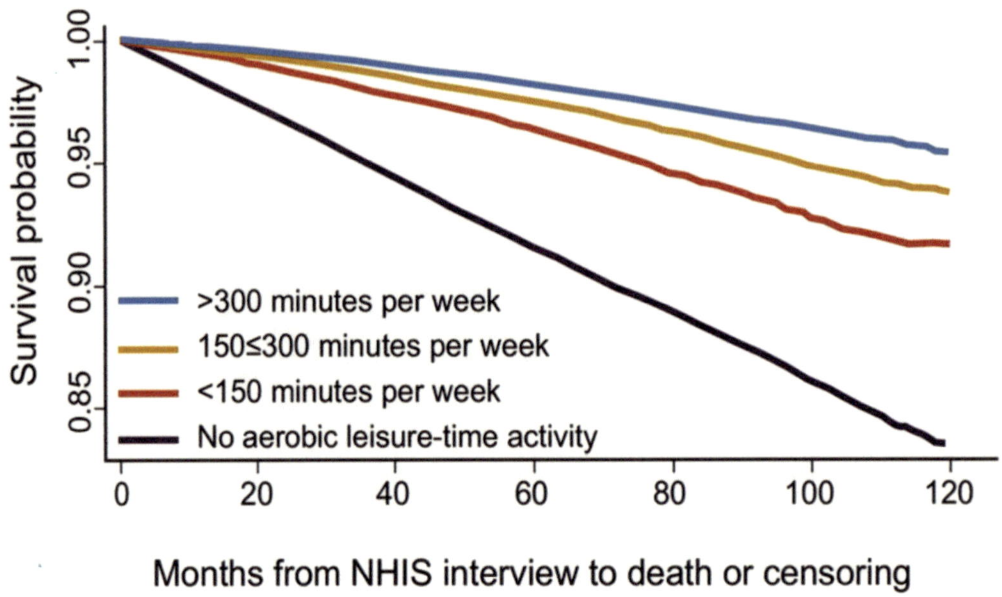

Note: U.S. adults aged ≥ 18 years (weighted); respondents not linked to death records were considered "censored", meaning they were presumed to be alive as of December 31, 2006. NHIS, National Health Interviews Survey, 1997-2004.

Adapted from Schoenborn and Stommel (2011).

Fig. 6. Survival probabilities by levels of adherence to 2008 aerobic physical activity guidelines.

Physical activity and the relationship with cardiovascular health was firstly studied in an epidemiologic basis by Morris and colleagues (1953a,b). Works were conducted to understand how both vocational and LTPA relate to fitness and risk of coronary heart disease (CHD). Authors studied London transit workers, and other occupations as postal service employees and civil servants. Initially they found bus conductors on London's double-decker omnibuses to be at lower risk than bus drivers; what disease the conductors did develop was less severe, and they were more likely to survive an attack. The conductors, who walked up and down stairs in a daily basis, often for decades, experienced roughly half the number of heart attacks and sudden death as the drivers. After that, Morris and colleagues (1990) studied a random sample of 3591 British civil servants during a follow-up of 8-year period ending in 1977, during which time 268 men died. Subjects were classified as having engaged in vigorous activities (>6 METs), or not. Of the subjects 22% reported some kind of vigorous exercise and their death rate was 4,2%. The remaining 78% reported no vigorous exercise and their mortality rate was 8,2%, i.e., twice as high. This differential in death rates persisted when controlling for age, smoking, obesity and successive intervals of follow up.

Several other populations have been studied for physical activity and physiological fitness in relation to health and specifically cardiovascular health (USDHHS, 1996). One of the most remarkable studies was conducted with 17549 men who entered Harvard College between

1916 and 1950 (Paffenbarger et al., 1978), and when aged 55–84 years responded to a questionnaire on their personal characteristics, health status and lifestyle habits like current and former physical activity, as participation in student sport whilst at university. These patterns have been related to cardiovascular disease mortality over a 16-year follow-up period (1962 to 1978), during which 1413 men died (Paffenbarger et al., 1986a,b).

Among Harvard alumni there were strong significant inverse associations between death rates and levels of each of the following physical activity: walking, stair climbing, sports play and combinations of these activities, measured in kJ/week. Gradients of benefit from more active lifestyles were consistent throughout, and maintained after controlling for age, smoking, hypertension and obesity. As compared with the one-third of least active men, the middle third experienced a 23 % reduction in death rate during follow-up and the one-third of most active men, a 32 % reduction. Light activities (<4METs), moderate activities (4–5METs), and vigorous activities (>6METs) each predicted lower death rates. Physical activity related inversely to total mortality, primarily to death due to cardiovascular or respiratory causes. Death rates declined steadily as energy expended on such activities increased from less than 500kcal/week to 3500kcal/week, beyond which rates increased slightly. This relationship was independent of the presence or absence of hypertension, cigarette smoking, extremes or gains in body weight, or early parental death (Figure 7).

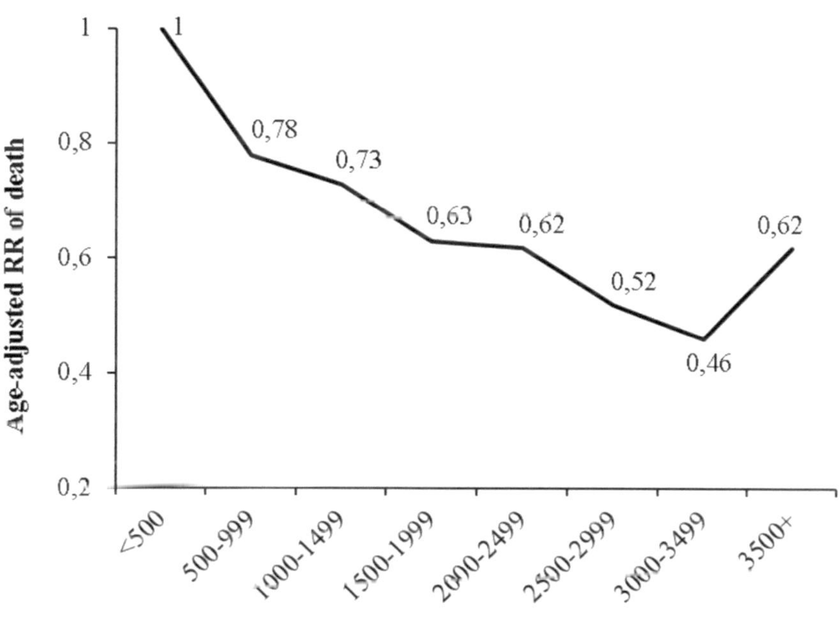

Source: Paffenbarger et al., 1986a.

Notes: Participated 16936 men. A total of 1413 alumni died during 12 to 16 years of follow-up (1962-1978). Exercise reported as walking, stair climbing, sports play, and combinations of these activities.

Fig. 7. Inverse association between weekly energy expenditure and RR of all-cause mortality.

Those men were studied for the effect on all-cause mortality from changing physical activity habits. Men who had increased or decreased their activity by less than 250kcal/week between the 1960s and 1977 were considered in an 'unchanged' category. Compared with their death rates, gradient reductions in mortality were observed with increased levels of physical activity, and gradient increases in mortality with decreased levels of activity. At the extremes of this gradient, men who had increased their energy expenditure by 1250kcal/week had a 20% lower risk of death than men in the unchanged category; men who decreased their activity by 1250kcal/week had a 26% higher risk (Paffenbarger et al., 1993, 1994).

Vigorous activity should be encouraged. Not only because in today's world, where time is a precious commodity, a short period of vigorous exercise expends as much energy as does moderate activity carried out for two or three times as long (Figures 8 and 9), but also because the kind of stimulation over tissues and systems could be more benefic to compensate lost, asymptomatic in an initial stage, that tends to occur with aging.

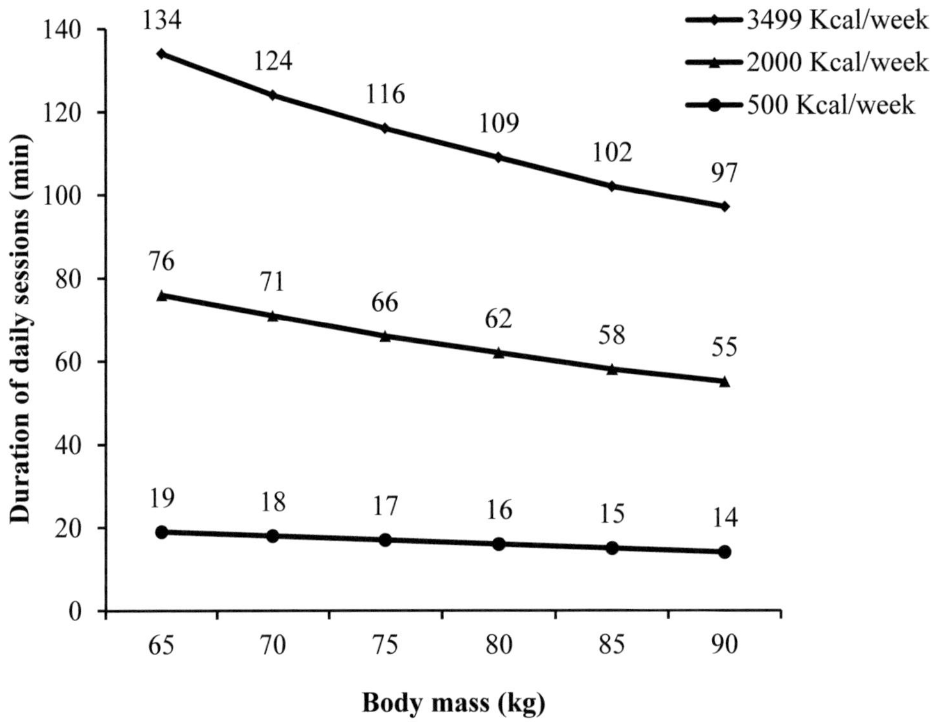

Fig. 8. Duration (min) of daily walking sessions, with moderate intensity (velocity of 80m/min; 3,3METs), for people with different body masses, to gain cardiovascular health (500kcal/week: RR=1,00; 2000kcal/week: RR≈0,62; 3499kcal/week: RR≈0,46).

Figure 8 illustrates time spent with walking at moderate intensity (velocity of 80m/min, or 4,8km/h) by people of different body masses, within the range 500-3499kcal/week (Paffenbarger et al., 1986a). A person weighting 75kg will needs to walk 116 minutes per each one of the 7 days of the week to maximize the potential benefits of physical activity on cardiovascular health, i.e. to spend 3499kcal/week (RR=0,46). In other words, and taking in account the work of Paffenbarger and colleagues (1986a) illustrated by the Figure 1, a person of 75kg will obtain progressive cardiovascular gain from 17 minutes of horizontal walking (RR=1,0) to 116 minutes of daily horizontal walking (RR=0,46). However, if that same person of 75kg of body mass decides to exercise at vigorous intensity (Figure 9), 40 minutes of horizontal running at 150m/min (9km/h) will be enough to maximize the potential gains on cardiovascular health.

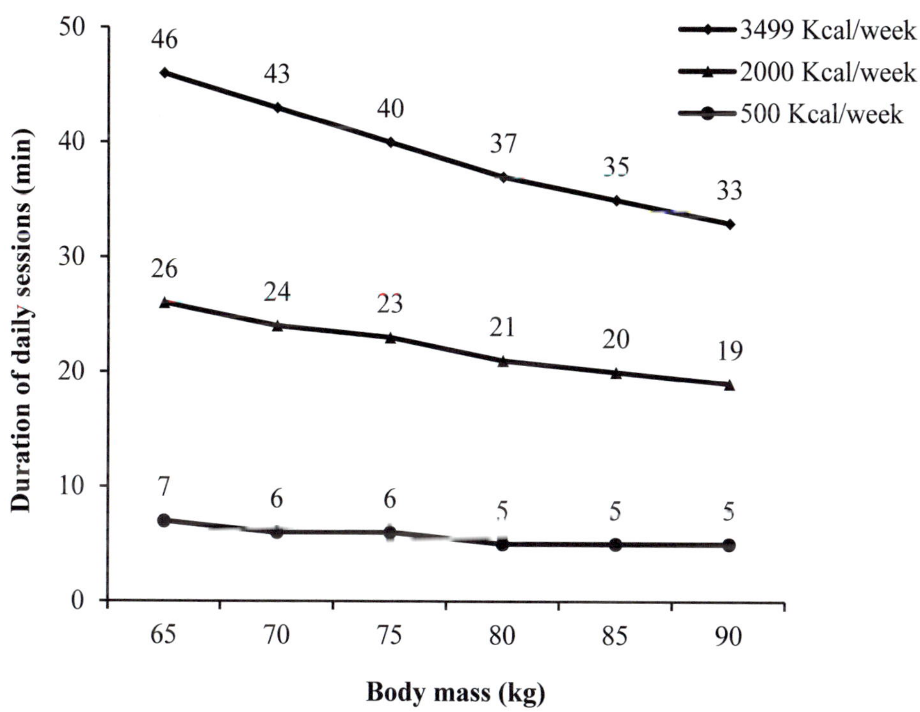

Fig. 9. Duration (min) of daily running sessions, with vigorous intensity (velocity of 150m/min; 9,6METs), for people with different body masses, to gain cardiovascular health (500kcal/week: RR=1,00; 2000kcal/week: RR≈0,62; 3499kcal/week: RR≈0,46).

7. Pro-inflammatory state and physical activity

Inflammation has emerged some years ago as a key pathophysiological event in vascular diseases and the consequent cardiovascular and cerebral injury. Inflammation is a complex process involving multiple cellular and molecular components, and is triggered by different pro-inflammatory mediators generated directly and indirectly by microbial invasion, endotoxins, immune complexes, and cytokines. Vascular endothelium is subjected to pro-inflammatory insults but fortunately is awarded with strong anti-inflammatory molecules that confer resistance to damage by transient pro-inflammatory attacks.

Inflammation is a natural response to infection or damage that intends to destroy or to inactivate the foreign agents permitting tissues repairing. Inflammation could be a local or systemic response, and the key mediators are the cells that act as phagocytes, with the most important being neutrophils, macrophages, and macrophages-like cells. The sequence of local events in a typical nonspecific inflammatory response includes: (i) vasodilatation of the microcirculation in the infected area, leading to increased blood flow; (ii) large increase in protein permeability of the capillaries and venules in the infected area, with resulting diffusion of protein and filtration of fluid into the interstitial fluid; (iii) chemotaxis: movement of leukocytes from the venules into the interstitial fluid of the infected area; (iv) destruction of bacteria in the tissue either through phagocytosis or by other mechanisms; (v) tissue repair (Widmaier et al., 2011). The events of inflammation, such as vasodilation, are induced and regulated by several chemical mediators including kinins, complement, products of blood clotting, histamine, eicosanoids, platelet-activating factors, cytokines, nitric oxide, C-reactive protein (CRP). CRP is an acute phase protein produced by the liver, always found at some concentration in the plasma, and act to minimize the extent of local tissue damage. CRP can bind nonspecifically to carbohydrates or lipids in the cell wall of microbes and facilitate opsonization to enhance phagocytosis.

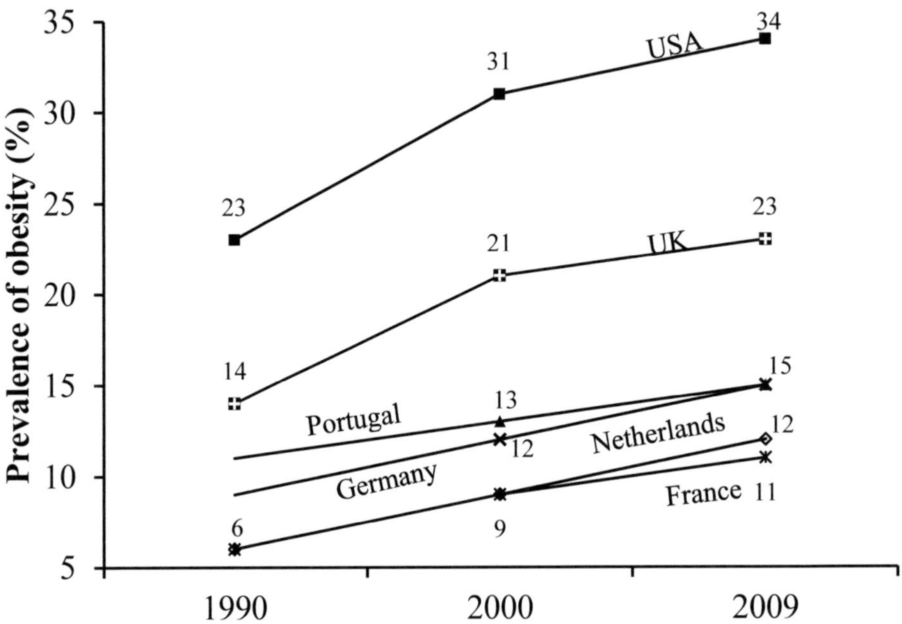

Source: OECD Health Data 2011. Extracted on 25 Oct 2011 from:

http://stats.oecd.org/Index.aspx?DataSetCode=HEALTH_LVNG

Notes: Data of Portugal are self-reported, in 1999 and 2006; data of France are self-reported, in 1990, 2000 and 2008; data of Germany are self-reported, in 1999 and 2009; data of UK are measured in 1991, 2000 and 2009; data of Netherlands are self-reported, in 1990, 2000 and 2009; data of USA are measured in 1991, 2000 and 2008.

Fig. 10. Decennial evolution of obesity (BMI ≥ 30kg/m^2) in % of total population.

There is scientific evidence indicating to atherosclerosis as an inflammatory disease (De Haro et al., 2008; Hamer & Stamatakis, 2008; Virani et al., 2008). In fact, some of the most prevalent risk factors for cardiovascular diseases have been shown to have a pro-inflammatory action including hypertension (Imatoh et al., 2007; Hamer & Stamatakis, 2008), diabetes (Porrini et al., 2007; Hwang et al., 2008), dyslipidemia (Kim et al., 2007), and overweight or obesity (Hamer & Stamatakis, 2008; Piestrzeniewicz et al., 2008). As high-sensitivity C-reactive protein (hs-CRP) is a sensitive marker of inflammation, it has been pointed as the golden marker of inflammation, with Berk and colleagues (1990) establishing for the first time a positive association between hs-CRP and angina pectoris. Other authors have also found positive association of the hs-CRP with risk of vascular disease (Koenig et al., 1999; Kuller et al., 1996; Ridker et al., 1998a; Ridker et al., 2002; Ridker et al., 2003). Since then, various investigations have concentrated on the effects of physical activity on hs-CRP (Church et al., 2002; Martins et al., 2010a; Martins et al., 2010b; Mora et al., 2006; Wannamethee et al., 2002).

Figure 10 illustrates decennial evolution of obesity, self-reported or measured, in different countries of Europe and North America. United States of America and United Kingdom attained higher values of obesity (BMI ≥ 30kg/m²) prevalence, according to the Organization for Economic Co-Operation and Development (OECD) 2011 health data, with 34% and 23% in 2009, respectively. The importance of this risk factor in this context is related with pro-inflammation action, as referred above. One would yet speculate that self-reported data by people in Portugal, France, Germany, and Netherlands are below to the real prevalence, which addresses for a rise of prevalence of obesity in these countries to values close to the measured ones in the USA and UK.

	Before	After
Body weight (kg)	73 (11)	72 (11)*
Waist circumference (cm)	94 (10)	91 (10)**
Body mass index (kg/m²)	30.6 (5.0)	30.3 (4.9)*
Blood pressure (mm Hg)		
Systolic	149 (21)	150 (19)
Diastolic	77 (10)	74 (9)*
Triglycerides (mmol/l)	1.35 (0.58)	1.20 (0.54)*
Total cholesterol (mmol/l)	5.64 (0.86)	5.29 (1.03)*
HDL-cholesterol (mmol/l)	1.31 (0.25)	1.37 (0.32)*
LDL-cholesterol (mmol/l)	2.36 (0.77)	2.05 (0.86)**
Total Cholesterol/HDL-cholesterol	4.40 (0.92)	4.02 (0.81)**
hs-CRP (mg/l)	5.4 (3.9)	4.0 (2.0)*
6-minute walk distance (m)	387 (76)	437 (83)**

Values are mean (SD). *$p<0.05$, **$p<0.01$ compared with before.

Source: Martins RA et al., (2010b).

Table 1. Exercising group.

Measurement of cholesterol by itself do not allow the recognition of about of the individuals who will present later with myocardial infarctions (Rifai & Ridker, 2001), and a number of studies (Ridker et al., 1998b; Ridker et al., 2001; Ridker et al., 2002; Onat et al., 2001; Torres & Ridker, 2003) reinforce the idea that introducing markers of inflammation in the models of diagnosis, beyond the lipid profile, result in more accuracy to predict atherogenic events, comparing with lipid-based models only. High serum levels of CRP have also been found not only in patients with elevated blood pressure but also in those with congestive heart failure (Barbieri et al., 2003; Torre-Amione, 2005), type 2 diabetes, metabolic syndrome and obesity (Das, 2001; Pradham et al., 2001; Ridker et al., 2003). Therefore, factors that may impact negatively hs-CRP levels, like physical activity, should be further studied, particularly in populations at increased risk of the above diseases.

	Before	After
Body weight (kg)	71 (12)	70 (13)
Waist circumference (cm)	93 (10)	91 (10)**
Body mass index (kg/m^2)	29.0 (4.4)	28.8 (4.7)
Blood pressure (mm Hg)		
Systolic	146 (20)	142 (24)
Diastolic	76 (9)	75 (13)
Triglycerides (mmol/l)	1.10 (0.35)	1.15 (0.35)
Total cholesterol (mmol/l)	5.14 (0.94)	5.27 (1.02)
HDL-cholesterol (mmol/l)	1.33 (0.28)	1.32 (0.29)
LDL-cholesterol (mmol/l)	2.39 (0.86)	2.27 (0.61)
Total Cholesterol/HDL-cholesterol	3.99 (0.98)	4.07 (0.83)
hs-CRP (mg/l)	5.5 (3.5)	5.1 (2.3)
6-minute walk distance (m)	342 (126)	343 (170)

Values are mean (SD). *$p<0.05$, **$p<0.01$ compared with before.

Source: Martins RA et al., (2010b).

Table 2. Control group.

Inflammatory processes have been positively associated with aging (Pedersen et al., 2003), with studies suggesting that physical activity would benefit atherosclerotic disease, at least partially, by reducing the inflammatory level (Wannamethee et al., 2002; Reuben et al., 2003). Serum CRP levels has been negatively associated with physical activity or physical fitness, but also with BMI and other adiposity measures (Church et al., 2002; Wannamethee et al., 2002; Mora et al., 2006; Martins et al., 2010b). These studies suggest that regular physical exercise might lower CRP levels, acting as an anti-inflammatory agent, by the effects over adipose tissue and/or by the effects on the muscle mass.

Martins and colleagues (2010b) present results (Table 1) showing beneficial effects of two exercising programs (i.e., aerobic and strength-based) in older adults with significant differences on body weight (-1%), waist circumference (-3%), BMI (-1%), diastolic blood pressure (-4%), triglycerides (-11%), total cholesterol (-6%), HDL-cholesterol (5%), LDL-cholesterol (-13%), total cholesterol/HDL-cholesterol relationship (-9%), hs-CRP (-26%), and 6-minute walk distance (13%), while the control group (Table 2) only had significant differences on waist circumference (-2%). At baseline, BMI correlated with total cholesterol ($r=0.35$, $p=0.007$), triglycerides ($r=0.38$, $p=0.004$), and hs-CRP ($r=0.46$, $p=0.001$). Waist circumference correlated with total cholesterol ($r=0.30$, $p=0.022$), triglycerides ($r=0.35$, $p=0.010$), hs-CRP ($r=0.38$, $p=0.010$), and total cholesterol/HDL-cholesterol ($r=0.38$, $p=0.005$). Finally, body weight also correlated with total cholesterol ($r=0.33$, $p=0.011$), triglycerides ($r=0.27$, $p=0.044$), hs-CRP ($r=0.40$, $p=0.006$), and total cholesterol/HDL-cholesterol ($r=0.33$, $p=0.016$).

Studies examining the effects on cardiovascular health by endurance and strength training have generally found either positive changes in lipid profile or no changes at all. More pronounced dyslipidemia at baseline has been pointed has having more favorable changes after training (Laaksonen et al., 2000), mediated by the reduction of body fat (Leon & Sanchez, 2001). On the other hand, older people are known to be under the effects of sarcopenia, which is characterized by loss of skeletal muscle mass and strength weakness. Sarcopenia has been associated not only with functional fitness impairment (Reid et al., 2008) but also with systemic inflammation (Visser et al., 2002). Resistance training (Marini et al., 2008) has been suggested to be an effective way to prevent the adverse outcomes of sarcopenia whereas the effects of aerobic training are not as clear.

The mechanisms underlying the positive effects of the physical activity on inflammation remain under discussion, being considered the hypothesis of reduction of body fat, and/or the increase of muscle mass. Some have hypothesized about changes in circulating inflammatory cytokine levels alter hs-CRP hepatic production. Reductions of serum IL-18, IL-6 and CRP have been reported after 10 months of aerobic exercise but not after flexibility/resistance exercise (Kohut et al., 2006). However, others failed to obtain exercise-induced effects in plasmatic inflammatory cytokines, including IL-6, TNF-α and IL-1β after 12 weeks of combined aerobic/resistance and flexibility training (Stewart et al., 2007). Additionally, TNF-α may contribute directly to sarcopenia once can disrupt the differentiation process in cultured muscle cells and promotes catabolism in mature muscle cells. Muscle mass is a primary site for glucose and triglyceride disposal (Dinneen et al., 1992) and the major determinant of metabolic rate (Zurlo et al., 1994). Age-related muscle loss may contribute to insulin resistance, dyslipidemia and increased adiposity. IL-6 protein is expressed in contracting muscle fibers and released from skeletal muscle during exercise whereas this is not the case for TNF-α (Steensberg et al., 2002). IL-6 is able to inhibit TNF-α, and IL-1 production stimulates the production of IL-1ra and IL-10 and the release of soluble TNF-receptors (Steensberg et al., 2003). In synthesis, a chronic training-induced reduction on hs-CRP concentrations in older adults is supported by various studies having as key factors increase in muscular mass and reduction in body fat.

8. Summary

Exercise and physical activity, or a wide concept of sport as defined by the Council of Europe, are cornerstones to act at different levels of prevention for cardiovascular health. Physical activity comprises any voluntary movement that substantially increases oxygen uptake above the resting level. Prevalence of sedentariness should be considered as a key point for public health initiatives across all ages, with particular emphasis in older adults because not only they have the higher prevalence of inactivity, but also the higher costs of health services. On the other side, energy expenditure related with occupational work has been diminishing, which addresses more importance to the leisure-time physical activity to the energy balance. Physical activity and cardiovascular fitness, i.e. oxygen uptake capacity, are both risk factors for cardiovascular health. Sometimes, questions arise about the most appropriate kind of exercise to burn energy and enhance oxygen uptake. However, the question seems to be easily answered since all fuel used in the body is ultimately processed by the aerobic energy pathways. This means that we can use the amount of oxygen consumed during the activity to calculate caloric burn. The impact of physical activity on fat mass is a sensitive point, and the question about the most appropriate intensity to burn fat also arises occasionally. Again, the answer seems to be very easy. Each individual should practice with the higher possible intensity, according to their risk stratification. The time necessary to reach the same level of energy expenditure is about one third when comparing vigorous intensity with moderate intensity, addressing for the lack of importance to discuss about the right zone to burn fat. Moreover, it is very well known that after about 2 minutes of exercising at high intensity the aerobic pathway (using fat free acids as fuel) becomes predominant over glycolytic pathway. Recent risk factors, as inflammation, have been considered. Again, exercise seems to be very promising in reducing the inflammatory processes, with the actual discussion centered on the acute and chronic effects of different modes of exercise, and on the underlying mechanisms.

9. References

Baptista F, Silva AM, Santos, DA, Mota J, Santos R, Vale S, Ferreira JP, Raimundo A, Moreira H (2011) Livro Verde da Actividade Física. Instituto do Desporto de Portugal, I.P. Lisboa

Barbieri M, Ferruci L, Corsi AM, Macchi C, Laurentani F, Bonafe M, Olivieri F, Giovagnetti S, Franceschi C, Paolisso G (2003) Is chronic inflammation a determinant of blood pressure in the elderly? American Journal of Hypertension 16:537-543

Berk BC, Weintraub WS, Alexander RW (1990) Elevation of C-reactive protein in "active" coronary artery disease. American Journal of Cardiology 65:168-172

Bonita R, Beaglehole R, Kjellstrom T (2006). Basic Epidemiology, 2nd edn. World Health Organization, Geneva

Bouchard C, Shephard RJ (1994) Physical activity, fitness, and health: the model and key concepts. In: Bouchard C, Shephard RJ, Stephens T (eds) Physical Activity, Fitness, and Health: International Proceedings and Consensus Statement. Human Kinetics Champaign, IL pp 77-88

Brownson RC, Boehmer TK, Luke DA (2005) Declining rates of physical activity in the United States: what are the contributors? Annual Review of Public Health 26:421-443

Center for Disease Control and Prevention (2008) U.S. Physical Activity Statistics: 1998–2007 No Leisure-Time Physical Activity Trend Chart, http://www.cdc.gov/nccdphp/dnpa/physical/stats/leisure_time.htm

Church TS, Barlow CE, Earnest CP, Kamper JB, Priest EL, Blair SN (2002) Associations between cardiorespiratory fitness and C-reactive protein in men. Arteriosclerosis, Thrombosis and Vascular Biology 22:1869-1876

Church TS, Thomas DM, Tudor-Locke C, Katzmarzyk PT, Earnest CP, Rodarte RQ, Martin CK, Blair SN, Bouchard C (2011) Trends over 5 Decades in U.S. Occupation-Related Physical Activity and Their Associations with Obesity. PLoS ONE 6:e19657. doi:10.1371/journal.pone.0019657

Commission of the European Communities (2007) White Paper on Sport. Commission of the European Communities, Brussels

Das UN (2001) Is obesity an inflammatory condition? Nutrition 17:953-966

De Haro J, Acin F, Lopez-Quintana A, Medina FJ, Martinez-Aguilar E, Florez A, March JR (2008) Direct association between C-reactive protein serum levels and endothelial dysfunction in patients with claudication. European Journal of Vascular Endovascular Surgery 35:480-486

Dinneen S, Gerich J, Rizza R (1992) Carbohydrate metabolism in non-insulin-dependent diabetes mellitus. New England Journal of Medicine 327:707-713

EC (2003) Special Eurobarometer 183-6 on Physical Activity / Wave 58.2. European Opinion Research Group EEIG, European Comission, Brussels

EC (2010) Special Eurobarometer 334 on Sport and Physical Activity / Wave 72.3. TNS Opinion & Social, European Comission, Brussels

Hamer M, Stamatakis E (2008) The accumulative effects of modifiable risk factors on inflammation and haemostasis. Brain, Behaviour and Immunity 22:1041-1043

Haskell WL, Lee IM, Pate RR, Powell KE, Blair SN, Franklin BA, Macera CA, Heath GW, Thompson PD, Bauman A (2007) Physical activity and public health: updated recommendation for adults from the American College of Sports Medicine and the American Heart Association. Medicine and Science in Sports and Exercise 39:1423–1434

Hwang JS, Wu TL, Chou SC, Ho C, Chang PY, Tsao KC, Huang JY, Sun CF, Wu JT (2008) Development of multiple complications in type 2 diabetes is associated with the increase of multiple markers of chronic inflammation. Journal of Clinical Laboratory Analysis 22:6-13

Imatoh T, Miyazaki M, Une H (2007) Does elevated high-sensitivity serum C-reactive protein associate with hypertension in non-obese Japanese males? Clinical Experimental Hypertension 29:395-401

Kim ES, Im JA, Kim KC, Park JH, Suh SH, Kang ES, Kim SH, Jekal Y, Lee CW, Yoon YJ, Lee HC, Jeon JY (2007) Improved insulin sensitivity and adiponectin level after exercise training in obese Korean youth. Obesity 15:3023-3030

Koenig W, Sund M, Fröhlich M, Fischer HG, Löwel H, Döring A, Hutchinson WL, Pepys MB (1999) C Reactive protein, a sensitive marker of inflammation, predicts future risk of coronary heart disease in initially healthy middle-aged men: results from the MONICA (Monitoring Trends and Determinants in Cardiovascular Disease) Augsburg Cohort Study, 1984 to 1992. Circulation 99:237-242

Kohut ML, McCann DA, Russell DW, Konopka DN, Cunnick JE, Franke WD, Castillo MC, Reighard AE, Vanderah E (2006) Aerobic exercise, but not flexibility/resistance exercise, reduces serum IL-18, CRP, and IL-6 independent of b-blockers, BMI, and psychosocial factors in older adults. Brain Behaviour and Immunity 20:201-209

Kuller LH, Tracy RP, Shaten J, Meilahn EN (1996) Relation of C-reactive protein and coronary heart disease in the MRFIT nested case-control study. Multiple Risk Factor Intervention Trial. American Journal of Epidemiology 144:537-547

Laaksonen DE, Atalay M, Niskanen LK, Mustonen J, Sen CK, Lakka TA, Uusitupa MI (2000) Aerobic exercise and the lipid profile in type 1 diabetic men: a randomized controlled trial. Medicine and Science in Sports and Exercise 32:1541–1548

Last JM (2001) A Dictionary of Epidemiology, 4th edn. Oxford University Press, Oxford

Lee MA, Mather M (2008) Population Bulletin: U.S. Labor Force Trends. www.prb.org

Leon AS, Sanchez OA (2001) Response of blood lipids to exercise training alone or combined with dietary intervention. Medicine and Science in Sports and Exercise 33:S502–S515, discussion S528–S529

Lollgen H, Bockenhoff A, Knapp G (2009) Physical activity and all-cause mortality: an updated meta-analysis with different intensity categories. International Journal of Sports Medicine 30:213–224

Marini M, Sarchielli E, Brogi L, Lazzeri R, Salerno R, Sgambati E, Monaci M (2008) Role of adapted physical activity to prevent the adverse effects of the sarcopenia. A pilot study. Italian Journal of Anatomy and Embryology 113:217-225

Martins RA, Neves AP, Coelho-Silva MJ, Veríssimo MT & Teixeira AM (2010a) High-sensitivity C-reactive protein, body fat and physical exercise in older people. European Journal of Applied Physiology 110:161-169

Martins RA, Veríssimo MT Coelho-Silva MJ, Cumming SP & Teixeira AM (2010b) Effects of aerobic and strength-based training on metabolic health indicators in older adults. Lipids in Health and Disease, 9:76

Mora S, Lee IM, Buring JE, Ridker PM (2006) Association of physical activity and body mass index with novel and traditional cardiovascular biomarkers in women. JAMA 295:1412–1419

Morris JN, Clayton DG, Everitt MG, Semmence AM, Burgess EH (1990) Exercise in leisure time: coronary attack and death rates. British Heart Journal, 63:325-334

Morris JN, Heady JA, Raffle PAB, Roberts CG, Parks JN (1953a) Coronary heart disease and physical activity of work. Lancet 2:1053–1057

Morris JN, Heady JA, Raffle PAB, Roberts CG, Parks JN (1953b) Coronary heart disease and physical activity of work. Lancet 2:1111–1120

Onat A, Sansoy V, Yildirim B, Keles I, Uysal O, Hergenc G (2001) C-reactive protein and coronary heart disease in western Turkey. American Journal of Cardiology 88:601-607

Paffenbarger RS, Wing AL & Hyde RT (1978) Physical activity as an index of heart attack risk in college alumni. American Journal of Epidemiology 108:161-175

Paffenbarger RS Jr, Hyde RT, Wing AL & Hsieh C-c (1986a) Chronic disease in former college students: XXX. Physical activity, all-cause mortality, and longevity of college alumni. New England Journal of Medicine 314:605–613

Paffenbarger RS Jr, Hyde RT, Wing AL, Hsieh C-c (1986b) Chronic disease in former college students: XXX. Physical activity, all-cause mortality, and longevity of college alumni. New England Journal of Medicine 315:399–401

Paffenbarger RS Jr, Hyde RT, Wing AL, Lee I-M, Jung DL, Kampert JB (1993) Chronic disease in former college students: XXXVII. The association of changes in physical activity level and other lifestyle characteristics with mortality among men. New England Journal of Medicine 328:538–545

Paffenbarger RS Jr, Kampert JB, Lee I-M, Hyde RT, Leung RW, Wing AL (1994) Chronic disease in former college students: LII. Changes in physical activity and other lifeway patterns influencing longevity. Medicine and Science in Sports and Exercise 26:857–865

Pate RR, Pratt M, Blair SN, Haskell WL, Macera CA, Bouchard C, Buchner D, Ettinger W, Heath GW, King AC, Kriska A, Leon AS, Marcus BH, Morris J, Paffenbarger RS, Patrick K, Pollock ML, Rippe JM, Sallis J, Wilmore JH (1995) Physical activity and public health. A recommendation from the CDC and the American College of Sports Medicine. JAMA 273:402–407

Pedersen M, Bruunsgaard H, Weis N, Hendel HW, Andreassen BU, Eldrup E, Dela F, Pedersen BK (2003) Circulating levels of TNF-alpha and IL-6-relation to truncal fat mass and muscle mass in healthy elderly individuals and in patients with type-2 diabetes. Mechanisms of Ageing and Development 124:495-502

Piestrzeniewicz K, Łuczak K, Komorowski J, Maciejewski M, Jankiewicz-Wika J, Goch JH (2008) Resistin increases with obesity and atherosclerotic risk factors in patients with myocardial infarction. Metabolism: Clinical and Experimental 57:488-493

Porrini E, Gomez MD, Alvarez A, Cobo M, Gonzalez-Posada JM, Perez L, Hortal L, García JJ, Dolores-Checa M, Morales A, Hernández D, Torres A (2007) Glycated haemoglobin levels are related to chronic subclinical inflammation in renal transplant recipients without pre-existing or new onset diabetes. Nephrology and Dialysis Transplantation 22:1994-1999

Pradhan AD, Manson JE, Rifai N, Buring JE, Ridker PM (2001) C-reactive protein, interleukin-6 and risk of developing type 2 diabetes mellitus. JAMA 286:327-334

Reid KF, Naumova EN, Carabello RJ, Phillips EM, Fielding RA (2008) Lower extremity muscle mass predicts functional performance in mobility-limited elders. Journal of Nutrition, Health and Aging 12:493-498

Reuben DB, Judd-Hamilton L, Harris TB, Seeman TE (2003) The associations between physical activity and inflammatory markers in high-functioning older persons: MacArthur Studies of Successful Aging. Journal of the American Geriatrics Society 51:1125-1130

Ridker PM, Buring JE, Cook NR, Rifai N (2003) C-reactive protein, the metabolic syndrome, and risk of incident cardiovascular events: an 8-year follow-up of 14719 initially healthy American women. Circulation 107:391-397

Ridker PM, Buring JE, Shih J, Matias M, Hennekens CH (1998a) Prospective study of C-reactive protein and the risk of future cardiovascular events among apparently healthy women. Circulation 25:731-733

Ridker PM, Glynn RJ, Hennekens CH (1998b) C-reactive protein adds to the predictive value of total and HDL cholesterol in determining risk of first myocardial infarction. Circulation 97:2007-2011

Ridker PM, Rifai N, Rose L, Buring JE, Cook NR (2002) Comparison of C-reactive protein and low-density lipoprotein cholesterol levels in the prediction of first cardiovascular events. New England Journal of Medicine 347:1557-1565

Ridker PM, Stampfer MJ, Rifai N (2001) Novel risk factors for systemic atherosclerosis: a comparison of C-reactive protein, fibrinogen, homocysteine, lipoprotein(a), and standard cholesterol screening as predictors of peripheral arterial disease. Journal of the American Medical Association 285:2481-2485

Rifai N, Ridker PM (2001) High-sensitivity C-reactive protein: a novel and promising marker of coronary heart disease. Clinical Chemistry 47:403-411

Schoenborn CA, Stommel M (2011) Adherence to the 2008 adult physical activity guidelines and mortality risk. American Journal of Preventive Medicine 40:514-521

Steensberg A, Keller C, Starkic RL, Osada T, Febbraio MA, Pedersen BK (2002) IL-6 and TNF-alpha expression in, and release from, contracting human skeletal muscle. American Journal of Physiology, Endocrinology and Metabolism 283:E1272-E1278

Steensberg A, Fischer CP, Keller C, Moller K, Pedersen BK (2003) IL-6 enhances plasma IL-1ra, IL-10, and cortisol in humans. American Journal of Physiology, Endocrinology and Metabolism 285:E433-E437

Stewart LK, Flynn MG, Campbell WW, Craig BA, Robinson JP, Timmerman KL, McFarlin BK, Coen PM, Talbert E, (2007) The influence of exercise training on inflammatory cytokines and C-reactive protein. Medicine and Science in Sports and Exercise 39:1714-1719

Torre-Amione G (2005) Immune activation in chronic heart failure. American Journal of Cardiology 95:3C-8C

Torres JL, Ridker PM (2003) Clinical use of high sensitivity C-reactive protein for the prediction of adverse cardiovascular events. Current Opinion in Cardiology 18:471-478

Troiano RP, Berrigan D, Dodd KW, Masse LC, Tilert T, McDowell M (2008) Physical activity in the United States measured by accelerometer. Medicine and Science in Sports Exercise 40:181-188

USDHHS (1996) Physical Activity and Health. A Report of the Surgeon General. USDHHS, CDC, National Center for Chronic Disease Prevention and Health Promotion, Atlanta GA

USDHHS (2000) Healthy People 2010: Understanding and Improving Health. 2nd ed. US Government Printing Office, Washington, DC

USDHHS (2010) Healthy People 2020. US Government Printing Office, Washington, DC

USDHHS (2011) Physical activity guidelines for Americans. USDHHS. Washington DC. www.health.gov/paguidelines/, accessed on October 19th

Virani SS, Polsani VR, Nambi V (2008) Novel markers of inflammation in atherosclerosis. Current Atherosclerosis Reports 10:164-170

Visser M, Pahor M, Taaffe DR, Goodpaster BH, Simonsick EM, Newman AB, Nevitt M, Harris TB (2002) Relationship of interleukin-6 and tumor necrosis factor-alpha with muscle mass and muscle strength in elderly men and women: the Health ABC Study. The Journals of Gerontology. Series A, Biological Sciences and Medical Sciences 57:M326-M332

Wannamethee SG, Lowe GD, Whincup PH, Rumley A, Walker M, Lennon L (2002) Physical activity and haemostatic and inflammatory variables in elderly men. Circulation 105:1785-1790

Welk GJ (2002) Physical Activity Assessments for Health-Related Research. Human Kinetics, Champaign, IL

Widmaier EP, Raff H, Strang KT, Vander AJ (2011) Vander's human physiology: the mechanisms of body function, 12th edn. McGraw-Hill Higher Education, New York

Zurlo F, Nemeth PM, Choksi RM, Sesodia S, Ravussin E (1994) Whole-body energy metabolism and skeletal muscle biochemical characteristics. Metabolism 43:481-486

14

Cardiovascular Disease Risk Factors

Reza Amani and Nasrin Sharifi
Ahvaz Jondishapour University of Medical Sciences, Iran

1. Introduction

Cardiovascular disease (CVD) is the leading cause of death not only in industrialized and developed countries but also in developing societies (WHO, 2008a). Changes in lifestyle of the population living in developing countries, which is due to the socioeconomic and cultural transition, are important reasons for increasing the rate of CVD. This observation has led to extensive research on prevention. Diagnosis the risk factors and predictors of CVD can help us detect high risk patients and prevent the disease, effectively.

Nowadays with a rapid progress in medical technology and diagnostic tools, more predictors are being added to the previous list of CVD risk factors. Therefore, we need to design updated risk assessment methods to screen high risk individuals early in their life span.

This chapter defines cardiovascular risk factors, classifies them, briefly describes how they interact, and discusses what strategies Should be implemented to prevent CVD progression.

2. Definitions

2.1 Coronary Heart Disease (CHD)

Coronary heart disease (CHD) is a condition in which the walls of arteries supplying blood to the heart muscle (coronary arteries) become thickened. This thickening, caused by development of lesions in the arterial wall, is called atherosclerosis; the lesions are called plaques. It can restrict the supply of blood to the heart muscle (the myocardium) and may manifest to the patient as chest pain on exertion (angina) or breathlessness on exertion. (Frayn 2005).

2.2 Cerebrovascular disease

Cerebrovascular disease involves interruption of the blood supply to part of the brain and may result in a stroke or a transient ischemic attack. The loss of blood supply to part of the brain may lead to irreversible damage to brain tissue. The blockage most commonly arises from the process of thromboembolism, in which a blood clot formed somewhere else (*e.g.* in the heart or in the carotid artery) becomes dislodged and then occludes an artery within the brain (cerebral arteries). Narrowing of the intracerebral arteries with atherosclerotic plaque may increase the risk, and may also lead to local formation of a blood clot. The etiology is similar to that of CHD (Frayn 2005).

2.3 Peripheral Vascular Disease (PVD)

Peripheral vascular disease (PVD) involves atherosclerotic plaques narrowing the arteries supplying other regions apart from the myocardium and brain. A common form involves narrowing of the arteries supplying blood to the legs. The result may be pain on exercise. In more severe cases, impaired blood supply leads to death of leg tissues, which requires amputation (Frayn 2005).

3. Epidemiology

3.1 Global and regional trends in CVD burden

In recent years, the dominance of chronic diseases as major contributors to total global mortality has emerged (WHO, 2008a). By 2005, the total number of cardiovascular disease (CVD) deaths (mainly coronary heart disease, stroke, and rheumatic heart disease) had increased globally to 17.5 million from 14.4 million in 1990(WHO, 2009a).

The World Health Organization (WHO) estimates there will be about 20 million CVD deaths in 2015, accounting for 30 percent of all deaths worldwide (WHO, 2005). Thus, CVD is today the largest single contributor to global mortality and will continue to dominate mortality trends in the future (WHO, 2009a).

Globally, there is an uneven distribution of age-adjusted CVD mortality that is mapped in Figure 1. The lowest age-adjusted mortality rates are in the advanced industrialized countries and parts of Latin America, whereas the highest rates today are found in Eastern Europe and a number of low and middle income countries(WHO, 2008a). The broad causes for the rise and, in some countries, the decline in CVD over time are well described. The key contributors to the rise across countries at all stages of development include tobacco use and abnormal blood lipid levels, along with unhealthy dietary changes (especially related to fats and oils, salt, and increased calories) and reduced physical activity(Hu, 2008;). Key contributors to the decline in some countries include declines in tobacco use and exposure, healthful dietary shifts, population-wide prevention efforts, and treatment interventions (Shafey et al, 2009; Davies et al, 2007).

4. Pathophysiology

Cardiovascular diseases, whether affecting the coronary, cerebral or peripheral arteries, share a common pathophysiology involving atherosclerosis and thrombosis (or clotting).

4.1 Atherosclerosis

Atherosclerosis is the most common cause of CVD and related mortality. The first observable event in the process of atherosclerosis is the accumulation of plaque (cholesterol from low-density lipoproteins [LDLs], calcium, and fibrin) in large and medium arteries.

This plaque can grow and produce ischemia either by insufficient blood flow if there is a high oxygen demand or by rupturing, forming a thrombus and occluding the lumen (Rudd et al., 2005). Only high-risk or vulnerable plaque forms thrombi. Characteristics of vulnerable

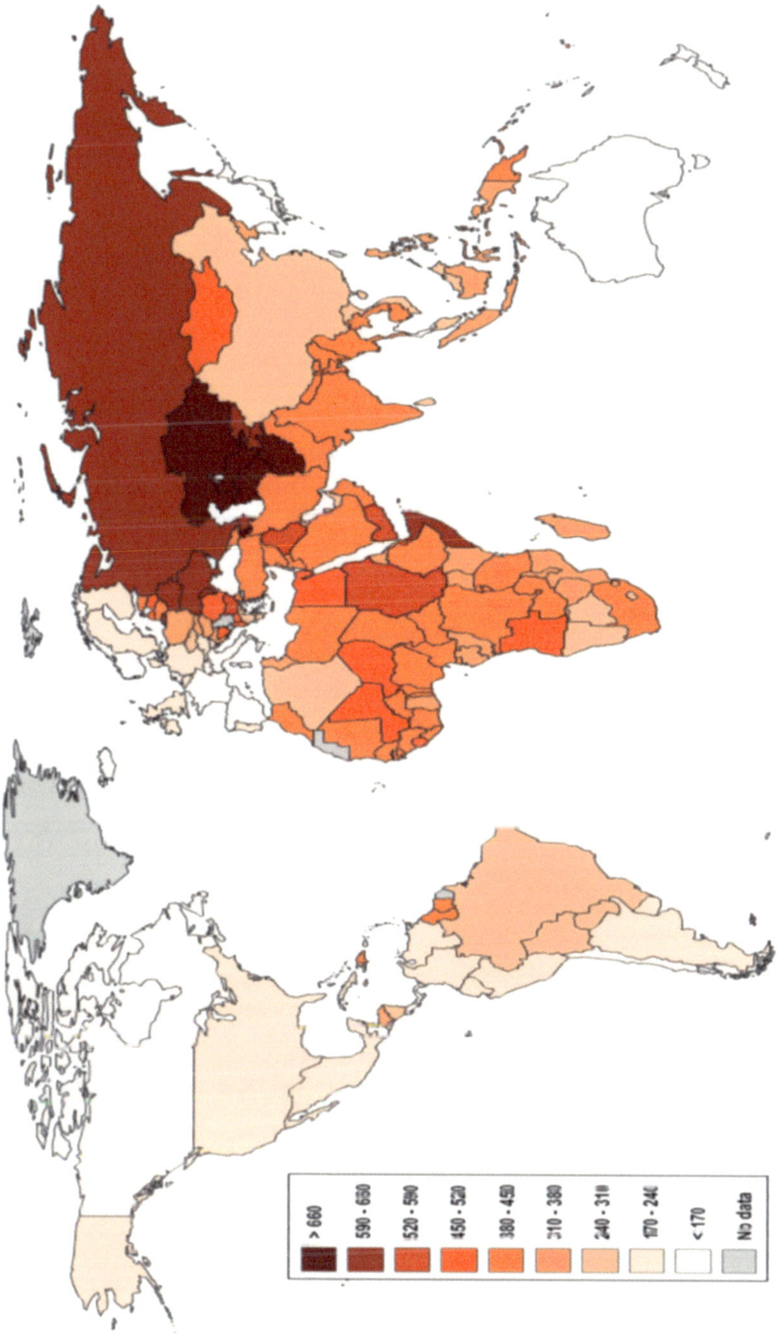

NOTE: Rates are age-standardized to WHO's world standard population.
SOURCES: WHO, 2009a

Fig. 1. Age-standardized deaths due to cardiovascular disease (rate per 100,000), 2004.

plaque are lesions with a thin fibrous cap, few smooth muscle cells, many macrophages (inflammatory cells),and a large lipid core(Figure 2) (Rudd et al., 2005). The site of plaque formation or atherogenesis is the endothelium in the artery wall. Normally the endothelium promotes dilation of the blood vessel ,less smooth muscle cell growth, and prevention of an anti-inflammatory response (Davignon and Ganz, 2004). In atherosclerosis the endothelium becomes dysfunctional before an atheroma or plaque, a more serious lesion, develops. This endothelial dysfunction results in the production of less nitric oxide, a key vasodilator, and the blood vessel becomes more constricted .It also becomes more permeable and allows LDL cholesterol to be taken up by macrophages, which then accumulate and form foam cells and eventually an early lesion known as a fatty streak.

5. Risk factors for cardiovascular disease

This section described the major risk factors for CVD in more detail. The section begins with lipid and inflammation-related factors, behavioral risk factors, including tobacco use, dietary factors, alcohol, and physical activity. This is followed by the major biological risk factors that mediate the role of these behaviors leading to CVD, including obesity, blood pressure, blood lipids, and diabetes.

5.1 Modifiable cardiovascular risk factors

5.1.1 Lipid-related factors

Lipid-related cardiovascular risk factors have attracted enormous attention over the past years, and consensus documents have been produced to implement treatment and preventive strategies. Essentially, this applies to the conventional risk factors such as high plasma total and low-density lipoprotein (LDL) cholesterol, low plasma high density lipoprotein (HDL) cholesterol and elevated plasma triglycerides.

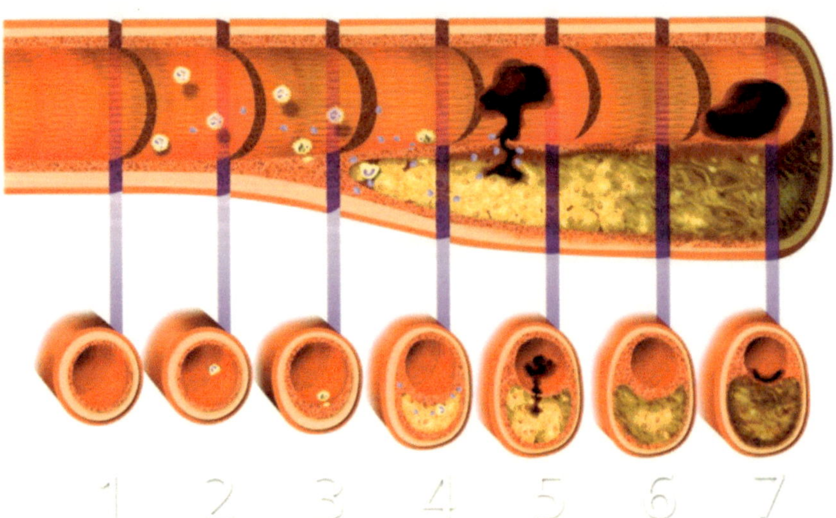

Fig. 2. Natural Progression of atherosclerosis

5.1.1.1 Atherogenic lipoproteins

A number of factors determine whether a cholesterol-containing lipoprotein particle resident in plasma has atherogenic properties. The size of the particle determines the ease by which the endothelium can be penetrated; small particles are more likely to be deposited in the arterial wall than large particles. The binding to the subendothelial matrix is also dependent on size, in which the smaller particles bind more avidly to proteoglycans (Anber *et al.*, 1997). The apoB protein, present as one molecule per lipoprotein particle, seems to be crucial. Firstly, lipoprotein particles without apoB are not atherogenic; secondly, apoB has multiple proteoglycan binding domains which enhance the retention of the particle in the subendothelial matrix (Skalen *et al.*, 2002). Finally, physicochemical and compositional characteristics, such as resistance factors against oxidative stress, are likely to be important in reducing the modification of lipoprotein particles.

5.1.1.2 Small, dense Low-Density Lipoprotein (LDL)

The formation of small, dense LDL particles is complex and can be seen as a genetic trait, but the major gene(s) responsible remain unknown. Environmental factors also play a major role, in that dietary factors can influence triglyceride as a major determinant. *In vitro* studies have shown that small, dense LDL particles are formed by sequential exchange of lipids between LDL and triglyceride-rich lipoproteins. The cholesteryl esters contained in the core of the LDL particle are exchanged for triglycerides by the cholesteryl ester transfer protein (CETP). Triglycerides entering the LDL particle are hydrolyzed by hepatic lipase and the core volume of the particle is reduced. The formation of small, dense LDL is limited by the availability of triglyceride-rich lipoproteins, as evidenced by the close positive correlation between plasma triglycerides and small, dense LDL. It is assumed that these processes take quite some time and the end product is therefore an aged particle that has lost its defense against free radical attack. The retention in plasma of the particle is partly due to the fact that small, dense LDL has a lower affinity for the LDL receptor than normal buoyant LDL (Nigon *et al.*, 1991). It is thought that a consequence of the altered chemical composition of the small, dense LDL particle is that it more avidly binds to the subendothelial matrix and upon challenge more easily undergoes oxidative modification thereby triggering foam cell formation (Tribble *et al.*, 1992; Chait *et al.*, 1993; Dejager *et al.*, 1993;).

The presence of triglyceride-rich lipoproteins is a principal modulator of small, dense LDL; the plasma concentration of the latter is strongly and positively related to the concentration of plasma triglycerides. In fact, all examples in which the triglyceride concentration has been altered to observe a change in the LDL profile are consistent: elevation of triglycerides leads to higher abundance of small, dense LDL; the opposite is observed when triglycerides are lowered, treated by diet or pharmacological agents. Low fat diets may lead to increased plasma triglyceride concentration; consequently a reduction in LDL size was observed in a study of 105 men switching from a high fat (46%) to a low fat (24%) diet (Dreon *et al.*, 1994). The total LDL cholesterol concentration was, however, reduced simultaneously, so the net effect on cardiovascular risk is not entirely clear.

In the Quebec Cardiovascular Study the cholesterol concentration in small dense LDL particle may give even more precise information. Again, in the Quebec heart study, the cholesterol concentration in small dense LDL particles showed the strongest association with the risk of CHD. These data suggest that the cholesterol within small dense LDL is particularly harmful. Therefore measurement of LDL particle size and possibly cholesterol content within these particles may enhance our capability to predict cardiovasular events (Lamarche *et al.*, 2001).

5.1.1.3 High-Density Lipoprotein (HDL)

HDL is another lipid profile fraction which is associated to the risk of CVD. Decreased levels of HDL-c correlated to increased risk of CVD. The atheroprotective role for HDL is mainly due to the pathway named *reverse cholesterol transport* (RCT). RCT is defined as the uptake of cholesterol from peripheral tissues back to the liver by HDL. Apo A1 is an apolipoprotein of the HDL that activates the enzyme lecithin-cholesteryl ester acyl-transferase (LCAT). The main function of LCAT is transferring cholesterol from cell to HDL. Both apo C and apo E on HDL are transferred to chylomicrons.

Apo E helps receptors metabolize chylomicron remnants and also inhibits appetite (Gotoh et al., 2006). Therefore high HDL levels are associated with low levels of chylomicrons; *very low density lipoprotein* (VLDL) remnants; and small dense LDLs and subsequently lower atherosclerotic risk. HDL has other potentially atheroprotective properties. The anti-oxidative activity of HDL is typically characterized by its ability to inhibit LDL oxidation. It has also been shown to inhibit the formation of reactive oxygen species. HDL can help to protect endothelial cells from apoptosis induced by mildly oxidized LDL. It can affect platelet function through the promotion of nitric oxide production (Chen et al, 1994; Suc et al 1997) and coagulation by the inhibition of several coagulation factors. There is considerable evidence for a direct protective role of HDL in inflammatory, oxidative, apoptotic, and thrombotic processes.

Major factors that increase HDL cholesterol level are exogenous estrogen, intensive exercise, loss of excess body fat, moderate consumption of alcohol and triglyceride lowering drugs such as fibrates and niacin. Treatment of low serum levels of HDL-C in at risk patients is an important therapeutic intervention and impacts rates of disease progression as well as cardiovascular events (Scanu and Edelstein , 2008).

5.1.2 Inflammation-related factors

Inflammation is a part of atherosclerosis process, beginning with the formation of fatty streak underlying the endothelium of large arteries. The infiltration of monocytes and lymphocytes occurs as a result of the expression of adhesion molecules by endothelial cells lining the artery wall. Several stimuli for the inflammatory response in atherosclerosis have been proposed in which oxidised low-density lipoprotein (LDL), is of most importance. Monocytes that have infiltrated the arterial intima and differentiated into macrophages take up oxidized LDL through scavenger receptors in an unregulated manner, accumulating large amounts of cholesterol and becoming foam cells. Macrophages eventually die, through necrosis and apoptosis, the lipid is deposited within the core of the developing plaque (Figure 3). Cytokines secreted by both lymphocytes and macrophages within the plaque exert pro- and anti-atherogenic effects on components of the vessel wall. Smooth muscle cells migrate from the medial portion of the arterial wall towards the intima and secrete extracellular matrix proteins that form a fibrous cap. The cap separates the highly thrombogenic contents of the plaque lipid core from the potent coagulation system contained within the circulating blood.

This chronic, low-grade inflammation is likely to be the result of cytokines secreted by monocytes and soluble adhesion molecules from the vessel wall into the circulation, where they subsequently act on the liver to induce the secretion of acute phase proteins, including C-Reactive Protein(CRP), fibrinogen and serum amyloid A (Frayn, 2005).

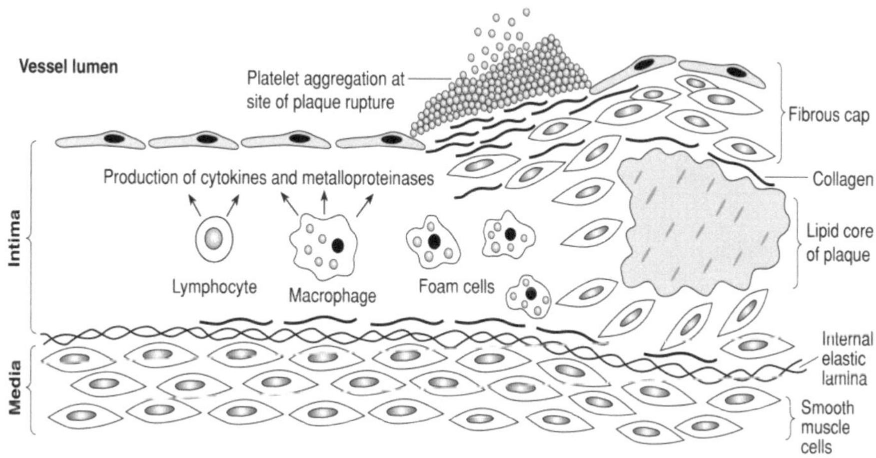

From Frayn 2005

Fig. 3. Schematic representation of the development of an atherosclerotic lesion, showing plaque rupture and platelet aggregation .

5.1.2.1 C-Reactive protein

Multiple studies have demonstrated that elevated levels of high-sensitivity C-reactive protein (hs-CRP) are associated with increased CVD risk. (Buckley et al.,2009; Musunuru et al., 2008). hs-CRP, previously considered to be an indicator of systemic inflammation, has recently received much attention in the scientific literature, not only as a potential marker of increased atherosclerotic risk, but also as a potential target of therapy for the prevention of atherosclerotic CVD. Evidence derived mainly from statin trials, supports the potential value of CRP as a therapeutic target for both primary and secondary prevention of CVD and CHD. The largest study to suggest an integral role for CRP as a target for therapy in primary prevention of CVD is the recent Justification for the Use of Statins in Prevention: An Intervention Trial Evaluating Rosuvastatin (JUPITER) trial. The investigators randomized 17,802 men ≥50 years of age and women ≥60 years of age with low LDL cholesterol levels < 130 mg/dL and hs-CRP ≥ 2 mg/L and no history of CVD or diabetes to 20 mg rosuvastatin daily or placebo. The primary end point was the first occurrence of MI, stroke, hospitalization for unstable angina, arterial revascularization, or CV death (Ridker et al; 2008). During the 1.9-year median follow-up duration (maximum follow-up period 5 years), rosuvastatin reduced LDL cholesterol by 50% and hs-CRP by 37%. Thus, JUPITER demonstrated a magnitude of effect larger than that of almost all prior statin trials (Ridker et al; 2009). Based on the results of the JUPITER study, the U.S. Food and Drug Administration (FDA) in February 2010 agreed to broader labeling for rosuvastatin. Rosuvastatin is currently approved for the reduction of risk for stroke, MI, and revascularization procedures in individuals who have normal LDL cholesterol levels and no clinically evident CHD but who do have an increased risk based on age, CRP levels, and the presence of at least one additional CVD risk factor. Accordingly, JUPITER not only demonstrated that hs-CRP successfully identified a population with "hidden risk" for CVD but also provided additional evidence for the potential utility of hs-CRP as a target for therapy in primary prevention of CVD disease.

Other inflammatory states such as obesity produce elevations in CRP even in young obese children (Blum et al., 2005). Body mass index (BMI) is moderately correlated ($r = 0.5$) to CRP levels (Rawson et al., 2003). Recently it was demonstrated that weight loss lowers CRP (Tchernof et al., 2002), which provides another physiologic benefit for weight management as a preventive strategy for CHD reduction. Currently it is known that elevated insulin levels in overweight children affect CRP. Physical activity did not appear to be related (Rawson et al., 2003). To date few studies have investigated the effects of dietary variables on CRP. In a cross-sectional study, higher intakes of fruits and vegetables were associated with lower CRP levels (Gao et al., 2004).

5.1.2.2 Fibrinogen

Fibrinogen is the precursor of fibrin. As the major clotting factor in the blood and a pro-inflammatory molecule, fibrinogen plays role in atherosclerosis. It is synthesized in the liver and, like CRP, is an acute phase protein, whose circulating levels can change during acute responses to tissue damage or infection. Thus Fibrinogen (Fg) is a biomarker of inflammation (Ross 1999), which, when elevated, indicates the presence of inflammation and identifies individuals with a high risk for cardiovascular disorders. Increased plasma Fg concentration typically accompanies hypertension development (Lominadze *et al.* 1998) and stroke (D'Erasmo *et al.* 1993). Factors associated with an elevated fibrinogen are smoking, diabetes, hypertension, obesity, sedentary lifestyle, elevated triglycerides, and genetic factors. Recent studies indicate that increased Fg content affects microcirculation by increasing plasma viscosity, RBC aggregation and platelet thrombogenesis (Lominadze et al; 2010). These changes lead to vascular dysfunction and exacerbate microcirculatory complications during cardiovascular diseases (figure 4).

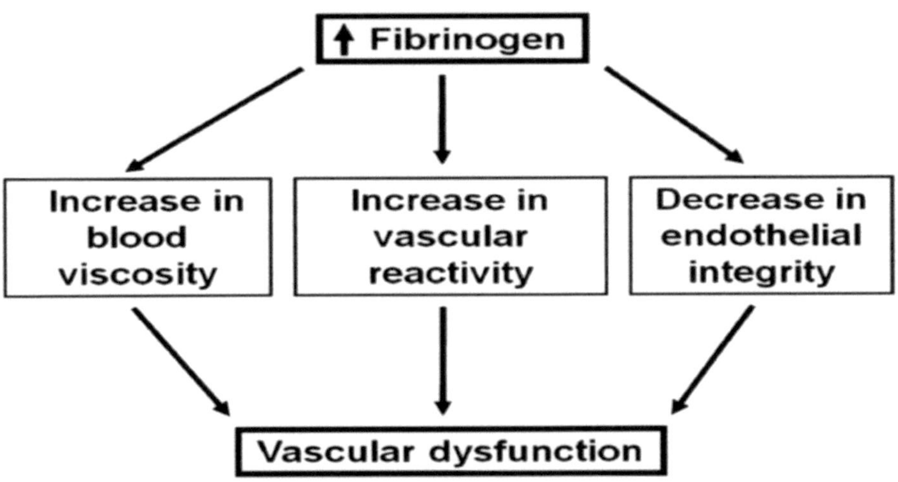

From Lominadze et al. 2010

Fig. 4. Schematic representation of fibrinogen-induced vascular dysfunction.

5.1.2.3 Serum amyloid A

Serum amyloid A (SAA) is a precursor of amyloid A protein and comprises both constitutive (apoSAA1, apoSAA2) and acute phase (apoSAA4) isoforms. The serum amyloid A proteins are a family of inflammatory apolipoproteins with a high affinity for HDL, and their production by the liver and other tissues is thought to be induced by IL-1 and IL 6. Their role in lipid metabolism is unclear, although they may be involved in HDL trafficking. A small number of studies have investigated the association between SAA and the incidence of CHD (Ridker *et al.*, 1998, 2000; Danesh *et al.*, 2000b). Taken together, these studies show that a comparison of individuals with values in the top third with those in the bottom third gives a combined risk ratio of 1.6 for CHD. However, further studies are required to determine whether the association is independent of possible confounders.

5.1.3 Behavioral and lifestyle risk factors

5.1.3.1 Tobacco

There are currently more than 1 billion smokers worldwide. Although use of tobacco products is decreasing in high income countries, it is increasing globally, with more than 80 percent of the world's smokers now living in low and middle income countries (Jha and Chaloupka, 1999).

In the Global Burden of Disease study, Lopez et al. (2006) estimated that in 2000, 880,000 deaths from CHD and 412,000 deaths from stroke were attributable to tobacco. Smoking cessation has been shown to have significant impacts on reducing CHD. In a major review of the evidence, Critchley and Capewell (2003) determined that successful smoking cessation reduced CHD mortality risk by up to 36 percent. Smoking cessation leads to significantly lower rates of reinfarction within 1 year among patients who have had a heart attack and reduces the risk of sudden cardiac death among patients with CHD (Gritz et al., 2007).

Two major trends are of real concern with respect to the future of tobacco-related CVD. First, in most parts of the world, the smoking rates are higher among the poorest populations (WHO, 2008b). The second worrisome trend is in smoking among girls (IOM, 2010).

In addition to active smoking, it has become increasingly apparent that exposure to secondhand smoke significantly increases cardiovascular risk. A recent IOM review of the effects of secondhand smoke exposure concluded that exposure to secondhand smoke significantly increases cardiovascular risk and that public smoking bans can significantly reduce the rate of heart attacks. The report concluded that secondhand smoke exposure increases cardiovascular risk by 25 to 30 percent and that there is sufficient evidence to support a causal relationship between secondhand smoke exposure and acute myocardial infarction (AMIs). This causality was reinforced by the report's conclusion that smoking bans significantly reduce the rate of AMIs, with declines ranging from 6 to 47 percent (IOM, 2009).

5.1.3.2 Dietary factors

The relationship between CVD and diet is one of the most studied relationships in epidemiology. Although nutritional research has traditionally focused on the effect of individual food groups or nutrients on CVD, there has been a shift in recent years toward comparing how different types of dietary patterns in their entirety affect CVD risk (IOM, 2010). The following sections reflect this shift by discussing research on dietary factors that have clear impacts on CVD risk.

5.1.3.2.1 Dietary fat

Healthy oils are those that contain no commercially introduced trans fatty acids, are low in saturated fatty acids, and are high in mono- and polyunsaturated fatty acids.

There is accumulating evidence that it is fat quality (the type of dietary fat), rather than the total amount of fat, that is particularly important for cardiovascular disease (Astrup, 2002).

5.1.3.2.1.1 Saturated Fatty Acids (SFA)

The predominant sources of SFAs are animal foods (meat and dairy). SFAs have the most potent effect on LDL cholesterol, which rises in a dose response fashion when increasing levels of SFAs are consumed. In our study, consumption of habitual hydrogenated fats and full-fat yoghurts (fat content more than 2.5%) increased the risk of CVD (OR = 2.12(1.23-3.64) and 2.35(1.32-4.18), respectively) (Amani et al, 2010). These foods are the major sources of SFAs. SFAs intake is the principal determinant of total cholesterol(TC) and CVD and substitution of 1% carbohydrate calories by SFAs increases TC by 1.5 mg/dL (Joseph et al, 2000). Of all the added fats in the diet, the most hypercholesterolemic promoting are palm kernel, coconut, and palm oils; lard; and butter. SFAs raise serum LDL cholesterol by decreasing LDL receptor synthesis and activity. Regardless of form, all fatty acids lower fasting triglycerides if they replace carbohydrate in the diet. In secondary prevention trials replacement of SFAs with MUFA, α-linolenic acid, and increased fruits and vegetables prevented fatal and nonfatal CVD events in persons with established disease (de Lorgeril, 1999). Thus fatty acids affect disease progression through lipids and other mechanisms and possibly through inflammation and thrombosis (Krummel, 2008).

5.1.3.2.1.2 Monounsaturated Fatty Acids (MUFA)

The American Heart Association (AHA) does not have any recommendation for the *cis* form of MUFAs (Lichtenstein et al., 2006). Oleic acid (C18:1) is the most prevalent MUFA in the American diet. Substituting oleic acid for carbohydrate has almost no appreciable effect on blood lipids; however, replacing SFAs with MUFA lowers serum cholesterol levels, LDL cholesterol levels, and triglyceride levels to about the same extent as polyunsaturated fatty acids (PUFAs) . The effects of MUFAs on HDL cholesterol depend on the total fat content of the diet. When intakes of both MUFA (>15% of total kilocalories) and total fat (>35% of kilocalories) are high, HDL cholesterol does not change or increases slightly compared with levels with a lower-fat diet (Krummel , 2008). Oleic acid as a part of the Mediterranean diet has been shown to have antiinflammatory effects. In epidemiologic studies high-fat diets of people in Mediterranean countries have been associated with low blood cholesterol levels and CHD incidence (Trichopoulou et al., 2003). Among other factors, the main fat source is olive oil, which is high in MUFA. Although higher-fat diets (low in SFA with MUFAs as the predominant fat) can lower blood cholesterol, they should be used with caution because of the caloric density of high-fat diets and the results of clinical trials, which have shown new atherosclerotic lesions in men who consume higher-fat diets. The negative association between the Mediterranean diet and CHD could be the result of factors other than MUFA intake. For example, these populations consume more fruits and vegetables, bread, cereals, fish, and nuts, and less red meat than many populations. Olive oil is the primary source of fat, and eggs are consumed from zero to four times per week (krummel, 2008).

5.1.3.2.1.3 Polyunsaturated Fatty Acids (PUFA)

The essential fatty acid linoleic acid (LA) is the predominant PUFA consumed in the American diet (Krummel, 2008). Population studies have demonstrated a negative correlation between LA intake and CHD rates (Wijendran and Hayes, 2004). Similarly, a meta analysis of 60 controlled human trials found that replacing PUFA for carbohydrate in the diet resulted in a decline in serum LDL cholesterol (Mensink et al., 2003). When SFAs are replaced with PUFAs in a low-fat diet, LDL and HDL cholesterol levels will be lowered. The lipid lowering effects of LA depend on the total fatty acid profile of the diet (Wijendran and Hayes, 2004). When added to study diets, large amounts of LA diminished levels of HDL cholesterol serum levels (Karmally, 2005). Studies suggest that high intakes of n-6 PUFAs may exert adverse effects on the function of vascular endothelium or stimulate production of proinflammatory cytokines. A low ratio of omega-6:omega-3 PUFA is recommended (Basu et al., 2006; Gibauer eial., 2006).

5.1.3.2.1.4 Omega-3 fatty acids

Fish oils, fish oil capsules, and ocean fish are rich source of the two main omega-3 fatty acids (i.e., eicosapentaenoic acid (EPA) and docosahexaenoic acid [DHA]). Many studies have shown that eating fish is associated with a decreased CVD risk. The recommendation for the general population for fish consumption is to eat fish high in omega-3 fatty acids (salmon, tuna, mackerel, sardines) at least twice a week (Psota et al., 2006). For patients who have CVD, 1 g of EPA and DHA combined is recommended from fish if possible but, if not, then from supplements (Lichtenstein et al., 2006). Patients who have hypertriglyceridemia need 2 to 4 g of EPA and DHA per day for effective lowering (Lichtenstein et a1.,2006). Omega-3 fatty acids lower triglyceride levels by inhibiting VLDL and apo B-100 synthesis and by decreasing postprandial lipemia.

α-Linolenic acid (ALA), an omega-3 fatty acid from vegetables, has anti-inflammatory effects. CRP levels were reduced when male patients consumed 8 g of ALA daily; similar results have not been observed for fish oil supplementation (Basu et a1.,2006). Omega-3 fatty acids also interfere with blood clotting by altering prostaglandin synthesis (Krummel, 2008).

5.1.3.2.1.5 Trans fatty acids

Trans-fatty acids are produced in the hydrogenation process used in the food industry to increase shelf life of foods and to make margarines, firmer (Krummel ,2008). The AHA (Lichtenstein et al., 2006) recommends no more than 1% of calories (about 1 3 g/day) from trans-fatty acids. These fatty acids raise LDL cholesterol; however, effects on inflammation have been conflicting (Basu et a1.,2006). Most trans-fatty acids intake comes from partially hydrogenated vegetable oils (krummel, 2008).

Mozaffarian et al (2007) showed that partially hydrogenated oils are extensively being used for cooking in Iranian homes with average per-person intake of 14 g/1000 kcal. Trans fatty acids (TFAs) accounted for 33% of fatty acids in these products, or 4.2% of all calories consumed (12.3 g/day). Consumption of hydrogenated fats was associated with higher

CAD risk (OR = 2.12(1.23-3.64)) in a study performed by Amani et al (2010). On the basis of TC:HDL-cholesterol effects alone, 9% of CHD events would be prevented by replacement of TFA in homes with *cis*-unsaturated fats (8% by replacement with saturated fats). On the basis of relationships of TFA intake with CHD incidence in prospective studies, 39% of CHD events would be prevented by replacement of TFA with *cis*-unsaturated fats (31% by replacement with saturated fats).

5.1.3.2.1.6 Dietary cholesterol

Dietary cholesterol raises total cholesterol and LDL cholesterol but to a lesser extent than SFAs. The AHA dietary patterns contain no more than 200 mg of cholesterol each day (Krummel; 2008). There is a threshold beyond which addition of cholesterol to the diet has minimal effects. When cholesterol intakes reach 500 mg/day, only small increments in blood cholesterol occur. Cholesterol responsiveness also varies widely among individuals. Some people are hyporesponders (i.e., their plasma cholesterol level does not increase after dietary cholesterol challenge), whereas others are hyperresponders (i.e., their plasma cholesterol level responds more strongly than expected to a cholesterol challenge). It has been suggested that hyperresponders may have the apo E-4 allele and poor rates of conversion of cholesterol to bile acids, which causes elevated LDL cholesterol. Feedings cholesterol to animals enriches lipoproteins, which are atherogenic beyond just the rise in serum cholesterol (Krummel, 2008).

SFAs and cholesterol synergistically affect LDL cholesterol level, decrease LDL receptor synthesis and activity, increase VLDLs enriched with apo E, increase all lipoproteins, and decrease chylomicron size (which is associated with CHD risk). The effect of dietary cholesterol on inflammatory factors has been inconsistent (Basu et a1.,2006).

5.1.3.2.2 Dietary sodium

There is evident that excessive sodium intake significantly increases CVD risk and that reduction in sodium intake at the population level decreases CVD burden (He and MacGregor, 2009, IOM, 2010). The most well-established mechanism by which sodium intake increases CVD risk is increasing blood pressure (BP). Numerous studies have found that there is a continuous and graded relationship between salt intake and blood pressure. In their recent major review of sodium trends and impact, He and MacGregor concluded that a reduction in salt from the current global intake of 9 to 12 g/day to the recommended levels of 5-6 g/day would have a major impact on BP and CVD (He and MacGregor, 2009; IOM, 2010). Salt's impact on CVD, however, extends beyond blood pressure. Animal and epidemiological studies have found that a diet high in sodium may directly increase the risk of stroke, which is independent and additive to salt's effect on BP (He and MacGregor, 2009 ; IOM, 2010).

5.1.3.2.3 Soy protein

In recent years, a great deal of interest has emerged in the role of soy-bean isoflavones in reducing heart diseases, and isoflavones might be responsible, in part, for the ability of soybean to lower the risk of CVD and atherosclerosis (Anderson et al, 1995) . Anderson suggested that about 60-70% of the cholesterol lowering effect of soy protein may be due to its isoflavone content (Anderson et al, 1995). Isoflavones are a group of phytoestrogens which occur mainly in soy and it is consumed for the purpose of both promoting health and preventing several chronic diseases, including coronary heart disease, cancers of reproductive organs and osteoporosis (Lichtenstein, 1998 ; Anerson et al, 1999). Aglycone forms of soy isoflavones especially genistein and daidzein have greatly been studied because of their greater estrogenic and antioxidant activities (Arora et al, 1998). Soy isoflavones have been shown to decrease total, VLDL and LDL cholesterol levels while increasing HDL cholesterol levels in peripubertal rhesus monkeys fed soy protein-based diets (Antony et al, 1996). It is claimed that purified isoflavones have no effect on plasma lipid and lipoprotein concentrations in normolipidemic subjects (Nestel et al, 1997; Hodgson et al, 1998). At present, there is no general agreement about the effect of soy protein isoflavones (SPI) on lipid profiles and moreover, it is not clear that which part of the soy protein has lipid-lowering effects. In a study, we designed animal model to assess the effect of SPI on serum lipid, lipoprotein profile, and blood sugar of experimentally- induced hypercholesterolemic rabbits,and to detect any dose-response effect of SPI on the above mentioned variables. In this research, the effect of soy protein containing 200 mg, 100 mg and a trace amount of both glycoside and aglycone forms of soy isoflavones were assessed in hypercholesterolemic male rabbits. Although the rabbits had a cholesterol-rich diet, the serum total and LDL-cholesterol remained unchanged in the SPI+ group (i.e. intact soy protein diet). The results have indicated that soy protein isoflavones maintained the serum lipid and lipoprotein levels in hypercholesterolemic rabbits kept on a high cholesterol diet, but alcohol-extracted (even half-dose isoflavones) soy protein diets do not have positive effect. Moreover, the hypocholesterolemic effect of isoflavones is not in a dose-response manner and it is suggested that isoflavones activity is closely related to soy protein (Amani et al, 2005).

5.1.3.2.4 Fiber

One of the potential ways by which soy protein might exert its effect on blood cholesterol is via its fiber content (about 6 g as non-starch polysaccharide per 100 g boiled beans), which is primarily soluble fiber. Soluble fiber (*e.g.* from oats) has been shown to lower plasma total and LDL-cholesterol, although the effect is small for those consuming moderate amounts (Truswell, 2002). In the meta-analysis by Brown *et al.* (1999) 2–10 g/day of soluble fiber was associated with a small but significant fall in total cholesterol (0.045 mmol/l per g fiber) and LDL-cholesterol (0.057 mmol/l per g fiber). Three apples or three (28 g) servings of oatmeal, providing 3 g soluble fiber, decreased total and LDL-cholesterol by about 0.13 mmol/l. The mechanism of this effect remains undefined. Suggestions include bile acid binding, resulting in an up-regulation of LDL receptors and thus increased clearance of LDL-cholesterol; inhibition of hepatic fatty acid synthesis byproducts of fermentation in the large bowel (*e.g.* propionate, acetate, butyrate); changes in motility or satiety; or slowed absorption of macronutrients resulting in improved insulin sensitivity (Brown *et al.*, 1999).

Consumption of diets rich in whole-grain cereals (*e.g.* whole-wheat cereals, whole meal bread and brown rice) has been associated with a lower risk of cardiovascular disease (Pietinen *et al.*, 1996; Jacobs *et al.*, 1999; Liu *et al.*, 1999; Truswell, 2002). Vitamin E, dietary fibre (Richardson, 2000), resistant starch and oligosacchrarides (Cummings *et al.*, 1992), as well as plant sterols (Jones *et al.*, 1997) are some of the components of whole-grain cereals that may contribute to a reduced risk of heart disease (Mc Kevith (2004) .

5.1.3.2.5 Antioxidant

Vitamins C, E, and B-carotene have antioxidant roles in the body. Vitamin E is the most concentrated antioxidant carried on LDLs and its major function is to prevent oxidation of

PUFA in the cell membrane (Krummel, 2008). Epidemiologic studies suggest that vitamin E and carotenoids are inversely related to CVD, but randomized trials have not supported these observations (Lee et al., 2005; Lichtenstein et al., 2006). Because data have not shown vitamin E to be protective, the AHA does not recommend vitamin E supplementation for CVD prevention (Lichtenstein et al., 2006). However, RRR-a-tocopherol, the natural form of vitamin E, shows promise as an antiinflammatory agent (Gasu et al., 2006). Foods with concentrated amounts of the phytonutrients catechins, have been found to improve vascular reactivity. These foods are red grapes, red wine, tea (especially green tea), chocolate, and olive oil, and should be worked into any CVD preventive eating plan (Kay et al., 2006). In our case - control study, drinking tea was significantly associated with lower risk of coronary events (Amani et al, 2010).

5.1.3.2.6 Stanols and sterols

Since the early 1950s plant stanols and sterols isolated from soybean oils or pine tree oil have been known to lower blood cholesterol (Lichtensteine et al., 2001). Recently they have been esterified and made into margarines. Consuming between 2 to 3 g/day lowers cholesterol by 9% to 20% (Lichtenstein et al., 2001). The mechanism for cholesterol lowering is by inhibiting absorption of dietary cholesterol. Adult Treatment Panel III (ATP-III) includes stanols as part of dietary recommendations for lowering LDL cholesterol in adults. Because these esters can also affect the absorption of and cause lower β-caroten , α-tocopherol, and lycopene levels, further safety studies are needed for use in normocholesterolemic individuals, children, and pregnant women (Krummel, 2008).

5.1.3.2.7 Dietary patterns

The effect on CVD risk of diets rich in whole grains and low in processed foods that are high in fat, sodium, and sugars has increasingly been investigated in both developed and developing countries. In parallel with economic development, radical dietary shifts toward Westernized diets that are high in animal products and refined carbohydrates and low in whole grains and other plant-based foods have occurred in many developing countries. For example in Iran, the results of Amani et al (2010) study showed that daily consumption of vegetable oils, tea and fish is significantly associated with lower risk of coronary events (odds ratio = 0.55(0.31-0.91), 0.3(0.15-0.65), 0.23(0.13-0.42), respectively). On the other hand, it was indicated that consumption of hydrogenated fats and full-fat yoghurt is associated with higher risk of coronary artery disease (OR = 2.12(1.23-3.64) and 2.35(1.32-4.18), respectively).

Substantial evidence has accumulated to support the notion that the traditional Mediterranean dietary pattern is protective against CVD . This pattern is characterized by an abundance of fruits, vegetables, whole grain cereals, nuts, and legumes; olive oil as the principal source of fat; moderate consumption of fish and lower consumption of red meat. It is important to note, however, that the dominance in research on the Mediterranean diet has come at the cost of research on other diets commonly consumed around the world that may also have heart health benefits (IOM , 2010).

5.1.3.2.8 Therapeutic life style change dietary pattern (TLC)

The ATP-III recommends the TLC dietary pattern for primary and secondary prevention of CHD. AHA recommends diet and lifestyle changes to reduce CVD risk in all people over the age of 2 years (Table 1) (Lichtenstein et al., 2006). SFA recommendations are less than 7% of calories; total fat content has a range of 25% to 35% of calories.

Consuming 30% to 35% of calories from fat while maintaining a low SFA and trans-fatty acid intake is the dietary pattern recommended for individuals with insulin resistance or metabolic syndrome. This higher fat intake, emphasizing PUFAs and monounsaturated fatty acids (MUFA), can be beneficial in lowering triglycerides and raising HDL cholesterol. Also, with a more liberal fat intake, LDL cholesterol can be lowered without exacerbating blood glucose levels. Increasing physical activity and decreasing energy intake to facilitate weight loss are critical to normalize multiple risk factors. Behavioral strategies for weight management to reduce cardiovascular risk have been provided by the AHA (Klein et al., 2004). Learning outcomes include planning meals that fit the TLC plan, reading food labels, modifying recipes, preparing or purchasing appropriate foods, and choosing healthier choices when dining out. Along with the TLC dietary pattern, the Dietary Approaches to Stop Hypertension (DASH) pattern is also appropriate for CVD prevention and treatment . Both of these dietary patterns emphasize grains, cereals, legumes, vegetables, fruits, lean meats, poultry fish, and nonfat dairy products.

Because animal fats provide about two thirds of the SFAs in diet, these foods are limited. High-fat choices are omitted, but low-fat choices can be included. Meat is limited to 5 oz/day, and eggs to four or fewer per week. Lean meats are high in protein, zinc, and iron; thus, patients who wish to consume meat, a 5-oz portion or less can be fit into the dietary plan if other low SFA choices are made. Neither food group has to be omitted; it is a matter of choice. Most people need to add the recommended two servings of fatty fish per week. Meeting sodium guidelines (1500 to 2300 mg daily) can be a challenge because lower-fat processed foods often contain salt to increase palatability. Patients may need to limit processed foods (Krummel 2008).

5.1.3.3 Alcohol

The global burden of diseases attributable to alcohol has recently been summarized; leading to the conclusion that alcohol is one of the largest avoidable risk factors in low and middle income countries (Rehm et al., 2009). Indeed, WHO estimates that the harmful use of alcohol was responsible for 3.8 percent of deaths and 4.5 percent of the global burden of disease in 2004 (WHO, 2009b). Excessive alcohol intake is associated with increased risk for hypertension, stroke, coronary artery disease, and other forms of CVD; however, there is also a robust body of evidence in a range of populations suggesting light to moderate intake of alcohol may reduce the risk of CHD. Indeed, research suggests that the relationship between alcohol intake and CVD outcomes follows a "J" curve, with the lowest rates being associated with low to moderate intakes of alcohol (Beilin and Puddey, 2006; Lucas et al., 2005). It is important to recognize that, as with any discussion of alcohol and health, the key issues are the quantity of alcohol consumed and the risk or benefit conferred by consumption. Although evidence indicates that low to moderate alcohol use can reduce the risk of CHD, excessive and harmful use clearly increases CVD risk (Beilin and Puddey, 2006; Lucas et al., 2005). It is important that approaches to reduce the burden of CVD not neglect the importance of reducing excessive alcohol consumption.

5.1.3.4 Physical activity

WHO and FAO have highlighted the importance of physical activity as a key determinant of obesity, CVD, and diabetes (Joint WHO/FAO Expert Consultation, 2003). For decades, evidences of the relationship between physical activity and CVD, independent of effects on weight and obesity, have been strengthened. Increasing physical activity—including brisk walking—has been shown to decrease the risk of chronic diseases such as CHD, stroke, some cancers (e.g., colorectal and breast cancer), type 2 diabetes, osteoporosis, high blood pressure, and high cholesterol (Physical Activity Guidelines Advisory Committee, 2008)

American Heart Association 2006 Diet Recommendations for Cardiovascular Disease Risk Reduction

- Balance calorie intake and physical activity to achieve or maintain a healthy body weight.
- Consume a diet rich in vegetables and fruits.
- Choose whole grain, high-fiber foods.
- Consume fish, especially oily fish, at least twice a week.
- Limit intake of saturated fat to <7% of energy, *trans*-fat to <1% of energy, and cholesterol to <300 mg/day by:
  - Choosing lean meats and vegetable alternatives.
  - Selecting fat-free (skim), 1%-fat, and low-fat dairy products.
  - Minimizing intake of partially hydrogenated fats.
- Minimize your intake of beverages and foods with added sugars.
- Choose and prepare foods with little or no salt.
- When consuming alcohol, do so in moderation.
- When eating food that is prepared outside of the home, follow the American Heart Association Diet and Lifestyle Recommendations.

Modified from Lichtenstein AH et al: Diet and lifestyle recommendations revision 2006: a scientific statement from the American Heart Association Committee, *Circulation* 114:83, 2006.

Table 1.

Regular physical activity and higher cardiorespiratory fitness are associated with lower overall mortality from CVD. Men and women who are physically active experience a lower risk of cardiovascular disease in general and CHD in particular (US Department of Health and Human Services, 1996; Wannamethee & Shaper, 2002). Furthermore, in the Nurses' Health Study, a large prospective study in the USA, both brisk walking and regular vigorous exercise were associated with a reduction in risk of coronary events by 30–40% (Manson *et al.*, 1999), and sedentary women who became active in middle age or later had a lower risk than their counterparts who remained sedentary . In one study performed among 145 women with central obesity, serum concentration of HDL-c was significantly higher in women who do more physical activity (Sharifi et al,2008). With overall mortality, the epidemiological literature for CHD indicates an inverse association and a dose response gradient between physical activity level or cardiorespiratory fitness and incidence of CHD. It helps to improve several risk factors for cardiovascular disease, including raised blood pressure, adverse blood lipid profile and insulin resistance.

5.1.4 Related diseases/syndrome

5.1.4.1 Overweight and obesity

Traditionally, obesity is defined as a BioPsychoSocial problem but in this chapter we rather intend to present it as an EcoBioPsychoSocioCutural issue.

Overweight and obesity have reached epidemic proportions, not only in developed but also in developing countries (Sassi et al., 2009). Even in low and middle income countries where undernutrition is still highly prevalent, overweight and obesity—especially among women—is a public health problem (Caballero, 2005; Hosseinpanah et al 2009). WHO and FAO reviewed the evidence on the relationship between obesity and the risk of CVD and concluded that overweight and obesity confer a significantly elevated risk of CHD (Joint WHO/FAO Expert Consultation, 2003). Increased body mass index (BMI) is also associated with greater risk of stroke in both Asian and Western populations (WHO/FAO, 2003). The association between obesity and CVD is partly mediated through hypertension, high cholesterol, and diabetes. Abdominal or central obesity measured by waist-to-hip ratio or waist circumference is associated with both CHD and stroke independent of BMI and other cardiovascular risk factors. Even in university educated women, obesity and central fat are also prevalent which increase the risk of heart disease. We studied 101female staff of the university, aged 20-45 years. Based on the bioelectrical impedance analysis (BIA) method, overweight and obesity rates were determined in 34.6 and 40.6 percent of women, respectively, and central obesity was prevalent in 27% of them (Amani, 2007a). It is worthy to note that to prevent erroneous classification, localization of cut-off points can be a more practical way to detect individuals at greater risk of chronic disease. In a sample of 637 married females, it was indicated that subjects in low BMI range tend to have higher fat percentages and they might represent a different category as overfat thin other than normal weight obese in Iranian women. (Amani, 2007b).

Obesity is also an independent risk factor for other cardiovascular outcomes, such as congestive heart failure and sudden cardiac death. Excess energy intake is one of the key contributors to obesity. The lack of data limits policy makers' abilities to focus attention on which dietary components lend to effective interventions that would reduce total calorie intake. One category that has been well studied in developed countries relates to sugar consumption, primarily in the form of sugar-sweetened beverages (including soft drinks, juice drinks, and energy and vitamin drinks). Recent NHANES data shows that up to 5.5 percent of dietary calories come from sugar-sweetened beverages in the United States (Bosire et al., 2009), which has led the American Heart Association to recommend an upper limit of 100 calories per day for women and 150 calories per day for men from added sugars, including soft drinks (Johnson et al., 2009). In some developing countries, consumption of sugar-sweetened beverages has increased dramatically in recent decades. Because of its excess caloric and sugar content, increasing consumption of sugar sweetened beverages may have important implications for obesity and cardiometabolic risk.

5.1.4.2 Hypertension

Hypertension is a risk factor for CHD, stroke, and heart failure. A recent review of the global burden of high blood pressure found that approximately 54 percent of stroke, 47 percent of IHD and 25 percent of other CVDs were attributable to hypertension. Among the major underlying risks for hypertension are sodium, body weight, and access to treatment. Primary prevention focused on sodium reduction, fruit and vegetable intake, weight control, and avoidance of excessive alcohol intake has been shown to make a difference (Krummel, 2008).

5.1.4.3 Diabetes

Around the world, diabetes is increasingly growing and is a significant contributor to CVD risk. People with diabetes have more than two-fold greater risk of CVD compared to non-diabetics (Asia Pacific Cohort Studies Collaboration, 2003). In fact, CVD is the leading cause of morbidity and mortality in people with diabetes (Booth et al., 2006; Kengne et al., 2007, 2009). Individuals without established clinical diabetes, but who are at increased risk of developing diabetes in the future, also have a higher risk of CVD (Asia Pacific Cohort Studies Collaboration, 2007). Women and younger individuals with diabetes have greater risk of CVD. Obesity is the single most important risk factor for type 2 diabetes, but unhealthy diet and physical inactivity also independently raise the population risk for diabetes (Schulze and Hu, 2005). According to the International Diabetes Federation's Diabetes Atlas 2010, the global estimated prevalence of diabetes for 2010 among people aged 20 to 79 years will be approximately 285 million people (6.4 percent of the global population), of which some 70 percent will be living in developing countries (International Diabetes Federation, 2010).

Diabetes is emerging as a particular concern in Asia, where more than 110 million individuals were living with diabetes in 2007, a large proportion of whom were young and middle aged. Asians tend to develop diabetes at a relatively young age and low BMI, and by 2025 the number of individuals with diabetes in the region is expected to rise to almost 180 million (Chan et al., 2009). Intensive glucose control reduces the risk of major cardiovascular events by approximately 10 percent, compared with standard treatment in people with diabetes. Interestingly, this benefit appeared to be independent of other cardiovascular risk factors (Kelly et al., 2009; Turnbull et al., 2009).

To sum up, as with the raising obesity epidemic, the prevalence of diabetes has increased dramatically worldwide. It is associated with serious health consequences and is a major risk factor for CHD and stroke. Therefore, prevention and management of diabetes are critical in reducing the global burden of CVD.

5.1.4.4 Psychosocial risk and mental health

Of all the psychosocial stressors associated with CVD, the link between depression and CVD is probably the best documented. There have been many published reviews and numerous meta-analyses have consistently found that depression and depressive symptoms are associated with an increased likelihood of developing CVD, a higher incidence of CVD events, poorer outcomes after CVD treatment and prevention efforts, and increased mortality from CVD. These associations remain consistent even after controlling for other CVD risk factors (Everson-Rose and Lewis, 2005; Frasure-Smith and Lesperance, 2006; Lesperance and Frasure-Smith, 2007; Lichtman et al., 2008).

Behaviors that increase CVD risks are more common in depressed patients. They are more likely to smoke, have poor diets, and be physically inactive. Furthermore, depression has been found to associate with the risk of non adherence to medical treatment regimens and lifestyle changes, making depressed patients with CVD or high CVD risk less likely to adhere to prevention efforts (Lichtman et al., 2008; Ziegelstein et al., 2000).

Chronic stress, most often studied by examining work-related stress, has been associated with negative behaviors such as low physical activity and poor diet, increased likelihood of recurrent CVD, as well as physiological consequences such as decreased heart rate variability. For instance, we found that the prevalence of overweight and obesity was higher in a sample of firefighters who may have chronic stress. Moreover they had high TC, TG and lipoprotein (a) and low HDL-C concentrations (Azabdaftari et al, 2009).

Acute stress from traumatic life events such as the death of a relative, earthquakes, or terrorist attacks have all been associated with significant temporal increases in the incidence of MI (Everson-Rose and Lewis, 2005; Figueredo, 2009).

It is clear that psychosocial factors play an important role in increasing CVD risk through both direct and indirect pathways. Continued research is needed to further explain the mechanisms by which psychosocial stressors and mental illness affect CVD risk. It is also important that clinicians are made aware of the effect of psychosocial factors on CVD risk, prognosis, and adherence to prevention efforts through improved training and knowledge expanding.

5.2 Nonmodifiable factors

5.2.1 Menopausal status

Loss of estrogen following natural or surgical menopause is associated with increased CVD risk. Endogenous estrogen has a protective role against CVD in premenopausal women, probably by preventing vascular injury. Rates of CHD in premenopausal women are low except in women with multiple risk factors. During the menopausal period total cholesterol, LDL cholesterol, and triglyceride levels increase; and HDL cholesterol level decreases, especially in women who are overweight or obese (Regitz-Zagrosek, 2006).

5.2.2 Age and gender

Age is a nonmodifiable risk factor for CHD. The increased risk for CHD parallels increase in age. Higher mortality rates from CHD are seen in both genders with increasing age.

Being older than 45 years of age is considered a risk factor for men (NCEP, 2002). For women the increased risk comes after the age of 55 years, which is after menopause for most women.

CVD prevalence, incidence, and mortality rates tend to be higher for men than for women. This finding has remained consistent historically (Lawlor et al., 2001) and across countries and regions (Allen and Szanton, 2005; Pilote et al., 2007; WHO, 2009).

Estrogen has a protective effect on the development of CVD risk factors and consequently is the reason most often cited for these gender differences (Regitz-Zagrosek, 2006). Estrogen is thought to contribute to premenopausal women's tendency to have lower systolic blood pressure, higher levels of HDL cholesterol, and lower triglyceride levels than men (Pilote et al., 2007).

The lower prevalence of smoking among women is another factor that could contribute to their decreased CVD incidence and mortality rates. Around the world, the prevalence of female smoking is lower than that of men (Pilote et al., 2007). Although rates of smoking, dyslipidemia, and hypertension are generally lower among women than men, women tend to have less favorable profiles for other key CVD risk factors. Worldwide, women are more likely to be sedentary than men (Guthold et al., 2008). Some researchers have suggested that women's social status in many cultures and their lack of leisure time due to childcare and other familial responsibilities likely contribute to their lower levels of physical activity (Brands and Yach, 2002; Pilote et al., 2007).

Another troubling gender difference is the increased prevalence of obesity among women. WHO data indicate that although overweight (BMI ≥ 25 kg/m2) is more common among men globally; obesity (BMI ≥30 kg/m2) is more common among women.

A number of different reasons have proposed by CVD researchers that why women might delay seeking medical attention, receive delayed treatment, and experience poorer outcomes during and after an MI or stroke. One often-cited reason that women tend to wait longer to seek treatment is that many do not perceive themselves as being at risk (Jensen and Moser, 2008).

Because of the robust evidence indicating gender differences in CVD incidence, morbidity, and outcomes, these differences, as well as the unique needs of women, should be considered when developing CVD research priorities, policies, and health service interventions.

6. Association between early life factors and subsequent risk for CVD

6.1 Low birth weight and adult cardiovascular disease

Ther is growing evidence in developing and developed countries ,based on cohort studies, that fetal and early childhood periods is important in the onset of CVD later in life (Victora et al., 2008; Walker and George, 2007; WHO, 2009c). The influences during this period include maternal factors during pregnancy, such as smoking, obesity, and malnutrition, and factors in infancy and early childhood, such as breastfeeding, low birth weight, and undernutrition.

Maternal smoking during pregnancy has been linked to CVD-related risk factors. It has been consistently associated with increased childhood obesity independent of other risk factors (Oken et al., 2008). A number of studies have examined the effects of maternal obesity on the body weight of their children; however, the evidence is inconsistent. Two cohort studies in the United States found that excessive weight gain or maternal obesity during pregnancy was associated with overweight and obesity in the children at ages 3 and 4 years (Gillman et al., 2008; Whitaker,2004). Similarly, a cohort study in Finland found that mothers' body mass index (BMI) was positively associated with their sons' BMI in childhood (Eriksson et al., 1999).

Another factor that appears to influence risk for long-term cardiovascular health is breastfeeding. Breastfeeding has been found to not only reduce childhood morbidity and mortality but also to be weakly protective against obesity later in life (Bhutta et al., 2008; Gluckman et al., 2008).

Undernutrition in infancy, especially when followed by rapid weight gain, is associated with increased risk of CVD and diabetes in adulthood (Barker and Bagby, 2005; Caballero, 2005; Gluckman et al., 2008). This phenomenon is known as the developmental origins theory of CVD. It means that if disruptions to the nutritional, metabolic, and hormonal environment at critical stages of development are happened, it may lead to permanent "programming" of the body's structure, physiology, and metabolism that translate into pathology and disease, including CVD, later in life (Barker, 1997, 1998, 2007). The exact physiological mechanisms through which this programming occurs are not yet fully elucidated; however, there is evidence that fetal and early postnatal undernutrition can cause metabolic, anatomic, and endocrine adaptations that affect the hypothalamic-pituitary-adrenal axis, lipoprotein profiles, and end organ glucose uptake, among other processes (Prentice and Moore, 2005). Support for the developmental origins theory of CVD comes from a number of retrospective, and more recently prospective, cohort studies in various populations. Studies in the United Kingdom, the United States, Finland, and India found that fetal undernutrition followed by a rapid catch-up growth from childhood to early adolescence was significantly associated with the later development of CVD in both men and women (Barker et al., 2005; Eriksson et al., 1999; Osmond and Barker, 2000). Early undernutrition followed by catch-up growth during childhood has also been associated with subsequent hypertension and type 2 diabetes (Barker, 1998; Osmond and Barker, 2000) This emerging data on the effects of rapid weight gain after early undernutrition have prompted some researchers to suggest a shift from the original "fetal origins" hypothesis to an "accelerated postnatal growth hypothesis" of CVD (Singhal et al., 2003, 2004).

The emerging evidence on the association between low birth weight followed by rapid growth in childhood and subsequent risk for CVD raises important considerations for addressing global CVD because low birth weight and exposure to undernutrition in utero and in infancy are common in many developing countries (Caballero, 2009; Kelishadi, 2007).

The acquisition and accumulation of risk for CVD continues in childhood and adolescence (Celermajer and Ayer, 2006). Unhealthful lifestyle practices such as consumption of high calorie and high fat foods, tobacco use, and physical inactivity begin in childhood, introducing major behavioral risks for CVD. Childhood adversity also influences adult cardiovascular health. In addition, there is also an emerging body of evidence on the presence of biological risk factors in children and youth, including pathophysiological processes associated with heart disease that can be seen as early as childhood.

6.2 Childhood obesity and CVD risk

Childhood obesity is associated with multiple risk factors for CVD, which are amplified in the presence of overweight and persist from childhood into adulthood. These risk factors include hyperlipidemia, high blood pressure, impaired glucose tolerance and high insulin levels, as well as metabolic syndrome. It has been estimated that 60 percent of overweight children possess at least one of these risk factors that can lead to CVD in adulthood (Freedman et al., 1999). This is especially important in terms of implications for global CVD because the prevalence of childhood obesity is increasing in developing countries (WHO, 2008a).

7. Public health approach to cardiovascular disease risk reduction

7.1 Cardiovascular disease as a public health problem

The prevention of cardiovascular disease is a major public health challenge for a number of years around the world. Although death rates have been falling in many westernized countries (*e.g.* USA, Australia, UK), rates are rising rapidly elsewhere.

7.2 Current dietary recommendations for primary prevention

Dietary recommendations tend to be country specific and are based on the available evidence.

The ATP-III recommends the TLC dietary pattern for primary and secondary prevention of CHD. In agreement, the AHA recommends diet and lifestyle changes to reduce CVD risk in all people over the age of 2 years (Lichtenstein et al., 2006).

As is evident, knowledge about the role of diet in risk factor reduction and reducing the risk of cardiovascular events themselves continues to expand. It is now recognized that CVD risk can be mediated through multiple biological pathways other than only serum total and LDL cholesterol or dietary factors. With this in mind, it is necessary to modify the dietary advice offered to those with an increased risk of CVD.

7.3 Health promotion in children and other subgroups of the population

Health aspects present in childhood, such as blood lipids, body weight and blood pressure may track into adulthood. Therefore, a useful health strategy is the adoption of sensible eating habits and an active lifestyle early in childhood. It is important to promote cardiovascular health in childhood by increasing physical activity and preventing or treating obesity, raised blood pressure, insulin resistance and type 2 diabetes (Williams *et al.*, 2002). Current nutritional recommendations for the general population are applicable for most children over 5 years and can be gradually applied from the age of 2 years. It is also recommended that all children and adolescents participate in physical activity for 1 hour daily which should be of at least moderate intensity (Fox & Riddoch, 2000). The implementation of guidelines and success of health strategies require input from the governments, health professionals, the food industry and teachers, as well as the children themselves and their parents. Moreover, social and cultural influences must be recognized when designing and implementing strategies.

8. Summary

- Cardiovascular disease is the leading cause of death worldwide, accounting for around 18 million deaths each year.
- Modifiable risk factors for cardiovascular disease include atherogenic lipoproteins, inflammatory related factors behaviors, lifestyle and chronic diseases such as obesity, diabetes and hypertension.
- Non modifiable risk factors include menopause, age and gender.
- There is evidence that a chronic, low-grade inflammation underlies atherosclerosis, although it is not clear whether this is a cause or effect phenomenon.
- The acute phase proteins, C-reactive protein (CRP), fibrinogen and serum amyloid A, appear to be associated with risk for cardiovascular disease.
- The advantages of a dietary pattern approach rather than individual dietary components can influence plasma cholesterol levels and may also affect other emerging risk factors.
- Physical activity has great impact on CVD risk reduction when it is accompanied by dietary pattern changes.
- Low birth weight and low weight gain during infancy are associated with an increased risk of adult cardiovascular disease, hypertension, type 2 diabetes and the insulin resistance syndrome.

9. Future research

Future research is required to establish the strength of the associations between the emerging risk factors described in this chapter and cardiovascular disease, in order to compare their predictive value with the established risk factors. For example, further work is required to evaluate the independence of many of the novel risk factors for cardiovascular disease and whether these associations are causal. In addition, more information is needed about how these novel risk factors might be modified by different aspects of the diet. As indicated in ancient Traditional Persian Medicine (TPM), understanding the effect of individual foods on the trend of heart disease and hyperlipidemias can be leading fields of study in the near future.

Moreover, local modified risk factors should be defined and addressed to track the patients at greater risks in more applicable ways.

10. References

Allen, J., & S. Szanton. 2005. Gender, ethnicity, and cardiovascular disease. *Journal of Cardiovascular Nursing* 20(1):1-6; quiz 7-8.

Amani R, Baghdadchi J & Zand-Moghaddam A, 2005. Effects of Soy Protein Isoflavones on Serum Lipids, Lipoprotein Profile and Serum Glucose of Hypercholesterolemic Rabbits. *Int J Endocrinol Metab* ; 2:87-92.

Amani R, noorizadeh M, Rahmanian S, Afzali N & Haghighizadeh M, 2010. Nutritional related cardiovascular risk factors in patients with coronary artery disease in IRAN:A case-control study. *Nutrition Journal*, 9:70.

Reza Amani, Fereshteh Boustani. 2007 a. Prevalence of obesity and dietary practices in Jondi-Shapour University female personnel, Ahvaz, Iran Pak J Med Sci;24(4):748-52.

Amani R, 2007 **b**. Comparison between bioelectrical impedance analysis and body mass index methods in determination of obesity prevalence in Ahvazi women. Eur J Clin Nutr ;61(4): 478-82.

Anber V, Millar JS, McConnell M, Shepherd J, Packard CJ& 1997. *Interaction of very-low-density, intermediatedensity, and low-density lipoproteins with human arterial wall proteoglycans. Arteriosclerosis, Thrombosis and Vascular Biology, 17, 2507–14.*

Anderson JW, Johnstone BM and Cook-Newell ME & 1995. Meta-analysis of the effects of soy protein intake on serum lipids. N Engl J Med. 3;333(5):276-82.

Anerson JJB, Anthony M, Messina M & Garner SC, 1999. Effects of phyto-oestrogens on tissues. *Nutr Res Rev*. 12: 75-116.

Anthony MS, Clarkson TB, Hughes CL Jr, Morgan TM & Burke GL, 1996. Soybean isoflavones improve cardiovascular risk factors without affecting the reproductive system of peripubertal rhesus monkeys. J Nutr. 126(1):43-50.

Arora A, Nair MG & Strasburg GM, 1998. Antioxidant activities of isoflavones and their biological metabolites in a liposomal system. *Arch Biochem Biophys*. 356(2):133-41.

Asia Pacific Cohort Studies Collaboration. 2003. The effects of diabetes on the risks of major cardiovascular diseases and death in the Asia Pacific region. *Diabetes Care* 26(2): 360-366.

Asia Pacific Cohort Studies Collaboration. 2007. Cholesterol, diabetes and major cardiovascular diseases in the Asia-Pacific region. *Diabetologia* 50(11):2289-2297.

Astrup A ,2002. *Dietary fat is a major player in obesity – but not the only one. Obesity Reviews, 3, 57– 8.*

Aygun A D et al,2005. Proinflammatoy cytokines and leptin are increased in serum of prepubertal obese children, *Mediators Inflamm* 3 :180.

Azabdaftari N, Amani R, Taha Jalali M, 2009. Biochemical and nutritional indices as cardiovascular risk factors among Iranian firefighters. *Ann Clin Biochem*. Sep;46(Pt 5):385-9

Barker, D. J. 1997. The fetal origins of coronary heart disease. *Acta Paediatrica Supplement* 422:78-82.

Barker, D. J. P. 1998. In utero programming of chronic disease. *Clinical Science* 95(2): 115-128.

Barker, D. J. P., & S. P. Bagby. 2005. Developmental antecedents of cardiovascular disease: A historical perspective. *Journal of the American Society of Nephrology* 16(9): 2537-2544.

Barker, D. J. P. 2007. The origins of the developmental origins theory. *Journal of Internal Medicine* 261(5):412-417.

Basu A et al,2006: Dietary factors that promote or retard inflammation, Arterioscler Thromb Vasc Biol, 26:995.

Beilin, L. J., & I. B. Puddey. 2006. Alcohol and hypertension: An update. *Hypertension* 47(6):1035-1038.

Bhutta, Z. A., T. Ahmed, R. E. Black, S. Cousens, K. Dewey, E. Giugliani, B. A. Haider, B.Kirkwood, S. S. Morris, H. P. S. Sachdev, & M. Shekar. 2008. What works? Interventions for maternal and child undernutrition and survival. *Lancet* 371(9610):417-440.

Blum CA et al,2005 . Low-grade inflammation and estimates of insulin resistance during the menstrual cycle in lean and overweight women. *J Clin Endocrinol Metab* 90:3230.

Booth, G. L., M. K. Kapral, K. Fung, & J. V. Tu. 2006. Recent trends in cardiovascular complications among men and women with and without diabetes. *Diabetes Care* 29(1):32-37.

Bosire, C., J. Reedy, & S. M. Krebs-Smith. 2009. *Sources of energy and selected nutrient intakes among the US population, 2005 -06 : A report prepared for the 2010 dietary guidelines advisory committee.* Bethesda, MD: National Cancer Institute.

Brands, A., & D. Yach. 2002. Women and the rapid rise of noncommunicable diseases *World Health Organization NMH Reader* (1):1-22.

Brown L, Rosner B, Willett WW& Sacks FM ,1999.) *Cholesterol lowering effects of dietary fibre: a meta-analysis.*

Buckley DI, Fu R, Freeman M, Rogers K & Helfand M. (2009). C-reactive protein as a risk factor for coronary heart disease: a systematic U.S. Preventive Services Task Force. *Ann Intern Med , 151,* 483-495.

Caballero, B. 2005. A nutrition paradox—underweight and obesity in developing countries. *New England Journal of Medicine* 352(15):1514-1516.

Caballero, B. 2009. Early undernutrition and risk of CVD in the adult. Presentation at Public Information Gathering Session for the Institute of Medicine Committee on Preventing the Global Epidemic of Cardiovascular Disease, Washington, DC.

Celermajer, D. S., & J. G. Ayer. 2006. Childhood risk factors for adult cardiovascular disease and primary prevention in childhood. *Heart* 92(11):1701-1706.

Chait A, Brazg RL, Tribble DL & Krauss RM ,1993. *Susceptibility of small, dense, low-density lipoproteins to oxidative modification in subjects with the atherogenic lipoprotein phenotype, pattern B. American Journal of Medicine, 94, 350–6.*

Chan, J. C., V. Malik, W. Jia, T. Kadowaki, C. S. Yajnik, K. H. Yoon, F. B. & Hu. 2009. Diabetes in Asia: Epidemiology, risk factors, and pathophysiology. *Journal of the American Medical Association* 301(20):2129 2140.

Chen , L. Y. , & J. L. Mehta . 1994 . Inhibitory effect of high-density lipoprotein on platelet function is mediated by increase in nitric oxide synthase activity in platelets. *Life Sci.* 55 : 1815 - 1821 .

Critchley, J., J. Liu, D. Zhao, W. Wei, and S. Capewell. 2004. Explaining the increase in coronary heart disease mortality in Beijing between 1984 and 1999. *Circulation* 110(10):1236-1244.

Cummings J, Bingham S, Heaton K, Eastwood M ,1992. *Fecal weight, colon cancer risk and dietary intake of non-starch polysaccharide (dietary fibre). Gastroenterology, 103, 1783–7.*

Danesh J, Whincup P, Walker M et al. ,2000. *Low grade inflammation and coronary heart disease: prospective study and update meta-analyses. British Medical Journal, 321, 199–203.*

Davies, A. R., L. Smeeth, and E. M. Grundy. 2007. Contribution of changes in incidence and mortality to trends in the prevalence of coronary heart disease in the UK: 1996-2005. *European Heart Journal* 28(17):2142-2147.

Davignon J, Ganz P, 2004. Role of endothelial dysfunction in atherosclerosis. *Circulation* ,109(23 suppl |):III27.

Dejager S, Bruckert E, Chapman MJ ,1993. *Dense low density lipoprotein subspecies with diminished oxidative resistance predominate in combined hyperlipidaemia. Journal of Lipid Research, 34, 295–308.*

de Lorgeril M et al,1999: Mediterranean diet, traditional risk factors, and the rate of cardiovascular complications after myocardial infarction, *Circulation,* 99 :779.

D'Erasmo E, Acca M, Celi F, Medici F, Palmerini T and Pisani D,1993. Plasma fibrinogen and platelet count in stroke. J Med;24:185–191.

Dreon DM, Fernstrom HA, Miller B, Krauss RM ,1994. Low-density lipoprotein subclass patterns and lipoprotein response to a reduced-fat diet in men. FASEB Journal, 8, 121–6.

Eriksson, J. G., T. Forsen, J. Tuomilehto, P. D. Winter, C. Osmond, and D. J. P. Barker. 1999. Catch-up growth in childhood and death from coronary heart disease: Longitudinal study. *British Medical Journal* 318:7181.

Everson-Rose, S. A., and T. T. Lewis. 2005. Psychosocial factors and cardiovascular diseases. In *Annual Review of Public Health* 26(1):469-500.

Figueredo, V. M. 2009. The time has come for physicians to take notice: The impact of psychosocial stressors on the heart. *American Journal of Medicine* 122(8):704-712.

Foster, R. K., and H. E. Marriott. 2006. Alcohol consumption in the new millennium—weighing up the risks and benefits for our health. *Nutrition Bulletin* 31(4):286-331.

Fox KR, Riddoch CJ (2000) *Charting the physical activity patterns of contempory children and adolescents. Proceedings of the Nutrition Society, 59, 497–504.*

Frasure-Smith, N., and F. Lesperance. 2006. Recent evidence linking coronary heart disease and depression. *Canadian Journal of Psychiatry—Revue Canadienne de Psychiatrie* 51(12):730-737.

Frayn K ,2005. *Cardiovascular disease diet, nutrition and emerging risk factors. Blackwell Publishing*. Oxford,UK.

Gao X et al,2004. Plasma C-reactive protein and homosysteine concentrations are related to frequent fruit and vegetable intake in Hispanic and non-Hispanic white elders . *J Nutr* ,134:913.

Gebauer SK et al, 2006. n-3 fatty acid dietary recommendations and food sources to achieve essentiality and cardiovascular benefits. Am J Clin Nutr 83(6 suppl):15262s.

Gillman, M. W., S. L. Rifas-Shiman, K. Kleinman, E. Oken, J. W. Rich-Edwards, and E. M. Taveras. 2008. Developmental origins of childhood overweight: Potential public health impact. *Obesity* 16(7):1651-1656.

Gluckman, P. D., M. A. Hanson, A. S. Beedle, and D. Raubenheimer. 2008. Fetal and neonatal pathways to obesity. In *Frontiers of hormone research*. Vol. 36. Edited by M. Korbonits. Basel: Karger. Pp. 61-72.

Gotoh K et al, 2006. Apolipoprotein A -IV interacts synergistically with melanocoftins to reduce food intake, *Am J Physiol Regul Integr Comp Physiol* 290 :R202.

Gritz, E. R., D. J. Vidrine, and M. Cororve Fingeret. 2007. Smoking cessation. A critical component of medical management in chronic disease populations. *American Journal of Preventive Medicine* 33(6 Suppl):S414-S422.

Guthold, R., T. Ono, K. L. Strong, S. Chatterji, and A. Morabia. 2008. Worldwide variability in physical inactivity—a 51-country survey. *American Journal of Preventive Medicine* 34(6):486-494.

Hadaegh F, Harati H, Ghanbarian A, Azizi F 2009. Prevalence of coronary heart disease among Tehran adults: Tehran Lipid and Glucose Study. *East Mediterr Health J.*;15(1):157-66.

He, F. J., and G. A. MacGregor. 2009. A comprehensive review on salt and health and current experience of worldwide salt reduction programmes. *Journal of Human Hypertension* 23(6):363-384.

Hodgson JM, Puddey IB, Beilin LJ, Mori TA and Croft KD,1998. Supplementation with isoflavonoid phytoestrogens does not alter serum lipid concentrations: a randomized controlled trial in humans. J Nutr.;128(4):728-32.

Hosseinpanah F, Barzin M, Eskandary PS, Mirmiran P, Azizi F, 2009. Trends of obesity and abdominal obesity in Tehranian adults: a cohort study.*BMC Public Health.* 23;9:426.

Hu, F. B. 2008. Globalization of food patterns and cardiovascular disease risk. *Circulation* 118(19):1913-1914.

IDF (International Diabetes Federation). 2006. The diabetes atlas. Brussels: IDF.

IDF. 2010. *The diabetes atlas.* Brussels: IDF.

IOM (Institute of Medicine). 2009. *Secondhand smoke exposure and cardiovascular effects: Making sense of the evidence.* Washington, DC: The National Academies Press.

IOM. 2010. *Promoting Cardiovascular Health in the Developing World: A Critical Challenge to Achieve Global Health.* Washington, DC: The National Academies Press.

Jacobs DR, Meyer KA, Kushi LH, Folsom AR ,1999. *Is whole grain intake associated with reduced total and cause-specific death rates in older women? The Iowa Women's Health Study. American Journal of Public Health, 89, 322–9.*

Jensen, L. A., and D. K. Moser. 2008. Gender differences in knowledge, attitudes, and beliefs about heart disease. *Nursing Clinics of North America* 43(1):77-104; vi-vii.

Jequier, E. 1999. Alcohol intake and body weight: A paradox. *American Journal of Clinical Nutrition* 69(2):173-174.

Jha, P., and F. J. Chaloupka. 1999. Curbing the epidemic: Governments and the economics of tobacco control. Washington, DC: World Bank.

Johnson, R. K., L. J. Appel, M. Brands, B. V. Howard, M. Lefevre, R. H. Lustig, F. Sacks, L. M. Steffen, J. Wylie-Rosett, P. A. American Heart Association Nutrition Committee of the Council on Nutrition, Physical Activity, and Metabolism, and the the Council on Epidemiology and Prevention. 2009. Dietary sugars intake and cardiovascular health: A scientific statement from the American Heart Association. *Circulation* 120(11):1011-1020.

Joint WHO/FAO Expert Consultation on Diet Nutrition and the Prevention of Chronic Diseases and World Health Organization Department of Nutrition for Health and Development.2003. *Diet, nutrition and the prevention of chronic diseases: Report of a joint WHO/FAO expert consultation, Geneva, January- February 2002, WHO technical report series.* Geneva: World Health Organization.

Jones PJ, MacDougall DE, Ntanios F, Vanstone CA ,1997. *Dietary phytosterols as cholesterol-lowering agents in humans. Canadian Journal of Physiology and Pharmacology, 75, 217–27.*

Joseph A, Kutty VR and Soman CR ,2000. High risk for coronary heart disease in Thiruvananthapuram City: A study of serum lipids and other risk factors. Indian Heart J 2000, 52:29-35.

Karmally W, 2005. Balancing unsaturated fatty acids: what is the evidence for cholesterol lowering ?*J Am Diet assoc* 105:1068.

Kay CD et al, 2006. Effects of antioxidant rich foods on vascular reactivity review of the clinical evidence Curr Atheroscer Rep 8:510.

Kelishadi, R. 2007. Childhood overweight, obesity, and the metabolic syndrome in developing countries. *Epidemiologic Reviews* 29:62-76.

Kelly, T. N., L. A. Bazzano, V. A. Fonseca, T. K. Thethi, K. Reynolds, and J. He. 2009. Glucose control and cardiovascular disease in type 2 diabetes. *Annals of Internal Medicine* 151(6):1-10.

Kengne, A. P., A. Patel, F. Barzi, K. Jamrozik, T. H. Lam, H. Ueshima, D. F. Gu, I. Suh, and M. Woodward. 2007. Systolic blood pressure, diabetes and the risk of cardiovascular diseases in the Asia-Pacific region. *Journal of Hypertension* 25(6):1205-1213.

Kengne, A. P., K. Nakamura, F. Barzi, T. H. Lam, R. Huxley, D. Gu, A. Patel, H. C. Kim, and M. Woodward. 2009. Smoking, diabetes and cardiovascular diseases in men in the Asia Pacific region. *Journal of Diabetes* 1(3):173-181.

Klein S et al, 2004. Clinical implications of obesity with specific focus on cardiovascular disease :a statement for professionals from the American Heart association Council on Nutrition, Physical Activity, and Metabolism: endorsed by the American College of Cardiology Foundation, *Circulation* 110; 2952.

Krummel DA 2008. Medical nutrition therapy for cardiovascular disease, In: *Krause's food & nutrition therapy* (2008). Mahan K & Scott-Stump S,pp(833-864) 12th ed. Philadelphia: Saunders; ISBN: 978-1-4160-3401-8

Lamarche B, St-Pierre AC, Ruel IL, Cantin B, Dagenais GR, Despres JP, 2001. A prospective, population based study of low density lipoprotein particle size as a risk factor for ischemic heart disease in men. Can J Cardiol; 17:859–65.

Lawlor, D. A., S. Ebrahim, and G. Davey Smith. 2001. Sex matters: Secular and geographical trends in sex differences in coronary heart disease mortality. *British Medical Journal* 323(7312):541-545: Erratum 325(7364):580.

Lesperance, F., and N. Frasure-Smith. 2007. Depression and heart disease. *Cleveland Clinic Journal of Medicine* 74(Suppl 1):S63-S66.

Lichtenstein AH,1998. Soy protein, isoflavones and cardiovascular disease risk. J Nutr. Oct;128(10):1589-92.

Lichtenstein AH et al,2001. Stanol/steroel ester-containing foods and blood cholesterol levels, *Circulation* 103:1177.

Lichtenstein AH et al, 2006. Diet and lifestyle recommendations revision 2006: a scientific statement from the American Heart Association Nutrition Committee, *Circulation* 114:82.

Lichtman, J. H., J. T. Bigger Jr., J. A. Blumenthal, N. Frasure-Smith, P. G. Kaufmann, F. Lesperance, D. B. Mark, D. S. Sheps, C. B. Taylor, and E. S. Froelicher. 2008. Depression and coronary heart disease: Recommendations for screening, referral, and treatment—a science advisory from the American Heart Association Prevention Committee of the Council on Cardiovascular Nursing, Council on Clinical Cardiology, Council on Epidemiology and Prevention, and Interdisciplinary Council on Quality of Care and Outcomes Research. *Circulation* 118(17):1768-1775.

Liu S, Stampfer MJ, Hu FB et al. ,1999. *Whole-grain consumption and risk of coronary heart disease: results from the Nurses' Health Study. American Journal of Clinical Nutrition, 70, 412–9.*

Lominadze D, Joshua I and Schuschke D, 1998. Increased erythrocyte aggregation in spontaneously hypertensive rats. Am J Hypertens;11:784–789.

Lominadze D, Dean WL, Tyagi SC and Roberts AM, 2010. Mechanisms of fibrinogen-induced microvascular dysfunction during cardiovascular disease. *Acta Physiol* ;198(1): 1–13.

Lopez, A. D., C. D. Mathers, M. Eszati, D. T. Jamison, and C. J. L. Murray. 2006. *Global burden of disease and risk factors.* Washington, DC: World Bank.

Lucas, D. L., R. A. Brown, M. Wassef, and T. D. Giles. 2005. Alcohol and the cardiovascular system research challenges and opportunities. *Journal of the American College Cardiology* 45(12):1916-1924.

Manson JE, Hu FB, Rich-Edwards JW et al. ,1999. *A prospective study of walking as compared with vigorous exercise in the prevention of CHD in women. New England Journal of Medicine, 341(9), 650–8.*

McKevith B ,2004. *Nutritional aspects of cereals. Nutrition Bulletin, 29, 111–42.*

Mensink RP et al, 2003. Effects of dietary fatty acids and carbohydrates on the ratio of serum total to HDL cholesterol and on serum lipids and apolipoproteins a: meta-analysis of 60 controlled trials, *Am J Clin Nutr* 77 :1146.

Mozaffarian D, Abdollahi M, Campos H, Houshiarrad A, Willett WC, 2007. Consumption of trans fats and estimated effects on coronary heart disease in Iran. *Eur J Clin Nutr,* 61(8):1004-10.

Mukamal, K. J., S. E. Chiuve, E. B. Rimm, K. J. Mukamal, S. E. Chiuve, and E. B. Rimm. 2006. Alcohol consumption and risk for coronary heart disease in men with healthy lifestyles. *Archives of Internal Medicine* 166(19):2145-2150.

Musunuru K, Kral BG, Blumenthal RS, et al. (2008). The use of high-sensitivity assays for C-reactive protein in clinical practice. *Nat Clin Pract Cardiovasc Med* , 5, 621-625.

National Cholesterol Education Program (NCEP): Expert Panel on Detection, Evaluation, and Treatment of High Blood Cholesterol in Adults (Adult Treatment Panel III final report, 2002. *Circulation* 106:3143.

Nestel PJ, Yamashita T, Sasahara T, Pomeroy S, Dart A, Komesaroff P, et al, 1997. Soy isoflavones improve systemic arterial compliance but not plasma lipids in menopausal and perimenopausal women. *Arterioscler Thromb Vasc Biol;* 17 (12):3392-8.

Oken, E., E. B. Levitan, and M. W. Gillman. 2008. Maternal smoking during pregnancy and child overweight: Systematic review and meta-analysis. *International Journal of Obesity* 32(2):201-210.

Osmond, C., and D. J. P. Barker. 2000. Fetal, infant, and childhood growth are predictors of coronary heart disease, diabetes, and hypertension in adult men and women. *Environmental Health Perspectives* 108(Suppl 3):545-553.

Pietinen P, Rimm EB, Korhonen P et al. ,1996. *Intake of dietary fibre and risk of coronary heart disease in a cohort of Finnish men. The Alpha-Tocopherol, Beta carotene Cancer Prevention Study. Circulation, 94, 2720–7.*

Pilote, L., K. Dasgupta, V. Guru, K. H. Humphries, J. McGrath, C. Norris, D. Rabi, J. Tremblay, A. Alamian, T. Barnett, J. Cox, W. A. Ghali, S. Grace, P. Hamet, T. Ho, S. Kirkland, M. Lambert, D. Libersan, J. O'Loughlin, G. Paradis, M. Petrovich, and V. Tagalakis. 2007. A comprehensive view of sex-specific issues related to cardiovascular disease. *Canadian Medical Association Journal* 176(6):S1-S44: Erratum 176(9):1310.

Rawson ES et al, 2001. Body mass index, but not physical activity, is associated with C-reactive protein, *Med Sci Sports Exerc* 35 :1160.=

Regitz-Zagrosek, V. 2006. Therapeutic implications of the gender-specific aspects of cardiovascular disease. *Nature Reviews Drug Discovery* 5(5):425-438.

Rehm, J., C. Mathers, S. Popova, M. Thavorncharoensap, Y. Teerawattananon, and J. Patra.2009. Global burden of disease and injury and economic cost attributable to alcohol use and alcohol-use disorders. *Lancet* 373(9682):2223-2233.

Richardson DP , 2000. *The grain, the wholegrain and nothing but the grain: the science behind the wholegrain and the reduced risk of heart disease and cancer. Nutrition Bulletin, 25, 353–60.*

Ridker PM, Buring JE, Shih J ,1998. *Prospective study of C-reactive protein and the risk of future cardiovascular events among apparently healthy women. Circulation, 97, 425–8*

Ridker PM, Hennekens CH, Buring JE, Rifai N ,2000. *Creactive protein and other markers of inflammation in the prediction of cardiovascular disease in women. N Engl J Med, 342, 836–43.*

Ridker PM, Danielson E, Fonseca FA, et al ,2008. Rosuvastatin to prevent vascular events in men and women with elevated C-reactive protein. *N Engl J Med*;359:2195–2207.

Ridker PM, Danielson E, Fonseca FA, et al ,2009.. Reduction in C-reactive protein and LDL cholesterol and cardiovascular event rates after initiation of rosuvastatin: a prospective study of the JUPITER trial. *Lancet* ;373:1175–1182.

Ross R ,1999. *Mechanisms of disease – atherosclerosis – an inflammatory disease. New England Journal of Medicine, 340, 115–26.*

Rudd JHF et al: Imaging of atherosclerosis-can we predict Plaque rupture?*Trends Cardiovasc Med* 15:17,2005.

Sassi, F., M. Cecchini, J. Lauer, and D. Chisholm. 2009. *Improving lifestyles, tackling obesity: The health and economic impact of prevention strategies.* Paris: OECD.

Scanu AM and Edelstein C, 2008. HDL: bridging past and present with a look at the future. *The FASEB Journal 22,* 4044-54.

Schulze, M. B., F. B. Hu. 2005. Primary prevention of diabetes: What can be done and how much can be prevented? *Annual Review of Public Health* 26:445-467.

Shafey, O., M. Eriksen, H. Ross, and J. Mackay. 2009. *The tobacco atlas.* 3rd ed. Atlanta: American Cancer Society.

Sharifi N, Mahdavi R, Ebrahimi-Mameghani M. Association between physical activity and lipid profile in a sample of women with central obesity. First National Congress of Metabolic Syndrome, Tabriz, Iran. 13-14 June, 2008.

Singhal, A., M. Fewtrell, T. J. Cole, and A. Lucas. 2003. Low nutrient intake and early growth for later insulin resistance in adolescents born preterm. *Lancet* 361(9363):1089-1097.

Singhal, A., T. J. Cole, M. Fewtrell, J. Deanfield, A. Lucas, A. Singhal, T. J. Cole, M. Fewtrell, J. Deanfield, and A. Lucas. 2004. Is slower early growth beneficial for long-term cardiovascularhealth? *Circulation* 109(9):1108-1113.

Skalen K, Gustafsson M, Knutsen Rydberg E et al , 2002. *Subendothelial retention of atherogenic lipoproteins in early atherosclerosis. Nature, 417, 750–4. susceptibility among six low density lipoprotein subfractions of differing density and particle size. Atherosclerosis, 93, 189–99.*

Trichopoulou et al, 2003. Adherence to a Mediterranean diet and survival in a Greek population, *N Engl J Med* 348:2599.

Truswell AS ,2002. *Cereal grains and coronary heart disease. European Journal of Clinical Nutrition, 56, 1–14.*

Turnbull, F. M., C. Abraira, R. J. Anderson, R. P. Byington, J. P. Chalmers, W. C. Duckworth, G. W. Evans, H. C. Gerstein, R. R. Holman, T. E. Moritz, B. C. Neal, T. Ninomiya, A. A. Patel, S. K. Paul, F. Travert, and M. Woodward. 2009. Intensive glucose control and macrovascular outcomes in type 2 diabetes. *Diabetologia.* DOI 10.1007/s00125-00009-01470-00120.

US Department of Health and Human Services ,1996. Physical Activity and Health: A Report of the Surgeon General. US Department of Health and Human Services, Centers for Disease Control and Prevention, Atlanta.

Victora, C. G., L. Adair, C. Fall, P. C. Hallal, R. Martorell, L. Richter, and H. S. Sachdev. 2008. Maternal and child undernutrition: Consequences for adult health and human capital. *Lancet* 371(9609):340-357

Walker, S., and S. George. 2007. Young@heart. USA: Fox Searchlight Pictures.

Wannamethee SG, Shaper AG , 2002. Physical activity and cardiovascular disease. Seminars in Vascular Medicine, 2, 257–65.

Whitaker, R. C. 2004. Predicting preschooler obesity at birth: The role of maternal obesity in early pregnancy. *Pediatrics* 114(1):e29-e36.

WHO.2003. *The world health report: 2003: Shaping the future.* Geneva: World Health Organization.

WHO.2005.*Preventing chronic diseases: A vital investment.* http://www.who.int/chp/chronic_disease_report/full_report.pdf (accessed April 23, 2009).

WHO. 2008a. *The global burden of disease: 2004 update.* Geneva: World Health Organization.

WHO. 2008b. *WHO report on the global tobacco epidemic, 2008 : The MPOWER package.* Geneva: World Health Organization.

WHO. 2009a. *World health statistics 09* . Geneva: World Health Organization.

WHO. 2009b. *Global health risks: Mortality and burden of disease attributable to selected major risks.* Geneva: World Health Organization.

WHO. 2009 c. *Aging and life course.* Geneva: World Health Oranization.

WHOSIS (World Health Organization Statistical Information System). 2009. World Health Organization.

Wijendran V and Hayes KC, 2004: Dietary n-6 and n-3 fatty acid balance and cardiovascular health. *Annu Rev Nutr* 24:597.

Willett WC, 1998. *Is dietary fat a major determinant of body fat? American Journal of Clinical Nutrition, 67, 556S–62S.*

Williams CL, Hayman LL, Daniels SR et al., *2002. Cardiovascular health in childhood: a statement for health professionals from the Committee on Atherosclerosis, Hypertension, and Obesity in the Young (AHOY) of the Council on Cardiovascular Disease in the Young, American Heart Association. Circulation, 106, 143–60.*

Ziegelstein, R. C., J. A. Fauerbach, S. S. Stevens, J. Romanelli, D. P. Richter, and D. E. Bush. 2000. Patients with depression are less likely to follow recommendations to reduce cardiac risk during recovery from a myocardial infarction. *Archives of Internal Medicine* 160(12):1818-1823.

15

Cardiovascular and Cerebrovascular Problems in the Development of Cognitive Impairment: For Medical Professionals Involved in the Treatment of Atherosclerosis

Michihiro Suwa
Department of Cardiology,
Hokusetsu General Hospital, Takatsuki, Osaka,
Japan

1. Introduction

When cognitive function declines at a rate greater than that expected based on the actual age, life circumstances and educational level, we define it as cognitive impairment (Blennow et al., 2006; Gauthier et al 2006). In the older generation, the neurodegenerative process is considered to occur several years before the development of clinically detectable cognitive impairment. Although aging is the most clear factor in the development of this disease process, several epidemiological studies have elucidated that cardiovascular risk factors, i.e., hyperlipidemia, hypertension, smoking and diabetes, are also associated with cerebrovascular disease processes that may deteriorate cognitive function and advance dementia (Casserly & Topol, 2004; Nash & Fillit, 2006; Whitmer et al., 2005). In this chapter, I would like to introduce the current positioning of cognitive impairment as a consequence of cardiovascular diseases as well as a form of cerebrovascular disease, to neurologists or psychiatrists as well as to general physicians or cardiologists.

2. Cognitive impairment

Currently, Alzheimer's disease is the most common form of dementia or cognitive impairment, but less than 20% of dementia patients exhibit the isolated form of Alzheimer's disease and around 50% of such patients exhibit a combination of Alzheimer's disease and intracerebral vascular disease. By contrast, the isolated vascular type only contributes 20% (Meguro et al., 2002). Therefore, various problems related to metabolic syndrome, i.e., hypertension, hyperlipidemia, diabetes, and smoking habit, contribute to the development or deterioration of cognitive impairment.

3. Cardiovascular problems in cognitive impairment

Furthermore, recent investigations have suggested that the incidence of cognitive impairment is higher in patients with congestive heart failure and that treatment for left ventricular (LV) systolic dysfunction may prevent or delay the development of dementia in elderly patients (Zuccala et al., 2003, 2005). An Italian investigation indicated that the incidence of congestive heart failure was markedly higher in subjects with Mini-Mental State Examination (MMSE) scores <24 (20.2%), compared with those with scores ≥24 (4.6%) (Zuccala et al., 2003). Also, the presence of cognitive impairment has been associated with increased in-hospital mortality in older patients with heart failure (Zuccala et al., 2005). These data may indicate that low cardiac output due to heart failure is related to the deterioration of cognitive function, although there have been no reports regarding the pathophysiology or etiology of heart failure in relation to cognitive impairment. Another investigation indicated an independent relation between the levels of b-type natriuretic peptide (BNP) and the degree of cognitive impairment in older subjects (>55years of age) with cardiovascular disease; despite the fact that the mechanism was unclear (Gunstad et al., 2006).

In patients with heart failure, more than half of them, especially in females, showed normal or preserved LV ejection fraction (EF), i.e., exhibited heart failure resulting from LV diastolic dysfunction (Hogg et al. ,2004). Also, in heart failure patients with cardiovascular risk factors, i.e., hyperlipidemia, hypertension, smoking and diabetes, heart failure with preserved EF is also common. Therefore, we evaluated the relationship between LV diastolic dysfunction and cognitive impairment in Japanese patients with cardiovascular diseases (Suwa & Ito, 2009).

In our study, patients were divided into 2 groups; those patients with normal cognitive function or mild cognitive impairment (MMSE>=24; n=68: group N) and those with depressed cognitive function (MMSE<24, n=13). Diastolic function was evaluated based upon the ratio of the early diastolic mitral flow velocity (E) by pulse-wave Doppler echocardiography to the early diastolic mitral annular myocardial velocity (e') by tissue Doppler echocardiography (Diastolic Doppler index: E/e'). BNP was also evaluated as an index of heart failure. Consequently, in depressed cognitive function, diastolic Doppler index, E/e', was deteriorated (6.1±1.3 vs. N: 4.6±1.3, $p<0.0003$) and BNP was higher (137±142 pg/ml vs. N: 60±49 pg/ml, $p<0.007$), compared with those with normal cognitive function. Furthermore, the number of patients with diabetes was also higher in depressed cognitive function than in normal cognitive function (46% vs. N: 18%). From these studies evaluating the relation between cardiac and cognitive function, heart failure due to LV systolic and diastolic dysfunction can affect the development and the deterioration of cognitive impairment.

Poor cerebral circulation:	Left ventricular systolic dysfunction Left ventricular diastolic dysfunction
Stroke:	Atrial fibrillation, Atherosclerotic vascular diseases including of carotid artery stenosis
Deep white matter hyperintensity in brain MRI:	Atherosclerotic abnormalities, due to hypertension, diabetes, hyperlipidemia, and smoking
Hippocampal atrophy in brain:	Senile process

MRI: magnetic resonance imaging

Table 1. Relationship between cardiovascular abnormalities and cerebrovascular diseases affecting the decline of cognitive function

The occurrence of atrial fibrillation (AF) is a risk of stroke, and stroke increases the risk of cognitive decline and dementia. Therefore, AF has been reported to be associated with cognitive decline and dementia (Jozwiak et al., 2006). Recently, even in stroke-free patients it has been shown that AF is a risk for cognitive impairment and hippocampal atrophy (Knecht et al., 2008). For these reasons, it was considered that AF was associated with abnormalities of hemostasis, endothelial damage, platelet dysfunction, and low cardiac output.

As another measurable index in the vascular system, the ankle to brachial index is also related to incidence of total dementia, vascular dementia and Alzheimer's disease, especially in carriers of the apolipoprotein E gene abnormality (Laurin et al. 2007).

4. Common interest between cardiovascular and cerebrovascular diseases

Brain magnetic resonance imaging is conducted to screen for cerebrovascular disease as well as cerebral disease, and hyperintensities in the deep white matter on T2-weighted images can be incidentally detected in 10-20% in adults aged 64 to 94% at age 82 in the general population (Fig.1 and Fig.2). At present, these white matter lesions are related to chronic hypoperfusion and disruption of the blood brain barrier due to small vessel disease in the lesion area (Debette & Markus, 2010). Also, white matter hyperintensities are more common in patients with cerebrovascular disease as well as cardiovascular disease, with risk factors affecting atherosclerosis, inclusive of hypertension (Hajjar et al., 2011). Furthermore, meta-analysis reveals that the white matter lesions predict an increased risk of stroke, dementia, and death. Although data that treatment for these risk factors reduces the progression of white matter hyperintensities are limited, it is also reported that antihypertensive therapy reduced the progression in patients with stroke (Saxby et al., 2008). Therefore, white matter hyperintensities may be important markers to not only detect the risk of stroke and dementia but also diagnose the atherosclerosis in cerebro-cervical vascular system. The progression of white matter lesions is independently related to baseline cerebral lesion, higher age, hypertension, and current smoking. Also, atherosclerotic processes in the carotid artery, connecting to the cerebral artery, are associated with the cerebral small vessel disease (Romero et al., 2009).

Modified Mini-Mental State Examination scale falls more according to the worsening of white matter grade (prominently in grade Two +). (Fig.3. Longstreth et al. 2005) (with permission, License No.2776831264727)

To date, some angiotensin receptor blockers have been reported to significantly reduce the incidence and progression of Alzheimer's disease and dementia, compared with the use of angiotensin converting enzyme inhibitors or other cardiovascular drugs, in a predominant male population (Saxby et al., 2008). Therefore, when prescribing antihypertensive drugs we may have to consider the contribution of such medicines.

At present, the CHADS2 score is widely used to validate the risk for stroke in patients with AF. A newer clinical study has shown that the CHADS2 score is useful to predict ischemic stroke in patients with stable coronary artery disease, even in those without baseline atrial fibrillation (Welles et al., 2011)

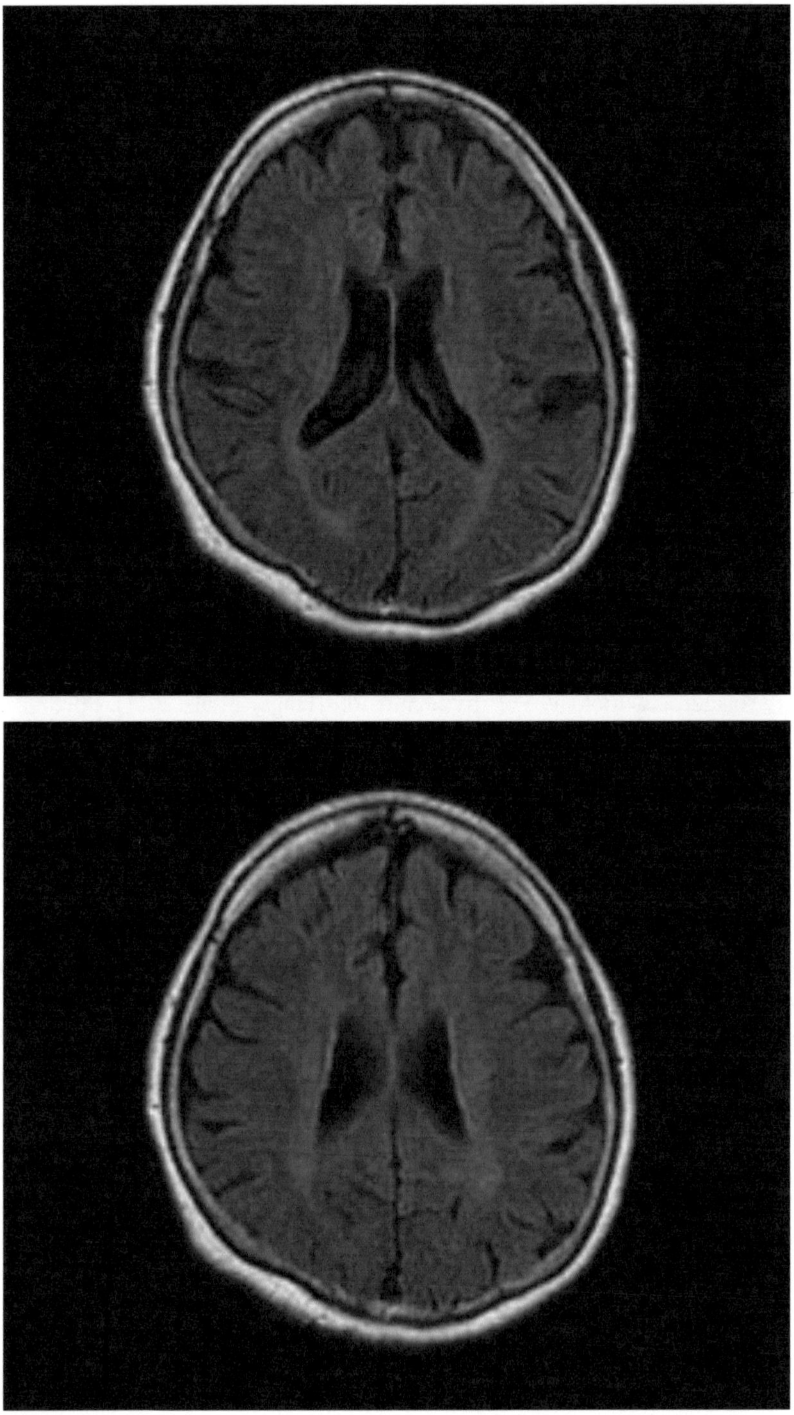

Fig. 1. Brain magnetic resonance imaging on T2 weighted images obtained from a 77 year old female without cognitive impairment and being under medication for hypertension. These images show somewhat brain atrophy but no white matter hyperintensities.

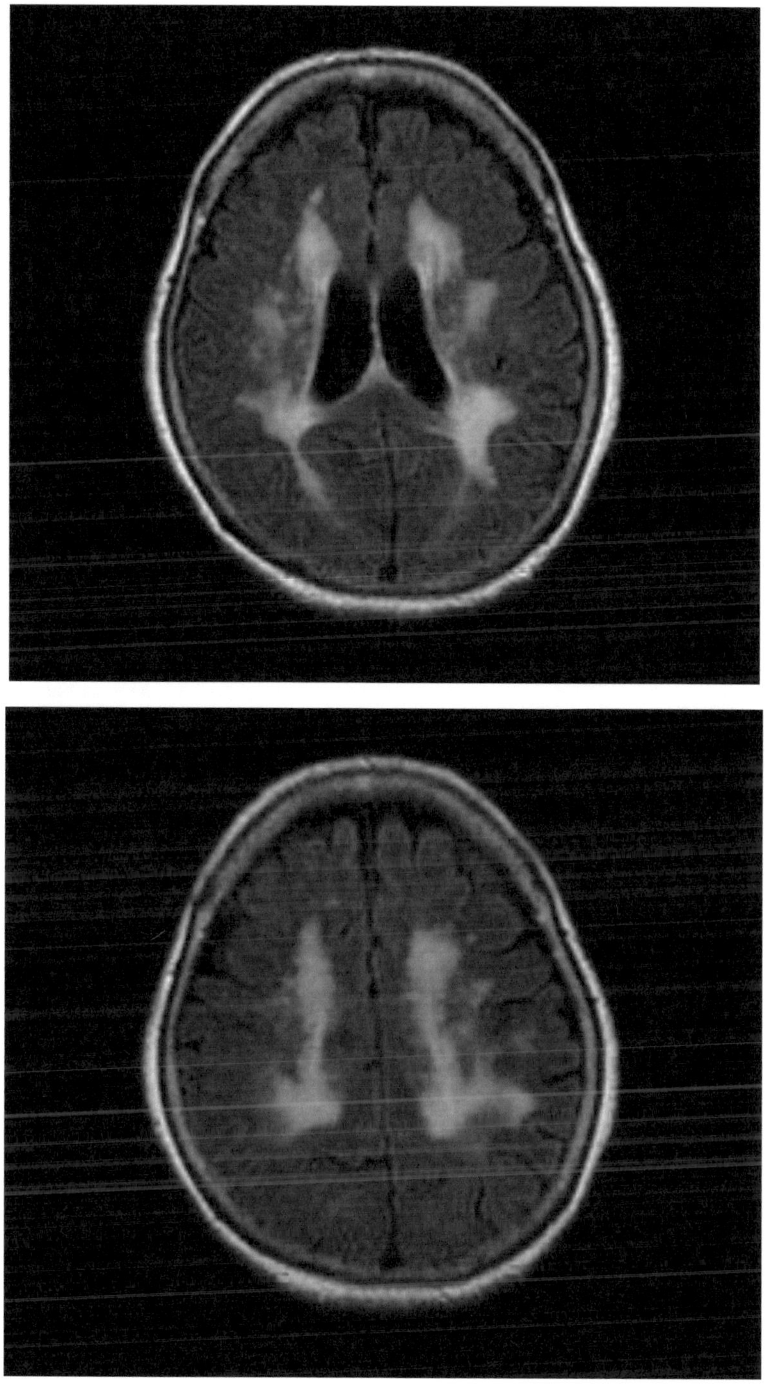

Fig. 2. White matter hyperintensities on brain magnetic resonance imaging from a 73 year old female with advanced cognitive impairment (score 18 on MMSE). Extensive hyperintensities can be seen in deep white matter, especially in periventricular region. She is under medication for hypertension and hyperlipidemia

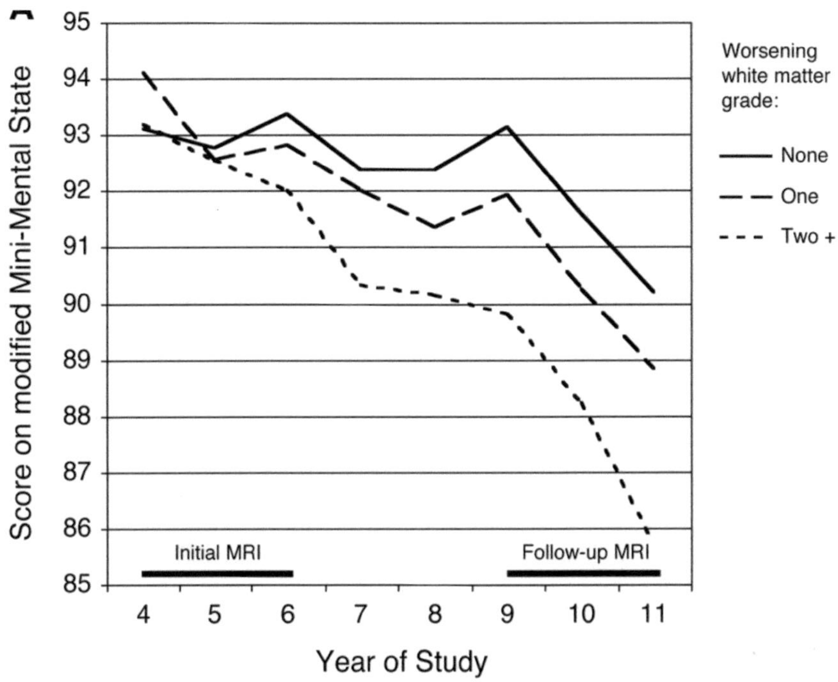

Fig. 3. Scores on modified Mini-Mental State Examination (vertical axis) for each year of study from initial to follow-up brain MRI scans (horizontal axis) by groups of participants (people aged 65 years and older) defined by worsening grade of white matter hyperintensity (three grade: None, grade One, and grade Two+).

Left ventricular systolic dysfunction:	Low left ventricular ejection fraction
Left ventricular diastolic dysfunction:	Reduced e′, Increased E/e′ ratio
B-type natriuretic peptide (BNP):	Increased BNP or N-terminal pro-BNP
Rhythm disturbance:	Development of atrial fibrillation
Ankle-brachial index (ABI):	Low ABI
Carotid ultrasonography	Internal carotid artery stenosis

e′: early diastolic mitral annular myocardial velocity by tissue Doppler echocardiography

E: early diastolic mitral flow velocity by pulse-wave Doppler echocardiography

Table 2. Cardiovascular indexes possibly to detect cognitive impairment

5. Relationship between echocardiographic parameters and age

Currently, LV diastolic function is evaluated based upon the following indices. Using pulse-wave Doppler echocardiography, the ratio of E velocity and the late diastolic transmitral flow velocity (A): (E/A ratio), and early diastolic flow deceleration time are measured. By tissue Doppler echocardiography of mitral annular motion, e′ myocardial velocity can be evaluated. Also, diastolic function was evaluated by the diastolic Doppler index (E/e′), and this index is also useful to evaluate LV end-diastolic pressure or left atrial pressure in patients with heart failure with depressed or normal LV EF (Ommen et.al., 2000).

Among the healthy subjects, the previous reports have evaluated the changes with age in various parameters. LV systolic function, obtained from LV EF by standard echocardiography or LV myocardial performance index using Doppler echocardiography, have shown minimum increments with age. However, LV diastolic function declined with age on echocardiographic parameters, i.e., E/A ratio and e' velocity decreased, and E/e' ratio increased (Munagala et al., 2003). Furthermore, LV wall thickness and LV mass increased gradually with age, and suggested depression of LV myocardial compliance (Daimon et al., 2008).

In some reports discussing the relationship between cognitive impairment and cardiovascular dysfunction, LV diastolic function was depressed with the deterioration of cognitive function, which may be more progressive than that with aging alone (Hogg et al. ,2004). Furthermore, in patients with heart failure, cognitive function is depressed, but there is no clear data as to whether LV systolic function is depressed with the decline of cognitive function and its decline is improved with the correction of systolic dysfunction.

6. Conclusion

While age is the most significant contributing factor to the development of cognitive impairment, several epidemiological studies have elucidated that cardiovascular risk factors, i.e., hyperlipidemia, hypertension, smoking and diabetes contribute to the deterioration of cognitive function. Furthermore, LV systolic and diastolic dysfunction, have been reported to cause cognitive impairment, likely as a result of the development of poor cerebral perfusion. Brain white matter hyperintensitiy and thromboembolic stroke due to atherosclerotic factors and atrial fibrillation are also related to producing cognitive impairment. Therefore, doctors and medical professionals, who are involved with medical treatment for cerebrovascular and cardiovascular diseases must keep in mind that atherosclerotic disease processes are also related to the development of cognitive impairment and progression of dementia.

7. References

Blennow, K et al (2006). Alzheimer's disease. Lancet, Vol.368, No.9533, pp. 387-403.

Casserly, I. & Topol, E. (2004). Convergence of atherosclerosis and Alzheimer's disease: inflammation, cholesterol, and misfolded proteins. Lancet, Vol. 363, No.9514, pp. 1139-46.

Daimon M et al. (2008). Normal values of echocardiographic parameters in relation to age in a healthy Japanese population: The JAMP Study. CIrc J Vol.72, No.11, pp. 1859-1866.

Debette S & Markus HS. (2010). The clinical importance of white matter hyperintensities on brain magnetic resonance imaging: Systemic review and meta-analysis. BMJ Vol.341, pp c3666 (on-line)

Gauthier, S et al (2006). Mild cognitive impairment. Lancet, Vol. 367: No. No.9518, pp.1262-70.

Gunstad J et al. (2006). Relation of brain natriuretic peptide levels to cognitive dysfunction in adults > 55 years of age with cardiovascular disease. Am J Cardiol Vol.98, No.4, pp. 538-40.

Hajjar I et al. (2011). Hypertension, white matter hyperintensities, and concurrent impairments in mobility, cognition, and mood: The cardiovascular health study. Circulation Vol. 123, No.8, pp. 858-865.

Hogg K et al. (2004). Heart failure with preserved left ventricular systolic function: Epidemiology, clinical characteristics, and prognosis. J Am Coll Cardiol Vol 43, No 3, pp.317-327

Jozwiak A et al. (2006) Association of atrial fibrillation and focal neurologic deficits with impaired cognitive function in hospitalized patients ≥65 years of age. Am J Cardiol Vol. 98, No.9, pp.1238-41.

Knecht S et al. (2008). Atrial fibrillation in stroke-free patients is associated with memory impairment and hippocampal atrophy. Eur Heart J Vol. 29, No.17, pp. 2125-2132.

Laurin D et al. (2007) Ankle-to-brachial index and dementia. Honolulu-Asia aging study. Circulation Vol. 116, No.20, pp. 2269-2274.

Longstreth WT Jr. et al. (2005). Incidence, manifestation, and predictors of worsening white matter on serial cranial magnetic resonance imaging in the elderly. The cardiovascular health study. Stroke 36, No. 1, pp56-61

Meguro K et al. (2002). Prevalence of dementia and dementing diseases in Japan: the Tajiri project. Arch Neurol. Vol. 59, No. 7, pp. 1109-1114

Munagala VK et al. (2003). Association of newer diastolic function parameters with age in healthy subjects: A population-based study. J Am Soc Echocardiogr Vol. 16, No.10, pp. 1049-56

Nash DT & Fillit H. (2006). Cardiovascular disease risk factors and cognitive impairment. Am J Cariol, Vol. 97, No.8, pp.1262-65.

Ommen SR et.al (2000). Clinical utility of Doppler echocardiography and tissue Doppler imaging in the estimation of left ventricular filling pressures. A comparative simultaneous Doppler-catheterization study. Circulation Vol. 102, No.15, pp. 1788 – 94.

Romero JR et al. (2009). Carotid artery atherosclerosis, MRI indices of brain ischemia, aging, and cognitive impairment. The Framingham study. Stroke Vol. 40, No.5, pp.1590-1596

Saxby BK et al. (2008). Candesartan and cognitive decline in older patients with hypertension. Neurology Vol. 70, No.19 pt2, pp.1858-1866.

Suwa M & Ito T (2009). Correlation between cognitive impairment and left ventricular diastolic dysfunction in patients with cardiovascular diseases. Int J Cardiol, Vol. 136, No. 3, pp. 351-354.

Welles CC et al. (2011). The CHADS2 score predicts ischemic stroke in the absence of atrial fibrillation among patients with coronary heart disease: Data from the Heart and Soul Study. ACC. 2011, J Am Coll Cardiol Vol.57, No.14, suppl S, E607.

Whitmer RA et al (2005). Midlife cardiovascular risk factors and risk of dementia in late life. Neurology, Vol.64, No.2, pp. 277-81.

Zuccala G et al. (2003). The effects of cognitive impairment on mortality among hospitalized patients with heart failure. Am J Med Vol. 115, No.2, pp. 98-103.

Zuccala G et al. (2005). Correlates of cognitive impairment among patients with heart failure: Results of a multicenter survey. Am J Med. Vol.118, No.5, pp. 496-502

16

French Paradox, Polyphenols and Cardiovascular Protection: The Oestrogenic Receptor-α Implication

Tassadit Benaissa[1], Thierry Ragot[2] and Angela Tesse[1]
[1]INSERM, UMR 915, Institut de recherche thérapeutique (IRT), Nantes,
[2]CNRS, UMR 8203, Institut de Cancérologie Gustave Roussy, Villejuif,
France

1. Introduction

Several epidemiological and clinical studies confirm an inverse correlation between a diet rich in vegetables, fruits, and red wine, in cancer development and chronic diseases such as cardiovascular diseases. This is linked to the presence in these aliments of high levels of nutrients of vegetal origin called phytonutrients. They are natural phytochemical compounds contained in plant food; they are not vitamins or minerals but they have beneficial effects on the health, sometimes acting in association with other essential nutrients. Phytonutrients are divided in three families: the terpenes, the sulfuric compounds, and the polyphenols which are the subject of this chapter.

Polyphenols are the most important group of phytonutrients. They are not only present in fruits and vegetables but also in seeds, spices, herbs and teas, at different concentrations and molecular structures in correlation with the aliment involved. The most studied polyphenolic compounds for their vascular action are resveratrol, delphinidin, quercetin and tannins contained in red wine. Indeed, the red wine is the beverage the most correlated to cardiac and vascular protection. It could reduce of 40% the risk of myocardial infarction, and of 25% the risk of vascular thrombotic events in brain.

Elevated content in polyphenols of red wine seems to play a benefic role in the mechanism of vascular and cardiac protection, not only by its anti-oxidant but also by its anti-thrombotic properties. Thus, more recently, research works were focused to study the vascular and cardiac effects of non-alcoholic fractions of red wine and have identified the oestrogenic receptor-α (ERα), as the preferential endothelial target of these molecules.

First, this chapter is focused on the "French Paradox" history. Then, we have described successively the composition and content of these compounds in food and beverages, and the epidemiological and fundamental studies showing how red wine polyphenolic compounds (RWPC) are able to improve endothelial function and cardiovascular protection. Finally, we explain the effects of oestrogens on the cardiovascular system and the implication of ERα in the beneficial cardiovascular effects of these natural molecules that could be used to prevent or treat cardiovascular diseases.

2. French paradox history

For a long time, it was suggested that a high fat intake is associated with an elevated risk of mortality for cardiovascular diseases in Anglo-Saxon populations. In contrast, several epidemiological studies have revealed a relatively low incidence of coronary heart diseases (CHD) in the French population, despite a high dietary intake of saturated fats. This was potentially attributable to the consumption of red wine (Renaud et al., 1999).

One of the first epidemiological studies conducted on 100,000 subjects in 1970 by Doctor Arthur Klatsky, a cardiologist of the Oakland Hospital in California, clearly evidenced that people following a diet with moderated consumption of red wine (1-3 glasses per day), showed a very little risk of death by CHD (Renaud et al., 1999). This was confirmed in 1979 by Doctor Saint-Léger which evidenced a negative correlation between wine consumption and mortality for CHD in men and women (from 55 to 64 years old), in more than 18 developed countries. Furthermore, Italy and France showed a lower level of mortality by myocardial infarction (about 3 or 5 folds less) compared to Anglo-Saxon populations such as Irish, North-American, and Scottish (Renaud et al., 1999). On the other hand, it has been demonstrated that to drink one glass of wine per day reduced death risk by CHD, but to drink more than three glasses of wine per day was associated with an increased death rate (Thun et al., 1997). In wine drinkers, the lower all-cause mortality was associated with a significant reduction in mortality from CHD, for about 45-48%, and other cardiovascular diseases (CVD), for about 39-40% (Renaud et al., 1999). Other studies have also suggested that both non-drinkers and heavy-drinkers have a higher risk of cardiovascular mortality than those who drink wine moderately (Providencia, 2006).

Then, numerous correlation studies concerning the strict relation between consumption of fat and CHD mortality have been conducted in various countries. In one of the most interesting ones, Artaud-Wild and colleagues examined the relation between CHD mortality and the intake of foodstuffs and nutrients in 40 different countries. After they have defined a cholesterol-saturated fat index (CSI), they studied this correlation in 100,000 men (aged 55 to 64 years) in all the countries studied. The findings of this epidemiological study evidenced that France had a CSI of 24 per 1000 kcal and a CHD mortality rate of 198; whereas Finland had a CSI of 26 per 1000 kcal and a CHD mortality rate of 1031 (Ferrières, 2004). The high consumption of saturated fatty acids suggests that French subjects could be exposed to a high risk of CHD (Renaud 1992), but it is in fact not the case considering the low rate of CHD mortality observed. Then, much attention has been focused on the possible superior protective effect of red wine consumption relative to those of other alcoholic beverages. So, the differential effects of wine, beer, and spirits have been examined. European research carried out in France and Denmark has shown that wine consumption was associated with a decrease of 24 up to 31% of all cause mortality; little to moderate wine drinking leads to a lower mortality rate from CVD than having an equivalent consumption of beer or spirits (Ferrières, 2004).

Nevertheless, alcohol consumption, from whatever sources, appears to have a J-shaped curve, whereby a modest intake is beneficial and either no intake or excess is harmful. This is confirmed by several studies: the Framingham study (Fuchs et al., 1995), the British Doctors study (Doll et al., 1994), the Cancer Prevention study of Thun and coworkers, conducted on about 490,000 persons (Thun et al., 1997), the Nurse Health study (Emberson et al., 2005), and other epidemiological investigations (Gaziano et al., 2000; Suh et al., 1992). It would take too long to report on all the studies dealing with the relations between alcohol and CHD.

The mechanisms involved in the protective role of red wine include anti-platelet, anti-coagulatory, improved glucose control, and anti-inflammatory effects as shown in MONICA (multinational MONItoring of trends and determinants in CArdiovascular disease) study (Imhof et al., 2004). The World Health Organization had collected all the results of these data, evidencing the protective role of moderated red wine consumption in cardiovascular disease development. Despite the high consumption of saturated fatty acids, why the French people do not develop a high CHD risk? This is the central question behind the "French Paradox" concept. The French epidemiologist Serge Renaud evidenced for the first time this "Paradox", which is defined as the light level of incidence of CVD in people following a diet containing a high quantity of saturated fatty acids, but also having a moderated red wine consumption (Pechanova et al., 2006, Renaud et al., 1999).

The results of Criqui and colleagues (Criqui & Ringel, 1994) were found in agreement with the French Paradox. In 21 developed countries, subjects in an age range of 35 to 74, without differences linked to gender, were studied and assessed at four time periods: 1965, 1970, 1980, and 1988, respectively. The independent variables chosen were: consumption of wine, beer, spirits, animal fats, vegetables, and fruits. Ischemic heart disease and all-cause mortality were finally assessed. Wine was the beverage most strongly negatively correlated with coronary diseases. Animal fat had a tendency to positive correlation, while fruits were negatively correlated. On the light of the numerous epidemiological studies, a protective activity of wine against CVD has been widely described, suggesting that moderated consumption of wine could reduce the risk of myocardial infarction and the risk of vascular thrombosis of brain vessels.

So many questions arose next. What were the elements that differentiate the wine (especially red wine) of other spirits? What were the processes responsible for the beneficial effect of wine consumption? What, in wine, promoted this effect?

3. Differences in polyphenolic compositions in food and beverages

Polyphenolic compounds are the biggest group of phytochemicals characterized by one or more phenolic rings associated with one or more hydroxyl groups, free or implicated in an ester, ether or eteroside function (Richter, 1993). This family of substances includes more than 8000 phenolic structures currently known, and among them, over 4000 flavonoids have been yet identified in plants and the list is constantly growing (Bravo, 1998; Cheynier, 2005; Harborne & Williams, 2000). Flavonoids contain a structural backbone C6-C3-C6, characterized by two C6 units of phenolic nature; while the non-flavonoids are phenolic acids divided in two main types, benzoic acid and cinnamic acid derivatives, based on C1-C6 and C3-C6 backbones, respectively (Tsao, 2010). The phenolic acids are usually contained as free molecules in fruits and vegetables. Phenolic acids could be also found in the bound form in grains and seeds (Chandrasekara & Shahidi, 2010).

Polyphenols are enrolled in numerous physiological functions in vegetal organisms: cell development, latent buds, blooming, and tuber formation. These substances are involved in the color of fruits, in particular they play a main role to confer the red color of ripe fruits, and in the savor and properties of food (Bahorun, 1997). Polyphenols include yellow, orange, red and blue pigments and various compounds implicated also in bitterness and astringency of unripe fruits, resulting from interaction of tannins with salivary proteins. Moreover, some volatile polyphenols, in particular vanillin and eugenol, are potent odorants and are responsible of the characteristic odor of cloves (Cheynier, 2005).

The content of polyphenolic compounds is particularly elevated in red wine but also in skin of red grapes, red fruits, cereals, several vegetables such as red onions, chocolate, tea, and coffee with different polyphenolic composition and percentage according to the kind of vegetal food or beverage (see Table 1) (Bravo, 1998; Tsao, 2010). Considering the diversity and wide distribution of polyphenols, they have been classified by their source of origin, biological function, and chemical structure. In plants, the majority of polyphenols exists as glycosides associated to sugar units or acylated sugars linked at different positions of the polyphenolic skeletons (Tsao, 2010).

Food	**Total polyphenols (mg/100 g of dry mutter)**	**Food**	**Total polyphenols (mg/100 g of fresh mutter)**
Cereals:		**Vegetables:**	
Barley	1200-1500	Onion	100-2025
Millet	590-1060		
Legumes:		**Fruits:**	
Black gram	540-1200	Apple	27-298
Green gram	440-800	Blackcurrant	140-1200
Pigeon peas	380-1710	Grapes	50-490
		Raspberry	37-429
Beverages	**Total polyphenols (mg/L)**	**Beverages**	**Total polyphenols (mg/L)**
Orange juice	370-7100	Tea	750-1050
Red wine	1000-6500	Coffee	1330-3670
White wine	200-300		

Table 1. Plant food and beverages with high levels of total polyphenolic compounds (from Bravo, 1998).

Some flavonoids such as the isoflavones are mostly found in plants of the leguminous family. Genistein and daidzein are the two main isoflavones found in soybeans and red clovers (Tsao et al., 2006). The flavonoid subgroup of the neoflavonoids is rarely present in food plants, but the open-ring chalcones are still found in fruits, in particular in apples and hops of beers (Tsao et al., 2003; Zhao et al., 2005). In contrast, other flavonoid subgroups such as flavones, flavonols, flavanones and flavanonols are most common and ubiquitous in the plant kingdom and in particular quercetin and kaempferol (Tsao, 2010). Flavanols or flavan-3-ols, also called catechins, are found in many fruits, the skin of grapes, apple and blueberries (Tsao et al., 2003). Catechin, epicatechin (isomer of catechin with *cis* configuration), and their derivatives, gallocatechins, are the major flavonoids contained in tea leaves and cacao beans and thus in chocolate (Si et al., 2006; Prior et al., 2001).

The red, blue and purple pigments of the majority of flower petals, fruits and vegetables and certain varieties of grains, for instance black rice, mainly contain anthocyanidins and in particular cyanidin, delphinidin, pelagonidin, and their methylated derivatives (composed up to 90% of anthocyanins). The color of these kinds of molecules can change with the pH and temperature: they are red in acidic and blue in basic conditions (Tsao, 2010). In grapes and apples, anthocyanins are found only in the red varieties (Cheynier, 2005).

Polyphenols are highly unstable species and, accordingly, their chemical structure can change during food and beverage processing and storage, leading to new compounds with different properties compared to their precursors (Xu et al., 2011). In particular, total catechin contents of fresh fruits can decrease of about 26% up to 58% after home preparation or industrial transformations (Cheynier, 2005).

Wine is a hydro-alcoholic acid solution. Indeed, its major component is water (80-90%) and ethanol (10-14%) implicated in the solubilization of polyphenols. The fraction of polyphenolic compounds contained in wine is high in red wine and its composition depends of the kind of wine. More precisely, generally red wine contains 1.2 gr/L of polyphenolic compounds while white wine contains only 0.2 gr/L of these compounds and, besides, does not contain the molecules involved in the red color such as the anthocyanidins and in particular delphinidin (see Table 2) (Pellegrini et al., 2000; Soleas et al., 1997). Interestingly, the level of these compounds in red wine is modified by the fermentation process used during wine production. Vinification variations and techniques are known to affect the phenolic composition of red wines. The fermentation of grape juice into wine is a complex microbial reaction, traditionally due to the sequential development of various species of yeast and lactic acid bacteria. In the past, wine was produced by natural fermentation of grape juice by yeasts originating from grapes and winery equipment (Ribereau-Gayon et al., 2000). Nowadays, another kind of fermentation process, the carbonic maceration, is more and more used to produce wine. With this method, freshly harvested bunches of grapes are allowed to ferment in carbonic anaerobiosis, in an atmosphere saturated with carbon dioxide (Navarro et al., 2000). The absence of oxygen is important to

Compounds (mg/L)	White young wine	White aged wine	Red young wine	Red aged wine
Total phenols	215	190-290	1300	955-1215
Non flavonoides	175	160-260	235	240-500
Flavonoides	30	25	1060	705
Catechins	25	15	200	150
Anthocyanins	0	0	200	20
Soluble tannins	5	10	550	450

Table 2. Polyphenolic compound contents in several types of wine (from Soleas et al., 1997).

reduce the oxidation of polyphenolic compounds, especially the monomeric anthocyanidins such as malvidin and delphinidin. The preservation of these molecules by this new carbonic process increases their final levels in wine compared to the traditional maceration of grapes (Pellegrini et al., 2000). Furthermore, the wine ageing could modify polyphenol composition and levels in white and red wines with a time-dependent reduction of catechins and anthocyanidins contents (see Table 2) (Pellegrini et al., 2000; Soleas et al., 1997).

It is interesting to note that, after food or beverage intake, the degradation and absorption of polyphenols within the gastrointestinal tract depend on the nature of the polyphenolic compound but also of the intestinal microflora, with subsequent fermentative effect on other dietary components. Thus, these molecules are modified by intestinal bacteria but they can influence in return microflora and its fermentative capacity (Bravo, 1998). Several recent studies are focused in how processing and beverage composition might influence phenolic profiles and bioavailability of an individual polyphenol. Specifically, they showed the impact of beverage formulations and the influence of digestion on stability, bioavailability, and metabolism of bioactive polyphenolic compounds from food and beverages. For example, the co-formulation with ascorbic acid and other phytochemicals may improve absorption of these health-promoting phytochemicals (Ferruzzi, 2010). Thus, it is critical to develop beverage products designed to deliver specific health benefits.

4. Beneficial effects of RWPC in cardiac and vascular functions

Evidences from different experimental studies has suggested the presence of molecules with anti-oxidant properties in red wine, such as tannins and other flavonoids. These molecules could be key factors in the protective effects observed (Vidavalur et al., 2006). Red wine, might provide, through the polyphenols (non-flavonoids and flavonoids), an anti-oxidant role, leading to additional protection mechanisms in coronary arteries (Liu et al., 2007). Thus, RWPC are able to decrease oxidative stress, enhance cholesterol efflux from the vascular wall, and inhibit lipoprotein oxidation. These components may also increase nitric oxide (NO) bioavailability, thereby antagonizing the development of endothelial dysfunction. Thus, RWPC are able to modify several factors involved in the development of CDV by a direct action on vascular cells and in particular in endothelium, thus playing a preventive role in the development of atherosclerosis, hypertension and myocardial infarction. One of the most studied molecules, the resveratrol, found in grapes and wine in significant amounts, is implicated in this beneficial action because of its ability to act as an anti-oxidant and an inhibitor of platelet aggregation (Kopp, 1998; Providencia, 2006).

On the light of several recent major studies, the consumption of RWPC reduces the incidence of CVD probably by their ability to change many factors and intermediate markers implicated in these diseases. A beneficial association between consumption of food rich in polyphenols, especially flavonoids, and other chronic diseases was also investigated. People with very low consumption of flavonoids showed a higher risk to develop chronic and degenerative diseases including cardiovascular disorders, diabetes, obesity and neurodegenerative disorders compared to people with a diet rich in polyphenols (Mojzisova and Kuchta, 2001). Thus, it is important to better identify factors that may affect the bioavailability of specific phenolic components from food and beverages and to better understand how these molecules are able to act positively on organism.

4.1 Role on nitric oxide production

RWPC are able to improve NO production and vascular endothelium-dependent relaxation. This is possible through their action to increase endothelial nitric oxide synthase (eNOS) expression and activation *in vitro* on endothelial cells and *ex vivo* on rodent vessels.

One of the earliest works on this purpose was conducted in 1993 by Fitzpatrick and coworkers. They found that extracts from grapes and wine containing polyphenols were able to induce an endothelial-dependent vasorelaxation, probably by NO production and elevated accumulation of guanosine 3',5'-cyclic monophosphate (cGMP) (Fitzpatrick et al., 1993). The mechanisms and the identification of the molecules involved in these vascular effects were still unknown. These findings were confirmed later by another study, in which it was evidenced an endothelial and NO-dependent relaxation induced by a non-alcoholic red wine extract, RWPC, and leucocyanidol administrated directly at low concentrations (from 10^{-4} to 10^{-2} g/L) *ex vivo* on noradrenaline pre-contracted rat aortic rings (Andiambeleson et al., 1997). This was associated with an enhanced NO generation and a seven-fold increase in cGMP accumulation. A non-relevant relaxant effect was found using the structurally closely related polyphenol, catechin, at the same concentrations on the same vessels. To better determine which group(s) of polyphenols were able to cause endothelial-dependent vasorelaxation, the same team separated RWPC by chromatography in 10 fractions. These fractions were tested separately for their capacity to induce the vascular relaxation on rat aortic rings with and without endothelium. In this study, it was shown that fractions containing high polymeric condensed tannins produced a moderate vasorelaxation, at relatively high concentrations (10^{-2} to 10^{-1} g/L) and flavan-3-ol, (+)-epicathtechin, also failed to produce endothelium-dependent vasorelaxation. In contrast, oligomeric condensed tannins and fractions containing anthocyanins, and in particular delphinidin, displayed strong vasorelaxant properties (maximal relaxation in the range of 59–77%) comparable to the original RWPC mixture (Andriambeloson et al., 1998).

The same endothelial-dependent relaxation was also found in small mesenteric arteries, but it was due to both NO and endothelium-derived hyperpolarizing factor (EDHF) and it was absent in vessels without endothelium. The NO component of the relaxation was linked to eNOS activity and absent when the NOS inhibitor, the N^G-nitro-L-arginine methyl ester (L-NAME), was used, while the EDHF component was abolished by partial depolarization with KCl. Thus, NO and EDHF are both required to promote endothelium-dependent relaxation produced by RWPC in mesenteric resistance arteries (Duarte et al. 2004).

Several studies conducted *in vitro* confirmed these results. In bovine aortic endothelial cells (BAECs) treated with RWPC (10^{-2} g/L), it was found an increased Ca^{2+}-dependent eNOS activation and a subsequent increased NO production. These required the presence of extracellular Ca^{2+}, although polyphenolic compounds were able to mobilize Ca^{2+} from intracellular stores and were also able to activate phospholipase C (PLC) and tyrosine kinase (TK) pathways. Provinols™, which contain similar types of polyphenols compared to the RWPC used by Andriambeloson and coworkers, and delphinidin displayed differences in the process leading to this increase in endothelial intracellular Ca^{2+}, thus illustrating multiple cellular targets of natural dietary polyphenolic compounds (Martin et al., 2002). This effect of RWPC in this cell model is associated with an increased superoxide ion (O_2^-) production in order to promote Ca^{2+} signaling (Duarte et al., 2004). Most recently, it was found that resveratrol, a stilbenoid contained in wine, used at nanomolar concentrations, rapidly activated extracellular-signal-regulated kinase (ERK)1/2 in BAECs and, in turn, activated eNOS (Klinge et al., 2005). The same effect of resveratrol was confirmed later in another model of endothelial cells, the human umbilical endothelial cells (HUVECs). The implication of ERα in the eNOS-pathway activation by resveratrol was also evoked (Klinge et al., 2008).

Interestingly, beneficial effects on hemodynamic parameters and on endothelial function were confirmed *in vivo* after a short-term oral administration of RWPC in normotensive rats at the dose of 20 mg/kg for 7 days. Indeed, these rats, after only 4 days of treatment, showed a significant decrease in blood pressure (129 ± 4 mmHg versus 141 ± 2 mmHg for control non-treated rats). This effect was associated, *ex vivo,* with an increased endothelium-dependent relaxation to acetylcholine in aortic rings, that was related to the enhanced endothelial NO activity. Nevertheless, RWPC induced at the same time gene expression of inducible NOS (iNOS) and inducible cyclooxigenase (COX-2), with subsequent endothelial thromboxane A_2 release in the arterial wall, maintaining unchanged agonist-induced contractility (Diebolt et al., 2001). The *in vivo* effects of Provinols™ (40 mg/kg per day) on hemodynamic and functional cardiovascular changes were also investigated during the inhibition of NO synthesis by L-NAME (40 mg/kg per day for 4 weeks) in rats. This model of hypertension evidenced that RWPC partially prevent L-NAME-induced hypertension, cardiovascular remodeling, and vascular dysfunction or accelerate the decrease of systolic blood pressure after L-NAME administration. These beneficial effects were mediated by the increased NO-synthase activity and the oxidative stress prevention (Bernatova et al., 2002; Pechanova et al., 2004). Nevertheless, most recently, the anti-hypertensive effects of RWPC, orally administered for 5 weeks at the dose of 40 mg/kg by gavage, was confirmed in female spontaneously hypertensive rats (SHR). The authors suggested that a chronic treatment with RWPC reduced hypertension and vascular dysfunction in this model of hypertension, rather through reduction in vascular oxidative stress (Lopez-Sepulveda et al., 2008). This findings revealed a major preventive role of these substances in cardiovascular complications linked to hypertension.

Polyphenol vascular activity in human vessels after food or beverage intake was confirmed by several studies that detected these molecules in human plasma at individual levels in the range of 0.5 to 1.6 μmol/L, comparable to the concentration required to induce 50% of the maximal relaxation, comprised between 1 and 10 μmol/L of active fractions (Paganga and Rice-Evans, 1997). Polyphenols detected in human plasma are in the range of 2.5 μg/ml after a 100 ml red wine intake (Duthie et al., 1998). Most interestingly, the vasorelaxant effect of polyphenols from red wine was confirmed also in men in which NO and normalized flow-mediated dilation were measured before and 30, 60, and 120 minutes after red wine consumption (Boban et al., 2006; Papamichael et al., 2004). Moreover, RWPC are not only able to improve NO production, for their anti-oxidant and anti-inflammatory properties but also increase the NO bioavailability in the vascular wall, by decreasing its transformation in peroxynitrite induced by O_2^- during oxidative stress.

Altogether, these findings suggest a possible beneficial effect of a diet rich in these vasoactive polyphenolic compounds to prevent hypertension as the effective concentrations of these molecules can be reached in human plasma and they might act on the endothelium *in vivo*. The RWPC responsible of this effect (resveratrol, delphinidin and tannins) could be used for hypertension treatment.

4.2 Protective role in cardiac function and ischemic diseases

RWPC, administrated in a preventive purpose way, are able to reduce cardiac or cerebral ischemic injuries in rat models of myocardial infarct and stroke, respectively. Left ventricular hypertrophy, myocardial fibrosis and vascular remodeling were investigated in rats during chronic inhibition of NOS activity by L-NAME. The *in vivo* treatment of rats with Provinols™ (40 mg/kg per day) reduced not only the increase in blood pressure caused by L-NAME treatment, but also protein synthesis in the heart and aorta caused by the chronic inhibition of NO synthesis, finally reducing myocardial fibrosis. These effects were associated with an increase of NOS activity, a moderate enhancement of eNOS expression and a reduction of oxidative stress in the left ventricule and aorta (Pechanova et al. 2004).

The protective cardiac effect of polyphenols was confirmed by another study, conducted in rats and observing, *ex vivo*, the effects of short-term oral administration of RWPC (20 mg/kg per day for one week) on cardiac responsiveness and ischaemia-reperfusion injury. The involvement of NO in the cardiac effects of RWPC was evaluated using L-NAME (2 mg/kg per day for one week), a dose which did not affect blood pressure, in a group of rats previously treated with polyphenols. Heart reactivity was studied in perfused isolated hearts by the Langendorff method. The hearts harvested from RWPC-treated rats showed a lower basal pressure, a greater heart rate and decreased inotropic responses to either isoprenaline or carbachol, the agonists of beta-adrenoceptors or muscarinic receptors, respectively. RWPC treatment did not modify cardiac expression of eNOS or Cu/Zn superoxide dismutase, a protein involved in oxidative stress protection. However, it was found increased nitrite levels in the coronary effluent from hearts harvested from RWPC-treated rats, suggesting an increased NO production. Most interestingly, in ischaemia-reperfusion protocols, RWPC treatment reduced infarct size, oxidative stress, and the myocardial content of end products resulting from lipid peroxidation, malondialdehyde and 4-hydroxynonenal, without affecting post-ischaemic contractile dysfunction. All these observed effects were prevented by L-NAME treatment, suggesting the involvement of NO in this protective role of RWPC on heart. In conclusion, these data showed that short-term treatment with RWPC could prevent the heart injury caused by cardiac ischemia through oxidative stress decrease and NO pathway improvement (Ralay-Ranaivo et al., 2004).

The presence of melatonin in red wine was demonstrated in most recent studies. Lamont and co-workers investigated the cardio-protective role of both melatonin and resveratrol. These molecules improve heart protection via the activation of the newly discovered survivor activating factor enhancement (SAFE) pathway. This pro-survival signaling pathway involves the activation of pro-inflammatory molecules such as tumor necrosis factor alpha (TNFα) and interleukin 6 (IL6) and the signal transducer and activator of transcription 3 (STAT3). They realized *ex vivo* studies in isolated perfused hearts from either wild type or total TNFα receptor 2-knockout or cardiomyocyte-specific STAT3-deficient mice. The protocols of heart injury by ischemia-reperfusion showed that both resveratrol and melatonin, at concentrations found in red wine, significantly reduced infarct size in wild-type mice (25% ± 3% versus 69 ± 3% in the control non treated mice) but failed to protect hearts in both knockout mice. Perfusion with either melatonin or resveratrol increased STAT3 phosphorylation prior to ischemia by 79% and 50% versus the control, respectively. These findings suggest that both melatonin and resveratrol contained in red wine, protect heart via the SAFE pathway, in an experimental model of myocardial infarction (Lamont et al., 2011).

Concerning cerebral ischemia, Ritz and co-workers investigated the beneficial effects of chronic or acute treatment of RWPC in rats submitted to an experimental model of stroke. Rats were treated for the chronic treatment with RWPC (30 mg/kg per day) dissolved in drinking water for one week, before being subjected surgically to a transient middle cerebral artery occlusion followed by reperfusion. The volume of the ischemic lesions was assessed 24 h after reperfusion and a proteomic analysis of brain tissues was performed, to study the effects of RWPC on expression of proteins involved in cerebral stroke injury. Treatment with RWPC partially or completely prevented the increased levels of excitatory amino acids (aspartate, glutamate and taurine) that characterized the response to ischemia in control rats, significantly reduced brain infarct volumes, and enhanced residual cerebral blood flow after brain ischemia. This was associated to lower basal concentrations of energy metabolites including glucose, lactate, and free radical scavengers such as ascorbate, in the brain parenchyma, compared with untreated rats. No difference in uric acid levels was found. These effects resulted in arterial vasodilatation, as the internal diameters of several arteries were significantly enlarged after RWPC treatment. Proteomic analysis revealed that RWPC could be able to modulate *in vivo* the expression of proteins involved in maintenance of neuronal caliber and axon formation, in protection against oxidative stress, and in energy metabolism (Ritz et al., 2008a). These data were confirmed in the second work of the same team, about the protective effects of an acute treatment with RWPC (a bolus of 0.1 mg/kg), realized by an intracerebral microdialysis started at the beginning of the stroke. In this study, RWPC induced increased residual blood flow after 10 minutes of the reperfusion following ischemia and reduced size of the cerebral ischemic infarct in both cortex and striatum. The acute treatment of rats with RWPC dramatically decreased the extracellular concentrations of excitatory amino acids and, concomitantly, increased the levels of free radical scavengers such as uric and ascorbic acids (Ritz et al., 2008b). Altogether these findings provide an experimental evidence of the advantage to use RWPC for the prevention, in patients with high risk to developing ischemic events, or in the acute treatment of patients during stroke.

Angiogenesis is a main process involved in the repair of ischemic injury. The role of RWPC in angiogenesis was also investigated and several studies evidenced that these molecules are able to modulate, at the molecular and cellular levels, several actors of the pivotal pathways involved in vascular cell proliferation and migration. Previous studies had demonstrated an anti-angiogenic role of polyphenols both *in vitro* and *in vivo* (Fotsis et al., 1998; Igura et al., 2001). In contrast, most recently, Baron-Menguy and co-workers evidenced a dose-dependent effect on angiogenesis of RWPC, and in particular of delphinidin, in a model of post-ischaemic neovascularization in rats submitted to femoral artery ligature. Indeed, high doses of RWPC (i.e. 7 glasses of red wine) reduced arterial, arteriolar, and capillary densities and blood flow, inhibited the phosphoinositol 3-kinase (PI3-K)/Akt/eNOS pathway, decreased vascular endothelial growth factor (VEGF) expression, and reduced metalloproteinase-2 (MMP-2) activation. In contrast, low doses of RWPC (i.e. 1/10th glass of red wine) increased neovascularisation in ischemic legs compared to control level in association with an increased blood flow. The angiogenic effect was linked to the overexpression of PI3-K/Akt/eNOS pathway and to increased VEGF production, without effect on MMP-2 activation. These anti- or pro-angiogenic effects of RWPC were reproduced when they used delphinidin, administrated alone at low or high doses. This dual dose-dependent effect of polyphenols in angiogenesis is particular interesting because of its potential applications both in the therapy of diseases requiring the block of angiogenesis such as in some cancers, and in the treatment of post-ischemic injuries to improve angiogenesis and ameliorate reperfusion of tissues, at high and low doses, respectively.

4.3 Role in metabolic diseases

It has been extensively evidenced the strict correlation between metabolic dysfunctions and the development of cardiovascular diseases. Endothelial dysfunction, an independent predictor of cardiovascular events, has been consistently associated with obesity and the metabolic syndrome in a complex interplay with insulin resistance. Deficiency of eNOS is considered as the primary defect that links insulin resistance and endothelial dysfunction (Cersosimo and Defronzo, 2006; Defronzo, 2006; Fornoni and Raij, 2005). Furthermore, several epidemiological studies have shown that patients affected by metabolic diseases are often also affected by hypertension and other cardio-vascular complications such as atherosclerotic plaque formation and increased levels of pro-thrombotic factors, associated to an elevated risk of mortality by vascular thrombotic events (Kopelman, 2000).

More recently, we have suggested a protective role of RWPC in metabolic syndrome (Agouni et al., 2009). In our study, Zuker fatty (ZF) rats (Fa/Fa), an experimental model of metabolic syndrome, or their "lean" littermates, received normal diet or a diet supplemented with Provinols™ for 8 weeks in food. This treatment significantly reduced the plasmatic levels of metabolic products such as glucose, fructosamine, total and LDL-cholesterol, and triglycerides, and finally improved cardiac and endothelial vascular functions. Regarding vascular function, Provinols™ corrected endothelial dysfunction in aortas and mesenteric arteries from ZF rats by improving endothelium-dependent relaxation in response to acetylcholine. This beneficial effect in endothelium was associated to an enhanced NO bioavailability due to increased NO production and eNOS activity, and reduced oxidative stress and O_2^- release. The effect on eNOS activity was associated to a decreased expression of caveolin-1, a protein known to inactivate eNOS by cell membrane sequestration, while the reduction of free radical production was linked to a decrease of Nox-1 (NADPH oxidase membrane sub-unit) expression (Agouni et al., 2009). In agreement with our work, this protective effect of RWPC in plasmatic metabolic parameters and oxidative stress linked to metabolic disorders was confirmed recently in hamsters submitted to high-fat diet (Suh et al., 2011)

Because of these interesting results, polyphenols might be good candidates for prevention and treatment of metabolic syndrome and cardiovascular risk reduction. This was previously suggested by another study of Napoli and coworkers who have shown that red wine consumption improved insulin resistance in type 2 diabetic patients (Napoli et al., 2005). Thus, RWPC could represent a new class of medicinal products against obesity-associated diseases.

5. The oestrogenic receptors in cardiovascular protection

Several epidemiological studies suggested a protective effect of oestrogens in premenopausal women in vascular and metabolic diseases development. These numerous studies showed that the incidence of hypertension and other cardiovascular diseases is significantly lower in premenopausal females compared to males and that, after the onset of menopause, the incidence increases dramatically, eventually approaching the level observed in age-matched males (Mendelsohn and Karas, 1999). This effect has been attributed to the fall in circulating oestrogen levels, contributing to a menopause-related increase in blood pressure, and thus to a greater predisposition to cardiovascular disease. Consistent with this, oestrogen replacement therapy has been reported to reduce the risk of cardiovascular disease, and in particular of hypertension and atherosclerosis, in postmenopausal women to that observed in premenopausal women (Barton et al., 2007; Mendelsohn and Karas, 1999). Oestrogens have been shown to have direct vasodilatory and anti-atherosclerotic effects via the oestrogen receptors expressed on human and rat arteries (Haas et al., 2007; Shaw et al., 2001). The mechanisms involved in the protective role played by these hormones is associated to vascular inflammation reduction (Nilsson, 2007), increased endothelial NO production (Chen et al., 1999) and the prevention of smooth muscle vascular cell proliferation (Pareet al., 2002). But the ability of oestrogens to elicit effects on autonomic functions involved in cardiac control appears also to constitute a major part of its beneficial effects (Spary et al., 2009). Despite wealth of evidences for its central autonomic role, the sites and mechanisms of oestrogenic action on the neural pathways of cardiovascular regulation are still poorly understood.

Oestrogens act on specific receptors which are transcription factors, the nuclear oestrogenic receptors (ERs). Two ERs have been described, ERα and ERβ, with several structurally and functionally conserved domains, and involved in genomic signaling mechanism or associated to plasma membrane, influencing cytosolic non-genomic signaling. ERα was first characterized in mid-1980 and the cloning of ERβ following in late 1995 (Kuiper et al., 1996). In addition, as a result of alternative splicing of the eight exons encoding rat ERβ, five different isoforms of this ER exist (β1, β2, β1δ3, β2δ3 and β1δ4) with a not yet completely determined role (Maruyama et al., 1998; Petersen et al., 1998; Price et al., 2000). It has been suggested that ERβ may modulate ERα gene transcription, acting in some conditions by opposite actions to ERα (Lindberg et al., 2003; Maruyama et al., 1998; Zhao et al., 2008).

In the absence of oestrogens, the receptors are conserved in an inactive state in a complex with one of the several chaperone molecules, such as heat shock protein 90 (Beato and Klug, 2000). Following binding to oestrogens, the receptor undergoes a conformational change, activating an intracellular cascade leading to the ER release from the chaperone. ER can forms homo- or hetero-dimers that interact with target gene promoters, inducing the up- or the down-regulation of several genes (Figure 1) (Hall et al, 2001). The ER subtypes have also been shown to interact differently with a range of other transcription factors, including activating protein-1 (Paech et al., 1997; Webb et al., 1999; Zhao et al., 2008). This genomic response usually occurs within hours after oestrogen exposure and is believed to be the result of a direct action, not involving the second messenger signaling pathways. In contrast, the non-genomic oestrogenic signaling is also possible but less well understood. It is associated to the cytosolic pathways with classical second messengers and occurs considerably faster than the genomic signaling (Kang et al., 2010). It is possible that these rapid non-genomic events are mediated by cytoplasmic, rather than nuclear ERα and ERβ, suggesting the involvement of another plasma membrane receptor, a particular G protein-coupled receptor (GPCR) which is not related to ERα or ERβ. To confirm this hypothesis more recently, another membrane-bound ER was emerged. This GPCR, the G protein coupled oestrogen receptor 1 (GPER1), also called GPR30, is able to bind with a high affinity to 17β-estradiol (E2), mediating oestrogenic signals in cardiovascular and metabolic regulations (Nilsson et al., 2011). GPER1 is expressed in different vascular segments and in the heart of several species. In rats, the mRNA of this receptor was found both in endothelial and in smooth muscle cells; but in mice and humans, it seems to be expressed primarily in endothelial cells of small systemic arteries, suggesting a direct role of GPER1 in endothelial function regulation, while the effects of its activation in vascular smooth muscle cells and vascular tone are indirect, via the endothelium (Nilsson et al., 2011). GPER1 is located to the endoplasmic reticulum of vascular cells mediating the rapid oestrogen signaling (Revankar et al., 2005).

The role of GPER1 activation by its specific agonist, G-1, on vascular tone was investigated in rat vessels. Several studies showed the involvement of this receptor in vascular relaxation by reducing angiotensin II (AngII) and/or endothelin-1 (ET-1)-induced vascular contractions. This was not influenced by the endogenous oestrogenic levels and it was gender independent (Haas et al, 2009, Lindsey et al., 2009; Meyer et al., 2010). This effect was not found in serotonin-dependent vascular contraction, suggesting a direct effect of GPER1 activation on the renin-angiotensin system, probably independent of NO production (Nillson et al, 2011). In contrast, another study suggests that GPER1 causes arterial relaxation via an endothelial and a NO-dependent mechanism (Broughton et al., 2010). Thus, the involvement of endothelial NO in this vascular relaxation cannot be excluded. Moreover, an hypotensive effect of GPER1 activation was observed in ovariectomized animals, in agreement with the hypertensive phenotype of GPER1 knock-out mice (Martensson et al., 2009). Furthermore, GPER1 activation could play a protective role in atherosclerosis and/or excessive angiogenesis during cancer, reducing vascular smooth muscle or endothelial cell proliferation, respectively (Haas et al., 2009; Holm et al., 2011).

If the non-genomic effects of E2 are realized through GPER1, ERα is the receptor implicated in the anti-atherogenic effects of oestrogens. Indeed, the ERα, when stimulated by E2, induces endothelial cell proliferation, vascular re-endothelialization, endothelial NO production, vascular inflammation attenuation, and reduction of smooth muscle cell proliferation (Brouchet et al., 2001; Pare et al., 2002; Vegeto et al., 2003). Nevertheless, studies conducted on vessels harvested from ERα or ERβ knockout mice showed that both these ERs are responsible for E2-dependent vascular relaxation (Guo et al., 2005). It was previously evidenced the association of a subpopulation of ERα with the endothelial membrane and the complex structure of caveolae (Chambliss and Shaul, 2002). The binding of E2 with ERα in caveolae leads to the MAPK/Akt pathway activation, resulting in eNOS phosphorylation and activation, and subsequent increased NO production (Figure 1) (Chambliss and Shaul, 2002). This beneficial effect on vascular function played by oestrogens was confirmed by epidemiological studies, in which the presence of endogenous oestrogens and their effect on cardiovascular homeostasis appear to be closely related to the degree of atherosclerosis progression throughout a woman's life (Clarkson 2007). Experimental studies suggest that in the mouse, ERα appears to be largely responsible for the protective effects of oestrogens against atherosclerotic vascular disease (Hodgin et al., 2001). In turn, according to some studies, the abundance of both ER subtypes, ERα and ERβ, in human aorta, decreases with the progression of atherosclerosis, aggravating the endothelial dysfunction of atherosclerotic vessels by the reduction of oestrogenic-dependent eNOS activation and NO release (Losordo et al., 1994; Nakamura et al., 2004).

On the light of the effect of E2 via ERα in eNOS pathway activation and NO production, a vascular role of oestrogens, similar to that evidenced for RWPC on endothelium, was evoked. Some researchers and our studies started to investigate if RWPC or one of the polyphenolic compounds contained in red wine, resveratrol or delphinidin, could play a role of phytoestrogens, interacting at high affinity with ERs and inducing their beneficial vascular effects via these endothelial receptors.

6. Oestrogenic receptor alpha and polyphenols

After the description of these encouraging findings, nobody exactly identified the pivotal compound responsible of RWPC vascular effects and, most important, how this molecule was able to interact with the vascular endothelium, thus improving endothelial function. It was previously described that resveratrol is able to enhance eNOS expression and activity, but the mechanisms by which this polyphenol induced these effects were still not well known (Wallerath et al., 2002). In a study conducted *in vitro* in BAECs, nanomolar concentrations of resveratrol induced ERK1/2 signaling activation, similar to that of E2, since this was dependent of ER activity triggering eNOS activation and NO release (Klinge et al., 2005). The same team, in another study *in vitro* (in HUVECs), better determined the mechanisms by which resveratrol was able to improve eNOS activation pathway. The authors of this work demonstrated for the first time that resveratrol increased interaction between ERα, Caveoline-1 (Cav-1) and proteins involved in eNOS activation such as Src, by a Gα-protein-coupled mechanism. A main role for ERα in the NO production induced by resveratrol in endothelial cells was suggested because they observed attenuated effects of resveratrol in cells in which ERα was depleted using a siRNA. Resveratrol and E2 did not stimulate ERβ/Cav-1 interaction (Klinge et al., 2008). Moreover ERα is 4.5 times more expressed then ERβ in HUVECs and no effect of a siRNA directed versus ERβ was found on resveratrol action in endothelium. This study implies that dietary intake of resveratrol might offer possible vascular protective effects via the activation of ERα *in vivo*.

In contrast, experiments conducted in rats did not evidence a role of oestrogen receptors in aorta endothelium-dependent relaxation to RWPC (Kane et al., 2009). The authors of this work showed that RWPC caused redox-sensitive PI3-K/Akt-dependent eNOS activation and NO-mediated relaxation in rat aortas *ex vivo*. This vascular effect was more pronounced in the aorta of female than male rats, but it was due most likely to increased expression levels of eNOS rather than activation of oestrogen receptors, because the inhibition of ER by the oestrogen antagonist, ICI 182780, did not modify the ability of RWPC to induce their vascular effects (Kane et al., 2009). Interestingly, another study conducted in female SHR rats evidenced that the chronic treatment with RWPC of ovariectomized rats induced reduction of arterial pressure and vascular dysfunction characterizing this hypertensive model in a manner independent of the ovarian function (Lopez-Sepulveda et al., 2008).

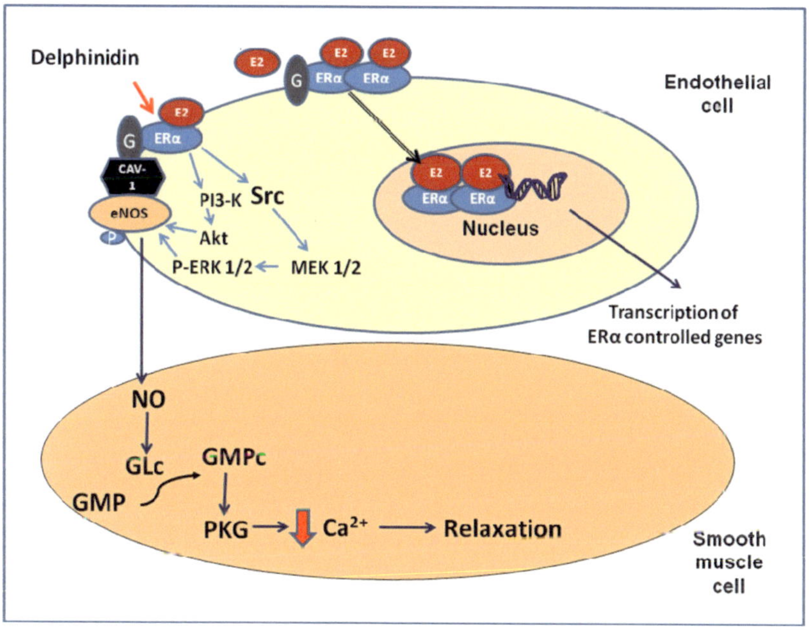

Fig. 1. ERα activation by polyphenols or oestrogens induces eNOS increased activity and NO production. Signaling pathway by which delphinidin or E2 interacting with ERα, activates rapidly eNOS and increases NO production in endothelial cells by PI3-K/Akt or via Src/ERK1/2 pathways. ERα is associated in endothelial cells caveolae with Cav-1 which links to the membrane the inactive form of eNOS. When ERα binds E2 or polyphenols, eNOS is phosphorylated in its active site, thus improving NO release. The same pathways implicated in delphinidin-ERα activation were proposed by Klinge and coworkers for endothelial cell stimulation by resveratrol at nanomolar concentrations (Klinge et al., 2008). NO is able to activate guanilyl-cyclase (GLc) in smooth muscle cells inducing increased levels of cyclic-GMP (GMPc) with subsequent protein-kinase G activation (PKG), reducing intracellular calcium and inducing vascular relaxation. On the right of the figure, is represented the homo-dimer formation and nuclear translocation of E2-activated ERα, inducing the genomic response.

Conversely, we investigated the hypothesis that ERα is one of the key targets involved *in vivo* in the vasculoprotective effects of RWPC (and in particular of delphinidin) interacting with the endothelium. Thus, the ERα implication in the French Paradox was first tested using ERα-deficient mice (Chalopin et al., 2010). We have shown the necessity of this oestrogenic receptor in the Provinols™- or delphinidin-induced endothelial-dependent relaxation, eNOS activation, and NO release. Indeed, no effect of these products on endothelium were observed in vessels harvested from ERα-deficient mice or in wild-type vessels without endothelium. The activation of ERα by RWPC or delphinidin alone induced the activation of the same pathway, evidenced by the previously described *in vitro* work of Klinge and colleagues with resveratrol. Indeed, E2 and the selective agonist of ERα, 1,3,5-tris(4-hydroxyphenyl)-4-propyl-1H-pyrazole (PPT), as well as Provinols™ and delphinidin, are able to activate molecular pathways involving Src, ERK1/2, eNOS and caveolin-1 phosphorylations (see Figure 1). The mechanism involved required ERα activation because of the absence of effect in vessels or cells from ERα-deficient mice, and after silencing, in wild-type endothelial cells, ERα activity or expression either with a pharmacological inhibitor (fulvestran) or with a siRNA, respectively. Moreover, using a binding assay and a docking study, we have shown that delphinidin fits on ERα's activation site, exerting 73% of specific inhibition against E2 on ERα, in the binding assay. Most importantly, ERα is also implicated in the *in vivo* effects observed in mice treated with Provinols™ administrated in the food, with respect to the improvement in endothelial function given by the concomitant increase in NO and decrease in O_2^- release in vessels. Indeed, these vascular and anti-oxidant effects of the *in vivo* treatment with Provinols™ were not found in ERα-deficient mice (Chalopin et al., 2010). Then, we have demonstrated for the first time the physiological relevance of ERα in the *in vivo* vascular effects of RWPC.

It is important to note that ERα, ERβ, and GPER-1 are all expressed in the arterial wall of both women and men (Meyer et al., 2006; Haas et al., 2007), and that E2 has potent dilator effects on vascular tone of human coronary and internal mammary arteries harvested from patients without gender differences (Haas et al., 2007; Mugge et al., 1993). These findings suggest a potential function for oestrogen receptor also in male cardiovascular system. Thus, RWPC could have the same protective vascular properties in both women and men through ERα. In line with the fact that ERα mediates atheroprotective effects, in a man with a disruptive mutation in the ERα gene, it was noted an impaired vascular function and a premature coronary artery disease (Sudhir et al., 1997). Thus, not only the female but also the male cardiovascular system appears to be an important target for oestrogens affecting vascular disease development (Haas et al., 2007; Meyer et al., 2008). Nevertheless, studies in humans comparing oestrogen plasma concentrations and the progression of cardiovascular diseases have revealed conflicting results (Meyer et al., 2008). Actually, there is doubt about the interest to treat male patients with oestrogen receptor agonists to interfere with atherosclerosis progression.

Finally, further works are needed to confirm if ERs are implicated in all the vascular and metabolic effects of RWPC or if ERα activation by RWPC induces only the eNOS pathway improvement. For instance, the role of ERs activation by RWPC in inhibition of endothelial cell proliferation and cell cycle progression or in angiogenesis has not been investigated yet.

7. Conclusion

The first epidemiological studies played a main role in the demonstration of a French Paradox existence, leading to the start of about forty years of scientific findings concerning the protective properties of polyphenols and, more particularly, those contained in red wine. Currently, the numerous data obtained *in vitro, ex vivo,* and *in vivo,* on their beneficial effects in heart and vessels, validly suggest a therapeutic potential for RWPC.

The last findings have identified in delphinidin and resveratrol some of the key molecules involved in the vascular effects of RWPC via ERα activation, adding a new piece to the puzzle explaining the French Paradox (Chalopin et al., 2010; Klinge et al., 2008). Indeed, despite a previous study (Kane et al., 2008), which evidenced no implication of ERs in RWPC-dependent vascular relaxation in rats, the last studies clearly showed that the beneficial endothelial effects of RWPC require ERα activation. This is followed by a rapid response to the polyphenolic stimuli in endothelial cells, involving the pathways associated to eNOS activation and subsequent NO release. Furthermore, the phytoestrogenic role of RWPC, and especially of delphinidin, was confirmed by binding experiences which found high affinity of delphinidin against ERα compared to its natural agonist E2 (Chalopin et al., 2010). Similar mechanisms and a phytoestrogenic role on ERα activation were suggested also for resveratrol on endothelial cells by Klinge and coworkers (Klinge et al., 2005, 2008).

In this chapter, we have focalized our attention on the red wine because it contains both, delphinidin and resveratrol, the main vasoactive compounds contained in non-alcoholic red wine extract. In particular, we wanted to explain the main mechanisms by which these compounds are able to induce cardiovascular protection against hypertension, cardiac ischemia, stroke and atherosclerotic plaque formation as one of the complications linked to metabolic syndrome. It is important to note that the effects of these substances could be different according to the concentrations employed as evidenced in experimental models of angiogenesis (Baron-Menguy et al., 2007). It is also relevant to remember of other beneficial properties of RWPC, as anti-oxidant, anti-inflammatory, anti-tumor or antithrombotic agents, that we have not extensively described here. Indeed, RWPC are also able to modulate the apoptotic, proliferative or migration processes in cells (Martin et al., 2003) by acting directly on vascular remodeling and angiogenesis (Brownson et al., 2002; Favot et al., 2003). Here, we have chosen to stress on strong properties of RWPC as vasodilators inducing endothelial NO production, because this effect implicates ERα activation as demonstrated in the last studies.

Furthermore, despite the favorable effect of some molecules contained in red wine in the prevention of several cardiovascular pathologies, alcohol is a serious problem of public health and, actually, it is important to remenber that these beneficial effects are due to the non-alcoholic fractions of red wine. Interestingly, in multinational studies it was shown an increased risk of mortality by myocardial infarction, especially in women who take no alcohol, but compared to moderate drinkers (Yusuf et al., 2004). Moreover, on the light of other epidemiological data, it seems to be developed the view that modest alcohol but neither zero nor more than modest intake reduces total mortality and cardiovascular risk by cardio and neuroprotection (Collins et al., 2009; Opie and Lecour, 2007).

According with the French Paradox, the moderate intake of wine (1 or 2 glasses per day) could be beneficial for health by reducing the risk of CVD mortality. As evidenced in Table 1, the content of these vasoactive substances is more relevant in red wine compared to other food and beverages. Finally on the light of all the epidemiological and fundamental studies analyzed in this chapter, and our works, we can suggest that RWPC, and in particular delphinidin and resveratrol, could be used for their therapeutic potential in the prevention and treatment of cardiovascular pathologies. We think that ERα activation might be the main molecular target triggering the beneficial effects of dietary supplementation of RWPC. Nevertheless, further studies are needed to verify the implication of ERα in other physiological effects of polyphenols and not only in NO release and vascular relaxation.

8. References

Agouni A., Lagrue-Lak-Hal A.H., Mostefai H.A., Tesse, A., Mulder P., Rouet, P., Desmoulin, F., H;eymes, C., Martinez, M.C., & Andriantsitohaina, R. (2009). Red wine polyphenols prevent metabolic and cardiovascular alterations associated with obesity in Zucker fatty rats (Fa/Fa). *PloS one,* Vol.4, No.5, (May 2009), pp. e5557.

Andriambeloson, E., Kleschyov, A.L., Muller, B., Beretz, A., Stoclet, J.C., & Andriantsitohaina, R. (1997). Nitric oxide production and endothelium-dependent vasorelaxation induced by wine polyphenols in rat aorta. *British J. Pharmacol.*, Vol.120, No. 6, (Mars 1997), pp. 1053-1058.

Andriambeloson, E., Magnier, C., Haan-Archipoff, G., Lobstein, A., Anton, R., Beretz, A., Stoclet, J.C., & Andriantsitohaina, R. (1998). Natural dietary polyphenolic compounds cause endothelium-dependent vasorelaxation in rat thoracic aorta. *J. Nutr.*, Vol.128, No.12, (December 1998), pp. 2324–2333.

Bahorun, T. (1997). Substances naturelles actives : La Flore Mauricienne, Une source d'aprovisionnement potentielle. In : *Proceedings of the Second Annual Meeting of Agricultural Scientists (AMAS)*, pp. 83-94, Food and Agricultural Research Council, Réduit, Mauritius, August 1997.

Baron-Menguy, C., Bocquet, A., Guihot, A.L., Chappard, D., Amiot, M.J., Andriantsitohaina, R., Loufrani, L., & Henrion, D. (2007). Effects of red wine polyphenols on postischemic neovascularization model in rats: low doses are proangiogenic, high doses anti-angiogenic. *FASEB J.*, Vol.2, No.13, (November 2007), pp. 3511-3521.

Barton, M., Meyer, M.R., & Haas, E. (2007). Hormone replacement therapy and atherosclerosis in postmenopausal women: does aging limit therapeutic benefits? *Arterioscler. Thromb. Vasc. Biol.*, Vol.27, No.8, (August 2007), pp. 1669-1672.

Beato, M., & Klug, J. (2000). Steroid hormone receptors: an update. *Hum. Reprod. Update*, Vol.6, No.3, (May-June 2000), pp. 225-236.

Bernatova, I., Penchanova, O., Babal, P., Kysela, S., Stvrtina, S., & Andriantstohaina, R. (2002). Wine polyphenols improve cardiovascular remodeling and vascular function in NO-deficient hypertension. *Am. J. Physiol. Heart Circ. Physiol.*, Vol. 282, No.3, (March 2002), pp. 942–948.

Boban, M., Modun, D., Music, I., Vukovic, J., Brizic, I., Salamunic, I., Obad, A., Palada, I., & Dujic, Z. (2006). Red wine induced modulation of vascular function: separating the role of polyphenols, ethanol, and urates. *J. Cardiovasc. Pharmacol.*, Vol.47, No.5, (May 2006), pp. 695-701.

Bravo, L. (1998). Polyphenols: chemistry, dietary sources, metabolism, and nutritional significance. *Nutr. Rev.*, Vol.56, No.11, (November 1998), pp. 317-33.

Brouchet, L., Krust, A., Dupont, S., Chambon, P., Bayard, F., & Arnal, J.F. (2001). Estradiol accelerates reendothelialization in mouse carotid artery through estrogen receptor-alpha but not estrogen receptor-beta. *Circulation*, Vol. 103, No.3, (January 2001), pp. 423-428.

Broughton, B.R., Miller, A.A., & Sobey, C.G. (2010). Endothelium-dependent relaxation by G protein-coupled receptor 30 agonists in rat carotid arteries. *Am. J. Physiol. Heart Circ. Physiol.*, Vol.298, No.3, (March 2010), pp. H1055-H1061.

Brownson, D.M., Azios, N.G., Fuqua, B.K., Dharmawardhane, S.F., & Mabry, TJ. (2002). Flavonoid effects relevant to cancer. *J. Nutr.*, Vol.132, No.11, (November 2002), pp. 3482S-3489S.

Cersosimo, E., & Defronzo, R.A. (2006). Insulin resistance and endothelial dysfunction: the road map to cardiovascular diseases. *Diabetes Metab. Res. Rev.*, Vol.22, No.6, (November-December 2006), pp. 423–436.

Chalopin, M., Tesse, A., Martínez, M.C., Rognan, D., Arnal, J.F., & Andriantsitohaina, R. (2010) Estrogen receptor alpha as a key target of red wine polyphenols action on the endothelium. *PLoS One,* Vol.5, No.1, (January 2010), pp. e8554.

Chambliss, K.L., & Shaul, P.W. (2002). Rapid activation of endothelial NO synthase by estrogen: evidence for a steroid receptor fast-action complex (SRFC) in caveolae. *Steroids,* Vol.67, No.6, (May 2002), pp. 413-419.

Chandrasekara, A., & Shahidi, F. (2010). Content of insoluble bound phenolics in millets and their contribution to antioxidant capacity. *J. Agric. Food Chem.,* Vol.58, No.11, (June 2010), pp. 6706-6714.

Chen, Z., Yuhanna, I.S., Galcheva-Gargova, Z., Karas, R.H., Mendelsohn, M.E., & Shaul, P.W. (1999). Estrogen receptor alpha mediates the nongenomic activation of endothelial nitric oxide synthase by estrogen. *J. Clin. Invest.,* Vol.103, No.3, (May 1999), pp. 401-406.

Cheynier, V. (2005). Polyphenols in foods are more complex than often thought. *Am. J. Clin. Nutr.,* Vol.81, No.1, (January 2005), pp. 223S-229S.

Clarkson, T.B. (2007). Estrogen effects on arteries vary with stage of reproductive life and extent of subclinical atherosclerosis progression. *Menopause,* Vol.14, No.3, (May-June 2007), pp. 373-384.

Collins, M.A., Neafsey, E.J., Mukamal, K.J., Gray, M.O., Parks, D.A., Das, D.K., & Korthuis, R.J. (2009). Alcohol in moderation, cardioprotection, and neuroprotection: epidemiological considerations and mechanistic studies. *Alcohol Clin. Exp. Res.,* Vol.33, No.2, (February 2009), pp. 206-219.

Criqui, M.H., & Ringel, B.L. (1994). Does diet or alcohol explain the French paradox? *Lancet,* Vol.344, No.8939-8940, (December 1994), pp. 1719-1723.

Defronzo, R.A. (2006). Is insulin resistance atherogenic? Possible mechanisms. *Atheroscler. Suppl.,* Vol.7, No.4, (August 2006), pp. 11–15.

Duarte, J., Andriambeloson, E., Diebolt, M., & Andriantsitohaina, R. (2004). Wine polyphenols stimulate superoxide anion production to promote calcium signaling and endothelial-dependent vasodilatation. *Physiol. Res.,* Vol.53, No.6, (2004), pp. 595-602.

Diebolt, M., Bucher, B., & Andriantsitohaina, R. (2001). Wine polyphenols decrease blood pressure, improve NO vasodilatation, and induce gene expression. *Hypertension,* Vol.38, No.2, (August 2001), pp. 159-165.

Doll, R., Peto, R., Hall, E., Wheatley, K., & Gray, R. (1994). Mortality in relation to consumption of alcohol: 13 years' observations on male British doctors. *B.M.J.,* Vol.309, No.6959, (October 1994), pp. 911-918.

Duthie, G.G., Pedersen, M.W., Gardner, P.T., Morrice, P.C., Jenkinson, A.M., McPhail, D.B., & Steele, G.M. (1998). The effect of whisky and wine consumption on total phenol content and antioxidant capacity of plasma from healthy volunteers. *Eur J. Clin. Nutr.,* Vol.52, No.10, (October 1998), pp. 733-736.

Emberson, J.R., Shaper, A.G., Wannamethee, S.G., Morris, R.W., & Whincup, P.H. (2005). Alcohol intake in middle age and risk of cardiovascular disease and mortality: accounting for intake variation over time. *Am. J. Epidemiol.,* Vol.161, No.9, (May 2005), pp. 856-863.

Favot, L., Martin, S., Keravis, T., Andriantsitohaina, R., & Lugnier, C. (2003). Involvement of cyclin-dependent pathway in the inhibitory effect of delphinidin on angiogenesis. *Cardiovasc. Res.,* Vol.59, No.2, (August 2003), pp. 479-487.

Ferrières, J. (2004). The French paradox: lessons for other countries. *Coronary disease,* Vol.90, No.1, (January 2004), pp. 107–111.

Ferruzzi, M.G. (2010). The influence of beverage composition on delivery of phenolic compounds from coffee and tea. *Physiol. Behav.,* Vol.100, No.1, (April 2010), pp. 33-41.

Fitzpatrick, D.F., Hirschfield, S.L., & Coffey, R.G. (1993). Endothelium-dependent vasorelaxing activity of wine and other grape products. *Am. J. Physiol.,* Vol.265, No.2, (August 1993), pp. H774-H778.

Fornoni, A., & Raij, L. (2005). Metabolic syndrome and endothelial dysfunction. *Curr. Hypertens. Rep.,* Vol.7, No.2, (April 2005), pp. 88–95.

Fotsis, T., Pepper, M.S., Montesano, R., Aktas, E., Breit, S., Schweigerer, L., Rasku, S., Wähälä, K., & Adlercreutz, H.(1998). Phytoestrogens and inhibition of angiogenesis. *Baillieres Clin. Endocrinol. Metab.,* Vol.12, No.4, (December 1998), pp. 649-666.

Fuchs, C.S., Stampfer, M.J., Colditz, G.A., Giovannucci, E.L., Manson, J.E., Kawachi, I., Hunter, D.J., Hankinson, S.E., Hennekens, C.H., & Rosner, B. (1995). Alcohol consumption and mortality among women. *N. Engl. J. Med.,* Vol.332, No.19, (May 1995), pp. 1245-1250.

Gaziano, J.M., Gaziano, T.A., Glynn, R.J., Sesso, H.D., Ajani, U.A., Stampfer, M.J., Manson, J.E., Hennekens, C.H., & Buring, J.E. (2000). Light-to-moderate alcohol consumption and mortality in the Physicians' Health Study enrollment cohort. *J Am Coll. Cardiol.,* Vol.35, No.1, (January 2000), pp. 96-105.

Guo, X., Razandi, M., Pedram, A., Kassab, G., & Levin, E.R. (2005). Estrogen induces vascular wall dilation: mediation through kinase signaling to nitric oxide and estrogen receptors alpha and beta. *J. Biol. Chem.,* Vol.280, No.20, (May 2005), pp. 19704-19710.

Haas, E., Bhattacharya, I., Brailoiu, E., Damjanović, M., Brailoiu, G.C., Gao, X., Mueller-Guerre, L., Marjon, N.A., Gut, A., Minotti, R., Meyer, M.R., Amann, K., Ammann, E., Perez-Dominguez, A., Genoni, M., Clegg, D.J., Dun, N.J., Resta, T.C., Prossnitz, E.R., & Barton, M. (2009). Regulatory role of G protein-coupled estrogen receptor for vascular function and obesity. *Circ. Res.,* Vol.104, No.3, (February 2009), pp. 288-291.

Haas, E., Meyer, M.R., Schurr, U., Bhattacharya, I., Minotti, R., Nguyen, H.H., Heigl, A., Lachat, M., Genoni, M., & Barton, M. (2007). Differential effects of 17beta-estradiol on function and expression of estrogen receptor alpha, estrogen receptor beta, and GPR30 in arteries and veins of patients with atherosclerosis. *Hypertension,* Vol.49, No.6, (June 2007), pp. 1358-1363.

Hall, J.M., Couse, J.F., & Korach, K.S. (2001). The multifaceted mechanisms of estradiol and estrogen receptor signaling. *J. Biol. Chem.,* Vol.276, No.40, (October 2001), pp. 36869-36872.

Harborne, J.B. & Williams, C.A. (2000). Advances in flavonoid research since 1992. *Phytochemistry,* Vol.55, No.6, (November 2000), pp.481-504.

Hodgin, J.B., Krege, J.H., Reddick, R.L., Korach, K.S., Smithies, O., & Maeda, N. (2001). Estrogen receptor alpha is a major mediator of 17beta-estradiol's atheroprotective effects on lesion size in ApoE−/− mice. *J. Clin. Invest.*, Vol.107, No.3, (February 2001), pp. 333-340.

Holm, A., Baldetorp, B., Olde, B., Leeb-Lundberg, L.M., & Nilsson, B.O. (2011). The GPER1 agonist G-1 attenuates endothelial cell proliferation by inhibiting DNA synthesis and accumulating cells in the S and G2 phases of the cell cycle. *J. Vasc. Res.*, Vol.48, No.4, (January 2011), pp. 327-335.

Igura K, Ohta T, Kuroda Y, & Kaji K. (2001). Resveratrol and quercetin inhibit angiogenesis in vitro. *Cancer Lett.*, Vol.171, No.1, (Septembre 2001), pp. 11-16.

Imhof, A., Woodward, M., Doering, A., Helbecque, N., Loewel, H., Amouyel, P., Lowe, G.D., & Koenig, W. (2004). Overall alcohol intake, beer, wine, and systemic markers of inflammation in western Europe: results from three MONICA samples (Augsburg, Glasgow, Lille). *Eur. Heart J.*, Vol.25, No.23, (December 2004), pp. 2092-2100.

Kane, M.O., Anselm, E., Rattmann, Y.D., Auger, C., & Schini-Kerth, V.B. (2009). Role of gender and estrogen receptors in the rat aorta endothelium-dependent relaxation to red wine polyphenols. *Vascul. Pharmacol.*, Vol.51, No.2-3, (August-September 2009), pp. 140-146.

Kang, L., Zang X, Xie, Y., Tu, Y., Wang, D., Liu, Z., & Wang, Z.Y. (2010). Involvement of estrogen receptor variant ER-alpha36, not GPR30, in nongenomic estrogen signaling. *Mol. Endocrinol.*, Vol.24, No.4, (April 2010), pp. 709-721.

Klinge, C.M., Blankenship, K.A., Risinger, K.E., Bhatnagar, S., Noisin, E.L., Sumanasekera, W.K., Zhao, L., Brey, D.M., & Keynton, R.S. (2005). Resveratrol and estradiol rapidly activate MAPK signaling through estrogen receptors alpha and beta in endothelial cells. *J. Biol. Chem.*, Vol.280, No.9, (March 2005), pp. 7460-7468.

Klinge, C.M., Wickramasinghe, N.S., Ivanova, M.M., & Dougherty, S.M. (2008). Resveratrol stimulates nitric oxide production by increasing estrogen receptor α-Src caveolin-1 interaction and phosphorylation in human umbilical vein endothelial cells. *F.A.S.E.B. J.*, Vol.22, No.7, (July 2008), pp. 2185-2197.

Kopelman, P.G. (2000). Obesity as a medical problem. *Nature,* Vol.404, No.6778, (April 2000), pp. 635–643.

Kopp, P. (1998). Resveratrol, a phytoestrogen found in red wine. A possible explanation for the conundrum of the French paradox? *Eur. J. Endocrinol.,* Vol.138, No.6, (June 1998), pp. 619–620

Kuiper, G.G., Enmark, E., Pelto-Huikko, M., Nilsson, S., & Gustafsson, J.A. (1996). Cloning of a novel receptor expressed in rat prostate and ovary. *Proc. Natl. Acad. Sci. U.S.A.,* Vol.93, No.12, (June 1996), pp. 5925-5930.

Lamont, K.T., Somers, S., Lacerda, L., Opie, L.H., & Lecour S. (2011). Is red wine a SAFE sip away from cardioprotection? Mecanisms involved in resveratrol and melatonin-induced cardioprotection. *J. Pineal Res.*, Vol.50, No.4, (May 2011), pp. 374-380.

Lindberg, M.K., Movérare, S., Skrtic, S., Gao, H., Dahlman-Wright, K., Gustafsson, J.A., & Ohlsson, C. (2003). Estrogen receptor (ER)-beta reduces ERalpha-regulated gene transcription, supporting a "ying yang" relationship between ERalpha and ERbeta in mice. *Mol. Endocrinol.,* Vol.17, No.2, (February 2003), pp. 203-208.

Lindsey, S.H., Cohen, J.A., Brosnihan, K.B., Gallagher, P.E., & Chappell, M.C. (2009). Chronic treatment with the G protein-coupled receptor 30 agonist G-1 decreases blood pressure in ovariectomized mRen2.Lewis rats. *Endocrinology.*, Vol.150, No.8, (August 2009), pp. 3753-3758.

Liu, B.L., Zhang, X ., Zhang, W., & Zhen, H.N. (2007). New enlightenment of French paradox resveratrol's potential for cancer chemoprevention and anti-cancer therapy. *Cancer Biology & Therapy,* Vol.6, No.12, (December 2007), pp. 1833-1836.

López-Sepúlveda, R., Jiménez, R., Romero, M., Zarzuelo, M.J., Sánchez, M., Gómez-Guzmán, M., Vargas, F., O'Valle, F., Zarzuelo, A., Pérez-Vizcaíno, F., & Duarte, J. (2008) Wine polyphenols improve endothelial function in large vessels of female spontaneously hypertensive rats. *Hypertension,* Vol.51, No.4, (April 2008), pp. 1088-1095.

Losordo, D.W., Kearney, M., Kim, E.A., Jekanowski, J., & Isner, J.M. (1994).Variable expression of the estrogen receptor in normal and atherosclerotic coronary arteries of premenopausal women. *Circulation,* Vol.89, No.4, (April 1994), pp. 1501-1510.

Maruyama. K., Endoh, H., Sasaki-Iwaoka, H., Kanou, H., Shimaya, E., Hashimoto, S., Kato, S., & Kawashima, H. (1998). A novel isoform of rat estrogen receptor beta with 18 amino acid insertion in the ligand binding domain as a putative dominant negative regular of estrogen action. *Biochem. Biophys. Res. Commun.,* Vol.246, No.1, (May 1998), pp. 142-147.

Martensson, U.E., Salehi, S.A., Windahl, S., Gomez, M.F., Swärd, K., Daszkiewicz-Nilsson, J., Wendt, A., Andersson, N., Hellstrand, P., Grände, P.O., Owman, C., Rosen, C.J., Adamo, M.L., Lundquist, I., Rorsman, P., Nilsson, B.O., Ohlsson, C., Olde, B., & Leeb-Lundberg, L.M. (2009). Deletion of the G protein-coupled receptor 30 impairs glucose tolerance, reduces bone growth, increases blood pressure, and eliminates estradiol-stimulated insulin release in female mice. *Endocrinology,* Vol.150, No.2, (February 2009), pp. 687-698.

Martin, S., Andriambeloson, E., Takeda, K., & Andriantsitohaina, R. (2002). Red wine polyphenols increase calcium in bovine aortic endothelial cells: a basis to elucidate signalling pathways leading to nitric oxide production. *Br. J. Pharmacol.,* Vol.135, No.6, (March 2002), pp. 1579-1587.

Martin, S., Giannone, G., Andriantsitohaina, R., & Martinez, M.C. (2003). Delphinidin, an active compound of red wine, inhibits endothelial cell apoptosis via nitric oxide pathway and regulation of calcium homeostasis. *Br. J. Pharmacol.,* Vol.139, No.6, (July 2003), pp.1095-1102.

Mendelsohn, M.E., & Karas, R.H. (1999). The protective effects of estrogen on the cardiovascular system. *N. Engl. J. Med.,* Vol.340, No.23, (June 1999), pp. 1801-1811.

Meyer, M.R., Baretella, O., Prossnitz, E.R., & Barton, M. (2010) Dilation of epicardial coronary arteries by the G protein-coupled estrogen receptor agonists G-1 and ICI 182,780. *Pharmacology,* Vol.86, No.1, (July 2010), pp. 58-64.

Meyer, M.R., Haas, E., & Barton, M. (2008). Need for research on estrogen receptor function: importance for postmenopausal hormone therapy and atherosclerosis. *Gend. Med.,* Vol.5, No.Suppl.A, (2008), pp. S19-S33.

Meyer, M.R., Haas, E., & Barton, M. (2006). Gender differences of cardiovascular disease: new perspectives for estrogen receptor signaling. *Hypertension,* Vol.47, No.6, (June 2006), pp. 1019-1026.

Mojzisová, G., & Kuchta, M. (2001). Dietary flavonoids and risk of coronary heart disease. *Physiol. Res.,* Vol.50, No.6, (2001), pp. 529-535.

Mügge, A., Riedel, M., Barton, M., Kuhn, M., & Lichtlen, P.R. (1993). Endothelium independent relaxation of human coronary arteries by 17 beta-oestradiol in vitro. *Cardiovasc. Res.*, Vol.27, No.11, (November 1993), pp. 1939-1942.

Nakamura, Y., Suzuki, T., Miki, Y., Tazawa, C., Senzaki, K., Moriya, T., Saito, H., Ishibashi, T., Takahashi, S., Yamada, S., & Sasano, H. (2004). Estrogen receptors in atherosclerotic human aorta: inhibition of human vascular smooth muscle cell proliferation by estrogens. *Mol. Cell. Endocrinol.*, Vol.219, No.1-2, (April 2004), pp. 17-26.

Napoli, R., Cozzolino, D., Guardasole, V., Angelini, V., Zarra, E., Matarazzo, M., Cittadini, A., Saccà, L., & Torella, R. (2005). Red wine consumption improves insulin resistance but not endothelial function in type 2 diabetic patients. *Metabolism*, Vol.54, No.3, (March 2005), pp. 306–313.

Navarro, S., Oliva, J., Barba, A., Navarro, G., Garcia, M.A., & Zamorano, M. (2000). Evolution of chlorpyrifos, fenarimol, metalaxyl, penconazole, and vinclozolin in red wines elaborated by carbonic maceration of Monastrell grapes. *J. Agric. Food Chem.*, Vol.48, No.8, (August 2000), pp. 3537-3541.

Nilsson, B.O. (2007). Modulation of the inflammatory response by estrogens with focus on the endothelium and its interactions with leukocytes. *Inflamm. Res.*, Vol.56, No.7, (July 2007), pp. 269-273.

Nilsson, B.O., Olde, B., & Leeb-Lundberg, L.M. (2011). G protein-coupled oestrogen receptor 1 (GPER1)/GPR30: a new player in cardiovascular and metabolic oestrogenic signalling. *Br. J. Pharmacol.*, Vol.163, No.6, (July 2011), pp. 1131-1139.

Opie, L.H., & Lecour, S. (2007). The red wine hypothesis: from concepts to protective signaling molecules. *European Heart Journal*, Vol.28, No.14, (July 2007), pp. 1683-1693.

Paech, K., Webb, P., Kuiper, G.G., Nilsson, S., Gustafsson, J., Kushner, P.J., & Scanlan, T.S. (1997). Differential ligand activation of estrogen receptors ERalpha and ERbeta at AP1 sites. *Science*, Vol.277, No.5331, (September 1997), pp. 1508-1510.

Paganga, G., & Rice-Evans, C.A. (1997). The identification of flavonoids as glycosides in human plasma. *F.E.B.S. Lett.*, Vol.401, No.1, (January 1997), pp.78-82.

Papamichael, C., Karatzis, E., Karatzi, K., Aznaouridis, K., Papaioannou, T., Protogerou, A., Stamatelopoulos, K., Zampelas, A., Lekakis, J., & Mavrikakis, M. (2004). Red wine's antioxidants counteract acute endothelial dysfunction caused by cigarette smoking in healthy nonsmokers. *Am. Heart J.*, Vol.147, No.2, (February 2004), pp. E5.

Pare, G., Krust, A., Karas, R.H., Dupont, S., Aronovitz, M., Chambon, P., & Mendelsohn, M.E. (2002). Estrogen receptor-alpha mediates the protective effects of estrogen against vascular injury. *Circ. Res.*, Vol.90, No.10, (May 2002), pp. 1087-1092.

Pechánová, O., Bernátová, I., Babál, P., Martínez, M.C., Kyselá, S., Stvrtina, S., & Andriantsitohaina, R. (2004). Red wine polyphenols prevent cardiovascular alterations in L-NAME induced hypertension. *J. Hypertens.*, Vol.22, No.8, (August 2004), pp. 1551-1559.

Pechanova. O., Rezzani, R.., Babal, P., Bernatova, I., & Andriantsitohaina R. (2006). Beneficial effects of provinols: cardiovascular system and kidney. *Physiol. Res.*, Vol.55, No.Suppl.1, (2006), pp. 17-30.

Pellegrini, N., Simonetti, P., Gardana, C., Brenna, O., Brighenti, F., & Pietta, P. (2000). polyphenol content and total antioxidant activity of *vini novelli* (young red wines). *J. Agric. Food Chem.*, Vol.48, No.3, (March 2000), pp. 732–735.

Petersen, D.N., Tkalcevic, G.T., Koza-Taylor, P.H., Turi, T.G., & Brown, T.A. (1998). Identification of estrogen receptor beta2, a functional variant of estrogen receptor beta expressed in normal rat tissues. *Endocrinology*, Vol.139, No.3, (March 1998), pp. 1082-1092.

Price, R.H. Jr, Lorenzon, N., & Handa, R.J. (2000). Differential expression of estrogen receptor beta splice variants in rat brain: identification and characterization of a novel variant missing exon 4. *Brain Res. Mol. Brain Res.*, Vol.80, No.2, (September 2000), pp. 260-268.

Prior, R.L., Lazarus, S.A., Cao, G., Muccitelli, H., & Hammerstone, J.F. (2001). Identification of procyanidins and anthocyanins in blueberries and cranberries (Vaccinium spp.) using high-performance liquid chromatography/mass spectrometry. *J. Agric. Food Chem.*, Vol.49, No.3, (March 2001), pp. 1270-1276.

Providencia, R. (2006). Cardiovascular protection by alcoholic beverages: scientific basis of the French paradox. *Rev. Port. Cardiol.*, Vol.25, No.11, (November 2006), pp. 1043-1058.

Ranaivo H.R., Diebolt M., & Andriantsitohaina R. (2004). Wine polyphenols induce hypotension, and decrease cardiac reactivity and infarct size in rats: involvement of nitric oxide. *British J. Pharmacol.*, Vol.142, No.4 (June 2004), pp. 671–678.

Renaud, S.C. (1992). What is the epidemiologic evidence for the thrombogenic potential of dietary long-chain fatty acids? *Am. J. Clin. Nutr.*, Vol.56, No.Suppl.4, (October 1992), pp. 823S-824S.

Renaud, S.C., Guéguen, R., Siest, G., & Salamon, R. (1999). Wine, beer, and mortality in middle-aged men from eastern France. *Arch. Intern. Med.*, Vol.159, No.16, (September 1999), pp. 1865-1870.

Revankar, C.M., Cimino, D.F., Sklar, L.A., Arterburn, J.B., & Prossnitz, E.R. (2005). A transmembrane intracellular estrogen receptor mediates rapid cell signaling. *Science*, Vol.307, No.5715, (March 2005), pp. 1625-1630.

Ribereau-Gayon, P., Dubourdieu, D., Donèche, B., & Lonvaud, A. (2000). Cytology, taxonomy and ecology of grape and wine yeast, In: *Handbook of Enology*, Vol.1, pp. 1-49, John Wiley & Sons.

Richter G. (1993). *Métabolisme des végétaux. Physiologie et biochimie*, Presses Polytechniques et Universitaires Romandes.

Ritz, M.F., Curin, Y., Mendelowitsch, A., & Andriantsitohaina, R. (2008b). Acute treatment with red wine polyphenols protects from ischemia-induced excitotoxicity, energy failure and oxidative stress in rats. *Brain Res.*, Vol.1239, (November 2008), pp. 226-234.

Ritz, M.F., Ratajczak, P., Curin, Y., Cam, E., Mendelowitsch, A., Pinet, F., & Andriantsitohaina, R. (2008a). Chronic treatment with red wine polyphenol compounds mediates neuroprotection in a rat model of ischemic cerebral stroke. *J. Nutr.*, Vol.138, No.3, (March 2008), pp. 519-525.

Shaw, L., Taggart, M., & Austin, C. (2001). Effects of the oestrous cycle and gender on acute vasodilatory responses of isolated pressurized rat mesenteric arteries to 17 beta-oestradiol. *Br. J. Pharmacol.*, Vol.132, No.5, (March 2001), pp. 1055-1062.

Si, W., Gong, J., Tsao, R., Kalab, M., Yang, R., & Yin, Y. (2006). Bioassay-guided purification and identification of antimicrobial components in Chinese green tea extract. *J. Chromatogr. A.*, Vol.1125, No.2, (September 2006), pp. 204-210.

Soleas, G.J., Diamandis, E.P., & Goldberg, D.M. (1997). Wine as a biological fluid: History, production, and role in disease prevention issue. *J. Clinical Laboratory Analysis*, Vol.11, No.5, (December 1998), pp. 287-313.

Spary, E.J., Maqbool, A., & Batten, T.F. (2009). Oestrogen receptors in the central nervous system and evidence for their role in the control of cardiovascular function. *J. Chem. Neuroanat.*, Vol.38, No.3, (November 2009), pp. 185-196.

Sudhir, K., Chou, T.M., Chatterjee, K., Smith, E.P., Williams, T.C., Kane, J.P., Malloy, M.J., Korach, K.S., & Rubanyi, G.M. (1997). Premature coronary artery disease associated with a disruptive mutation in the estrogen receptor gene in a man. *Circulation*, Vol.96, No.10, (November 1997), pp. 3774-3777.

Suh, I., Shaten, B.J., Cutler, J.A., & Kuller, L.H. (1992). Alcohol use and mortality from coronary heart disease: the role of high-density lipoprotein cholesterol. The Multiple Risk Factor Intervention Trial Research Group. *Ann. Intern. Med.*, Vol.116, No.11, (June 1992), pp. 881-887.

Suh, J.H., Virsolvy, A., Goux, A., Cassan, C., Richard, S., Cristol, J.P., Teissèdre, P.L., & Rouanet, J.M. (2011). Polyphenols prevent lipid abnormalities and arterial dysfunction in hamsters on a high-fat diet: a comparative study of red grape and white persimmon wines. *Food Funct.*, Vol.2, No.9, (September 2011), pp. 555-561.

Tsao, R. (2010). Chemistry and biochemistry of dietary polyphenols. *Nutrients*, Vol.2, No.12, (December 2010), pp. 1231-1246.

Tsao, R., Papadopoulos, Y., Yang, R., Young, J.C., & McRae, K. (2006). Isoflavone profiles of red clovers and their distribution in different parts harvested at different growing stages. *J. Agric. Food Chem.*, Vol.54, No.16, (August 2006), pp. 5797 5805.

Tsao, R., Yang, R., Young, J.C., & Zhu, H. (2003). Polyphenolic profiles in eight apple cultivars using high-performance liquid chromatography (HPLC). *J. Agric. Food Chem.*, Vol.51, No.21, (Octobre 2003), pp. 6347-6353.

Thun, M.J., Peto, R., Lopez, A.D., Monaco, J.H., Henley, S.J., Heath, C.W., & Doll, R. (1997). Alcohol consumption and mortality among middle-aged and elderly U.S. adults. *N. Engl. J. Med.*, Vol.337, No.24, (December 1997), pp. 1705–1714.

Vegeto, E., Belcredito, S., Etteri, S., Ghisletti, S., Brusadelli, A., Meda, C., Krust, A., Dupont, S., Ciana, P., Chambon, P., & Maggi, A. (2003). Estrogen receptor-alpha mediates the brain antiinflammatory activity of estradiol. *Proc. Natl. Acad. Sci. U.S.A.*, Vol.100, No.16, (August 2003), pp. 9614-9619.

Vidavalur, R., Otani H., Singal, P.K., & Maulik N. (2006). Significance of wine and resveratrol in cardiovascular disease: French paradox revisited. *Exp. Clin. Cardiol.*, Vol.11, No.3, (Fall 2006), pp. 217-225.

Wallerath T., Deckert G., Ternes T., Anderson H., Li H., Witte K., & Förstermann U. (2002). Resveratrol, a polyphenolic phytoalexin present in red wine, enhances expression and activity of endothelial nitric oxide synthase. *Circulation*, Vol.106, No.13, (September 2002), pp. 1652-1658.

Webb, P., Nguyen, P., Valentine, C., Lopez, G.N., Kwok, G.R., McInerney, E., Katzenellenbogen, B.S., Enmark, E., Gustafsson, J.A., Nilsson, S., & Kushner, P.J. (1999). The estrogen receptor enhances AP-1 activity by two distinct mechanisms with different requirements for receptor transactivation functions. *Mol. Endocrinol.*, Vol.13, No.10, (October 1999), pp.1672-1685.

Xu, Y., Simon, J.E., Welch, C., Wightman, J.D., Ferruzzi, M.G., Ho, L., Passinetti, G.M., & Wu, Q. (2011). Survey of polyphenol constituents in grapes and grape-derived products. *J. Agric. Food Chem.*, Vol.59, No.19, (October 2011), pp. 10586-10593.

Yusuf, S., Hawken, S., Ounpuu, S., Dans, T., Avezum, A., Lanas, F., MacQueen, M., Budaj, A., Pais, P., Varigos, J., & Lisheng, L. (2004). Effect of potentially modifiable risk factors associated with myocardial infarction in 52 countries (the INTERHEART study); case-control study. *Lancet*, Vol.364, No.9438, (September 2004), pp. 937-952.

Zhao, C., Dahlman-Wright, K., & Gustafsson, J.A. (2008). Estrogen receptor beta: an overview and update. *Nucl. Recept. Signal.*, Vol. 6, (February 2008), pp. e003.

Zhao, F., Watanabe, Y., Nozawa, H., Daikonnya, A., Kondo, K., & Kitanaka, S. (2005). Prenylflavonoids and phloroglucinol derivatives from hops (Humulus lupulus). *J. Nat. Prod.*, Vol.68, No.1, (January 2005), pp. 43-49.

17

Importance of Dermatology in Infective Endocarditis

Servy Amandine, Jones Meriem
and Valeyrie-Allanore Laurence*
*Department of Dermatology,
Hôpital Henri Mondor, Créteil,
France*

1. Introduction

Infective endocarditis (IE) is a rare affection with an annual incidence of between 15 to 60 cases per million. If untreated, IE is fatal, and the overall mortality is evaluated above 20%. IE is an endovascular microbial infection of intracardiac structures. The early characteristic lesion corresponds to variable sized vegetation leading to valvular destruction and abscess formation.

Epidemiologic profile evolved progressively with decreasing proportion of IE on abnormal native valve compensated by an increased proportion of prosthetic valve IE and native valve IE with previously unrecognized predisposing conditions. Among causative microorganisms, the responsibility of staphylococci is more frequently observed. Diagnosing IE remains a clinical challenge because evolution is insidious and symptoms are polymorphous. This diagnosis must be systematically considered in the presence of purpura, distal necrosis but also in patients who had have chronic dermatosis which correspond to an underestimated potential source of IE.

2. Pathophysiology

Secondary to damage of endothelium, extracellular matrix proteins are exposed leading to development of non-bacterial thrombotic endocarditis (NBTE) with fibrin and platelets. Endothelial damage can occur after mechanical lesions (devices, repeated intravenous injection of particulate material), turbulent blood flow (congenital heart disease, prosthetic valves…), inflammation (chronic rheumatic fever) or degenerative lesions (European society of cardiology [ESC], 2009). NBTE facilitates micro-organism adherence and infection of endothelium (Figure 1).

International specialists (American Heart Association [AHA], 2007; ESC, 2009) no longer differentiate acute, subacute and chronic IE based on usual progression of untreated disease. Indeed, although clinical manifestations are more insidious in subacute IE, severe

*Corresponding Author

complications can occur and it is currently difficult to determine the onset of the disease. Presently, IE are classified depending on the type of valve damage (right/left-sided, native/prosthetic valve).

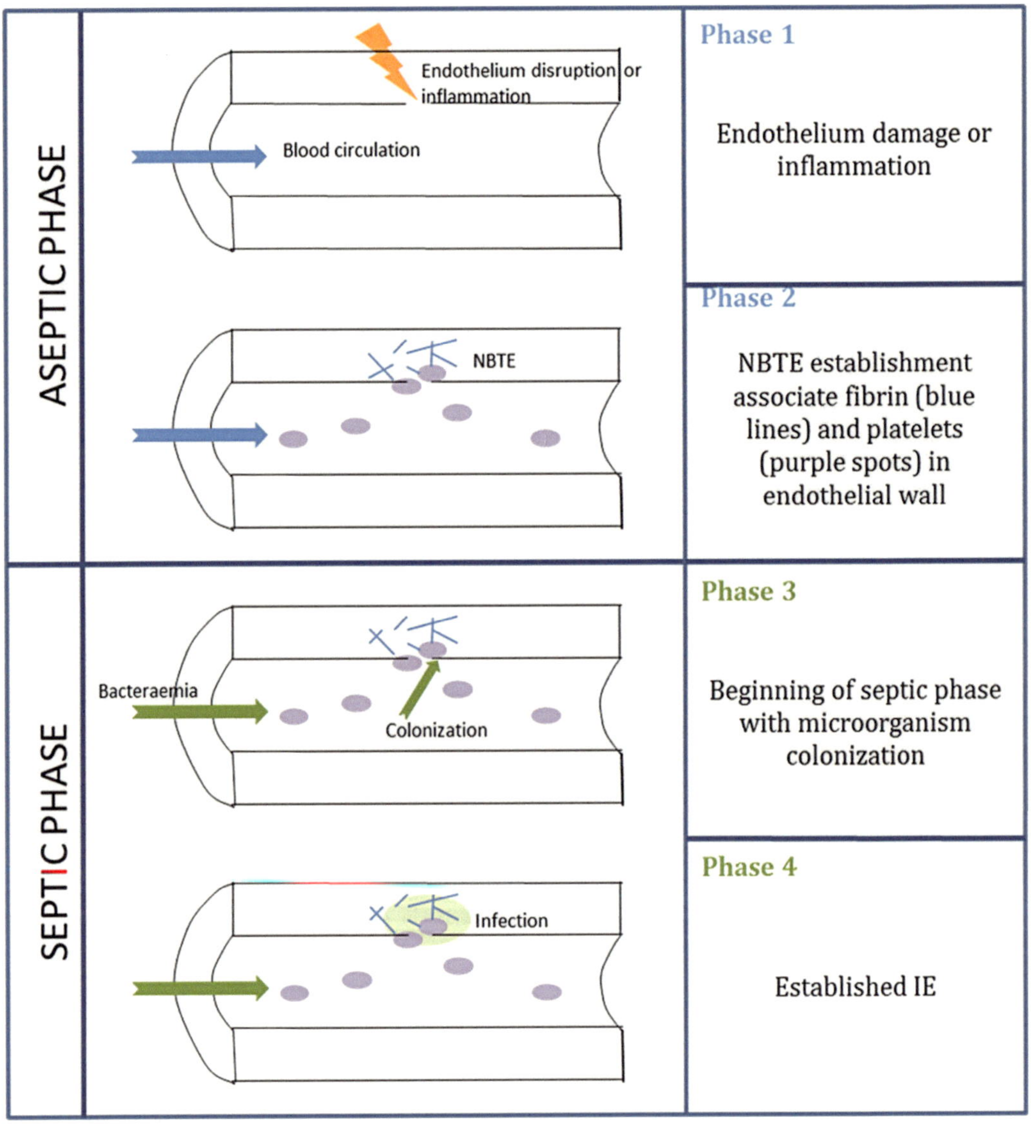

Fig. 1. Pathophysiology of IE with aseptic and septic phases (A. Servy; August 2011). NBTE: non- bacterial thrombotic endocarditis

3. Epidemiology

3.1 Incidence

IE is a rare disease with 2 to 6 per 100 000 persons affected per year (Que, 2011). Classically described in young patients after chronic rheumatic heart disease. Its incidence in industrialized countries is more elevated in at-risk groups, mainly persons older than 65 years old (15 per 100 000 per year). At present, the average is 57 years old (Que, 2011; ESC, 2009).

Native valve IE is the most frequent. Left-sided native valve IE represents 70% of disease incidence and the mortality is evaluated at 15% (25-45% with healthcare-associated). 5-10% of IE affect right-sided native valve, mainly in intravenous-drug users, and patients with congenital heart disease or devices. *Staphylococcus spp* is most frequently involved in right-sided native valve IE and mortality is less than 10% (Que, 2011).

Prosthetic valve IE is also increasing (10-30% of IE), mechanical and bioprosthetic equally. The prevalence of valve prostheses IE is above 6% (0.3-1.2% per year). Left-sided prosthetic valve endocarditis (20% of IE) is the most severe with 20 to 40% mortality. The main germs involved in early prosthetic valve IE (less than one year after cardiac surgery) include staphylococci, fungi and Gram-negative bacilli, whereas late IE is associated with staphylococci, oral streptococci, *S. bovis* and enteroccoci (ESC, 2009).

3.2 Risk factors

3.2.1 Characteristics of patient

The main risk factor is age (median age above 60) (Murdoch, 2009) due to degenerative valve, immunosuppressive conditions and multiple comorbidities. However, edentate people have a lower risk of IE. Digestive portal of entry is frequent in this population, mainly in *S. bovis* and enterococcus IE and should be researched.

Many comorbidities increase the risk of IE, leading to heart diseases. At present, in industrialized countries, chronic rheumatic heart disease has become exceptional and the proportion of degenerative valve lesion and congenital heart disease is more important as well as their responsibility for IE (Moreillon, 2004). Chronic immunosuppressive therapy (chemotherapy, topical corticosteroid…) or affections are predisposing conditions, mainly diabetes mellitus (16% of IE), hemodialysis (8%), cancer (8%) and HIV infection (2%) (Murdoch, 2009). Physicians should be aware of the risk of EI in cases of acute or chronic dermatosis. Chronic bacteria carriers, wounds, and percutaneous invasive procedure increase significantly the risk of bacteremia.

3.2.2 Situations at risk

All iatrogenic invasive procedures are at risk of bacteremia such as catheter, urinary surgery, and endoscopy (Table 1). Nevertheless, intravenous drug users are more at risk (10% of IE) due to poor hygiene. Indeed 55% of active heroin, cocaine and methamphetamine injection drug users report a lifetime history of skin infection mainly in cases of intramuscular injection or frequent heroin or speedball injection (Phillips, 2010). In these cases, *S. aureus* and fungi must be suspected and treated. Dental treatments are too easily suspected (AHA, 2007; Strom, 1998) whereas most of the time, no procedure or situation at risk are identified and daily bacteremia is often involved (AHA, 2007). In a recent French study (Association pour l'Etude et la Prévention de l'Endocardite Infectieuse [AEPEI], 2002), 63% of IE cases had no situation at risk identified.

Risk factors of IE		
Patient characteristics		Situations at risk
Age		Invasive procedures: - percutaneous (drug, catheter...) or - dental Daily bacteremia - Brushing teeth - Chewing ...
Comorbidities	Heart disease and prosthetic valve Diabetes mellitus Chronic renal failure Immunosuppressive affection	
Treatment	Immunosuppressive therapy	

Table 1. Procedures and situations at risk of bacteremia.

3.3 Causal microorganisms

Distribution of causative microorganisms of IE is different, depending on the patient's characteristics (Table 2) and portal of entry. Gram-positive bacteria are the most frequent microorganisms. They are responsible for more than 80% of IE because they have greatest ability to adhere and colonize damaged valves (Que, 2011).

Microorganisms (%)	Valve affected			
	Native valve IE		Intracardiac device IE	
	Drug abusers	Others patients	Prosthetic valve	Others
Staphylococcus aureus	68	28	23	35
Coagulase-negative staphylococcus	3	9	17	26
Viridans group streptococci	10	21	12	8
Streptococcus bovis	1	7	5	3
Enterococcus ssp	5	11	12	6
HACEK	0	2	2	1
Fungi	1	1	4	1
Polymicromial	3	1	0.8	0
Negative culture findings	5	9	12	11

Table 2. Microbiologic etiology of IE depend on patient's characteristics (Murdoch, 2009). HACEK: Haemophilus (parainfluenzae, aphrophilus, paraphrophilus and influenza), Actinobacillus actinomycetemcomitans, Cardiobacterium hominis, Eikenella corrodens, Kingella (kingae and dentrificans).

Although increasing involvement of oral streptococci, streptococcaceae remain the main pathogen (nearly 60% of IE). In streptococci group, group D (*S. bovis*...) are found in 25%, oral streptococci in 17% and pyogenic streptococci (*S. agalactiae, S. pyogenes*) in 6% of IE.

Enterococci (mainly *E. faecalis*) are also frequent (8%), mainly in elderly people and prosthetic valve carriers (AEPEI, 2002). Urinary and digestive portal of entry (including colon cancer, and diverticulitis) must be researched with colonoscopy and imaging. Presence of *S. bovis* equally implies digestive portal of entry.

The role of Staphylococcaceae is increasing (20-34% of IE) with 23% of IE due to *S. aureus* and 6% to coagulase-negative staphylococci (AEPEI, 2002; Miro, 2005). Staphylococcus IE is more frequent in intravenous drug users, HIV patients, right-sided IE and iatrogenic infection. The prevalence of IE in patients with *Staphylococcus aureus* bacteremia is elevated (22%) and some authors recommend a systematic echocardiography in this situation (Rasmussen, 2011).

The responsibility of others germs is lesser and unusually several microorganisms are associated in rare instances (less than 5%). No germ is identified in 5% of cases (AEPEI, 2002).

3.4 Portals of entry

Any site of infection can be responsible of IE. However, some portals of entry are more frequent and must be investigated. Cutaneous portal of entry is frequent (20%) and often misdiagnosed by physicians. In these cases, IE mainly developed on traumatic or chronic wounds, infected or inflammatory dermatosis, intravenous drug use, percutaneous iatrogenic procedures… Dental portal of entry is observed in 9% of cases (poor dental condition, dental procedure). Genitourinary and digestive portal of entry are observed respectively in above 2-11% and 5-9% (AEPEI, 2002; Tornos, 2005).

4. Diagnosis

4.1 Clinical manifestations

Clinical diagnosis of IE is often difficult because of various clinical manifestations and insidious evolution. Moreover, atypical presentation is usual in elderly, immunocompromised patients (lack of fever) and carriers of prosthetic valve, mainly in earlier phase (less than one 1 year after surgery). In fact, in this last group, blood cultures are frequently negative, echocardiography is difficult (ESC, 2009) and inflammatory syndrome and fever is classical even in absence of IE. So, clinical suspicion of IE should be systematically discussed in these cases, and complementary investigations performed.

4.1.1 General signs

Fever is the most frequent sign (approximately 90%) and usually temperature normalizes within 1 week (5-10 days) under adaptive antibiotherapy. An impaired general health condition can be observed with weight loss, fatigue and anorexia.

4.1.2 Cardiological signs

Cardiological manifestations are nearly constant. Heart murmurs are found in up 85% of IE (ESC, 2009) but occurrence of new ones (48%) or increasing of an older murmur (20%) are more evocative (Murdoch, 2009). Clinical manifestations of heart complications can be added (mainly heart failure).

4.1.3 Extracardiac manifestations

Extracardiac manifestations are also frequent, particularly in right-sided IE (78% versus 52% in left-sided IE) with 68% of pulmonary embolism (AEPEI, 2002).

If IE is suspected, dermatological manifestations should be systematically searched and discussed despite rarity (5 to 25% of IE present skin manifestations) not only for diagnosis but also for prognostic (Table 5). They can easily lead to suspicion of IE. In our recent study (unpublished data), we demonstrated a link between the presence of cutaneous signs and embolic events (18.4% of embolic events in lack of cutaneous sign versus 33%) without higher mortality. Dermatological manifestations (Figures 2 and 3) seem to be also less frequently observed with enteroccoci infection (14.5% versus 27.1%) (Martínez-Marcos, 2009).

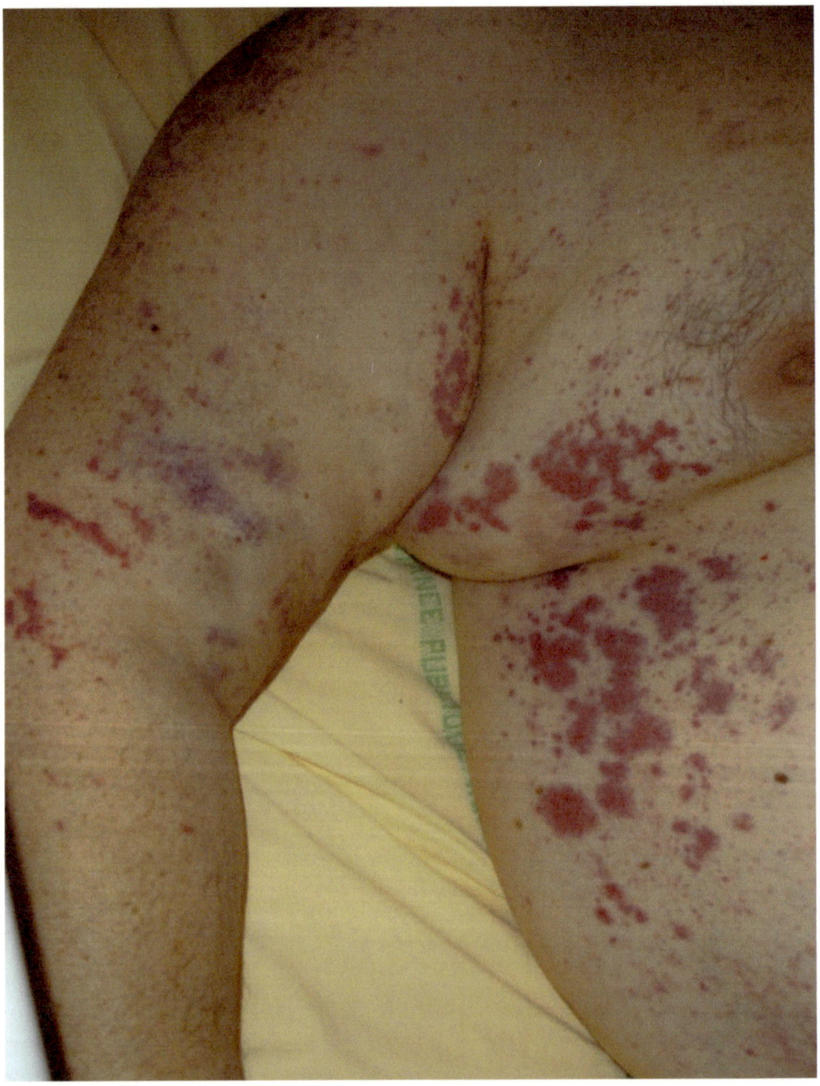

Fig. 2. Vascular purpura on trunk and arms during IE.

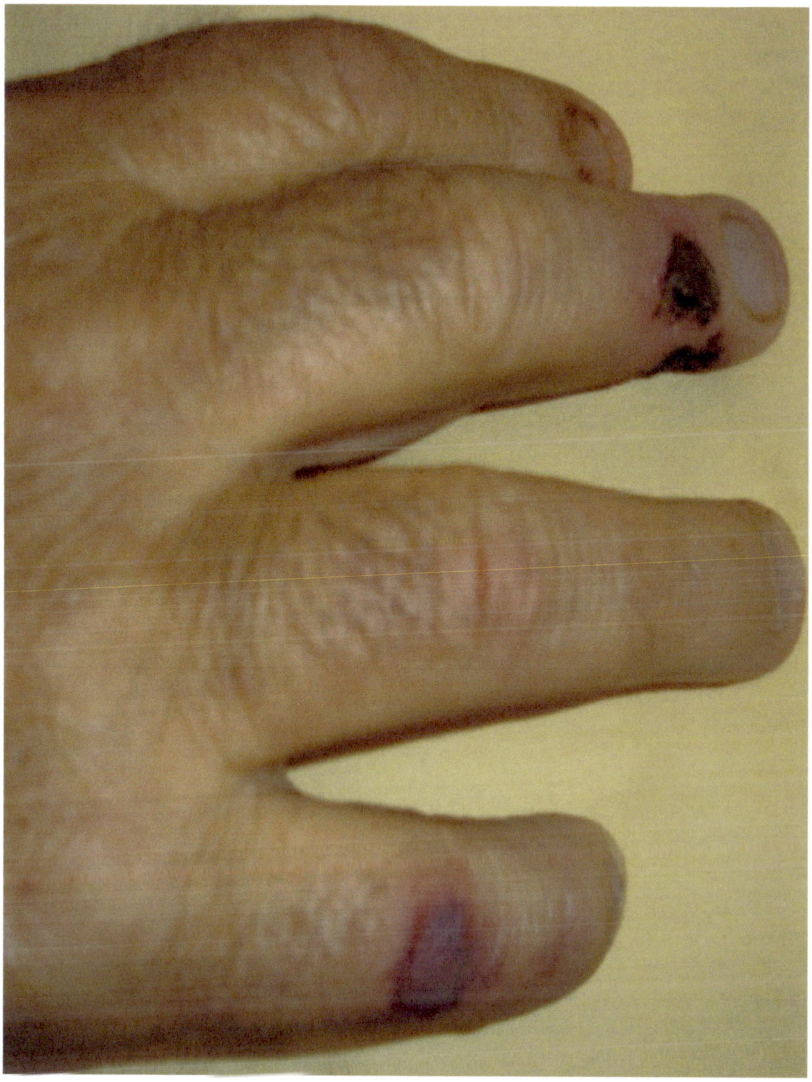

Fig. 3. Necrotic lesions of fingers (same patient): old Janeway lesion or purpura lesion.

- **Osler's lesions** are specific and described as purple painful nodes on palms, soles, fingertips, pulp of the toes or sometimes on ears (Farrior, 1976). Unfortunately, prevalence is low (3-3.6%) (AEPEI, 2002; Murdoch, 2009) and lesions disappear in a few days without sequelae. In a study including 43 intravenous-drug users IE, Osler's nodes were observed in 50% of left-sided IE whereas none were noticed in right-sided IE (33 right-sided). Moreover, bacteriological study of nodes revealed the same microorganisms as in blood (*S. aureus*).
- **Janeway lesions** are small non tender erythematous and painless macular (sometimes nodular!) localized on palms or soles (2-5% of IE) (AEPEI, 2002; Murdoch, 2009). These lesions are equally specific and their differenciation difference with Osler nodes is often as difficult, clinically as histologically.

- **Purpura** is more frequent (7.3%) (AEPEI, 2002) but not specific. Its pathophysiology is still unclear including often septic embolism and/or leucocytoclastic cutaneous vasculitis by complex immune depositions (Lévesque 1999). Vascular purpura is characterized by red lesions that don't blanch on applying pressure, caused by erythrocyte extravasation. Lesions are localized on lower parts of the body (legs, back). In IE, lesions are also described on the neck and near the clavicles. IE mucosal purpura is often observed on conjunctivae and mouth (Heffner, 1979).
- **Splinter haemorrhages** are common in many diseases and found in 8 to 14% of IE (Konstantinou, 2009; Murdoch, 2009).

30% of IE (ESC, 2009) has at least one vascular or immunological phenomenon. Vascular phenomenon includes systemic arterial embolism (17-33%) (AEPEI, 2002; Murdoch, 2009), infectious embolism (septic pulmonary infarct, infectious aneurysm) and classically Janeway lesions. Immunological manifestations are mainly represented by Osler's nodes and Roth spots (2%) (Murdoch, 2009).

Musculoskeletal symptoms are common with mainly arthralgia (14%) (Murdoch, 2009), myalgia and back pain. In the presence of, spondylodiscitis (3-15%) (ESC, 2009) mainly observed in streptococci IE must be systemically discussed. Splenomegaly is less frequently noticed (11%) (Murdoch, 2009).

4.2 Laboratory studies

4.2.1 Biology findings

- Inflammatory syndrome

In most cases, unspecific inflammatory syndrome is observed, including neutrophils hyperleucocytosis, elevated erythrocyte sedimentation rate (ESR) and C-reactive protein.

- Microbiological diagnosis

Three sets of blood cultures, including at least one aerobic and one anaerobic samples and spaced of at least 30 minutes, should be obtained from a peripheral vein before beginning any antimicrobial therapy. The blood cultures are positive in 85% of cases (ESC, 2009). However, blood culture can be negative in cases of prior antibiotherapy or specific microorganisms (Table 3). In this last case, other bacteriological investigations are performed, such as serologies, specific PCR and culture on surgical material, catheter and device (pacemaker, defibrillator…) or embolus samples.

Negative blood culture	
Frequently	Constantly: bacteria intracellular
Fastidious Gram-negative bacilli of HACEK group Nutritionally variant streptococci Brucella Fungi	Coxiella burnetii Bartonella Chlamydia Trophynema whipplei

Table 3. Microorganisms and negative blood culture. HACEK group: Haemophilus (parainfluenzae, aphrophilus, paraphrophilus and influenza), Actinobacillus actinomycetemcomitans, Cardiobacterium hominis, Eikenella corrodens, Kingella (kingae and dentrificans).

- Rheumatoid factor is an immunological phenomenon, not specific but found in 5% of IE (Murdoch, 2009).

4.2.2 Histologic findings

Valvular histology after cardiac surgery is the gold standard for diagnosis of IE and observed vegetations, microorganisms and/or valvular inflammation (Greub, 2005).

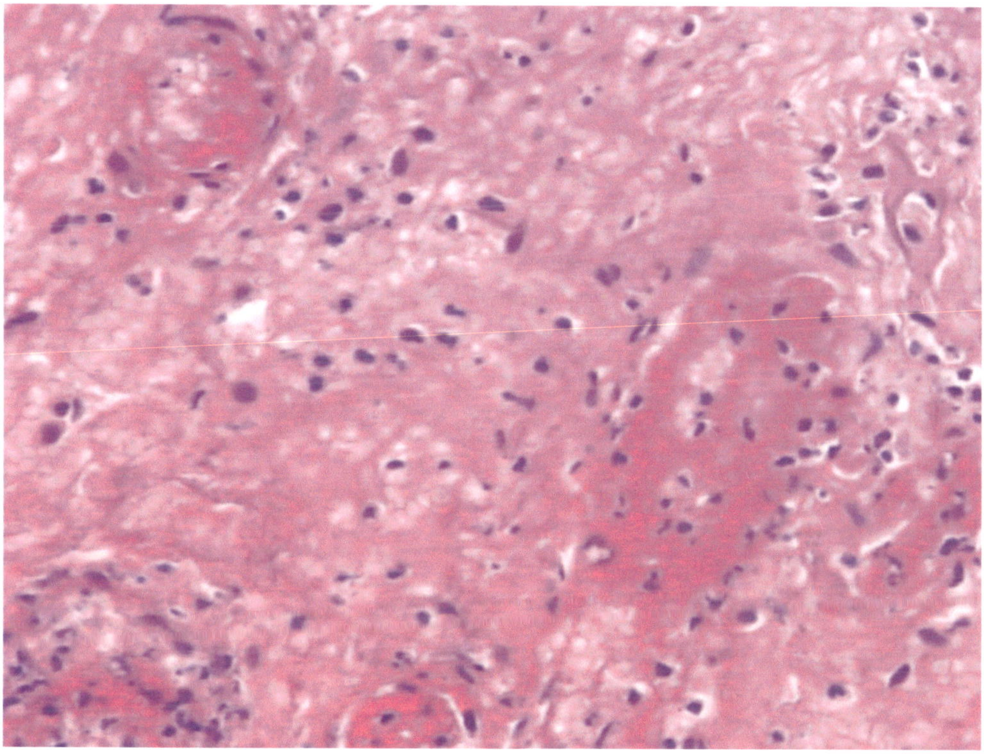

Fig. 4. Cutaneous leucocytoclastic vasculitis (H&E stain; x200).

Kidney fragments can reveal different unspecific lesions including glomerulonephritis or interstitial lesions.

Skin biopsies for histological study are often performed. Osler's nodes are classically explained by immune complex deposition, mainly responsible of leucocytoclastic vasculitis. Janeway lesions are associated with septic emboli, however, all histological findings can be observed in both lesions (Cardullo, 1990; Kerr, 1979; Loewe, 2009; Espinosa Parra, 2002).

4.3 Imaging studies

4.3.1 Echocardiography

Echocardiography is the second fundamental examination for IE diagnosis and its heart complications. In first-line, transthoracic echocardiography (TTE) must be systematically performed in case of suspicion. Its sensibility only ranges from 40 to 63%. So, in cases with negative examination, poor quality of the exam, prosthetic valve… transoesophageal echocardiography (TEE) is recommended if there is high clinical suspicion. In the other cases, a second echocardiography must be performed 7-10 days later if suspicion remains (ESC, 2009). Evocative signs of IE are vegetations (mobile echogenic masses implanted in the endothelium in the trajectory of valvular regurgitation or implanted in prosthetic material), abscess and new dehiscence of a valvular prosthesis (Evangelista, 2004). However, echocardiography does not permit differentiation between septic and aseptic vegetations; so lesions persisting after effective treatment must not be interpreted as a clinical recurrence of the disease unless supported by clinical features and bacteriological evidence.

Echocardiography is repeated as soon as new complications are suspected or at completion of antibiotic therapy for evaluation of cardiac and valve function.

4.3.2 Other imaging

Computed tomography can be used in second intention to diagnose (good evaluation of valvular abnormalities) IE (Feuchtner, 2009) and its systemic complications.

Magnetic resonance imaging is also useful for detection of complications such as cerebral emboli.

4.4 Duke criteria

Various manifestations of IE exist and diagnosis is often difficult. Therefore, the Duke criteria combining clinical and biological criteria have been proposed (Table 4) (Li, 1999).

5. Differential diagnoses

IE is an insidious disease associated with a clinical polymorphism. Differential diagnoses are multiple and it is impossible to give an exhaustive list. Suspicion of IE must be systematically discussed in cases of unexplained fever until proof of contrary. Note echocardiographic differential diagnoses: aseptic vegetations in Libman-Sacks endocarditis (in systemic lupus erythematosus and antiphospholipid syndrome) and marantic endocarditis associated with gastric and pulmonary adenocarcinoma.

6. Severe complications

6.1 Morbidity

6.1.1 Heart complications

Heart failure is the most frequent complication (50 to 60% of IE) mainly on aortic native valve IE (29%). It can be explained by valve insufficiency after native valve destruction causing acute regurgitation (chordal rupture, leaflet rupture or perforation) or prosthesis dehiscence. Other causes of heart failure include intracardiac fistulae, myocarditis, pericarditis (in *S. aureus* infection mainly) or valve obstruction by big vegetations. Surgery is often indicated (Table 5) in emergency because this complication is the worst predictive factor of in-hospital and 6-month mortality.

Definition of term used				
Pathologic criteria	**Microorganisms** demonstrated by culture or histologic examination of a vegetation, a vegetation that has embolized, or an intracardiac abscess specimen			
	Pathologic lesions showing active IE: vegetation or intracardiac abscess confirmed by histologic examination			
Clinical criteria	Major criteria	**Blood culture positive for IE**	Typical microorganisms consistent with IE from 2 separate blood culture	• Viridans streptococci • *Streptococcus bovis* • HACEK group • *Staphylococcus aureus* • Community-acquired enteroccoci in the absence of a primary focus
			Microorganisms consistent with IE from persistently positive blood culture	At least 2 positive cultures of blood samples drawn > 12h apart
				All of 3 or a majority of ≥ 4 separate cultures of blood (with first and last sample drawn at least 1h apart)
			Single positive blood culture for *Coxiella burnettii* or antiphase I IgG antibody titer >1:800	
		Evidence of endobacterial involvment	Echocardiogram positive for IE TEE recommended in patients with prosthetic valves rated at least "possible IE" by clinical criteria or complicated IE (paravalvular abscess) TTE as first test in others patients	Oscillating intracardiac mass on valve or supporting structures in the path of regurgitant jets or on implanted material in the absence of an alternative anatomic explanation
				Abscess
				New partial dehiscence of prosthetic valve
			New valvular regurgitation (worsening or changing of pre-existing murmur not sufficient)	
	Minor criteria	Predisposition, predisposing heart condition or injection drug use		
		Fever, temperature >38°C		
		Vascular phenomena, major arterial emboli, septic pulmonary infarcts, mycotic aneurysm, intracranial hemorrhages, Janeway's lesion		
		Immunologic phenomena: glomerulonephritis, Osler's nodes, Roth's spots, rheumatic factor		
		Microbiological evidence: positive blood culture but does not meet a major criterion, serological evidence of active infection with organism consistent with IE		

Definition of IE		
Definite IE	Pathologic criteria	≥1
	Clinical criteria	2 major criteria
		1 major + 3 minor criteria
		5 minor criteria
Possible IE	1 major + 1 minor criteria	
	3 minor criteria	
Rejected	Firm alternative diagnosis explaining evidence of IE	
	Resolution of IE syndrome with antibiotic therapy for ≤ 4 days	
	No pathologic evidence of IE at surgery or autopsy, with antibiotic therapy for ≤ 4 days	
	Does not meet criteria for possible IE as above	

Table 4. Modified Duke criteria (Li, 1999) (TEE: transesophageal echocardiography; TTE: transthoracic echocardiography)

Perivalvular complications should be suspected in case of persistent fever, unexplained or occurrence of atrioventricular block. They included abscess (most common in aortic and prosthesis IE), pseudoaneurysms, fistulae and signed uncontrolled infection. *Staphylococcus aureus* is most often implicated. Despite surgical treatment, 41% of patients die during hospitalization (ESC, 2009).

6.1.2 Uncontrolled infection

Resistant microorganisms, persisting systemic infection, other sites of infection, septic shock etc … can explain locally uncontrolled infection leading to acute coronary syndrome and third degree atrioventricular block. Indication of surgery should be discussed in these cases. Persisting fever, after 7-10 days of antibiotherapy, may discuss uncontrolled infection, adverse reaction to antibiotic, perivalvular complication, thrombosis, emboli… A complete infectious investigation with blood sample examination and intravenous line replacement and cultures, should be performed as well as echocardiography.

6.1.3 Systemic embolism

Migration of cardiac vegetations is responsible for systemic embolism (20-50% of IE) mainly in brain and spleen in left-sided IE and lung in native right-sided and pacemaker lead IE (ESC, 2009). However, all organs can be affected in case of patent foramen ovale. Embolisms are not uncommonly silent (20%) and often life-threatening. The incidence of embolic events increases during the first 2 weeks after the onset of antibiotherapy. Risk factors of embolism are individualized (Table 5) and prompt antibiotherapy can limit its occurrence (Thuny, 2005). Addition of antithrombotic therapy (thrombolytic drugs, anticoagulant or antiplatelet therapy) doesn't appear helpful in preventing whereas cardiac surgery during the first week of antibiotherapy (embolic risk peak) seems beneficial.

Risk factors of embolism		
Vegetation characteristics	Location	Mitral valve
		Multivalvular IE
	Size	>10mm
	Mobility	Increasing or decreasing under antibiotherapy
Microorganisms	Bacteria	Staphylococci
		Streptococcus bovis
	Fungi	*Candida spp*
Past history	Previous embolism	
Biology	Elevated C-reactive protein	

Table 5. Risk factors of embolism in IE (Durante Mangoni, 2003; ESC, 2009)

6.1.4 Neurological complications

Neurological damages after vegetation embolism are observed in 20 to 40 % of IE, mainly due to *Staphylococcus aureus* infection. These complications include stroke, infectious aneurysm (or mycotic aneurysm), brain abscess, meningitis, toxic encephalopathy and seizure and are associated with poor prognosis (mainly ischaemic or haemorragic strokes) (ESC, 2009; Thuny, 2007). Cerebral imaging (computed tomography or better magnetic resonance imaging) should be performed in the presence of neurological signs or headaches (infectious aneurysm).

Only poor neurological prognostic factors (coma, severe comorbidities and severe brain damage) can prohibit cardiac surgery (Table 5). In case of haemorragic stroke, cardiac surgery must be postponed for at least 1 month. In emergency cardiac situation, cooperation with neurosurgeon is mandatory. The best way to prevent these complications is to quickly start antibiotherapy (ESC, 2009).

For patients with previous antithrombotic treatment and in the absence of stroke, oral anticoagulant therapy should be replaced by unfractionned heparin for a period of 2 weeks, mainly in case of *S. aureus* IE (higher risk of bleeding). In case of an ischaemic stroke, the same schema of replacement is proposed. Anticoagulation has to be stopped in case of a haemorragic stroke and a mechanical valve; unfractionned heparin should be reinitiated as soon as possible. Previous antiplatelet therapy must be stopped only in the occurrence of major bleeding (ESC, 2009).

6.1.5 Metastatic infection

Infectious aneurysms (3% of IE) (AEPEI, 2002) are secondary to arterial septic embolism, mainly in the brain. Most of them are silent but rupture is associated with poor prognosis. No predicting factor has been individualized, however treatment (neurosurgery or endovascular surgery) is proposed in case of large, enlarging or already ruptured aneurysms. After specific antibiotherapy, most of unruptured infectious aneurysms resolve.

Systemic abscesses (other than cerebral) are rare and should be suspected in case of persistent fever and bacteremia. Clinical criteria and imaging investigation help to find the site of the infection s (tomography, ultrasound etc). Treatment can be completed by surgery or percutaneous drainage in case of partial response to antibiotics. All organs can be affected: spleen, bone (spondylodiscitis 3-15%) etc (ESC, 2009).

6.1.6 Renal complications

Acute renal failure is frequent (30%) but often reversible. Causes are multiple: glomerulonephritis by immune complex deposition, renal infarction, haemodynamic impairment and antibiotic or contrast agent toxicity (ESC, 2009).

6.1.7 Recurrences: Relapses and re-infections

Relapse is mainly observed after inadequate antibiotic treatment (insufficient duration, resistant microorganisms, empirical antibiotherapy in IE with negative blood culture) or persistent focus of infection. Conversely, re-infection is a new IE with different microorganism(s) and mainly includes patients with previous IE, intravenous drug abusers, prosthetic valve carriers and chronic dialysis patients. Re-infection increases risk of death and of valve surgery (ESC, 2009).

6.2 Mortality

In-hospital mortality varies from 9.6 to 26%. Prognosis is influenced by many factors (Table 6) but the mortality is higher (79%) in presence of heart failure associated with periannular complications and Staphylococcus infection (Chu, 2004; ESC, 2009). Operative mortality is also significant (16%) mainly in patients with prosthetic valves (Fayad, 2011).

Predictors of a poor prognostic			
Patient characteristics	Presence of complications	Microorganisms	Echocardiographic findings
- Older age - Prosthetic valve IE - Previous IE (= reinfection) - Insulin-dependent diabetes mellitus - Comorbidities	- Heart failure - Renal failure - Stroke - Septic chock - Periannular complications	- *S. aureus* - Fungi - Gram-negative bacilli	- Periannular complications - Severe left-side valve regurgitation - Low left-ventricular ejection fraction - Large vegetation - Severe prosthetic dysfunction - Premature mitral valve closure and other signs of elevated diastolic pressure

Table 6. Predictors factor of a poor prognosis in IE (ESC, 2009)

7. Treatment: Prolonged antimicrobial therapy and infectious source eradication

7.1 Medical treatment

Medical treatment should be started quickly after carrying out of bacteriological samples, in particular blood cultures (3 independent sets at 30 minutes intervals). Antimicrobial therapy is first empirical (Table 7) and as soon as possible, it is adapted to micro-organism sensitivity (ESC, 2009). In all the cases, this treatment should be prolongated for several weeks and toxicity should be followed-up. As soon as possible, portal of entry and complications should be found and treated. Symptomatic care is usual and classical.

7.2 Surgical treatment

Cardiac surgery is often necessary to treat or prevent complications or eradicate infectious sites (Table 8). Surgery is more frequently necessary in some types of IE such as native valve IE (87% of IE operated with 57% in aortic IE and 50% for mitral IE), Staphylococci and Streptococci IE (respectively 35 and 33% of IE operated) (Fayad, 2011).

With the exception of an emergency, extracardiac infections must be eradicated before surgery. Coronary angiography is also recommended in patients at risk (men older than 40, post-menopausal women, patients with at least one cardiovascular risk factor or a history of coronary disease) excluding emergency or cases with large aortic vegetation (risk of dislodgment during examination). Repair and replacement of the valve are possible but the last technique is preferred in complex cases. Intra operative transoesophageal echocardiography is precious to guide surgeons. The operative mortality is moderate (16%) and is more frequent with prosthetic valve carriers (ESC, 2009).

Characteristics of patient		Antibiotherapy suggested for adults patients		
		Association of antibiotics	Dosage	Duration (weeks)
• Native valve or • Prosthetic valve since more than 12 months		Ampicillin-sulbactam IV	12g/day (in 4 doses)	4-6
		Gentamicin IV or IM	3mg/kg/day (in 2 or 3 doses)	4-6
	Allergy to β-lactams	Vancomycin IV	30mg/kg/day (in 2 doses)	4-6
		Gentamicin IV or IM	3mg/kg/day (in 2 or 3 doses)	4-6
		Ciprofloxacin	1000 mg/day (in 2 doses) po or 800mg/day (in 2 doses) IV	4-6
Prosthetic valve since less than 12 months		Vancomycin IV	30mg/kg/day (in 2 doses)	6
		Gentamicin IV or IM	3mg/kg/day (in 2 or 3 doses)	2
		Rifampicin po	1200mg/day (in 2 doses)	2

Table 7. Proposed antibiotic regimens for initial empirical treatment (po: *per os*/ IM: intramuscular/ IV intravenous). Be careful with chronic use of gentamicin and vancomycin. Serum levels of these antibiotics should be measured once a week for both and additional renal function testing should be performed for gentamicin.

7.3 Follow-up

Complications are usual and should be searched for regularly. This requires a daily clinical examination during the first weeks. Electrocardiogram should be performed frequently (mainly in aortic or prosthesis IE) looking for new atrioventricular block or ischemia signs. Bacteriological samples should be analyzed until their negativity. Heart failure and death can occur after several months, so echocardiography is recommended in case of cardiological signs but also after antibiotic treatment and should be repeated regularly during the first year (at 1, 3, 6 and 12 months) (ESC, 2009).

Recurrence is frequent. Consequently, patients should be informed about this risk and prevention rules should be applied closely.

8. Prevention

8.1 Antibiotic prophylaxis

In recent years, antibiotic prophylaxis has become more and more limited. In fact, no antibiotic permit disappearance of bacteremia after at-risk at-risk procedures. Until now, no study has proven the benefit of prophylactic treatment in the prevention of IE. At present, only antibiotic prophylaxis is recommended by ESC (ESC, 2009) for highest risk dental procedures in patients with highest risk cardiac conditions (Table 9). AHA (AHA, 2007) also recommends antibiotic prophylaxis for procedures on the respiratory tract or on infected skin in patients with highest risk of IE. Prophylaxis is associated with a small risk of death by anaphylaxis but no case has been reported to date and the main risk is microbial resistance development.

<table>
<tr><th colspan="3" rowspan="2">Indica-tions</th><th colspan="3">Location of IE</th></tr>
<tr><th>Left-sided native valve IE</th><th>Prosthetic valve IE (PVE)</th><th>Right-sided IE</th></tr>
<tr><td rowspan="8">Heart complications</td><td rowspan="8">Heart failure</td><td rowspan="6">+</td><td>Severe acute regurgitation or valve obstruction causing refractory oedema pulmonary or cardiogenic shock</td><td>Severe prosthetic dysfunction (dehiscence or obstruction)</td><td rowspan="6">Right heart failure secondary to severe tricuspid regurgitation with poor response to diuretic therapy</td></tr>
<tr><td>Emergency</td><td>Emergency</td></tr>
<tr><td colspan="2">Fistula into a cardiac chamber or pericardium causing refractory pulmonary oedema or shock</td></tr>
<tr><td colspan="2">Emergency</td></tr>
<tr><td>Severe acute regurgitation or valve obstruction and persisting heart failure or echocardiographic signs of poor haemodynamic tolerance (early mitral closure or pulmonary hypertension)</td><td>Severe prosthetic dysfunction and persisting heart failure</td></tr>
<tr><td>Urgent</td><td>Urgent</td></tr>
<tr><td rowspan="2">-</td><td>Severe regurgitation and no heart failure</td><td>Severe prosthetic dehiscence without heart cardiac</td><td rowspan="2"></td></tr>
<tr><td>Elective</td><td>Elective</td></tr>
<tr><td colspan="3" rowspan="8">Uncontrolled infection</td><td colspan="2">Locally uncontrolled infection (abscess, false aneurysm, fistula, enlarging vegetation)</td><td rowspan="8">Microorganisms difficult to eradicate (persistent fungi…) or bacteremia for > 7 days (S. aureus, P. aeruginosa…)</td></tr>
<tr><td colspan="2">Urgent</td></tr>
<tr><td colspan="2">Persisting fever and positive blood cultures > 7-10 days</td></tr>
<tr><td colspan="2">Urgent</td></tr>
<tr><td colspan="2">Fungi or multiresistant organisms</td></tr>
<tr><td colspan="2">Urgent / Elective</td></tr>
<tr><td rowspan="2"></td><td>Staphylococci or Gram negative bacteria (most of cases of early PVE)</td></tr>
<tr><td>Urgent/Elective</td></tr>
<tr><td colspan="3" rowspan="6">Prevention of embolism</td><td>Large vegetation (>10mm) following one or more embolic episodes despite appropriate antibiotic therapy</td><td>Recurrent emboli despite appropriate antibiotic treatment</td><td rowspan="6">Persistent tricuspid valve vegetation > 20mm after recurrent pulmonary emboli with or without concomitant heart failure</td></tr>
<tr><td>Urgent</td><td>Urgent</td></tr>
<tr><td colspan="2">Large vegetation (>10mm) and other predictors of complicated course
(heart failure, persistent infection, abscess)</td></tr>
<tr><td colspan="2">Urgent</td></tr>
<tr><td colspan="2">Isolated very large vegetation (>15mm)</td></tr>
<tr><td colspan="2">Urgent</td></tr>
</table>

Table 8. Indications and timing of surgery (ESC, 2009). Emergency: within 24 hours. Urgent: within a few days. Elective: after 1 -2 weeks of antibiotic treatment.

<table>
<tr><th>Cardiac conditions at highest risk of IE</th><th colspan="2">Dental procedures at high risk</th></tr>
<tr><td rowspan="4">• Prosthetic cardiac valve or material used for cardiac valve repair
• Previous IE
• Some congenital heart disease (CHD)
  • Cyanotic CHD
- without surgical repair or
- with residual defects, palliative shunts or conduits
  • CHD with complete repair with prosthetic material whether placed by surgery or by cutaneous technique, up to 6 months after the procedure
  • CHD when a residual defect persists at the site of implantation of a prosthetic material or device by cardiac surgery or percutaneous technique</td><td colspan="2">• Manipulation of gingival region
• Manipulation of periapical region of the teeth
• Perforation of oral mucosa</td></tr>
<tr><td colspan="2">Antibiotic prophylaxis</td></tr>
<tr><td colspan="2">Single dose 30-60 minutes before procedure</td></tr>
<tr><td>• Adults
  • Amoxicillin 2g po or IV
  • If allergy: Clindamycin 600mg po or IV</td><td>• Children
  • Amoxicillin 50mg/kg po or IV
  • If allergy: Clindamycin 20mg/kg po or IV</td></tr>
</table>

Table 9. Recommendations for antibiotic prophylaxis of IE for patients undergoing dental procedures (ESC, 2009) (po: *per os*/ IV: intravenous)

8.2 Hygienic rules

Most IE occurs without history of procedure more at-risk situation of bacteremia (Strom, 1998).

Daily activities like chewing or tooth brushing carry transient but significant bacteremia and can cause IE (AHA, 2007). Consequently, it is recommended to maintain a good oral hygiene for all population.

For patients and drug users, disposable intravenous material is mandatory.

8.3 Others rules

In medical practice, percutaneous iatrogenic procedures should be avoided especially on skin injuries and topical corticosteroid should be used with caution. Regular bacteriological skin analysis is recommended during the follow-up of erosive dermatosis because it allows quick adapted antibiotherapy in the case of secondarily advent IE. Of course, all prospective portals of entry and all comorbidities have to be searched and supported.

9. Conclusion

Infective endocarditis (IE) is a severe disease the diagnosis of which remains difficult due to clinical polymorphism and frequent insidious evolution over several days or months. Skin manifestations are very useful for diagnosis but should alert practitioners for presence of embolic complications. Epidemiologic profile of IE has changed in recent years and so has prophylactic and therapeutic recommendations. IE concerns all practitioners and we have to keep it in mind with any patient.

10. Acknowledgment

Thank you to Pr Olivier Chosidow (Department of dermatology, Hôpital Henri Mondor, Créteil; France) and Dr Nicolas Ortonne (Department of pathology, Hôpital Henri Mondor, Créteil; France) for histological pictures.

11. References

Cardullo, AC.; Silvers, DN. & Grossman, ME. (1990). Janeway lesions and Osler's nodes: a review of histopathologic findings. *J Am Acad Dermatol,* Vol.22, No.6, (June 1990), pp. 1088-90, ISSN 2370335

Chu, VH. et al (2004). Early predictors of in-hospital death in infective endocarditis. *Circulation,* Vol.109, No.14, (March 2004), pp. 1745-9, ISSN 1503 7538

Durante Mangoni, E. et al (2003). Risk factors for "major" embolic events in hospitalized patients with infective endocarditis. *Am Heart J,* Vol.146, No.2, (August 2003), pp. 311-6, ISSN 1289 1201

Espinosa Parra, FJ. et al (2002). Diagnostic utility of Osler's nodules in infectious endocarditis among parenteral drug users. *An Med Interna,* Vol. 19, No.6, (June 2002), pp. 299-301, ISSN 1215 2389

Evangelista, A. & Gonzalez-Alujas, MT. (2004). Echocardiography in infective endocarditis. *Heart,* Vol.90, No.6, (June 2004), pp. 614-7, ISSN 1514 5856

Farrior, JB. & Silverman, ME. (1976). A consideration of the differences between a Janeway's lesion and an Osler's node in infectious endocarditis. *Chest,* Vol.70, No.2, (August 1976), pp. 239-43, ISSN 947688

Fayad, G. et al (2011). Characteristics and prognosis of patients requiring valve surgery during active infective endocarditis. *J Heart Valve Dis,* Vol.20, No.2 (March 2011), pp. 223-8, ISSN 2156 0826

Feuchtner, GM. et al (2009). Multislice computed tomography in infective endocarditis: comparison with transesophageal echocardiography and intraoperative findings. *J Am Coll Cardiol,* Vol.53, No.5, (February 2009), pp. 436-44, ISSN 1917 9202

García-Porrúa, C. & González-Gay, MA. (1999). Bacterial infection presenting as cutaneous vasculitis in adults. *Clin Exp Rheumatol,* Vol.17, No.4, (July 1999), pp. 471-3, ISSN 1046 4561

Greub, G. et al (2005). Diagnosis of infectious endocarditis in patients undergoing valve surgery. *Am J Med,* Vol.118,No.3, (March 2005), pp. 230-8, ISSN 1574 5720

Habib, G. et al; ESC Committee for Practice Guidelines (2009). Guidelines on the prevention, diagnosis, and treatment of infective endocarditis (new version 2009): the Task Force on the Prevention, Diagnosis, and Treatment of Infective Endocarditis of the European Society of Cardiology (ESC). Endorsed by the European Society of Clinical Microbiology and Infectious Diseases (ESCMID) and the International Society of Chemotherapy (ISC) for Infection and Cancer. *Eur Heart J* , Vol.30, No.19, (October 2009), pp. 2369-413, ISSN 1971 3420

Heffner, JE. (1979). Extracardiac manifestations of bacterial endocarditis. *West J Med*, Vol.131, No.2, (August 1979), pp. 85-91, ISSN 516715

Hoen, B. et al; Association pour l'Etude et la Prévention de l'Endocardite Infectieuse (AEPEI) Study Group (2002).Changing profile of infective endocarditis: results of a 1-year survey in France. *JAMA*, Vol.288, No.1, (July 2002), pp. 75-81, ISSN 1209 0865

Kerr, A Jr. & Tan, JS. (1979). Biopsies of the Janeway lesion of infective endocarditis. J Cutan Pathol, Vol.6, No.2, (April 1979), pp. 124-9, ISSN 479431

Konstantinou, MP. et al (2009). Infective endocarditis in dermatological unit. Ann Dermatol Venereol, Vol.136, No.12, (December 2009), pp. 869-75, ISSN 2000 4311

Lévesque, H. & Marie, I. (1999). Infection and vascular purpura. *J Mal Vasc*, Vol.24, No.3, (June 1999), pp. 177-82, ISSN 1046 7526

Li, JS. et al (2000). Proposed modifications to the Duke criteria for the diagnosis of infective endocarditis. *Clin Infect Dis*, Vol.30, No.4, (April 2000), pp. 633-8, ISSN 1077 0721

Loewe, R.; Gattringer, KB. & Petzelbauer, P. (2009). Janeway lesions with inconspicuous histological features. *J Cutan Pathol*, Vol.36, No.10, (October 2009), pp. 1095-8, ISSN 1918 7106

Martínez-Marcos, FJ. et al; Grupo para el Estudio de las Infecciones Cardiovasculares de la Sociedad Andaluza de Enfermedades Infecciosas (2009). Enterococcal endocarditis: a multicenter study of 76 cases. *Enferm Infecc Microbiol Clin*, Vol.27, No.10, (December 2009), pp. 571-9, ISSN 1947 7041

Miro, JM. et al; International Collaboration on Endocarditis Merged Database Study Group (2005). Staphylococcus aureus native valve infective endocarditis: report of 566 episodes from the International Collaboration on Endocarditis Merged Database. *Clin Infect Dis*, Vol.41, No.4, (August 2005), pp. 507-14, ISSN 1602 8160

Moreillon, P. & Que, YA. (2004) Infective endocarditis. *Lancet*, Vol.363, No.9403, (January 2004), pp. 139-49, ISSN 1472 6169

Murdoch, DR. et al; International Collaboration on Endocarditis-Prospective Cohort Study (ICE-PCS) Investigators(2009). Clinical presentation, etiology, and outcome of infective endocarditis in the 21st century: the International Collaboration on Endocarditis-Prospective Cohort Study. *Arch Intern Med, Vol. 169, No.5, (March* 2009), pp. 463-73, ISSN 1927 3776

Phillips, KT. & Stein, MD (2010). Risk practices associated with bacterial infections among injection drug users in Denver, Colorado. *Am J Drug Alcohol Abuse*, Vol.36, No.2, (March 2010), pp. 92-7, ISSN2033 7504

Que, YA. & Moreillon, P. (2011). *Infective endocarditis. Nat Rev Cardiol*, Vol.8, No.6, (June 2011), pp. 322-36, ISSN 2148 7430

Rasmussen, RV. et al (2011). Prevalence of infective endocarditis in patients with Staphylococcus aureus bacteraemia: the value of screening with echocardiography. *Eur J Echocardiogr*, Vol.12, No.6, (June 2011), pp. 414-20, ISSN 2168 5200

Strom, BL. et al (1998). Dental and cardiac risk factors for infective endocarditis. A population-based, case-control study. *Ann Intern Med*, Vol.129, No.10, (November 1998),pp. 761-9, ISSN9841581

Strom, BL. et al (2000). Risk factors for infective endocarditis: oral hygiene and nondental exposures. *Circulation*, Vol.102, No.23, (December 2000), pp. 2842-8, ISSN 1110 4742

Thuny, F.et al. (2005). Risk of embolism and death in infective endocarditis: prognostic value of echocardiography: a prospective multicenter study. *Circulation*, Vol.112, No.1, (July 2005), pp. 69-75, ISSN .1598 3252

Thuny, F.et al. (2007). Impact of cerebrovascular complications on mortality and neurologic outcome during infective endocarditis: a prospective multicentre study. *Eur Heart J*, Vol.28, No.9, (May 2007), pp. 1155-61. ISSN 1736 3448

Tornos, P. et al (2005). Infective endocarditis in Europe: lessons from the Euro heart survey. *Heart*, Vol.91, No.5, (May 2005), pp. 571-5, ISSN 1583 1635

Wilson, W. et al; American Heart Association Rheumatic Fever, Endocarditis and Kawasaki Disease Committee, Council on Cardiovascular Disease in the Young; Council on Clinical Cardiology; Council on Cardiovascular Surgery and Anesthesia; Quality of Care and Outcomes Research Interdisciplinary Working Group; American Dental Association (2007). Prevention of infective endocarditis: guidelines from the American Heart Association: a guideline from the American Heart Association Rheumatic Fever, Endocarditis and Kawasaki Disease Committee, Council on Cardiovascular Disease in the Young, and the Council on Clinical Cardiology, Council on Cardiovascular Surgery and Anesthesia, and the Quality of Care and Outcomes Research Interdisciplinary Working Group. *J Am Dent Assoc*, Vol.138, No.6, (June 2007), pp. 739-45 and 747-60, ISSN 1754 5263

18

Cardiovascular Risk Factors: Implications in Diabetes, Other Disease States and Herbal Drugs

Steve Ogbonnia
Department of Pharmacognosy,
University of Lagos, Lagos,
Nigeria

1. Introduction

The danger and the increasing prevalence of heart diseases world wide are now of a great concern and are attributed to the cardiovascular risk factors. Cardiovascular risk factors have been identified to be the underlying latent or potent causes of death in all heart diseases and also in many other disease states such as diabetes. Reduction in the risk factors with synthetic drugs or drugs of natural products origin in the course of treatment of some disease states where implicated has been found to improve tremendously the health of the patient.

Cardiovascular risk factors include triacylglycerols (triglycerides), cholesterol, cholesteryl esters, very low density lipoprotein–cholesterol (VLDL-c), low density lipoprotein-cholesterol (LDL-c), and anti-athrogenic high density lipoprotein–cholesterol (HDL-c) and are collectively referred to as plasma lipids. An increase in plasma lipids concentrations beyond certain level give rise to physiological condition known as "Hyperlipidemia". Hyperlipidemia is, therefore, characterized by abnormal elevation in plasma triglyceride, cholesterol and low density lipoprotein-cholesterol (LDL-c) and very low lipoprotein - cholesterol (VLDL-c) and has also been reported to be the most prevalent indicator for susceptibility to atherosclerotic heart disease (Maruthapan and Shree, 2010). Managing cardiovascular disease states, therefore, requires drugs that would be capable of lowering blood plasma lipids in order to reduce mortality and morbidity associated with the cardiovascular complications (Hasimun et al., 2011). It has been reported in epidemiological studies that a strong positive correlation exists between increase in the blood cholesterol level and incidence of cardiovascular heart disease (CHD) (Hamed et al., 2010; Imafidon 2010; Maruthapana and Shree 2010), and also increase in the incidence of atherosclerosis(Hasimun et al., 2011). A strong relationship between increase in C-reactive protein (CRP) and cardiovascular risk factors has also been reported as well as increase in myocardial infection and coronary artery disease among individuals with angina pectoris (Ghayour –Mobarhan et al. 2007).

Atherosclerosis arises from the deposition of fatty substances, cellular waste products, calcium and fibrin in the arteries, resulting in clotting (Lewis et al., 2002) and is considered one of the major causes of coronary heart disease. It is recognized as a common threat to life, usually seen in individuals consuming high quantities of cholesterol and saturated fats in their diets. It has also been established in animal studies that raising dietary cholesterol alone could increase atherosclerosis susceptibility (Madhumathi et al., 2006). Atherosclerosis is characterized by endothelia dysfunction, muscular inflammation resulting from build up of plasma lipids which tantamount to vascular remodeling, acute and chronic luminal obstruction, abnormalities in the blood flow and diminished oxygen supplies to target organs (Madhumathi et al., 2006). The development of atherosclerosis could also be attributed to other factors such as oxidative stress which is responsible for the oxidation of low-density lipoprotein-cholesterol (LDL-c) and is considered as one of the first steps of atherosclerotic pathogenesis. Local inflammatory processes have also been identified to play a crucial role in the transition from reversible accumulation of cholesterol in the arterial wall to irreversible damage of the arteries (Brunner-La Rocca1, et al., 2005). Many factors contributing to etiology of atherosclerosis in addition to diet include diabetes mellitus, psychological factors and the presence of glucocorticoids.

Diabetes mellitus (DM) is a major degenerative disease in the world today afflicting many lives both in the developed and developing countries (Ogbonnia et al., 2011). It has been succinctly described as the common metabolic disorder of carbohydrate and fat metabolism, which is due to absolute or relative lack of insulin and is characterized by hyperglycaemia and hyperlipidemia (Sharon and Marvin, 1975; Walter, 1977). Diabetes is a multiple disease state and has been defined as "a state of premature cardiovascular death that is associated with chronic hyperglycemia and also associated with blindness and renal failure" (Fisher and Shaw, 2001). This assertion was to draw attention and to encourage multiple clinical approaches that would altogether help reduce cardiovascular risk factors in diabetic patients (Ogbonnia et al., 2011). Diabetes especially the type 2 model might be postulated to occur primarily due to underlying abnormality of insulin resistance - that is resistance of the body to the biological actions of insulin. The consequences of insulin resistance lead to hyperinsulinaemia and are associated with CRFs - dyslipidaemia including athrogenic lipid profile with increase in low and very-low density lipoprotein-cholesterols (LDL-c and VLDL-c) and reduction in the anti-athrogenic high density lipoprotein-cholesterol (HDL-c). Cardiovascular risk factors have been implicated and even occur at a frequency much higher than expected in some other disease states such as benign prostatic hyperplasia (BPH). Benign prostatic hyperplasia is a neoplastic enlargement of the prostate gland and is common in elderly men (Ejike and Ezeanyika, 2010). Epidemiological studies have demonstrated that many of the risk factors associated with cardiovascular diseases are the same as found in BPH (Dharmananda, 2011), and these risk factors include obesity, hypertension and diabetes. The diabetes connection may be considered very strong and the risk centers on the non-insulin dependent diabetes mellitus (NIDDM) which most often involves excessive insulin levels, a possible direct contributor to the growth of the prostrate (Hammarten and Hogstedt, 2011). The treatment of BPH became a medical issue mainly in 1970s at the same time that the cardiovascular disease therapy came to fore and the incidence of the disease has become higher (Dharmananda, 2011). Herbal or phytomedicines are now being investigated with some recorded successes for the management of cardiovascular risk factors with the accompanied disease states. Herbal remedies with active components understood to be sterols, such as beta-sitosterol has been used as a therapeutic agent for BPH (Bombardelli and Morazzoni, 1997).

2. Cardiovascular risk factors

Cardiovascular risk factors consisting mostly of plasma lipids including triacylglycerol (triglycerides), cholesteryl esters and cholesterol are synthesized by the liver and adipose tissues and may also be absorbed from the diet (Stryer, 1988). They are also efficiently synthesized from carbohydrate diets largely in the intestinal epithelia tissues in addition to the liver (Metzler, 1974), and are transported between various tissues and organs for utilization and storage. These plasma lipids like other lipids are generally insoluble in water and pose a transportation problem in aqueous blood plasma. This problem is overcome by associating the nonpolar lipids comprising triacylglycerol (triglycerides) and cholesteryl esters with amphipatic lipids such as phospholipids, cholesterol and proteins to produce water-miscible lipoproteins (Conn and Stumpf, 1976; Stryer, 1988). A lipoprotein is a particle consisting of core hydrophobic lipids surrounded by a shell of polar lipid and apoprotein and mediates the cycle by transporting lipids from the intestine as chylomicrons - and from the liver as very low density lipoproteins-cholesterol (VLDL-c) - to most tissues for oxidation and to adipose tissue for storage. Lipoproteins are grouped according to increasing densities by centrifugation as follow:

i. Chylomicrons which incorporate intestinal absorbed triacylglycerol from intestinal absorption of triacylglycerol and other lipids.
ii. Very low density lipoprotein-cholesterol (VLDL-c, or pre – β- Lipoprotein), are derived from the combination of newly synthesized triacylglycerol together with small amounts of phospholipids and cholesterol and apolipoproteins all synthesized in the liver (Stryer, 1988).
iii. Intermediate density lipoprotein (IDL)
iv. Low density lipoprotein-cholesterol (LDL-c) (LDL-c or β-Lipoproteins), representing a final stage in the catabolism of VLDL-c, and

High density lipoproteins-cholesterol (HDL-c, or α-Lipoproteins), involved in cholesterol transport and also in VLDL-c and chylomicron metabolism.

Major groups of lipoproteins have been identified to be physiologically important and are used in clinical diagnosis. The primary role of LDL-c appears to be the transport of esterified cholesterol to tissue while that of the high density lipoproteins-cholesterol (HDL-c) is to carry excess cholesterol away from most tissues to the liver. The size of the lipoprotein particles also varies from a 200 – to 500 –nm diameter for chylomicrons to as little as 5 nm for the smallest HDL particles (Metzler, 1974).

Lipoprotein is made up of triacylglycerol (16%) which is the predominant lipid in chylomicrons and VLDL-c, while phosholipids (30%) and cholesterol (14%) are the predominant lipids of HDL c and LDL-c respectively and cholesterol esters (36%) (Stryer, 1988). It also contains much smaller fraction of unesterified long chain fatty acids (free fatty acids) which are metabolically the most active of plasma lipids. These constitute what is collectively known as 'Cardiovascular Risk Factors' which are implicated in many disease states as potent or latent causes of death. Lipoproteins may be separated according to their electrophoretic properties into: α-, β-, and pre -β- Lipoproteins (Holme and Peck, 1998).

The protein moiety of a lipoprotein is known as apolipoprotein or apoprotein constituting nearly 70% of HDL-c and as little as 1% of chylomicrons. Some apolipoproteins are integral and can not be removed, whereas others are free to transfer to other lipoprotiens. Seven principal apoprotein, A – 1, A – 2, A – 4, B – 48, B – 100, C and E have been isolated and characterized. They are synthesized and secreted by the liver and the intestine and generally have two principal roles: they solubilize highly hydrophobic lipid and also they contain signals that regulate the movement of particular lipid into and out of specific target cells and tissues.

Lipoprotein	Source/major core lipid	Diameter (nm)	Density (g/mL)	Composition	Main Lipid Components		Mechanism of lipid delivery
				Protein (%)	Lipid (%)	< 0.95	
Chylomicrons	Dietary triacylglycerol Intestine	90-1000	< 0.95	1-2	98-99	< 1.006	Hydrolysis by lipoprotein lipase
Chylomicrons remnants	Dietary cholesterol esters Chylomicrons	45-150	< 1.006	6-8	92-94	0.95-1.006	Receptor-mediated endocytosis by liver
VLDL	Endogenous triacylglycerols Liver (Intestine)	30-90	0.95-1.006	7-10	90-93	1.006-1.019	Hydrolysis by liproprotein lipase
IDL	Endogenous cholesterol esters VLDL	25-35	1.006-1.019	11	89	1.019-1.063	Receptor-mediated endocytosis by liver and conversion to LDL
LDL	Endogenous cholesterol esters VLDL	20-25	1.019-1.063	21	79		Receptor-mediated endocytosis by liver and other tissues
	Endogenous cholesterol esters						Transfer of cholesterol esters to IDL and LDL

Table 1. Composition of the Lipoproteins in plasma of humans.

Each apolipoproteins carry out one or more distinct roles.

i. The apo B, stabilizes lipoproteins micelles and as the sole protein of LDL-c serves the function of solubilizing cholesterol within LDL-c complex which in turn increases the transport capacity of LDL-c for subsequent deposit on arterial wall (Madhumathi et al., 2006).
ii. They are enzyme cofactors. The apoC-II has specific function of activating the lipoprotein lipase that hydrolyses triacylglycerols of chylomicrons and VLDL. Lack of either C-II or the lipase results in a very high level of triacylglycerol in the blood.
iii. They act as ligands for interaction with lipoprotein receptors in tissues, e.g apoB-100 and apo E for the LDL receptors, apo E for the LDL receptor– related protein (LRP) which has been identified as the remnant receptor, and apo A-1 for the HDL-c receptor. The function of Apo A-IV and apo D, however, are not yet clearly defined, although apo D, is believed to be an important factor in human neurodegenerative disorders.

2.1 Cholesterol

Cholesterol is physiologically very essential for all animal life, and is primarily synthesized from simpler substances within the body. It is an amphipathic waxy steroid of fat that is manufactured in the liver or intestines. It constitutes essentially structural component of membrane required in establishing proper membrane permeability and fluidity and is also a constituent of the outer layer of plasma lipoproteins. Cholesterol is the principal sterol synthesized by animals and transported in the blood plasma of all mammals (Leah, 2009). It is also an important component implicated in the manufacture of bile acids, steroid hormones, and vitamin D (Jain, 2005; Maxifield and Tabas, 2005; Hasimun, 2011). The hydroxyl group on cholesterol interacts with the polar head groups of the membrane phospholipids and sphingolipids, while the bulky steroid and the hydrocarbon chain are embedded in the membrane, alongside the nonpolar fatty acid chain of the other lipids. In this structural form, cholesterol reduces the permeability of the plasma membrane to protons (positive hydrogen ions) and sodium ions.

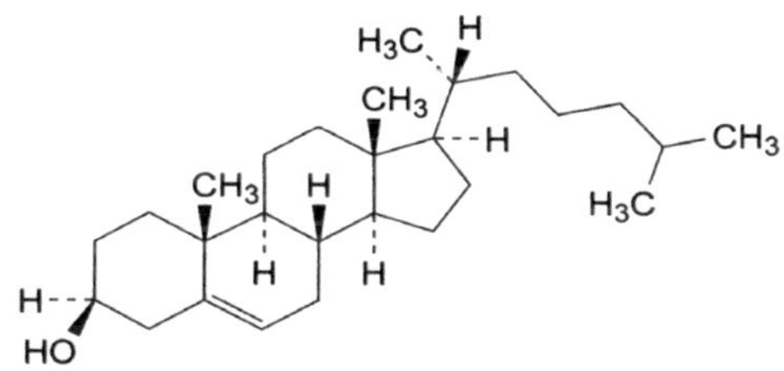

Fig. 1. Chemical structure of cholesterol

Most cholesterol is carried in the blood by low density lipoprotein (LDL), which delivers it directly to cells where it is needed. Both a 74-kDa cholesteryl ester transfer protein and a phospholipid transfer protein are also involved in this process. Cholesterol esterases, which release free cholesterol, may act both on lipoproteins and on pancreatic secretions. The LDL-cholesterol complex binds to LDL receptors on the cell surfaces. These receptors are specific for apolipoprotein B-100 present in the LDL. The occupied LDL-receptor complexes are taken up by endocytosis through coated pits; the apolipoproteins are degraded in lysosomes, while the cholesteryl esters are released and cleaved by a specific lysosomal acid lipase to form free cholesterol.

Animal fats are complex mixtures of triglycerides, with fewer amounts of phospholipids and cholesterol. As a consequence all food containing animal fats contain cholesterol to varying extent. Plasma cholesterol concentration elevation is, therefore ,one of the important CRFs as its transportation within lipoprotein is affected and is strongly associated with progression of atherosclerosis.

2.2 Triacylglycerols

Triacylglycerols (figure 2b see the figure below) serve as biochemical energy reserves in the cell and may be oxidized in the liver to provide energy or deposited as depot fat in characteristic regions of the animal where they act as a long-term food store and insulator (Plummer, 1998). They are the neutral and saponifiable lipids found in most organisms. Triacylglycerols (triglycerides) which are chemically fatty acid esters of the trihydroxy alcohol, glycerol (Figure 2a), are compounds that usually make up the bulk of ingested lipids and are transported to the blood via the lymphatic system in the form of chylomicrons. Triacylglycerols synthesized endogenously as against those obtained from the diet, are carried by VLDL produced primarily by the liver (Styer, 1988). Studies have suggested that triacylglycerol (TG)-rich lipoprotein(TRL) plays an important role in the development of atherosclerosis because both coronary artery disease and myocardial infarction have been associated with abnormal postprandial lipoprotein pattern (Moreno-Luna et al., 2007)

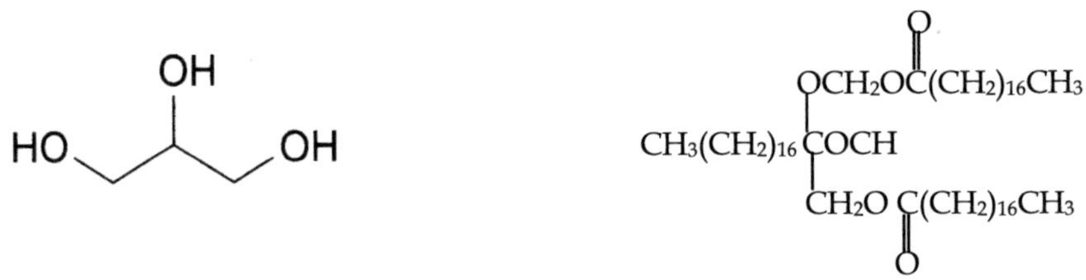

A triacylglycerol (Tristearin)

(a) (b)

Fig. 2. (a) Chemical structure of cholesterol (b) chemical structure of triacylglycerol

Most of the fatty acids synthesized or ingested by an organism are either transformed into triacylgylcerols and stored for metabolism to give energy or incorporated into phospholipids components of the membrane. Triacylgylcerols have as precursor fatty acyl-CoAs and glycerol-β-phosphate but many enzymatic steps are involved in their biosynthesis in animal tissues. Although the triglycerides have been found to be important predictors of CVD in many studies, no clinical trial data has established that lowering triglycerides in individuals with or without diabetes independently leads to lowering of CVD occurring rates even after changes in HDL-cholesterol are adjusted for. From the foregoing, it is evident that elevated cholesterol, low HDL-c, high TG and high LDL-c are all risk factors for CVD. The pattern of occurrence of these abnormalities in type 2 DM especially has been severally reported in both developed and developing economies (Idogun et al., 2007; Williams et al., 2008).

2.3 Very Low Density Lipoprotein-cholesterol (VLDL-c or preβ- lipoproteins)

VLDL-c is synthesized in the liver and contains primarily triglycerides in their lipid cores for their export and also some cholesterol ester (Botham and Mayes, 2006). As their triglycerides are cleaved by endothelial lipoprotein lipase and transferred to hepatic tissues, the VLDL (very-low-density lipoprotein) particles lose most of their apolipoprotein C and become intermediate-density lipoproteins. VLDL is one of the five major groups of lipoproteins which functions to enable fats and cholesterol to move within the water-based solution of the bloodstream. VLDL-c particles have a diameter of 30-80 nm each and transports endogenous products such as triglycerides, phospholipids, cholesterol, and cholesteryl esters, whereas chylomicrons transport exogenous (dietary) products. It functions as the body's internal transport mechanism for lipids.

2.4 Low Density Lipoprotein-cholesterol (LDL-c)

The primary role of LDL-c appears to be the transport of esterified cholesterol to tissues (Guyton and Hall, 2006). Low density lipoprotein results when triacylglycerols are released from VLDL-c by the action of the same lipase that acts on chylomicrons and the remnants which are rich in cholesterol esters are called intermediate density lipoprotein (IDL). IDL particles have two fates as half of them are taken up by the liver and the other half converted into LDL which is the major carrier of cholesterol in blood (Styer, 1988). LDL-c or β- lipoprotein represent the final stage in the metabolism of VLDL. Originally, LDL-cholesterol was determined by a lengthy, laborious process called ultracentrifugation of serum. A much more rapid test became available based on the following Friedwald equation: Total cholesterol = LDL-cholesterol + HDL-cholesterol + VLDL-cholesterol (VLDL-cholesterol = triglycerides/5). One can rapidly and easily do a lipid profile by enzymatically measuring the important lipids—total cholesterol, HDL- cholesterol, and triglycerides. Dividing triglycerides by five gives the relatively unimportant, but hard to measure, VLDL-cholesterol, which is useful in then calculating the very important LDL cholesterol (Holme and Peck, 1998).

2.5 High Density Lipoprotein-cholesterol (HDL-c or ⟨-lipoprotein)

HDL-c is involved in the cholesterol transport and in VLDL and chylomicron metabolism. Unlike LDL which primary role appears to be the carriage of esterified cholesterol to the tissues, HDL functions to carry excess cholesterol away from most tissues to the liver. The apoA-I present in the HDL-c particle binds lipid and also activates lecithin cholesterol acyltransferase (LCAT), which catalyzes formation of cholesteryl esters which migrate into the interior of the HDL-c and are carried to the liver (Metzler, 1974). Recent studies on patients with LCAT deficiency have shown a modest but significant increase in incidence of cardiovascular disease consistent with a beneficial effect of LCAT on atherosclerosis (Rousset et al., 2009) HDL particles compared to other lipoproteins, are assembled outside of cells from lipids and proteins, some of which may be donated from chylomicrons or other lipoprotein particles. HDL has higher protein content than other lipoproteins and is more heterogeneous. The major HDL protein is apolipoprotein A-I, but many HDL particles also contain A-II, and apolipoproteins A-IV, D, and E may also be present. A low plasma level of HDL-cholesterol is associated with a high risk of atherosclerosis.

3. Implicated disease states

3.1 Diabetes

Diabetes mellitus is a major global health problem and is now recognized as one of the leading causes of death in the developing countries, where the high prevalence of the disease could be attributed to improved nutritional status coupled with a gross lack of modern facilities for the early diagnosis of the disease (Uebanso et al., 2007; Ogbonnia et al., 2008[a]). Diabetes mellitus (DM) is a complex disease characterized by abnormal pattern of fuel usage resulting from over production of glucose and its under utilization by other organs (Stryer, 1988). Diabetes has been succinctly described as the common metabolic disorder of carbohydrate and fat metabolism, which is due to absolute or relative lack of insulin and is characterized by hyperglycaemia (Walter, 1977; Shah et al., 2008 and Sharma et al., 2010; Dinesh et al., 2011).

Diabetes mellitus is therefore a multifactorial disease associated with hyperglycemia, (Shah et al., 2008; Sharma et al., 2010); lipoprotein abnormalities, raised basal metabolic rate and high oxidative stress inducing damage to beta cells. The abnormalities in carbohydrates and lipid metabolism in diabetes also result in excessive production of reactive oxygen species (ROS) and defect in ROS scavenging enzymes in addition to oxidative stress. The low level of insulin associated with diabetes has been found to increase the activity of anti-enzyme, fatty acyl Coenzyme A oxidase, which initiates the β-oxidation of the fatty acids, resulting in lipid peroxidation (Shah et al., 2008). Increased lipid peroxidation has also been found to impair membrane function by decreasing membrane fluidity and changing the activity of the membrane-bound enzyme and receptors. The resulting lipid radicals and lipid peroxides are harmful to the cell in the body and are associated with atherosclerosis and brain damage.

Chronic hyperglycemia which occurs in diabetes causes glycation of body proteins which in turn leads to secondary complications affecting eyes, kidneys, nerves and arteries (Mishra and Garg, 2011). These may be delayed, lessened or prevented by maintaining blood glucose values close to normal in modern medicine, though no satisfactory effective therapy is available for total cure of diabetes mellitus.

Diabetes mellitus is also associated with hyperlipidaemia with profound alteration in the concentrations and compositions of plasma lipid. Changes in the concentration of the lipids in diabetes contribute to the development of vascular disease. Excessive levels of blood cholesterol accelerate atherogenesis and lowering high blood cholesterol reduces the incidence of CHD (Grundy, 1986). One of the risk factors for coronary heart disease is elevated total cholesterol (TC), low density lipoprotein-cholesterol (LDL-c) and lowered high density lipoprotein-cholesterol (HDL-c). The development of cardiovascular disease in DM is often predicted by several factors which include central obesity, hypertriglyceridemia and hypertension. Hypertriacylglyceridemia and low high-density liopoproteinaemia are two components of the atherogenic profile seen in DM. Elevated low density lipoprotein-cholesterol (LDL-c) has also been found to be an independent risk factor for the development of cardiovascular disease and is often reported to be the commonest lipid abnormality found in patients with DM (Udawat and Goyal, 2001; Idogun et al., 2007).

3.2 Atherosclerosis

Atherosclerosis or arteriosclerosis is a disease of large and medium size muscular arteries and is characterized by endothelial dysfunction vascular inflammation and build up of lipids, cholesterol, calcium and cellular debris within intima of vessel wall. This build up results in plaque formation, vascular remodeling, acute and chronic luminal obstruction, abnormalities in the blood flow and diminished oxygen supply to the target organ. (Madhumathi et al., 2006). Atherosclerotic disease has been found to be the most common cause of myocardial ischemia. Myocardium is said to be ischaemic when the pumping capability of the heart is impaired as a result of fall in the coronary blood flow which could not meet up with the metabolic need of the heart. In artherosclerotic disease, there is a localised lipid deposits called plaques develop within the arterial walls. In the severe cases of the disease these plaques become calcified and are so large that they physically narrow the lumen of the arteries producing stenosis (Mohrman and Heller, 2006). umerous studies have revealed important risk factors for the development of arthrosclerosis and these include diseases such as diabetes mellitus, arterial hypertension, and also smoking and elevated blood cholesterol

Current concepts in atherosclerosis suggest that oxidation of LDL-c is involved in its pathogenesis. The critical role of oxidized LDL-c in atherogenesis may be due to its rapid uptake by the foam cells lining the arterial intima, which are thought to have macrophage-like properties. When LDL-c is oxidized chemotactic effect is exerted on monocytes and this increase the uptake of LDL-c leading to the formation of arterial plaque. Lipid oxidation can be inhibited by the use of antioxidants such as vit E which inhibit the formation of lesions in hypercholesterolemic rabbits (Chein and Frishman, 2003).

Hypercholesterolemia has also been implicated in the process of atherogenesis and a curvilinear relationship has been documented between increasing cholesterol and increasing incidence of CVD (Brunzell et al., 2008). The role of LDL-c in the development of CVD cannot be overemphasized as there is documented evidence that high levels of LDL-c not only cause atherosclerosis but pharmacological interventions that reduce LDL-c are associated with stabilization and regression of atherosclerosis in proportion to the cholesterol lowering achieved (O'Keefe et al., 2004). Low levels of HDL-c have been consistently reported in cardiovascular diseases (Idogun et al., 2007; Sani-Bello et al., 2007, Singh et al., 2007). Primary treatment of coronary artery disease (and atherosclerosis in general) should include attempts to lower blood lipid by dietary and pharmacological techniques to prevent and possibly reverse further deposit of plaques.

3.3 Benign Prostatic Hyperplasia (BPH)

Benign Prostatic Hyperplasia (BPH) is a neoplastic enlargement of the prostate gland, and is a common problem among aging men (Ejike and Ezeanyika, 2010, Dharmananda, 2011). The etiology of this disease is still poorly understood, but it has been proposed to have two phases:

One of the phases involves no clinical sign but there maybe some microscopic changes while the other manifests as the disorder of urination caused by the obstruction of the urinary tract by an enlarged prostate gland (Dharmananda, 2011).

Epidemiological studies have demonstrated that many of the risk factors associated with cardiovascular diseases apply also as risk factors for BPH. The problems associated with diabetic may be considered very strong as the risk in non-insulin dependent diabetes (NIDDM); which most often connected with insulin resistance may be a possible direct contributor to the growth of BPH (Dharmananda, 2011). NIDDM which arises from either impairment of insulin utilization or dysfunction on the metabolism of carbohydrates, fats and protein or both culminates in hyperlipidemia- hence elevation in plasma cardiovascular risk factor. BPH is therefore associated with metabolic syndrome (Kasturi et al., 2006; Ozden, 2007).

4. Herbal drugs used to control CRF in the disease states

Herbal medicines may be described as medicines prepared either with a single plant part or combinations of different plant parts either fresh,dried or as extract are now recognized as potent therapeutic agents. Plants derived medicines commonly referred to as "phytomedicines" have been effectively employed in the management of variety of pathological conditions and are associated with fewer side effects (Nirmala et al., 2011; Ogbonnia et al, 2011). In recent years, they have been found to be effective both as hypoglycaemic and hypolipidemic agents (Ogbonnia et al., 2008[c]; 2010[b]) and have also been empirically used by many people from various cultures to lower cholesterol levels (Hamed, et al., 2010). Herbal medicines owe their therapeutic activities to the presence in them of secondary organic compounds or natural products constituents called the 'active constituents'.

4.1 Herbal active constituents

Herbal drugs contain natural products or secondary metabolites as the active constituents responsible for their physiological and pharmacological activities. The physiological and pharmacological activities have been found amongst alkaloids, phenolics and flavonoid compounds, glycosides (steroidal and saponins), and terpenoids, and is brought about through one or combination of two or more of the mechanisms that are the same as in the disease state they are being used. The mechanisms of their antidiabetic and antilipidemic activities which contribute to lowering of plasma lipids are the same mechanisms responsible for lowering of cardiovascular risk factors. These include the following: Glycosidase (Glucosidase) inhibition mechanism; alpha-amylase inhibition mechanism; antioxidant activities mechanism; inhibition of hepatic glucose metabolizing enzymes mechanism and inhibition of glycosylation of haemoglobin mechanism. These different mechanisms of activities are briefly discussed below

4.2 Possible mechanism of actions

The different classes of secondary product active constituents present in different herbal medicines may act through one or different mechanisms to bring about lowering or clearing of cardiovascular risk factors in a patient which may be probably the same mechanism through which they act exert their pharmacological action to control the disease state in question. Notably some of these possible mechanisms of actions may include:

4.2.1 Glycosidase (Glucosidase) inhibitor mechanism

One of the earliest features of type II diabetes and also observed in pre-diabetic phase is the loss of early phase secretion of insulin. Early phase insulin secretion is seen after a meal or after oral or intravenous ingestion of glucose and it is responsible for inhibition of hepatic glucose output and its absence results in postprandial hyperglycemia. (Ogbonnia and Anyakora 2009[c]). The α-glucosidase inhibitors category of drugs have been found to decrease postprandial glucose level by interfering with carbohydrate digestion and delaying gastrointestinal absorption of glucose . Slowing down digestion and breakdown of starches may have beneficial effects on insulin resistance and glycaemic index control on people suffering from diabetes. In this group some cryptic or water soluble alkaloids especially polyhydroxy alkaloids, have been identified to be potent glucosidase inhibitor (Kameswara et al., 2001). This as a whole comprises of relatively simple monocyclic pyrrolidine and piperidine alkaloids, necines, amino alcohols which are derivatives bicyclic pyrrolizidine, and are mostly esters of amino alcohols and of aliphatic carboxylic acids.

4.2.2 Inhibition of hepatic glucose metabolizing enzymes mechanism

Synthesis of glucose by the liver and kidney from non carbohydrate precursor such as lactate, glycerol and amino acid constitutes a process known as gluconeogenesis. The liver hydrolytic enzymes glucose-6-phosphatase and fructose-1, 6- diphoshatase have been shown to play a crucial role in gluconeogenesis contributing to hyperglycaemic condition found in diabetes. Herbal drug products may act by binding with the enzymes. Treatment with an herbal drug has been observed to decrease the activities of these liver enzymes significantly with a concomitant decrease in blood sugar level (Lazar, 2006).

4.2.3 Antioxidants effects

Phenolics and polyphenolics are associated with antioxidant properties and have been reported to categorically reduce the oxidation of the LDL-c (Kar, 2007). Flavonoids in hawthorn extract have been found to reduce wall tension in normal and sclerotic blood vessels. These chemicals are also presumed to stimulate beta-2-receptors and thus widen coronary arteries and blood vessels in skeletal muscle . Flavonoids and other antioxidants act to destroy free radicals which are particles that can damage cell membranes, interact with genetic material and possibly develop heart diseases and cancer. They have also been found to decrease two other markers of cardiovascular disease, homocysteine and C-reactive protein. C-reactive protein (CRP) has been reported to be associated with increased risk of cardiovascular disease, myocardial infection (MI) coronary artery disease mortality among individuals with angina pectoris.

Oxidative stress has been reported to increase in diabetic patients and is regarded as common pathway by which many classical cardiovascular disease (CVD) risk factors and postprandial dysmetabolism may initiate and promote atherosclerosis (WHO 1985). Studies have shown that treatment with antioxidant reduces diabetic complications (Negappa et al., 2003). Flavonoids have been shown to scavenge reactive oxygen species (ROS) that are produced under severe stress conditions and protect plant cell and animal cell from oxidative stress and may have important role in human health.

4.2.4 Inhibition of glycosylation of haemoglobin mechanism

It has now become apparent that both fasting and postprandial hyperglycaemia contributes to overall glycaemic burden and therefore total glycosylation of haemoglobin, HbA., Many studies have shown that there is substantial evidence and a very strong correlation between hyperglycaemia and the risk of developing cardiovascular disease and mortality. Postprandial hyperglycemia has been found to occur together with postprandial hyperlipidaemia which is also associated with increased oxidative stress and endothelia dysfunction. However, one could therefore postulate that herbal drug products that are effective in the reduction of postprandial hyperglycaemia may not only play a role in managing type II diabetes but could also offer a tantalizing possibility of reducing cardiovascular risk.

S/no	Plant/Herbal Drugs	Work Done	Reference
1.	Alstonia congensis Engler (Apocynaceae) bark and Xylopia aethiopica (Dunal) A. Rich (Annonaceae) fruits	Evaluation of acute in mice and subchronic toxicity	Ogbonnia et al., 2008[a]
2	Leone Bitters, a Nigerian polyherbal formulation	Antimicrobial evaluation, acute and subchronic toxicity studies	Ogbonnia et al., 2008[a], 2010[a]
3.	Parinari curatellifolia Planch, (Chrysobalanaceae) seeds	Assessing plasma glucose and lipid levels, body weight and acute toxicity following oral administration of an aqueous ethanolic extract.	Ogbonnia et al., 2008[b]
4.	poly-herbal formulation	on alloxan- induced diabetic rats	Ogbonnia et al., 2008[b], 2010[b]
5.	Treculia africana Decne and Bryophyllum pinnatum Lam	Evaluation of Hypoglycaemic and Hypolipidaemic Effects of Aqueous Ethanolic Extracts	Ogbonnia et al., 2008[c]
6.	Stachytarpheta angustifolia	Evaluation of acute and subchronic toxicity in animals and phytochemical profile	Ogbonnia et al., 2009a
7.	Parinari curatellifolia Planch (Chrysobalanaceae) seeds	Evaluation of acute in mice and subchronic toxicity	Ogbonnia et al., 2009[b]
8.	Parinari curatellifolia and Anthoclista vogelli	Diabetes and cardiovascular factors	Ogbonnia et al., 2011
9.	Azadirachta indica	Diabetes Mellitus and hypolipidemic effects	Dinesh et al., 2011
10.	Holarrhena antidysenterica	Diabetes	Ali et al., 2009
11.	Annona muricata Linn Centratherum anthelmintica	Diabetes Diabetes	Shah et al., 2008
12.	Grape seed extract	cholesterol	http://www.nativeremedies.com/article/cholesterol-education-heart-disease.html
13.	Red yeast rice contains a natural form of lovastatin	cholesterol	
14.	Vilis vinifera extract and Oroxylum indicum	cholesterol	D'Mello et al., 2011
15.	Garlic	Cholesterol, antithrombic Cardiovascular diseases	Hoareau and DaSilva,1999
16.	Hawthorn leaf and flower		

17.	Cinnamomic camphoric aetherolleum	Coronary artery disease (CAD)	
18.	Rosmarini folium (Rosemary leaf)		
19.	Pini aetheroleum(pine neddle)		
20.	Eucalypti folium (Eucalyptus leaf)		
21.	Menthae aetheroleum (menthol)		
22.	Bacopa monnieri Linn	Diabetes	Ghosh et al., 2006
23.	Feronia elephantum Corr	Diabetes	Mishra and Garg, 2011
24.	Achilleamellifolium (yarrow) Convallaria majalis (lilly of the valley)Cratcgeus laevigata (hawthorn) Cynarascolymus (globeantichoke) Gingko biloba (gingko) Vibumum opulus	Cardiovascular diseases	Hoareau and DaSilva, 1999

Table 2. Some researched plants and plant medicines found to have lowering effects on cardiovascular risk factors.

5. Summary

- The danger and the increasing prevalence of heart diseases world over are now of a great concern
- These diseases could be attributed to the cardiovascular risk factors which also have been identified to be the underlying latent or potent causes of death in heart diseases in particular and also in many other disease states
- Cardiovascular risk factors include triacylglycerols (triglycerides), cholesterol, cholesteryl esters, very low density lipoprotein - cholesterol (VLDL-c), low density lipoprotein-cholesterol (LDL-c), and anti-athrogenic HDL which are collectively referred to as plasma lipids
- Cholesterol is a fat-like substance that is present in cell membranes and is a precursor to steroid hormones and bile acids.
- Coronary atherosclerosis is the deposition of cholesterol and fibrin complexes within the lumen of a coronary artery that narrows the lumen, thereby limiting blood flow.
- Coronary heart disease (CHD) is atherosclerosis of one or more coronary arteries that has resulted in symptomatic disease such as angina pectoris, myocardial infarction, or congestive heart failure, or has required coronary artery surgery or coronary angioplasty.
- Lipoproteins are lipid-containing proteins in the blood that transport cholesterol throughout the body.
- Disease states with underlying cardiovascular risk factors include diabetes, atherosclerosis and benign prostatic hyperplasia.

6. References

Ali, K M., Chatterjee K, De D. Bera TK and Ghosh D. 2009. Efficacy of aqueous extract of seed of Holarrhena antidysenterica for the management of diabetes in experimental model rat: A correlative study with antihyperlipidemic activity. International Journal of Applied Research in Natural Products. Vol. 2 no 3: 13-21.

Bombardelli E and Morazzoni, P. 1997. Prunus africana, Phytotherapy Vol.68 no3:205-218.

Botham MK and Mayes AP. 2006. Lipid Transport and Storage. In Murray KM, Granner KD and Rodwell WV Eds. Happers Illustrated Biochemistry. 27th edn. McGraw Hill Singapore: 217-229.

Brunzell JD, Davidson M, Furberg CD, Goldberg RB, Howard BV, Stein J, Witztum JL. 2008. Lipoprotein management in patients with cardiometabolic risk. Consensus statement from the American Diabetes Association and the American college of Cardiology Foundation. Diabetes Care, 31:811-822.

Chein C. P and Frishman H. W. 2003. Lipid disorders. In. Grawford H. Michael Ed. Current Diagnosis and Treatment in Cardiology 2nd edition. International edition. Large medical Books/McGraw Hill. New York. 17

Conn E E and Stumpf PK. 1976. Lipids. In: Outline of Biochemistry. 4th edn. John Wiley& Sons Inc. New York, London Sidney and Toronto pp 57-72

D'Mello PM, Darji KK, Shetgiri PP. 2011. Evaluation of antiobesity activity of various Plant extracts. Pharmacognosy Journal, Vol. 3 no 21:56-59

Dharmananda S, 2011. Herbal therapy for Benign prostatic hyperplasia. Clin. Exp. Pharmacol. Physiol., 33: 808-812.

Dinesh k B, Analava M, Manjunatha M. 2011. Azadirachtolide: An anti-diabetic and hypolipidemic effects from Azadirachta indica leaves Pharmacognosy Communications www.phcogcommn.org Vol. 1 no 1:78- 84

Ejike ECC C and Ezeanyika US L, 2010. Hormonal Induction of Benign Prostatic Hyperplasia in Rats: Effects on Serum Macromolecular Metabolism. International Journal of Current Research. Vol 6: 065-067.

Fisher M, Shaw KM. 2001. Diabetes- a state of premature death. Pract.Diab.Vol.18 no6: 31-37

Ghayour –Mobarhan M, Yaghootkar H, Lanham-New SA, Lamb DJ and Ferns GA 2007. Association between serum CRP concentration with dietary intake in healthy and dyslipidaemic patients. Asia Pac J. Clin Nutr. Vol. 16 no.2 262-268 (http://herbaltreatment.us/index.php/cardiovascular-disease/coronary-artery-disease).Flavonoids

Ghosh T, Maity KT, Sengupta P, Dash KD and Bose A, 2006. Antidiabetic and In Vivo Antioxidant Activity of Ethanolic Extract of Bacopa monnieri Linn. Aerial Parts: A Possible Mechanism of Action. Iranian Journal of Pharmaceutical Research. Vol. 7no.1: 61-68

Grundy, S.M., 1986. Comparison of monounsaturated fatty acid and carbohydrates for lowering plasmacholesterol. N. Eng. J. Med. Vol.314: 745-748.

Guyton C A and Hall E J+. 2006. Lipid Metabolism In: Medical Physiology. 11th International edition Elsevier Inc. Philadelphia, Pennsylvania: 540-851. ISBN 0-8089-2317X

Hamed M Raouf, Hassanein, MA Nahed Ali A Azza and. EL-Nahhas M.Y Toqa 2010. An Experimental Study on the Therapeutic Efficacy of the Combined Administration of Herbal Medicines with Atorvastatin against Hyperlipidemia in Rats Journal of Applied Sciences Research, Vol. 6 no.11: 1730-1744.

Hammarsten J and Hogstedt B. 2001. Hyperinsulinemia as a risk factor for developing benign prostatic hyperplasia, European Eurology, Vol.39 no 2: 151-158

Hasimum P., Sukandar E.., Adnyana I.K., and Tjahjono DH. 2011. A simple method for screening Antihyperlidemic Agents. International Journal of pharmacology. Vol 7, no 1: 74-78 doi:10. 3923/ij p.2011.74.78

Hoareau L and DaSilva J. E. 1999. Medical plants: are emerging health and plant Biotechnology vol 2 no 2: 1-5

Holme J. D and Peck H. 1998. Lipid. In Analytical Biochemistry. 3rd Edn Addison Wesley Longman Ltd. ISBN 058229438-X: pp 403 – 433 – 450.

Idogun ES, Unuigbe EP, Ogunro PS, Akinola OI, Famodu AA. 2007. Assessment of serum lipids in Nigerians with type 2 diabetes mellitus complications. Pak J Med Sci Vol. 23:708-712.

Imafidon K E. 2010. Tissue lipid profile of rats administered aqueous extract of Hibiscus Rosa-Sinensis, Linn. Journal of Basic and Applied Sciences Vol. 6, no. 1: 1-3,

Jain J, L, Jain S and Jain N. 2005. Pyruvate oxidation and citric acid cycle. In: Fundamentals of Biochemistry Reprint S. Chgnd and Company Ltd, New Delhi-India : 481-521.

Kameswara, R.B.; Kesavulu, M.M.; Apparao, C. 2001. Journal of Ethnopharmacology, Vol. 78: 67-71

Kar A. 2007. Nutriceuticals. In: Pharmacognosy and Pharmacobiotechnology.2nd edn. New Age International Publisher, New Delhi: 735-778

Kasturi S, Russell S and McVary KT. 2006. Metabolic syndrome and lower urinary tract symptoms secondary to benign prostatic hyperplasia. Curr Urol Rep., Vol. 7:288-292.

Lazar, F.G.; Saltiel, R.A. 2006. Nature Review: Drug Discovery, Vol.15,no4: 333-342.

Leah Emma 2009. "Cholesterol". Lipidomics Gateway doi:10.1038/lipidmaps.2009.3 http://www.lipidmaps.org/update/2009/090501/full/lipidmaps.2009.3.html

Lewis R, Gaffin D, Hoefnagels M and Paker B. 2002. Circulatory System Spare Parts. In Life.4th edn., McGraw –Hill Higher Education, a division of the McGraw –Hill Companies, ISBN 0-07-027134-8 pp 680-699

Madhumathi BG, Venkataranganna MV, Gopumadhavan S, Rafiq M and Mitra SK. 2006. Induction and evaluation of atherosclerosis in New Zealand white rabbits. Indian J Exp Biol.Vol.44 : 203-208

Maruthapan, V., Shree K. Sakthi. 2010. Antihyperlipidemic potential of a polyherbal dug (Geriforte) on atherogenic diet induced hyperlipidemia: A Comparison with Ayurslim. International Journal of Chemical and Analytical Science Vol. 1. no 3:37-39

Maxfield FR and Tabas I. 2005 Roles of cholesterol and lipid organization in disease. Nature., 438: 612-621 metabolic syndrome. *Am J Cardiovasc Drugs* 2005, 5(6):379-387.

Metzler E. David 1974. Specific Aspects of Lipid Metabolism. In Biochemistry: The chemical reactions of living cells. 2nd Edition.. Elsevier Academic Press. Vols 1 & 2:1180- 1225

Mishra A and Garg P G, 2011. Antidiabetic activity of fruit pulp of Feronia elephantum Corr Pharmacognosy Journal Vol 3 no 20: 27-32

Mohrman. E. David and Heller Jane Lois. 2006 Cardiovascular disease. In Cardiovascular physiology. 6th edition. McGraw Hill, Boston: 205-221

Moreno-Luna, Rafael, Perez-Jimenez Francisco, Marin Carmen, Perez-Martinez Pablo, Gomez Purification, Jimenez-Gomez Yolanda, Delgado-Lista Javier, Moreno Junan A., Tanaka Toshiko, Orodovas Jose M and Lopez-Miranda J. 2007. Two Independent Apolipoprotein A5 Haplotypes Modulate Postprandial Lipoprotein Metabolism in a Healthy Caucasian Population. Journal of Clinical Endocrinology & Metabolism, diol: 10. 1210/jc.2006-1802, Vol. 92, no. 6: 2280-2285.

Nagappa, A.N.; Thakurdesai, P.A.; Venkat, R.N.; Singh, J. 2003. Antidiabetic activity of Terminalia catappa Linn fruits. Journal of Ethnopharmacology, Vol. 88: 45-50

Nirmala A. Saroja S Gayathri Devi. G. 2011. Antidiabetic Activity of Basella rubra and its Relationship with the Antioxidant Property. British Biotechnology Journal. Vol. 1 no1: 1-9.

Ogbonnia S, Adekunle A A, Bosa M.K, and Enwuru VN. 2008[a]. Evaluation of acute and subacute toxicity of Alstonia congensis Engler (Apocynaceae) bark and Xylopia aethiopica (Dunal) A. Rich (Annonaceae) fruits mixtures used in the treatment of diabetes. African Journal of Biotechnology. Vol. 7 no.6:701-705

Ogbonnia S, Adekunle A, Olagbende- Dada S, Anyika EN, Enwuru NV, Orolepe M. 2008[b]. Assessing plasma glucose and lipid levels, body weight and acute toxicity following oral administration of an aqueous ethanolic extract of Parinari curatellifolia Planch, (Chrysobalanaceae) seeds in alloxan-induced diabetes in Rats. African Journal of Biotechnology vol.7 no.8: 3520-3525

Ogbonnia Steve O., Odimegwu Joy I. Enwuru Veronica N. 2008[c]. Evaluation of Hypoglycaemic and Hypolipidaemic Effects of aqueous ethanolic extracts of Treculia africana Decne and Bryophyllum pinnatum Lam. and their Mixture on Streptozotocin (STZ)-induced diabetic rats. African Journal of Biotechnology Vol.7no 15: 2535-2539 (http://www.umm.edu/altmed/articles/garlic-000245.htm

Ogbonnia SO, Nkemehule FE, Anyika EN. 2009[a]. Evaluation of acute and subchronic toxicity in animals and phytochemical profile of aqueous ethanolic extract of Stachytarpheta angustifolia (Mill) Vahl (Fam. Verbanaceae) plant. Journal of Biotechnology vol.8 no.9: 3213-2539.

Ogbonnia SO, Olayemi SO, Anyika EN, Enwuru VN, Poluyi O.O. 2009[b]. Evaluation of acute in mice and subchronic toxicity of hydroethanolic extract of Parinari curatellifolia Planch (Chrysobalanaceae) seeds in rats. Journal of Biotechnology vol.8 no.9: 3245-3251

Ogbonnia SOand Anyakora C 2009[c] Chemistry and Biology Evaluation of Nigerian Plant with anti-Diabetic Properties. Juliani H.R., Simon J.E and Ho C-T. (Eds.). In African Natural Products: new discoveries and challenges in chemistry and quality American Chemical Society, Washington DC. ISBN 978-0-8412-6987-3

Ogbonnia SO, Mbaka G. O, Igbokwe NH, Anyika E, A lli P, Nwakakwa N. 2010[a]. Antimicrobial evaluation, acute and subchronic toxicity studies of Leone Bitters, a Nigerian polyherbal formulation in rodents. Agriculture and Biology Journal of North America, Vol. 1 no. 3: 366-376. ISSN Print: 2151-7517, ISSN Online: 2151-7525 Science Huβ, http://www.scihub.org/ABJNA

Ogbonnia SO, Mbaka G. O, Adekunle A, Anyika E. N, Gbolade O. E, Nwakakwa N. 2010b Effect of a poly-herbal formulation, Okudiabet, on alloxan-induced diabetic rats. Agriculture and Biology Journal of North America, Vol.1no.2: 139-145. ISSN Print: 2151-7517, ISSN Online: 2151-7525 Science Huβ, http://www.scihub.org/ABJNA

Ogbonnia, S.O.; Mbaka, G.O.; Anyika, E.N.; Ladiju, O.; Igbokwe, H.N.; Emordi, J.E. and Nwakakwa, N. 2011. Evaluation of Anti-diabetics and Cardiovascular Effects of Parinari curetellifolia Seed Extract and Anthoclista vogelli Root Extract Individually and Combined on Postprandial and Alloxan-Induced Diabetic Albino Rats. British Journal of Medicine & Medical Research 1(3): 146-162.

O'Keefe JH, Cordain L, Harris WH, Moe RM, Vogel R., 2004. Optimal lowdensity lipoprotein is 50 to 70 mg/dl: lower is better and physiologically normal. J Am Coll Cardiol Vol.43:2142-2146.

Ozden C, Ozdal OL, Urganioglu G, Kovuncu H, Gokkaya S and Mermis A. 2007. The correlation between metabolic syndrome and prostatic growth in patients with benign prostatic hyperplasia. Eur Urol., Vol. 51:199-206.

Plummer T. D, 1998. Lipids. In: An introduction of practical Biochemistry. 3rd edn. Tata McGraw – Hill Educational Private Limited. New Delhi- India: pp 189-204. ISBN – 13:978–0–07–099487-4, ISBN-10: 0-07-099487-0.

Rousset X, Vaisman B, Amar M, Sethi A A and Remalev AT. 2009. Lecithin: cholesterol acyltranferease…from biochemistry to role in cardiovascular disease. Current Opinion Endocrinology Diabetes Obesity Vol.16 no.2:163-171.

Sani-Bello F, Bakari AG, Anumah FE. 2007. Dyslipidaemia in persons with type 2 diabetes mellitus in Kaduna, Nigeria. Int J Diabetes and Metabolism Vol.15:9-13.

Shah JG, Patel MS, Patel KV and Gandhi TR 2008. Evaluation of Anti-diabetic and Anti-oxidant Activity of Centratherum anthelmintica in STZ-induced Diabetes in Rats. The International Internet Journal of Pharmacology, Vol.6 no1:1-10.

Sharma VK, Kumar S, Patel HJ and Hugar S. 2010. Hypoglycemic activity of Ficus glomerata in alloxan induced diabetic rat. International Journal of Pharmaceutical Sciences Review and Research, Vol. 1 no 2:18-22.

Sharon, G. B., Marvin, R. B. (1975). Synthesis and evaluation of potential hypoglycaemic agents I: carnitine analogs, J Pharm. Sci., 64(12), 1949-1952.

Singh IM, Shishehbor DO. 2007. Ansell BJ: High-density lipoprotein as a therapeutic target: a systematic review. *JAMA* 298:786-798.

Stryer L. 1988. Biosynthesis of Membrane Lipids and Steroids Hormones. In: Biochemistry.3rd edn. W.H. Freeman and Company, New York, USA: 547-574

Udawat H, Goyal RK. 2001. Lipid lowering effect of simvastatin in patients of type 2 DM. *Indian Heart J* 53:172-176.

Uehanso T, Arai H, Taketani Y, Fukaya M, Yamamoto H, Mizuno A, Uryu K, Hada T and Takeda E, 2007. Extracts of Momordica charantia Suppress Postprandial Hyperglycemia in Rats. J Nutr Sci Vitaminol, 53, 482 – 488.

Walter, B.J. (1977). An introduction to the principles of disease. W.B. Saunders Company. Philadelphia USA, pp. 374-377.

WHO Expert Committes. In WHO Technical Report Series of Diabetes Mellitus, 1985, 727.

Williams K, Tchernof A, Hunt KJ, Wagenknecht LE, Haffner MS, Sniderman AD. 2008. Diabetes, abdominal adiposity and atherogenic dyslipoproteinaemia in women compared with men. *Diabetes* 57:3289-3296.

19

Morphology and Functional Changes of Intestine, Trophology Status and Systemic Inflammation in Patients with Chronic Heart Failure

G.P. Arutyunov and N.A. Bylova
The Russian State Medical University (RSMU), Russia

1. Introduction

1.1 Morphological and functional changes of the small intestine in patients with different classes of chronic heart failure

Current understanding prompts to view chronic heart failure (CHF) as a systemic condition. Traditionally, the following organs are considered the target organs of CHF: heart, kidneys, brain. However, low cardiac output and increased activity of the renin-angiotensin-aldosterone system (RAAS), which lead to vasospasm and ischemia, are bound to have effect on functions of other organs, including small intestine, large intestine, and adipose tissue. The increased activity of RAAS is likely to have effect on morphological restructuring of the intestine as well. It can be assumed that accumulation of collagen in the intestinal wall, as well as development of edema and ischemia, decrease the functional activity of the intestinal wall and are a major factor of the malabsorption syndrome, which, in its turn, leads to progressive loss of body mass. This results in progression of certain clinical manifestations in patients with CHF, such as: weakness, fatigue, and progressive decrease of exercise tolerance, which cannot be explained by changes in peripheral circulation alone. The incidence of these complaints is known to increase as the NYHA class of the CHF grows, and it reaches its peak in patients with class IV (Harrington & Anker, 1997).

Loss of body mass means a significantly worse prognosis for the patients with CHF. According to SOLVD study, ≥6 % decrease of body mass in patients with CHF is a potent predictor of negative impact on survival along with other factors such as age, gender, LV ejection fraction, NYHA class (Anker et al., 2003).

Therefore, decrease of body mass should be considered an important sign, equal in significance to such symptoms as dyspnea and edema.

Obviously, a search for new methods to correct the nutritional status in patients with CHF is necessary. The method of nutritional support may be one of these promising options to treat and stop development the malabsorption syndrome, as this method constitutes a system with pathogenesis-based rationale that implies prescription of balanced nutritive mixtures characterized by maximum degree of absorption even in the setting of morphological changes in the intestine.

1.2 Materials and methods

This was an open-label prospective study approved by the Ethics Committee of the Russian State Medical University. All of the patients participating in this study had signed the informed consent.

The study included 110 patients with New York Heart Association (NYHA) class I-IV ischemic CHF, with history of CHF for more than 24 months. Age of the patients was 45 to 65 years, mean age was 58.7±5.3 years. All of the patients were allocated to different groups based on the severity of their CHF. The control group included 38 patients (24 male and 14 female), 45 to 65 years old (mean age 60.6±2.6), in which no signs of CHF were found after testing. The patient populations had comparable basic parameters at baseline.

All of the patients with the signs of CHF received standard basic therapy, which included ACE inhibitors, β-blockers, loop diuretics or thiazide diuretics, cardiac glycosides, nitrates, aspirin, and aldosterone antagonists. Patients in the control group received therapy for their main condition.

Patients were investigated using the following sets of tests:

- Endoscopy with biopsy of the small intestine (the samples were taken 10 cm below the plica duodenojejunalis). Preparation and analysis of microscopic specimens were performed in the Pathology Department of the Bakulev Scientific Center of Cardiovascular Surgery.
- Assessment of functional activity of the small intestine (measurement of excretion of fat in feces, biochemical measurement of total protein and protein fractions in feces via nitrogen content, measurement of carbohydrate absorption in the small intestine using the D-xylose test).

Statistical analyses of the results were performed using standard statistical formulas with Microsoft Excel 7.0 and BIOSTAT software. Arithmetic means of values in the sample population (M) and standard deviations (σ) were determined. The significance of differences between groups was determined using Student test at $p < 0.05$. Relationship between parameters was assessed by calculating the correlation coefficient (r) with the level of errorless prognosis at 95 % ($p<0.05$).

1.3 Results

1.3.1 Morphological changes of the small intestine in patients with NYHA class I-IV CHF

The photographs of microscopic specimens (Fig. 1) demonstrate the pattern of the mucosa of the small intestine typical for patients with NYHA class IV CHF (a) and healthy individuals (b). Collagen fibers are stained pink.

These photographs demonstrate that in patients with NYHA class III-IV CHF the collagen fibers stained pink take up a significant area of the small intestine mucosa, while in patients without signs of CHF only solitary collagen fibers are present.

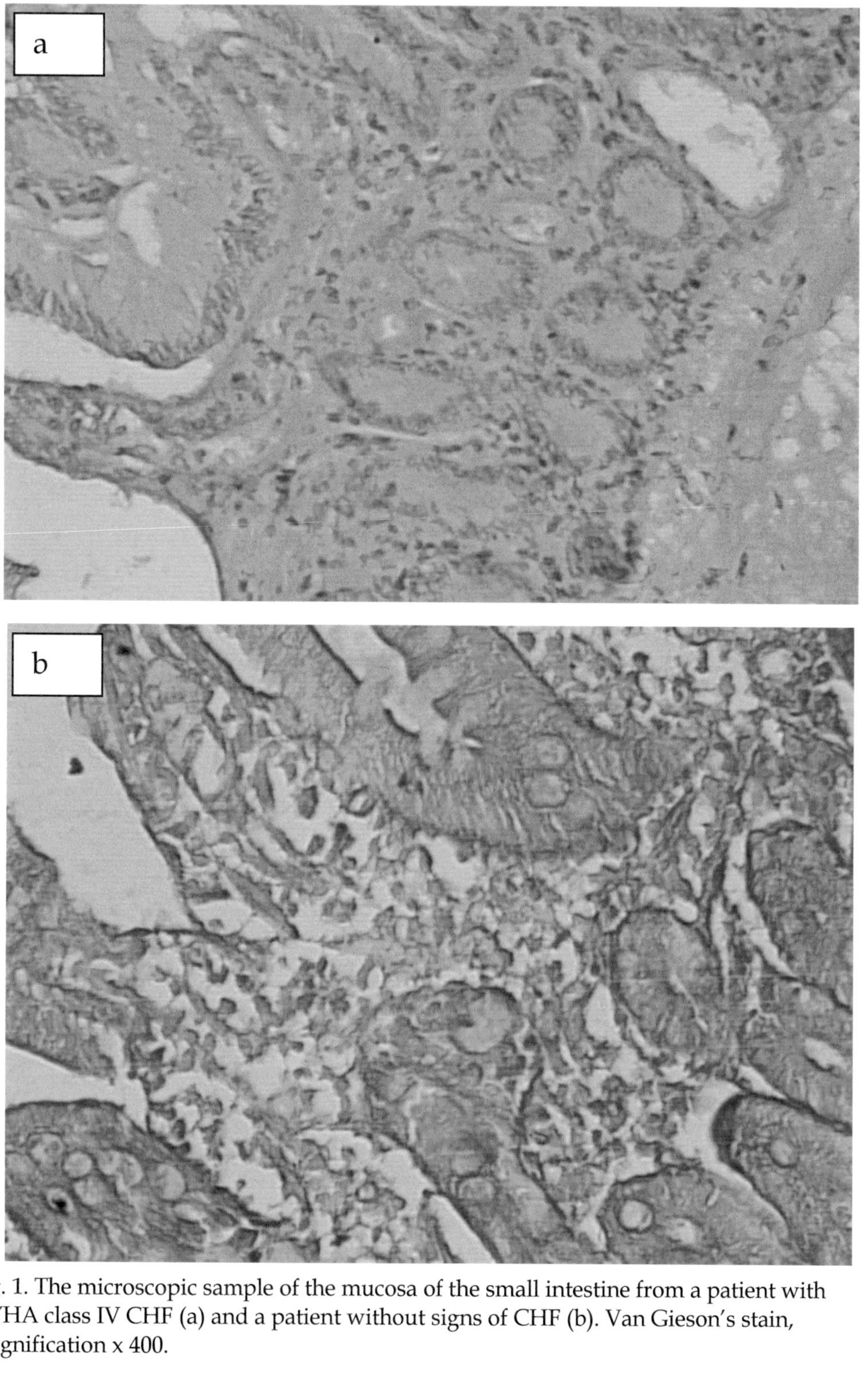

Fig. 1. The microscopic sample of the mucosa of the small intestine from a patient with NYHA class IV CHF (a) and a patient without signs of CHF (b). Van Gieson's stain, magnification x 400.

Collagen deposition level in patients with NYHA classes III and IV was significantly different from values measured in patients with NYHA classes I or II and in patients without signs of CHF. Comparison of collagen relative density between patients without CHF and with NYHA class I or II CHF did not reveal significant differences. However, a clear trend towards increase of collagen level in the latter was noted. Also, the difference in the amount of collagen between CHF patients with NYHA classes III and IV was not significant.

When assessing the microscopic specimens of the small intestine, high amount of collagen was observed to mechanically push enterocytes away from a capillary vessel. This increases the intestine-blood barrier and may have an impact on nutrient absorption.

The measured data are presented in Table 1.

Groups	Distance between EBM and a capillary vessel, µm	Significance of difference between groups
1. No CHF	8.4±0.7	p1-2 >0.05; p1-3>0.05; p1-4<0.05; p1-5<0.05
2. NYHA class I	10.1±1.2	p2-3>0.05; p2-4>0.05; p2-5>0.05
3. NYHA class II	11.3±1.1	p3-4<0.05; p3-5<0.05
4. NYHA class III	18.6±1.4	p4-5>0.05
5. NYHA class IV	19.1±1.2	

Table 1. Distance between EBM (enterocyte basal membrane) and the capillary wall

Even primary assessment of microscopic photographs revealed atrophy of villi of the small intestine mucosa in patients with NYHA class III-IV CHF. Fig. 2 shows pattern of the mucosa in a patient with NYHA class IV CHF (a) compared to a patient from the control group (b).

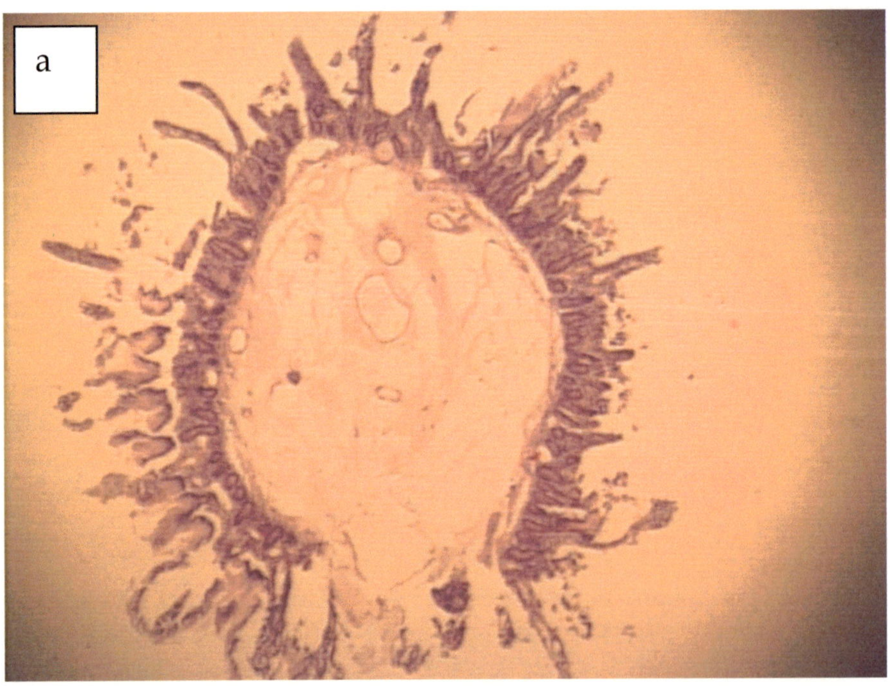

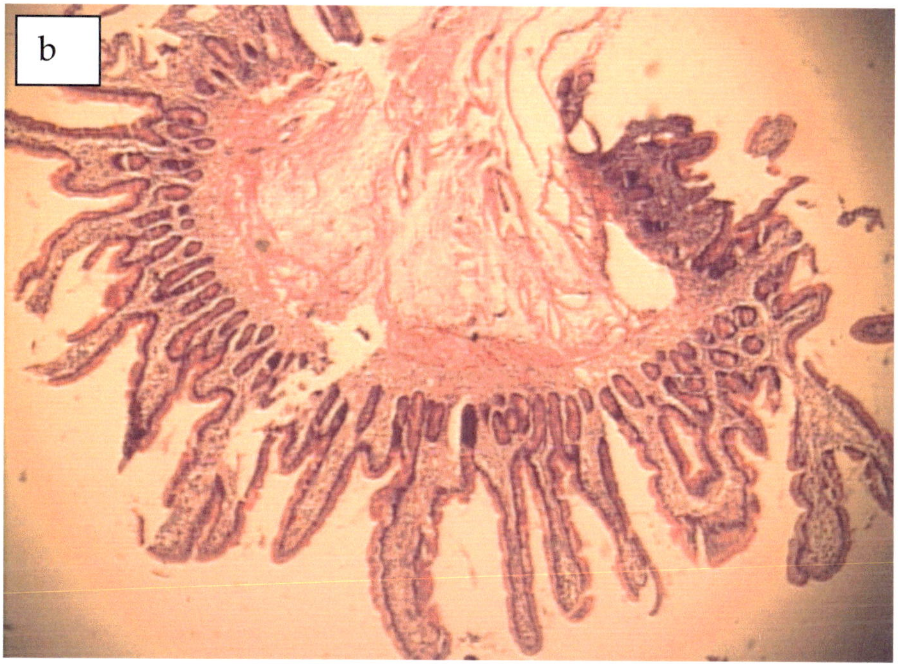

Fig. 2. Villi of the small intestine mucosa in a patient with NYHA class IV CHF (a) and a patient without CHF (b).Magnification x100. Hematoxylin-eosin stain.

Quantitative values describing changes in the villi of the small intestine in patients with different classes of CHF are shown in the Table 2.

Groups	Mean length of a villus, μm	Mean width of a villus, μm	Significance of difference between groups
No CHF	372±9.9	98±4.4	p1-2>0.05; p1-3>0.05; p1-4<0.05; p1-5<0.05
Class I CHF	369±7.4	94±3.5	p2-3>0.05; p2-4>0.05; p2-5>0.05
Class II CHF	374±6.9	91±6.1	p3-4<0.05; p3-5<0.05
Class III CHF	254±5.5	65±3.1	p4-5>0.05
Class IV CHF	223±6.1	59±3.0	

Table 2. Length and width of mucosal villi in the small intestine of patients with CHF.

To conclude, analysis of the small intestine mucosa biopsy samples demonstrated significant morphological changes, which worsen with the severity of CHF. Increase of intestine-blood barrier and decrease of the absorbing area of the villi determined further study of nutrient absorption, which, supposedly, should have decreased significantly in patients with CHF.

1.3.2 Functional changes of the small intestine in patients with NYHA class I-IV CHF

Analysis of protein absorption parameters revealed the following pattern: in patients with NYHA class I CHF, losses of total nitrogen were virtually below the upper limit of normal range, reaching 7.1±0.2 % of daily consumption. No significant differences were found between the patients of the control group (5.9±0.21 %) and classes I or II ($p>0.05$). With NYHA class IV CHF, the loss of protein was significantly higher - 18.6±1.3 %; this was on average 3.1 times higher than in the group of patients without CHF ($p<0.05$). In the group of patients with NYHA class III, the loss of protein was 16.7±1.8 %. Comparison of the protein loss levels in CHF patients with NYHA class III and IV vs. the protein loss levels in patients with NYHA class I and II showed a significant difference ($p>0.05$).

Levels of total fat loss were most pronounced in CHF patients with NYHA class III and IV (22.4±2.1 % and 24.1±2.12 % of the daily consumption, respectively) and exceeded the levels in patients without CHF (5.5±0.86 %) 4-fold on average. For NYHA classes I and II, fat loss levels were at the upper limit of normal (6.1±1.1 and 7.2±0.9 % of daily consumption, respectively) and were not significantly different from the values in the group of patients without CHF ($p>0.05$).

Analysis of D-xylose test results demonstrated a dependency similar to the one observed for absorption of proteins and fats. In patients with NYHA class IV CHF, the 5-hour excretion of D-xylose was 0.89±0.05 g. This was 1.4 times lower than the values for the control group. For NYHA class III CHF, D-xylose excretion was 0.96±0.03 g. This was also significantly different from normal values. Patients with NYHA class I and II did not show significant differences compared to the control group.

To conclude, patients with CHF experience deterioration of absorption for all basic nutrients, and the absorption reduction demonstrates dependence upon the severity of the CHF.

1.4 Attempts for correction

Taking into consideration the pronounced changes of the small intestine in patients with severe CHF that lead to development of malabsorption syndrome and protein-energy insufficiency, such patients demand specific correction of their nutritional status. Naturally, raw nutrients will hardly be utilized in the intestine that underwent these changes. A possibility to use specifically treated nutrients in the form of standard mixes for oral feeding was the objective that we assessed in the second phase of this study.

This part was an open-label, randomized, prospective, 24-week study.

Patients with NYHA class III and IV CHF were screened for this study. Total number of subjects was 74 (46 males, 28 females).

Randomization was performed using a random number method, with even numbers corresponding to the standard-of-care group (Group 1), and odd numbers corresponding to the nutritional support group (Group 2). The number of patients assigned to Group 1 was 36. Group 2 included 38 patients.

Figure 3 shows the study design.

Subjects in Group 1 (n=36) received standard basic therapy and their usual nutrition within the standard diet for cardiovascular patients.

Subjects in Group 2 (n=38), in addition to the basic therapy and standard diet, received a balanced nutritive mix, comprising 25 % of daily calories.

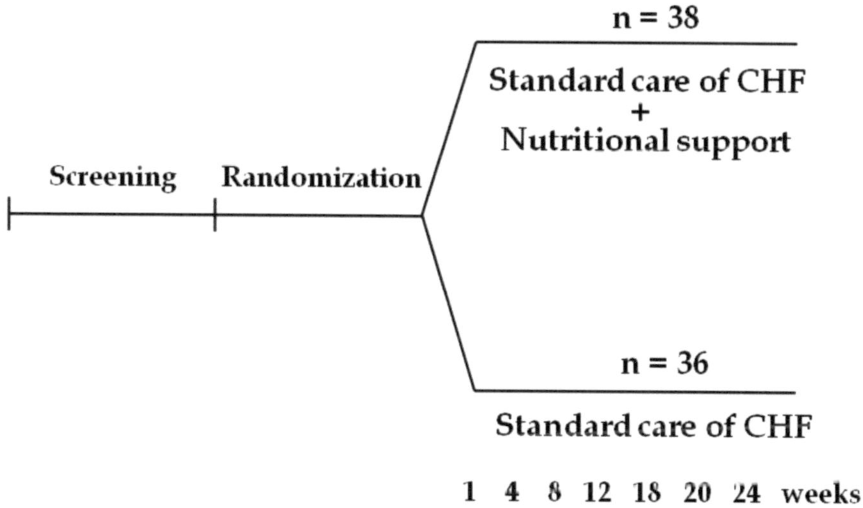

Fig. 3. Study Design.

The absolute majority of the patients were male and had history of ischemic origin of their disease. Their mean age was over 60 years. Mean NYHA class within these groups was 3.5 and 3.4, respectively. The resulting groups were identical in structure by gender, age and other clinical characteristics, warranting their comparability. The following tests were performed during this study: 6-minute test, echocardiography (LVEF), diet review, measurement of body mass and BMI, estimation of body fat mass and lean body mass, total protein, albumin, absolute lymphocyte count, hand dynamometry, assessment of absorption for proteins, fats, and carbohydrates, morphometric study of small intestine mucosa biopsy specimens, count of hospitalizations due to CHF progression.

Estimations of energy and nutrient demands were performed for all subjects before therapeutic diet and nutritional support were prescribed.

Subjects in Group 2 had 25 % of their energy demands (daily energy consumption) covered using balanced nutritive mixes, and the remaining 75 % were covered using the standard diet. All patients maintained dietary diaries, which allowed us to control the amount of energy they have received with their usual diet.

The balanced nutritive mixes used for nutritive support were Peptamen (Nestle, Switzerland), Berlamin Modular (Berlin-Chemie, Germany), Unipit and Nutrien-standard (Nutritek, Russia).

Assessment of nutritional support efficacy included change of 6-minute test parameters over time, change of LBM over time, and number of hospitalizations due to CHF progression compared between the experimental group and the control group.

During 24-week observation, a total of 11 patients died in 2 groups: 4 males and 2 females in Group 1 (standard-of-care), and 3 males and 2 females in Group 2 (oral nutritional support). Total number of hospitalization events throughout 24 weeks was 54 and 42 in Group 1 and Group 2, respectively. Table 3 shows causes of death and hospitalization.

Cause	Hospitalization		Death	
	Group 1	Group 2	Group 1	Group 2
CHF progression	36 (66,7%)	28 (66,7%)	4 (66,7%)	3 (60%)
Recurrent MI	6 (11,1%)	7 (16,7%)	1 (16,7%)	2 (40%)
Pneumonias	10 (18,5%)	6 (14,3%)	1 (16,7%)	0
Other	2 (0,4%)	3 (0,7%)	0	0
Total	54	42	6	5

Table 3. Causes of death and hospitalization for Groups 1 and 2.

Three patients chose to withdraw from study: 2 of them were from the standard-of-care group, and another one from the nutritional support group (the reason was moving to another city). Compliance was assessed using patient diaries, where their adherence to basic therapy and to nutritional support was recorded. Compliance below 80 % was reported for 2 subjects in Group 1 and 2 subjects in Group 2 (these subjects were excluded from the final analysis). As a result, in the standard-of-care group 26 patients completed the study, and in the nutritional support group 30 patients completed the study.

1.4.1 Changes of 6-minute test parameters over time

The trend for growth of the parameters in Group 2 was noticeable starting from Week 2. The curves of 6-minute test for the 2 groups diverged significantly starting from Week 8. After 24 weeks, the exercise tolerance in patients receiving standard nutrition decreased significantly (p=0.025). The baseline values for 6-minute test in this group were 85 to 243 m, mean 203.4±41.6 m. After 24 weeks, the mean distance walked in 6 minutes decreased by 19 % (164.7±48.1 m).

Six patients with NYHA class III CHF experienced substantial deterioration of their health – worsening of dyspnea, weakness, edema, i. e. their condition progressed to NYHA class IV.

In the group of patients receiving the nutritional support, the baseline for the 6-minute test was 182.2±45.6 m (range 34 m to 221 m), and Week 24 mean was 231.3±41.1 m (75 m to 295 m), i. e. a statistically significant (p=0.015) increase in exercise tolerance was observed. In this group, progression of NYHA class III to class IV was recorded for 2 patients only.

To conclude, in patients receiving the standard diet, Week 24 exercise tolerance decreased significantly, whereas in patients receiving nutritional support, significant increase of the exercise tolerance was observed. Statistical significance for the difference between the groups was p=0.021.

1.4.2 Change of hand dynamometry measurements over time

After 24 weeks of monitoring, no significant differences were found for dynamometry variables when comparing pre-treatment and post-treatment values; however, there was a trend towards increase for these variables in the nutritional support group (mean increase 0.2 kg, p=0.084). In the standard-of-care group, the variables decreased, with mean change of 0.4 kg; this change was not statistically significant (p=0.09).

1.4.3 Change of LBM over time

For most of the patients receiving nutritional support, a significant increase of LBM was shown (mean change 5.8±1.2 kg or 8.9 %, p=0.038). For 2 patients, a progressive decrease of LBM was recorded on treatment (the LBM decreased by 2.1 kg and 3.4 kg). In the standard nutrition group, 23 patients experienced statistically significant decrease of their LBM (mean decrease 3.6±0.7 kg or 4.9 %, p=0.036). The LBM did not change significantly in 2 patients, and an increase of LBM (+1.7 kg) was reported for 1 patient.

To conclude, long-term nutritional support leads to statistically significant increase of LBM, while in the standard nutrition group the LBM continues to decrease progressively. The differences between groups were statistically significant (p=0.04).

1.4.4 Changes of laboratory variables over time (absolute lymphocyte count and serum albumin)

In the nutritional support group, a statistically significant increase of nutritional status was demonstrated: the absolute lymphocyte count increased from 1590 to 1710 x109 (+12.5 %, p=0.04), and the albumin level increased from 25.1 to 29.4 g/L (+17.1 %, p=0.045). In the standard-of-care group, no significant changes were observed after 24 weeks of monitoring for the lymphocyte count and albumin. The differences between groups were statistically significant (p=0.04).

To conclude, the nutritional support demonstrated a favorable effect for all basic nutritional status variables.

1.4.5 Other variables

For the effect of nutritional support on protein, fat and carbohydrate absorption variables see Table 4.

Absorption variables	Group 1		Group 2	
	Baseline	Week 24	Baseline	Week 24
Total protein loss, % of daily consumption	18.1±0.3	17.9±0.2	17.9±0.2	15.48+0.9
Total fat loss, % of daily consumption	22.5±0.6	21.6±0.4	23.4±0.4	20.7±1.3
D-xylose excretion with urine, g/5 h	0.81±0.05	0.85±0.04	0.82±0.04	0.83±0.04

Table 4. Absorption of nutrients in patients with NYHA class III-IV CHF, pre-treatment and post-treatment.

No statistically significant changes were demonstrated in either group for morphometric variables during the treatment period of 24 weeks.

1.5 Conclusion

The study of the small intestine condition revealed marked changes of structure and functional activity of the intestine in all patients with CHF. The degree of the small intestine impairment directly depends on the severity of the CHF. This suggests direct impact of heart failure on gastrointestinal restructuring.

We consider the oral nutrition system involving prescription of balanced nutritional mixes to be one of the promising options to treat cardiac cachexia, as it has a pathogenesis-based rationale. This study was an attempt to evaluate the efficacy of the nutritional support during CHF progression.

2. Morphological and functional changes of the large intestine in patients with different classes of chronic heart failure

2.1 Introduction

Current understanding acknowledges the role of the following factors in the pathogenesis of CHF: neuroendocrine imbalance with excessive production of neurohormones, impairment of various target organs (cardiac muscle, kidneys, skeletal muscles, small intestine). However, many authors observed increased level of pro-inflammatory cytokines in CHF patients that cannot be explained by neuroendocrine activation. A number of authors reported a correlation between cytokine levels and blood plasma concentration of the endotoxin (lipopolysaccharide of gram-negative bacteria).

In an attempt to find the origin of the endotoxin, various bacteria were considered, particularly the bacteria of upper and lower respiratory tract, H. pylori, microorganisms of urinary tract and intestine. The strongest changes were found in the flora of the large intestine, where increase of the total number of microorganisms was observed, predominantly gram-negative. However, there were no reports of detailed analysis of the intestinal flora composition, and the parietal mucin layer flora was not taken into account.

The data on flora changes suggested potential methods of correction, particularly the selective decontamination method. However, according to literature reports, a course of selective decontamination reduces the number of microorganisms in the large intestine in the phase of antibacterial treatment only, while as early as 6 weeks after their discontinuation characteristics of the flora return to baseline. This shows lack of efficacy of the selective decontamination alone in CHF patients with high NYHA classes.

From our perspective, there are two possible approaches to correct the endotoxemia that leads to systemic inflammation: (1) development of methods that act on the intestinal wall by decreasing its permeability to the endotoxin, and (2) treatment that has direct effect on the intestinal flora towards normalization of both numbers and the composition of the flora.

2.2 Materials and methods

Laboratory tests.

Quantitative assay of endotoxin level using Kinetic-QCL test №50-650 U "Bioscience Cambrex Wallkersville", USA.

Quantitative assay of IL-6 (IL-6 Human ELISA Kit (1 x 96 Well Plate), Cytokine company, Russia), TNF-alpha (TNF alpha Human ELISA Kit (1 x 96 Well Plate), Cytokine company, Russia), CRP (C Reactive Protein Human ELISA Kit - 1 x 96 Well Plate, Abcam, USA) plasma levels using solid phase ELISA.

2.3 Assessment of the microbial landscape, large intestine wall structure, endotoxin levels, and pro-inflammatory cytokines in CHF patients with different NYHA classes

To study these variables, three consecutive groups were enrolled: Group 1: 65 patients with NYHA class III-IV CHF; Group 2: 60 patients with NYHA class I-II CHF; Group 3: 56 patients, control group (patients with ischemic heart disease and arterial hypertension without signs of CHF).

2.3.1 Changes in lumen flora of the large intestine in CHF patients with different NYHA classes and in the control group

Comparison of the first and the second study groups revealed statistically significant differences ($p<0.05$) for the following variables: total number of enterobacteria was 10^9 colony-forming units (CFU)/g in Group 1 vs. 10^7 CFU/g in Group 2. Enterobacteria pool growth was predominantly formed by *E. coli* (10^7 CFU/g in NYHA I-II group vs. 10^9 CFU/g in NYHA III-IV group, $p<0.0001$), various *Klebsiella sp.* (10^5 CFU/g in NYHA I-II group vs. 10^7 CFU/g in NYHA III-IV group, $p<0.005$), and citrate-assimilating enterobacteria (10^6 CFU/g in NYHA I-II group vs. 10^8 CFU/g in NYHA III-IV group, $p<0.005$). Differences in concentrations of *Citrobacters, Enterococci* and *Candida* yeasts were also statistically significant.

Comparison of the results for Group 1 (NYHA class III-IV) and control group subjects showed differences similar to the comparison of Group 1 versus Group 2, with the exception of differences in Clostridia populations (lecithinase- and hydrogen sulfide-positive strains): 10^7 CFU/g in CHF patients with NYHA III-IV vs. 10^5 CFU/g in the control group ($p<0.05$).

Comparison of Group 2 (NYHA I-II CHF) versus control group demonstrated minimal changes in the gut microbiome. Statistically significant differences were shown for *Bacteroides* only (10^9 CFU/g in NYHA class I-II patients vs. 10^{10} CFU/g in the control group, $p<0.05$). In CHF patients with NYHA class III-IV the levels of *Bacteroides* were not significantly different from results reported for the control group; therefore, from our perspective, these data can be ignored in practice.

Statistically significant differences were demonstrated for *Clostridia* (hydrogen sulfide-positive, lecithinase-positive): 10^5 CFU/g in the control group vs. 10^7 CFU/g in CHF patients with NYHA class III-IV, as well as for *Enterococci* and *Candida* yeasts ($p<0.05$). No statistically significant differences between groups were demonstrated for other microorganisms.

Conclusion: the higher is NYHA class of CHF, the stronger are the changes in the large intestine flora due to growth of gram-negative species.

2.4 Changes of the parietal mucin layer flora in CHF patients with NYHA class I-IV

The microorganisms located in the parietal mucin layer have the most significant impact on the host. Therefore, our objective was to study the changes in parietal mucin layer flora in CHF patients with NYHA class I-IV.Taking into account the minimal changes in lumen flora between NYHA class I-II patients and the control group, and considering technical difficulties associated with parietal flora studies, we decided to skip investigation of parietal mucin layer flora in the large intestine for the control group.We decided to approximate the results from biopsies of CHF patients with NYHA class I-II as normal.

Biopsy studies showed changes similar to those reported for feces. A statistically significant changes of the enterobacteria population in CHF patients with NYHA class III-IV was demonstrated (10^8 CFU/g vs. 10^5 CFU/g in patients with NYHA classes III-IV and I-II, respectively; $p<0.0001$).These changes were due to growth of *E. coli* (10^8 CFU/g vs. 10^5 CFU/g in NYHA III-IV vs. NYHA I-II, respectively; $p<0.0001$), *Klebsiella* (10^8 CFU/g vs. 10^5 CFU/g in NYHA III-IV vs. NYHA I-II, respectively; $p<0.005$), and citrate-assimilating enterobacteria (10^8 CFU/g vs. 10^5 CFU/g in NYHA III-IV vs. NYHA I-II, respectively; $p<0.005$).No statistically significant differences were found in the biopsy specimens for *Clostridia, Enterococci,* as well as for *Candida* yeasts. However, statistically significant differences were demonstrated for the population of *Bifidobacteria*: 10^3 CFU/g vs. 10^6 CFU/g in NYHA III-IV vs. NYHA I-II, respectively ($p<0.05$).

Conclusion: the parietal mucin layer flora changes corresponded to the changes of the lumen flora: the higher is NYHA class, the greater is the population of gram-negative microorganisms. No changes in the population levels of gram-positive flora was demonstrated for lumen flora, while in the parietal mucin layer a decrease of *Bifidobacteria* population was reported.

2.5 Changes in the structure of the intestinal wall in CHF patients with NYHA class I-IV

Changes found in the microbial landscape of both lumen flora and parietal mucin layer flora prompted us to study the large intestine wall structure in CHF patients with NYHA class I-IV.

In Group 2, no changes were observed in the biopsy specimens of large intestine mucosa. In Group 1, hyperemic vessels and focal dense lymphoid-cellular infiltrates were reported in the lamina propria of the large intestine mucosa (Fig. 4). This pattern is consistent with marked chronic inflammation.

To confirm the lymphoid nature of the infiltrates, OLA reaction (common lymphocytic antigen) was performed (Fig. 5).

A strong positive infiltrate (derivates of white blood cell line) was observed in the lamina propria of the large intestine mucosa. Particularly, intraepithelial lymphocytes were seen clearly. CD8+ staining (Fig. 6) revealed intraepithelial CD8+-positive T-lymphocytes in the superficial layer of the large intestine mucosa.

Ki67 reaction revealed positive cells of gland epithelium (Fig. 7) in the proliferation phase. At the same time, there were solitary cells positive for Muc5 reaction (i. e. containing mucin 5) in the superficial epithelium of the large intestine mucosa.

Histopathology also revealed a large number of siderophages (Fig. 8), suggesting chronic congestion in the large intestine vessels. We considered these changes to be a sign of the chronic heart failure.

Conclusion: the CHF patients with NYHA class III-IV showed signs of marked chronic inflammation in the large intestine mucosa, along with tissue edema and venous congestion. The severity of these changes increased with higher NYHA class and the severity of CHF decompensation symptoms.

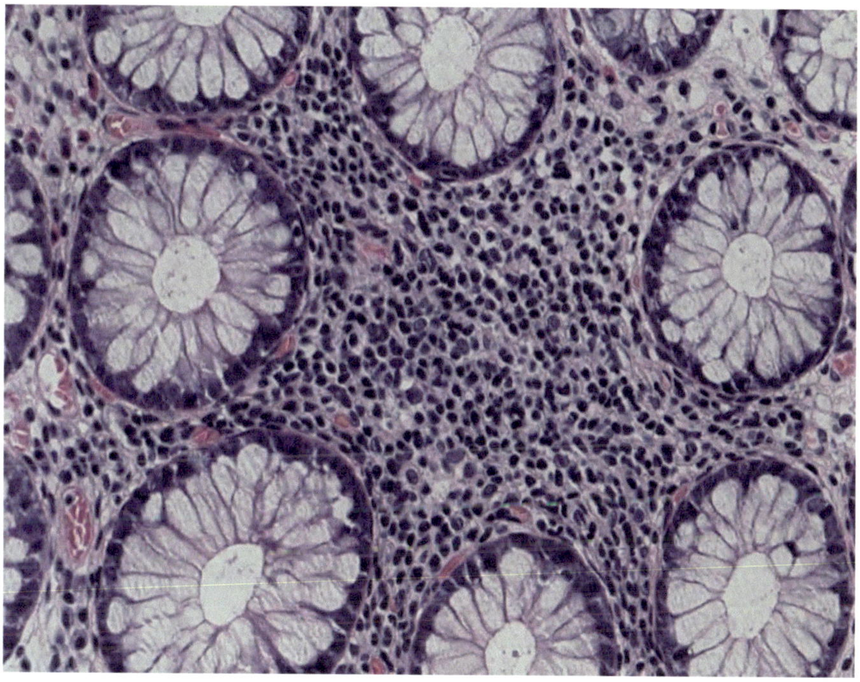

Fig. 4. Biopsy sample of the large intestine mucosa. Hematoxylin-eosin stain.

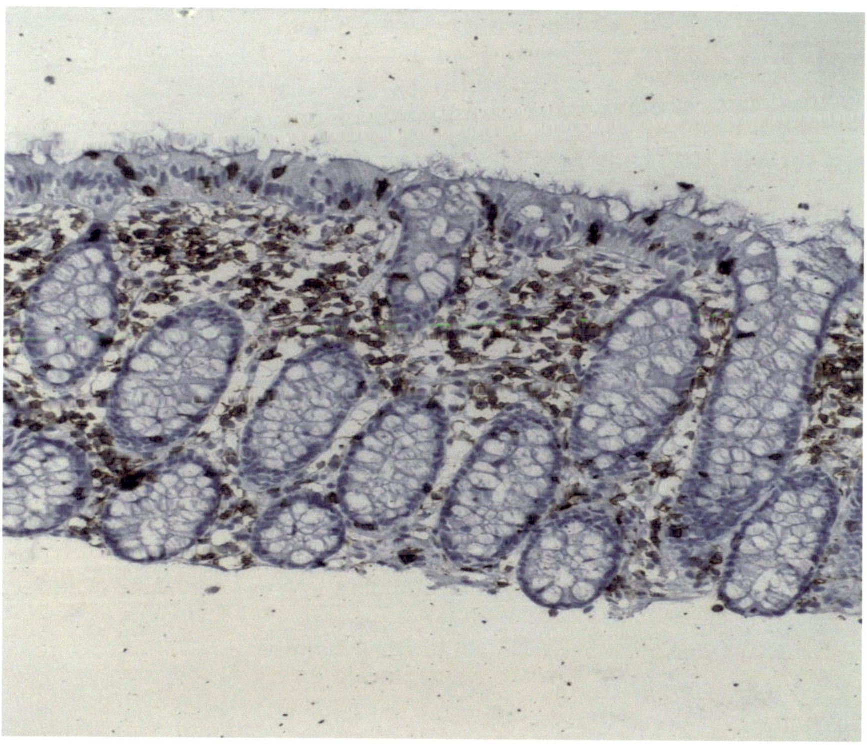

Fig. 5. Biopsy sample of the large intestine mucosa. OLA reaction.

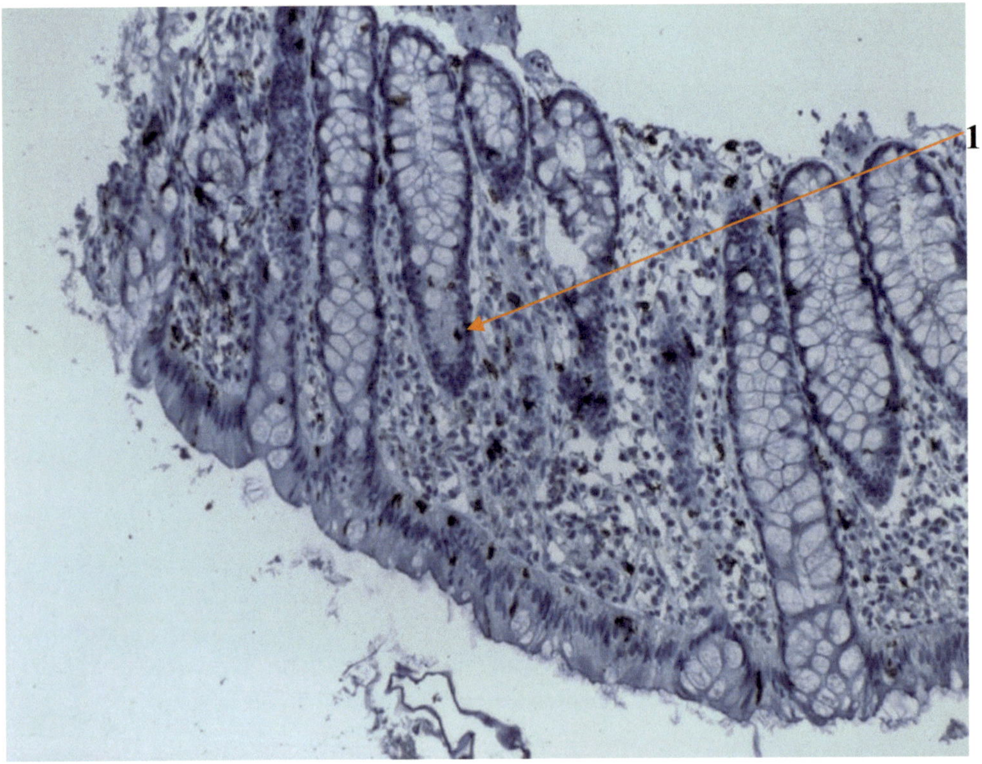

Fig. 6. Biopsy sample of the large intestine mucosa, CD8+ lymphocyte stain. 1 - CD8+ lymphocytes.

2.6 Endotoxin level assessment

Plasma levels of the endotoxin were 1.2±0.03 EU/L in NYHA class III-IV subjects and 0.46±0.01 EU/L in NYHA class I-II subjects (EU - endotoxin units). The level of the endotoxin in the control group subjects was 0.35±0.02 EU/L. Notably, plasma endotoxin levels directly correlated with the changes in population numbers of the large intestine gram-negative flora.

The CHF patients with NYHA class III-IV had levels of IL-6 at 11.5±0.3 U/L, TNF-alpha at 6.6±0.4 U/L, and CRP at 8±0.65 mg/ml. The CHF patients with NYHA class I-II had levels of IL-6 at 4.6±0.3 U/L, TNF-alpha at 3.7±0.4 U/L, and CRP at 5.5±0.29 mg/ml. The levels of these pro-inflammatory cytokines in the control group were within normal limits: : IL-6 was 2 U/L, TNF-alpha was 1.5 U/L, and CRP was 2.9 mg/ml. The identified changes prompted us to suggest two approaches to correction of these conditions:

1. Targeting the large intestine wall using different diuretic regimens, including agents with tissue activity.
2. Selective decontamination in combination with probiotics.

2.7 Use of different diuretic regimens

Figure 9 shows the study design.

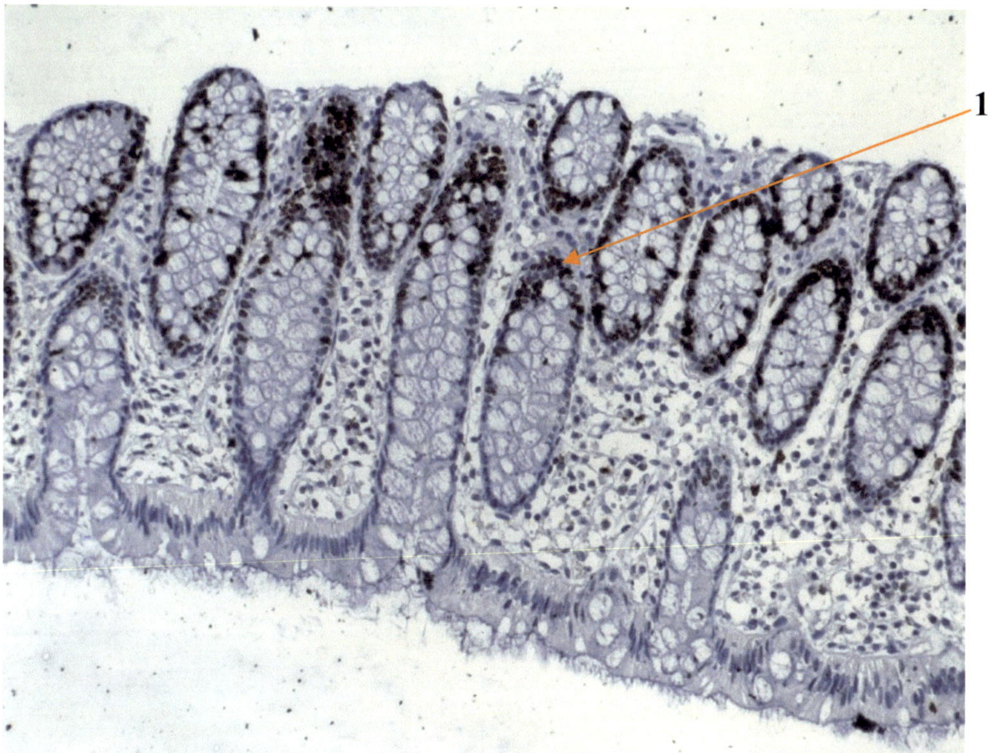

Fig. 7. Biopsy sample of the large intestine mucosa, Ki67 reaction.

1 proliferating epithelial cells of a gland.

The study drugs were prescribed for the first 5 days after the screening visit. After that, the study drug was discontinued and patients remained on the standard-of-care therapy for the 30 days of follow-up (until compensation of their clinical status).

The following tests were performed in this study:

- body mass and the volume of excreted fluid,
- results of 6 minute test,
- Clinical Status Assessment Scale score (points),
- plasma levels of the endotoxin,
- feces flora composition and enzyme activity of the microorganisms,
- results of colonoscopy with cecum biopsy and further histopathology and histochemistry of the obtained samples.

These tests were performed on Day 1, Day 6 and Day 30 of the study.

After the study treatment period, all patients were switched to the supportive care regimen and received the standard-of-care therapy; this phase lasted for 30 days.

One patient died while on study (CHF decompensation was the cause of death).

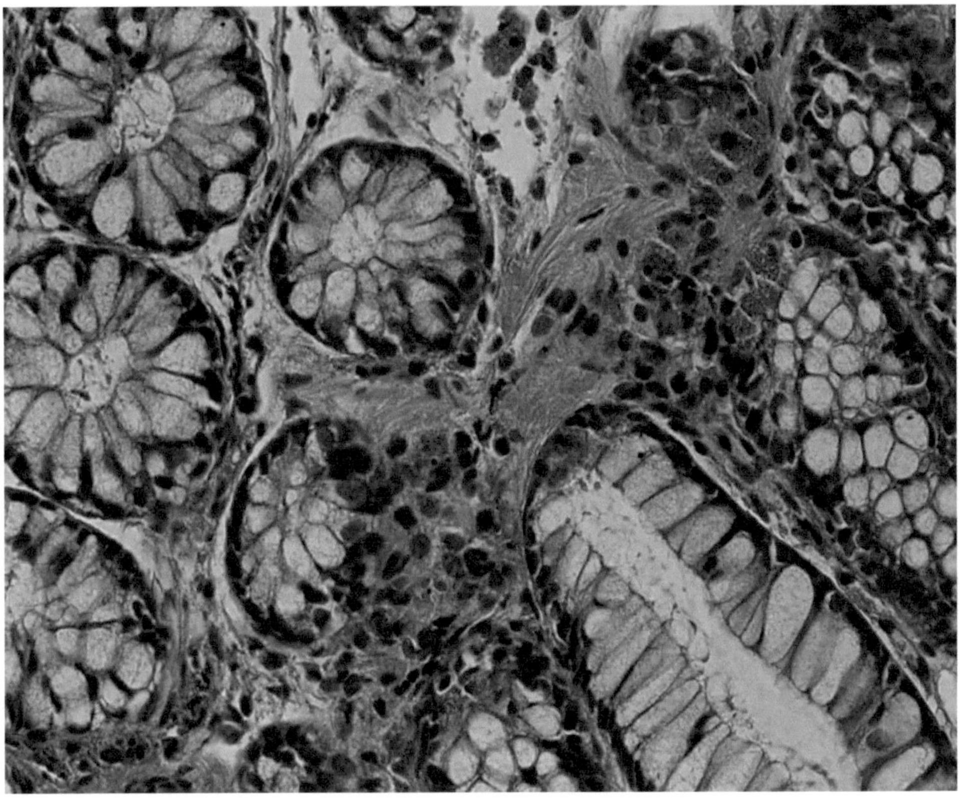

Fig. 8. Biopsy sample of the large intestine mucosa. Hematoxylin-eosin stain. 1 – siderophage.

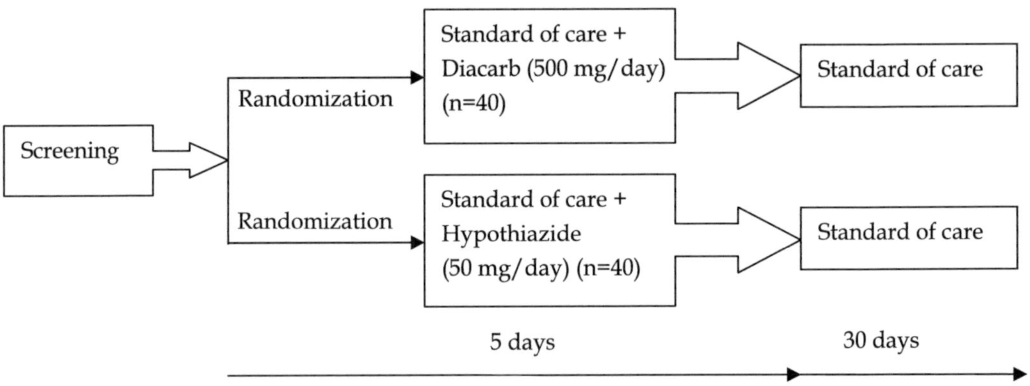

Fig. 9. Study design for the assessment of efficacy of Diacarb (acetazolamide) and Hypothiazide (hydrochlorothiazide) in comprehensive therapy of CHF patients with NYHA III-IV.

Data from 79 subjects who completed the study was therefore used for the analysis of study results.

During the study, 15 adverse reactions were reported, but none of these caused discontinuation of the study treatment.

No statistically significant differences between groups were demonstrated for the main variables.

2.8 Changes of body mass and volume of excreted urine over time

To determine efficacy of each study diuretic regimen, changes of the body mass and the volume of excreted urine were evaluated throughout the study. After the first five days, a decrease of body mass to 83±0.5 kg and 83.1±0.36 kg was demonstrated in both Group 1 and Group 2, respectively. The decrease was statistically significant against the baseline body mass of 87 kg, but the difference between groups was not statistically significant ($p=0.872$).

The volume of excreted urine in the study groups was the highest on the first day of treatment, comprising 2.51±0.1 L and 2.5±0.25 L for Group 1 and Group 2, respectively. This effect decreased proportionally during the following five days in both groups. Notably, no statistically significant difference was detected between groups both in terms of body mass change ($p=0.99$) and in terms of the volume of excreted urine.

2.9 Changes of endotoxin levels over time

Substantial decrease of endotoxin levels on the follow-up Day 21 (1.2±0.02 EU/L to 0.2±0.01 EU/L) was demonstrated in all groups. However, in the Diacarb group, this process was substantially faster: as early as on Day 5, the endotoxin levels were at 0.4±0.02 EU/L, whereas in the thiazide diuretic group the levels were at 0.78±0.01 EU/L ($p=0.012$). Notably, while the diuretic effects in the Hypothiazide and Diacarb groups were almost identical, the latter group demonstrated faster decrease of the endotoxin level.

This is probably due to tissue pH change caused by Diacarb, which facilitates fast dehydration of the large intestine wall and decreases its permeability for the endotoxin. To support this hypothesis, we performed histopathology and histochemistry studies using the biopsy samples from the large intestine at Day 1 and Day 5. To exclude the role of the large intestine flora, we also monitored its composition throughout the study.

2.10 Assessment of diuretic regimen effects on structural changes in the large intestine wall over time

Assessment of the histological and histochemical patterns in the large intestine mucosa during Diacarb or Hypothiazide treatment demonstrated the following changes.In the thiazide group (Fig. 10 and Fig. 11), there were signs of reduced mucosal edema on treatment (Day 6); however, a rise of local inflammatory reaction was also evident (lymphoplasmocytic infiltration, increased number of segmented WBCs, predominantly eosinophils).This may be a relative effect caused by reduction of edema and shortening of intercellular distances rather than an absolute growth of the inflammatory infiltration.

A decrease of edema on Day 6 was also seen in the Diacarb group (Fig. 12, Fig. 13), but, in addition to that, the level of local inflammation decreased (the infiltration by lymphoid cells is consistent with low-intensity chronic inflammation).

Most probably, the difference between Diacarb and Hypothiazide in their effects on large intestine wall edema causes different permeability of the wall for the endotoxin, which results in different kinetics of blood endotoxin level reduction in the CHF patients with NYHA class III-IV. These findings may result from changes in pH of the intestinal wall, better microcirculation, and consequent decrease of infiltration. Another possibility is that Diacarb, a carbonic anhydrase inhibitor, blocks alpha-carbonic anhydrase of gram-negative bacteria, depressing their pathogenic effect on the intestinal wall.

2.11 Assessment of effects of diuretic regimens on changes of flora over time

No statistically significant changes in concentration of gram-negative bacteria both in feces and in biopsy material were demonstrated, regardless of the treatment regimen.

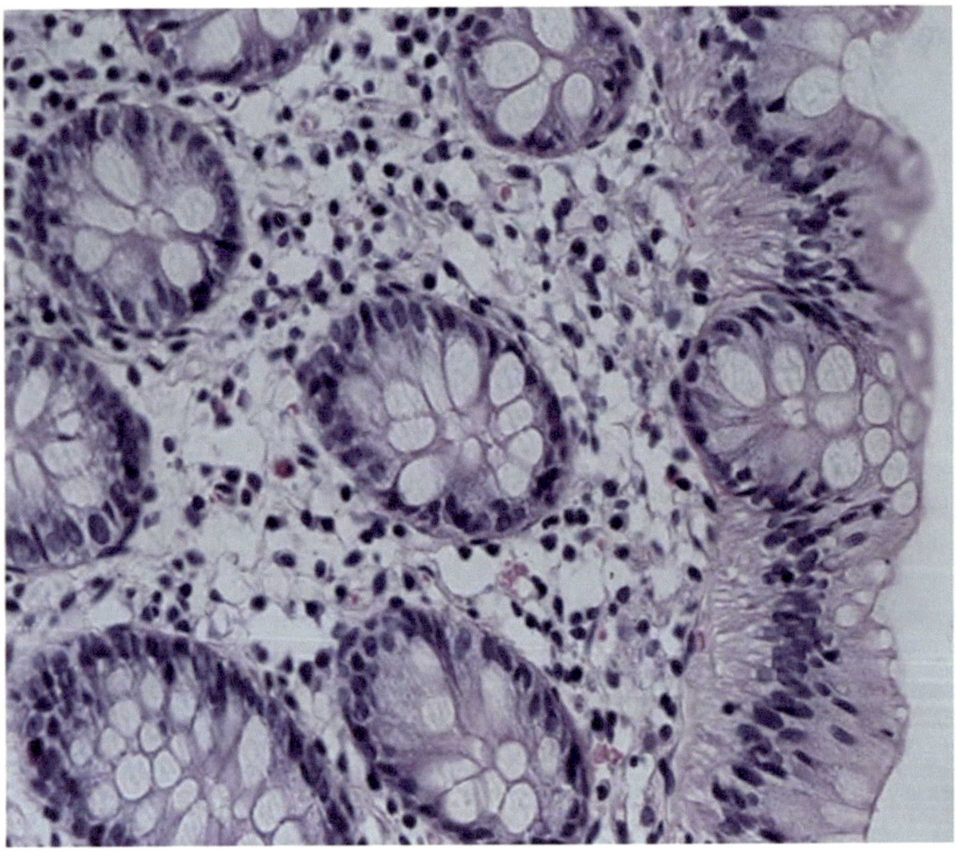

Fig. 10. Magnification x 400 (good), hematoxylin and eosin stain.Before treatment, "fuzzy" lymphoid-cellular infiltration and solitary eosinophils were noted in the *lamina propria* of the large intestine mucosa.

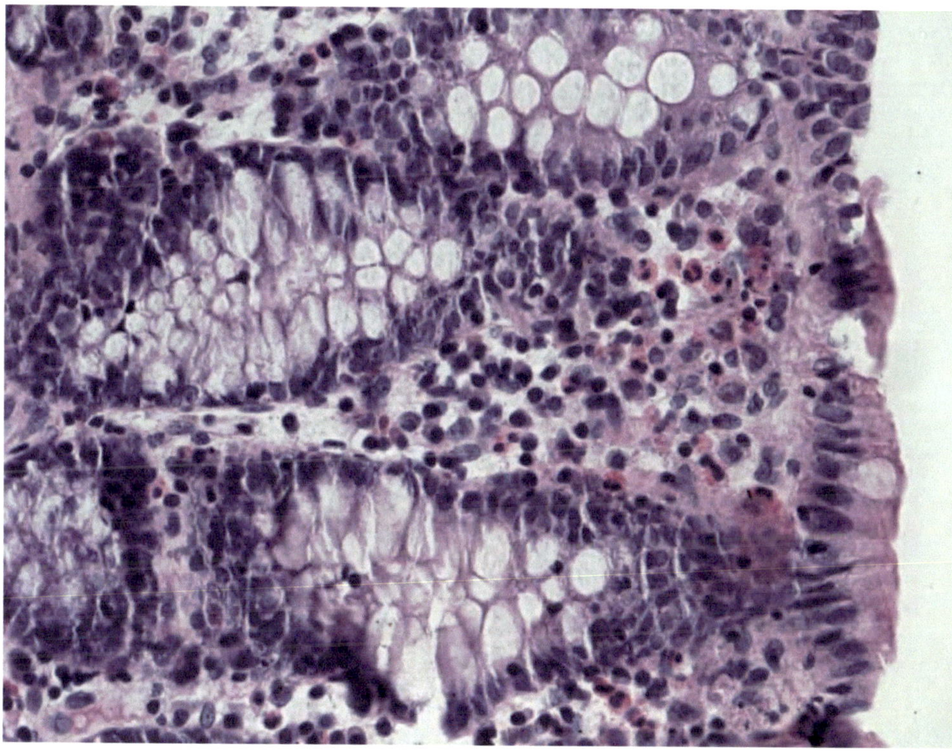

Fig. 11. Magnification x 400 (good), hematoxylin and eosin stain.Day 6 of the treatment period.Lymphoplasmocytic infiltration increases. The population of segmented WBCs, particularly eosinophils, increases significantly.

These results demonstrate that plasma endotoxin levels in CHF patients with NYHA class III-IV are affected not only by the gram-negative flora population in the intestine, but also by the severity of edema, and therefore by the degree of decompensation of patient's clinical status.The endotoxin levels in this case are probably affected by the increase of the intestinal wall permeability for the endotoxin caused by the edema.

As patient's status improves towards compensation, the endotoxin levels decrease to normal values. This process is faster with the use of Diacarb compared to the use of Hypothiazide. However, this is not accountable to their diuretic effects, because there were no statistically significant differences in the changes of body mass and the volume of excreted urine between Diacarb and Hypothiazide.It is likely that Diacarb improves microcirculation by changing tissue pH, and causes not only improvement of renal urine filtration, but also faster shrinking of tissues, particularly shrinking of the intestinal wall, which decreases its permeability for the endotoxin.

Differences in the inflammatory infiltrate intensity between Hypothiazide and Diacarb groups were discovered (in addition to decreased edema, Diacarb reduces the inflammation in the large intestine mucosa). This effect is probably accountable to improved microcirculation in the intestinal wall in the Diacarb group, as well as carbonic anhydrase inhibition produced by Diacarb leading to block of alpha-carbonic anhydrase of gram-negative bacteria, which reduces their pathogenic effect on the intestinal wall.

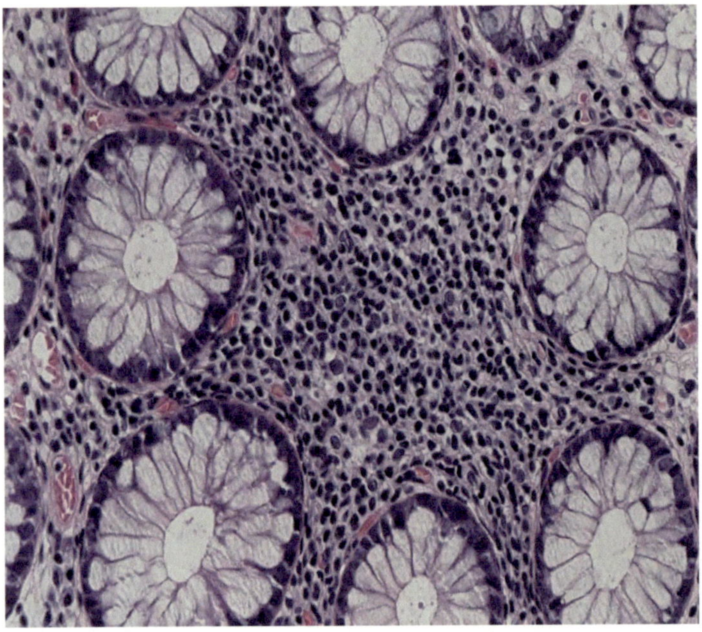

Fig. 12. Magnification x 400 (good), hematoxylin and eosin stain.Before treatment, there were hyperemic vessels and focal dense lymphoid-cellular infiltration in the *lamina propria* of the large intestine. This pattern is typical for strong chronic inflammation.

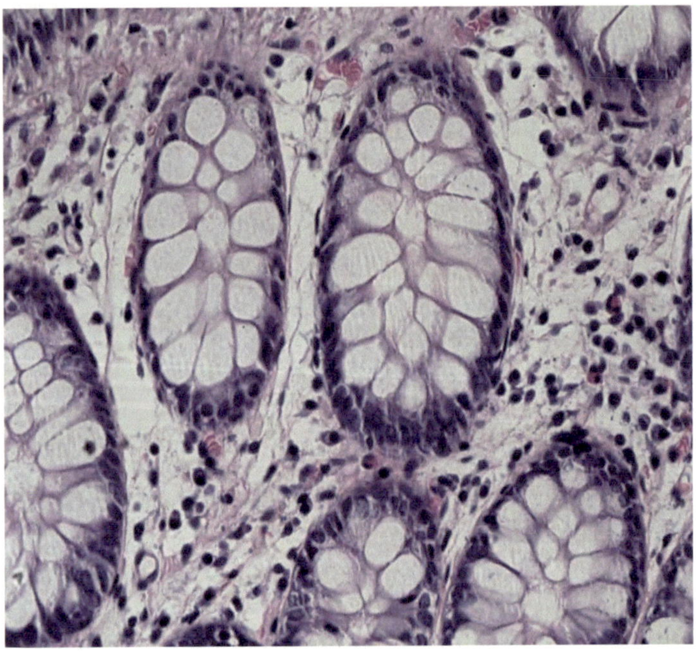

Fig. 13. Magnification x 400 (good), hematoxylin and eosin stain. Day 6 of the treatment period."Fuzzy" lymphoid-cellular infiltration is seen in the *lamina propria* of the large intestine mucosa, which is consistent with the pattern of weak chronic inflammation.

Conclusion: administration of Diacarb facilitates faster decrease of plasma endotoxin levels, which allows for faster compensation of patient's clinical status.

2.12 Use of selective decontamination alone vs. selective decontamination in combination with probiotics in comprehensive therapy of NYHA class III-IV CHF

All patients included in this phase of the study received standard-of-care therapy, including:

- ACE inhibitors/ angiotensin receptor blockers (mean daily dose of 10 mg/160 mg);
- beta-blockers (prescribed from Day 5 after the start of the therapy, dose titration from the minimum therapeutic dose, mean daily dose was 50 mg of metoprolol per day);
- digoxin 0.00025 g per day (in case of atrial fibrillation with tachycardia or LVEF below 25 %);
- aspirin 125 mg/day (secondary prophylaxis method);
- Cordarone 200 mg/day (in case of ventricular disturbances with risk of high Lown grades);
- loop diuretics (Lasix) with mean daily dose of 70 mg/day.

The following drugs were chosen for the study:

- antibacterial fluoroquinolone: ciprofloxacin with daily dose of 1000 mg;
- probiotic: Primadophilus Bifidus, 1 capsule per day.

At the study start, all patients received a 5-day selective decontamination with oral ciprofloxacin 1000 mg/day.After that, patients were randomized into two groups:

- Group 1 (n=45) received standard-of-care;
- Group 2 (n=45) received the probiotic - Primadophilus Bifidus, 1 capsule per day for 14 days.

After the completion of probiotic treatment, both groups received standard-of-care.

The following study variables were evaluated on Day 1, Day 5, and Day 21:

- results of 6-minute test,
- Clinical Status Assessment Scale score (points),
- plasma levels of the endotoxin,
- feces flora composition and enzyme activity of the microorganisms.

In this phase, 2 deaths occurred in the group receiving selective decontamination alone.In the Primadophilus Bifidus group, one patient experienced adverse effects leading to patient's decision to discontinue the drug.

Data from 87 subjects who completed the study was therefore used for the analysis of study results.

Ten cases of adverse reactions were reported during the study. Only one of these cases caused the patient to stop the drug.

The resulting groups had comparable basic characteristics.

2.13 Changes of the large intestine flora over time with the use of selective decontamination alone or selective decontamination combined with the probiotic

By Day 5 of the study, a statistically significant decrease was demonstrated in Group 1 for total population of both gram-negative microorganisms (baseline value was $10^{12\pm0.1}$ CFU/g, the value after the selective decontamination was $10^{6\pm0.4}$ CFU/g; p=0.000) and gram-positive microorganisms (baseline value was $10^{6\pm0.56}$ CFU/g, the value after the selective decontamination was $10^{4\pm0.32}$ CFU/g; p=0.000)However, on Day 21 study visit, gram-negative and gram-positive populations returned to their baseline levels ($10^{11.9}$ CFU/g and $10^{6.1}$ CFU/g, respectively; p=0.000). These results support literature reports of low efficacy of the selective decontamination used alone.

In the group where probiotics were prescribed after the course of selective decontamination, Day 5 populations decreased similarly to Group 1, both for gram-negative (baseline $10^{12.05\pm0.6}$ CFU/g, post-decontamination $10^{6.3\pm0.4}$ CFU/g; p=0.000) and gram-positive (baseline $10^{5.2\pm0.5}$ CFU/g, post-decontamination $10^{4.2\pm0.2}$ CFU/g; p=0.000) microorganisms.However, after Primadophilus Bifidus administration for 14 days, gram-positive flora population grew to $10^{8.02\pm0.1}$ CFU/g, and an insignificant growth of gram-negative flora to $10^{7.27\pm0.1}$ CFU/g was demonstrated, which is consistent with normal values for gram-negative population in the large intestine.

Conclusion: administration of probiotics after a course of selective decontamination normalizes large intestine flora levels, whereas decontamination alone leads to reduction of microbial populations for a short term only.

2.14 Changes of the endotoxin level over time

In Group 1, Day 5 endotoxin levels decreased from baseline significantly (baseline: 1.2±0.9 EU/L, Day 5: 0.55±0.06 EU/L; p=0.000), which corresponded to the reduction of gram-negative population in the large intestine. However, at Day 21, as the gram-negative population in the large intestine grew, the plasma endotoxin levels returned to their baseline values (1.18±0.05 EU/L); on Day 30, the endotoxin concentration remained high (1.21±0.045 EU/L).

In Group 2, after the selective decontamination was completed and the gram-negative population in the large intestine reduced, the plasma endotoxin levels also declined (baseline: 1.24±0.01 EU/L, Day 5: 0.67±0.03 EU/L, p=0.000). A trend towards decline of plasma endotoxin levels and achievement of normal values was demonstrated subsequently (Day 21: 0.56±0.02 EU/L, Day 30: 0.26±0.08 EU/L). These results can be explained by the reduction of the gram-negative populations in the large intestine due to administration of the selective decontamination followed by probiotic.

2.15 Assessment of changes in plasma pro-inflammatory cytokine levels over time

With the use of the selective decontamination alone, the decrease of the following variables on Day 5 was demonstrated: IL-6 to 4.1±0.03 U/L (baseline 4.9±0.01 U/L), TNF-alpha to 5±0.09 U/L (baseline 5.7±0.04 U/L), and CRP to 4 mg/ml (baseline 8.6 mg/ml).However, as early as on Day 12, these cytokine variables were shown to return to their baseline levels, which persisted till Day 30. This demonstrates poor efficacy of the selective decontamination alone for the system inflammation marker endpoints.

When the selective decontamination was used in combination with the probiotic, decrease in the population of enterobacteria in the large intestine and decrease of plasma endotoxin levels were reported.However, while levels of the pro-inflammatory cytokines decreased by Day 5 (CRP: 4.2±0.1 mg/ml on Day 5 vs. baseline 7.82±0.05 mg/L; IL-6: 3.9±0.05 U/L on Day 5 vs. baseline 5±0.01 U/L; TNF-alpha: 5.01±0.02 U/L on Day 5 vs. baseline 5.8±0.02 U/L), but on Day 21 they already rebounded above the baseline levels, and on Day 30 there was a trend towards further growth of their levels.

This is probably accountable to the decrease of gram-negative flora population in the large intestine due to the antibacterial treatment, and consequent decline of plasma levels of the endotoxin.Normal population numbers of the gram-negative flora are further maintained by the administration of the probiotic. However, the probiotic contains gram-positive microorganisms, which bind to the Toll-like receptors, initiating the synthesis of pro-inflammatory cytokines in the large intestine enterocytes, leading to further exacerbation of the systemic inflammation.

These results demonstrate lack of efficacy for the selective decontamination used alone.When the selective decontamination was combined with the probiotic, normalization of the intestinal flora and plasma endotoxin levels was reported. However, a significant growth of the pro-inflammatory cytokine levels occurs with this regimen, which affects patient's status and is likely to require additional correction.

These data demonstrated that comprehensive therapy for CHF combined with the selective decontamination alone (i. e. without probiotic) caused to a short-term decline of gram-negative flora population, while the population numbers of gram-positive flora remained almost unaffected. A short-term decline in plasma levels of the endotoxin and pro-inflammatory cytokines was also reported. However, as early as one week after the discontinuation of the antibacterial treatment, gram-negative flora population numbers returned to their baseline levels, accompanied by the increase in plasma levels of the endotoxin and the pro-inflammatory cytokines. A potential explanation for this pattern is that CHF patients with NYHA class III-IV develop significant restructuring of their large intestine walls, providing favorable conditions for domination of gram-negative flora.Isolated use of the selective decontamination, neither supported by any agents that repair large intestine wall structure, nor combined by any probiotics, fails to provide stable, long-term changes in the large intestine flora.

However, administration of probiotics added to the antibacterial treatment demonstrated persistent effect: normalization of gram-negative flora levels and plasma endotoxin levels. Notably, with the use of the probiotic, blood CRP levels increased, which is probably accountable to the presence of gram-positive flora in the probiotic, prompting the host to produce more antibodies. Unfortunately, the CRP levels were not followed for a longer period of time, and the time needed for the CRP to reach normal levels remained unknown.It can only be assumed that this period should not take too much time, because the subjects were exposed to the probiotic for 2 weeks only. However, if a long-term, persistent growth of the CRP levels in blood do occur, decompensated CHF patients with NYHA class III-IV might benefit from administration of statins.

3. Clinical significance of adipose tissue changes over time in patients with chronic heart failure of ischemic origin. Treatment options

3.1 Introduction

Syndrome of cardiac cachexia is one of the most severe complications of chronic heart failure. Among the latest advancements in the field of immunology is the concept of cytokine activation system and its role in the pathogenesis of chronic heart failure and development of cardiac cachexia. Currently, two main classes of cytokines are known to participate in the development of heart failure:vasoconstrictive cytokines (endothelin-1 and big endothelin) and vasodepressive cytokines (TNF-α, IL-1, IL-6, IL-8). Patients with signs of cardiac cachexia are known to have higher levels of inflammation markers than patients with normal body mass (Francis, 1998; Monteiro, 2007). Notably, adipose tissue is one of the sources of cytokines.In addition to leptin and adiponectin, adipose tissue was demonstrated to participate in production of TNF-α and IL-6 (Moses, 2004; Nagaya, 2001; Springer, 2010).

We assumed that one of the methods to decrease the activities of pro-inflammatory cytokines could be the increase of dry body mass (body muscle mass, body fat mass) (Dostalova et al., 2003). Therefore, one of the options to correct the levels of inflammatory markers in this category of patients could be nutritional support.

From our perspective, there are two possible approaches to correct the systemic inflammation:development of methods that can increase the mass of the adipose tissue and methods that have direct effect on the synthesis of pro-inflammatory cytokines.

3.2 Assessment of body composition, levels of leptin, adiponectin, and pro-inflammatory cytokines in patients with different NYHA classes of CHF

To study these variables, three consecutive groups were enrolled in the first part of the study: Group 1 included chronic heart failure patients with NYHA class I-II, Group 2 included chronic heart failure patients with NYHA class III-IV (subgroup A: without cachexia; subgroup B: with cachexia), Group 3 was a control group.Patient screening was performed in the population of patients with history of CHF of ischemic origin with NYHA class I-IV for more than 6 months, older than 40 years of age, admitted to a general internal medicine department or a cardiology department (n=197).The control group included outpatients of the Consultation and Diagnostics Polyclinic (n=52).

Clinical characteristics of the patients:

Age:these three groups were comparable in terms of patients' age.

From the results of analysis of associated clinical conditions, diabetes mellitus was reported in 57.1 % of CHF patients with NYHA class III-IV with cachexia and in 48.6 % without cachexia, as well as in 14 % of patients with NYHA class I-II.

Analysis of concomitant medications: CHF patients with NYHA class III-IV with/without cachexia were on ACE inhibitors or ARB in 64.2 %/63.8 %, on beta-adrenoblockers in 82.1 %/80 %, on digoxin in 75 %/76.1 %, on diuretics in 35.7 %/34.3 %, and on Cordarone in 28.6 %/19.5 % of cases, respectively.For NYHA class I-II patients, the corresponding variables were: on ACE inhibitors/ARB 51.6 %, on beta-adrenoblockers 59.4 %, on digoxin 9.3 %, on diuretics 45.3 %, on Cordarone 3.1 %.

3.3 Comparison of methods used to evaluate body composition in patients with CHF of different NYHA class and the control group patients

Two methods were used to study body composition: caliper measurement and bioimpedance analysis.Comparison of these methods in all three groups did not reveal any statistically significant differences between the values obtained using caliper measurements and bioimpedance analyzer.However, the method of caliper measurements is subjective and is not suitable for patients with decompensated heart failure (i. e. with severe edema syndrome).Moreover, unlike caliper measurements, bioimpedance analyzer of body composition allows to estimate not only the body fat mass, but also total fluid content, which is important for the assessment of the body composition in patients with decompensated chronic heart failure.

Comparison of Group 1 vs. Group 2 revealed statistically significant differences in the adipose tissue mass, which was 29.7±2.2 kg in Group 1 and 22.2±2.1 kg in Group 2 ($p<0.001$), as well as in the lean body mass, which was 54.8±6.9 kg in Group 1 and 59.7±6.1 kg ($p<0.001$) in Group 2. This was associated with changes in total fluid content, which was 38.2±3.1 kg in Group 1 vs. 48.8±3.3 kg in patients with NYHA class III-IV ($p<0.001$).BMI did not differ significantly between groups.

Comparison of the study results between Group 2 (NYHA III-IV) and the control group revealed changes similar to those between Group 1 and Group 2.

Comparison of Group 1 (NYHA I-II) vs. the control group revealed statistically significant differences in the body fat mass, which was 29.7±2.2 kg in Group 1 vs. 32.6±2.4 kg in Group 3 ($p<0.001$), and statistically significant differences in total fluid content, which was 38.2±3.1 kg in Group 1 vs. 25.6±2.9 kg in Group 3 ($p<0.001$).

In patients with cachexia, a significantly lower LBM of 55.2±4.9 kg and body fat mass of 15.65±1.8 kg were reported. Notably, the total fluid content levels in these patients was greater than levels of this variable in patients without cachexia, but the differences of this variable were not statistically significant.

Conclusion: the higher is NYHA class of CHF, the stronger are changes of body composition; with higher NYHA class, adipose tissue mass declines, total fluid content grows.These changes were stronger in patients with cachexia.

3.4 Levels of leptin, adiponectin, and pro-inflammatory cytokines in patients with different NYHA classes and in the control group

The patients with NYHA III-IV were found to have adiponectin levels at 18.6±4.9 μg/mL, leptin levels at 43.8±8.3 ng/mL, IL-6 levels at 11.7±0.3 U/L, TNF-α levels at 6.6±0.2 U/L, CRP levels at 8.8±0.4 mg/ml. These values were significantly higher than values reported for patients with NYHA class I-II and for patients in the control group, who had their levels of adipokines and pro-inflammatory cytokines within normal range.

Comparison of patients with NYHA class III-IV with and without cachexia demonstrated the following differences: leptin levels were significantly higher in patients without cachexia (47.9±4.2 ng/mL), while levels of adiponectin, IL-6, TNF-α, and CRP were significantly higher in patients with cachexia.

Conclusion: the higher is NYHA class of CHF, the stronger is the intensity of chronic inflammation. While this may be an effect of growing intoxication in patients with advanced stages of CHF, this could also be associated with the role of the adipose tissue in production of pro-inflammatory cytokines and biologic agents that stimulate cytokine production. Higher classes of NYHA are associated with lower adipose tissue mass, which leads to increase of adiponectin plasma levels.However, the levels of leptin in patients with NYHA class III-IV are also high, which may be accountable to big dimensions of adipocytes. Patients with cachexia have significantly lower levels of leptin when compared to patients without cachexia; this is probably associated with shrinking of the lipid droplet in the adipocyte.

3.5 Evaluation of visceral and subcutaneous tissue structure in patients with different CHF classes

To study this variable, autopsies of deceased patients (with NYHA class I-IV chronic heart failure diagnosed before their death) were performed. Patients were allocated into two groups: Group 1: before death, patients were diagnosed with NYHA I-II chronic heart failure; Group 2: before death, patients were diagnosed with NYHA III-IV chronic heart failure. Patients of Group 2 were divided in two subgroups: patients with cachexia and patients without cachexia. All patients were admitted to GKB no. 4 (City Clinical Hospital no. 4) before death. For NYHA I-II patients, the main reasons for hospitalization were: unstable angina, acute myocardial infarction, hypertensive crisis, heart rhythm disorder, cerebrovascular accident; for NYHA III-IV patients, the main reasons for hospitalization were: decompensation of CHF, acute/recurrent myocardial infarction, heart rhythm disorder, cerebrovascular accident.The postmortem assessment included measurement of the subcutaneous fat, measurement of the omentum mass, morphometric study of the subcutaneous fat, omental fat and pericardial fat.

Of 118 subjects total, 50 subjects were in the first group, 56 subjects were in the second group, and 12 subjects belonged to the third group. These three groups were comparable in terms of patients' age. The main cause of death for NYHA I-II patients was the acute myocardial infarction (46.0 %), and for NYHA II-III patients (both with cachexia and without cachexia) the main cause of death was post-infarction cardiosclerosis (58.3 %, 48.2 %, respectively). The most frequent complication leading to death in patients with NYHA class I-II CHF was acute heart failure; in patients with NYHA class III-IV the most frequent complication leading to death was CHF decompensation. Pneumonia incidence in patients with NYHA class III-IV was higher (22 %) than in NYHA I-II patients (4 %). Multiple complications were reported for 22.0 % patients with NYHA I-II, 46.4 % patients with NYHA III-IV without cachexia, and 100 % of patients with NYHA III-IV with cachexia.

During autopsy, the following investigations were performed: measurement of subcutaneous fat thickness 2 cm below the navel, measurement of omentum weight; autopsy samples of subcutaneous fat, omental fat, and pericardial fat at the apex of the heart were collected.

There were no statistically significant differences between patients with NYHA I-II and NYHA III-IV without cachexia in the thickness of subcutaneous fat: it was 5.3±1.7 cm and 5.1±2.2, respectively ($p=0.6$).In CHF patients with NYHA III-IV with cachexia, the difference in thickness of subcutaneous fat (2.4±1.1 cm) was statistically different from NYHA III-IV patients without cachexia ($p<0.001$).

In CHF patients with NYHA class III-IV, omentum weight was significantly lower than in patients with NYHA I-II (387±134 g vs. 521±142 g, respectively; $p<0.001$).In CHF patients with NYHA classes III and IV, the omentum weight was 164±87 g, which is significantly lower than in patients without cachexia ($p<0.001$).

The morphometric analysis of the samples showed the following changes.In the subcutaneous fat, lymphocytic infiltration was the strongest in patients with NYHA class III-IV with cachexia (average 12.4±4.7 %); in patients with NYHA class I-II this variable was 3.8±2.2 % (comparison: $p<0.001$), and in NYHA III-IV patients without cachexia it was 4.3±2.4 % (comparison: $p<0.001$).No significant differences in the proportion of fibrous tissue in the subcutaneous fat was found between the groups.The percentage of fibrous tissue was 3.8±1.9 % in NYHA class I-II patients, 4.1±2.3 % in NYHA class III-IV patients without cachexia, and 4.6±2.6 % in NYHA class III-IV patients with cachexia ($p_{1-2}=0.469$, $p_{1-3}=0.229$, $p_{2-3}=0.506$). See Fig. 14, 15, 16.

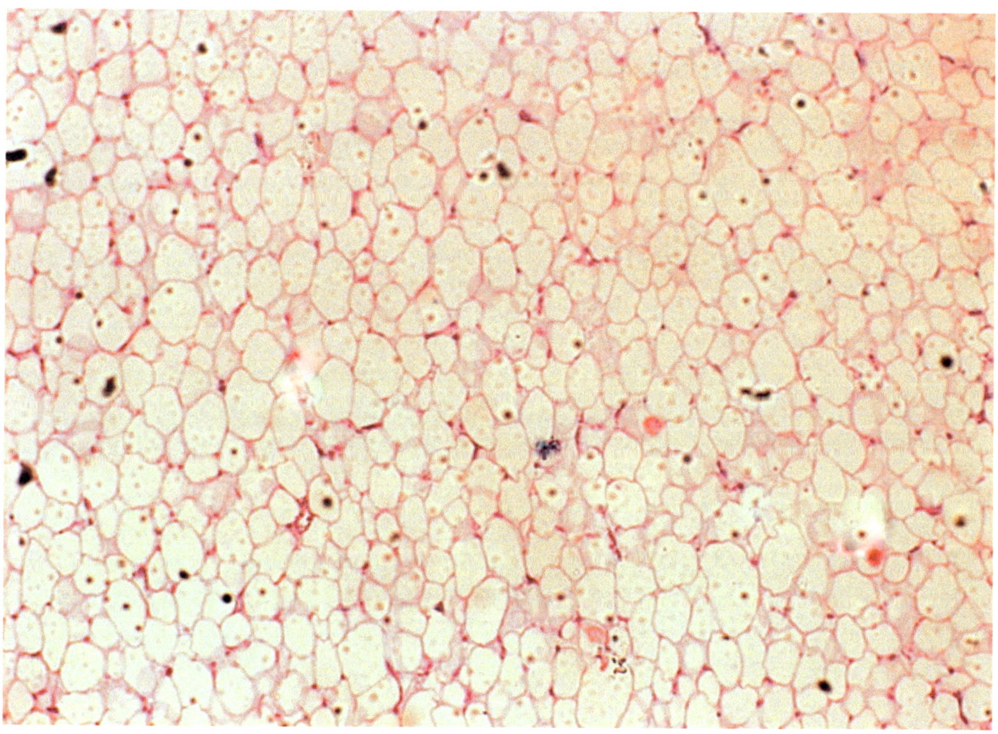

Fig. 14. Subcutaneous fat in a CHF patient with NYHA class I. Romanowsky-Giemsa stain.

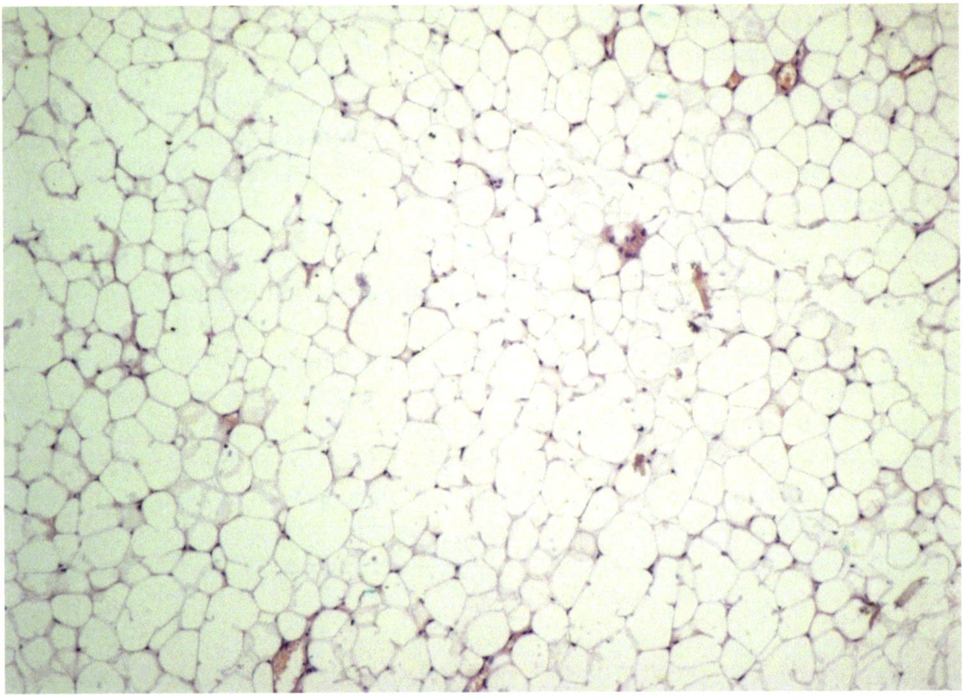

Fig. 15. Subcutaneous fat in a CHF patient with NYHA class III.

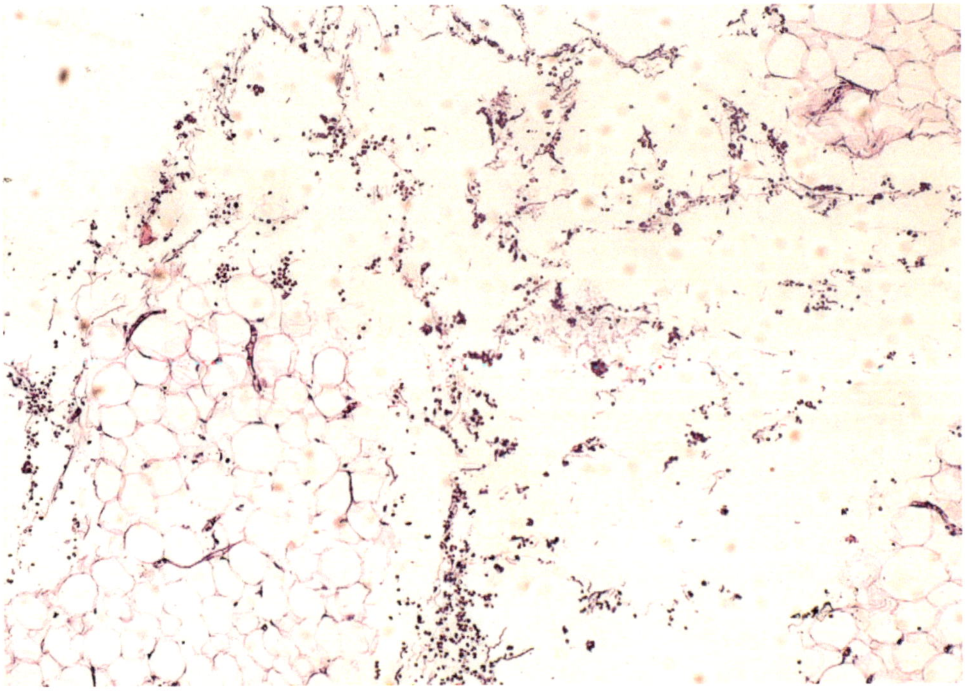

Fig. 16. Subcutaneous fat in a CHF patient with NYHA class IV with cachexia. Romanowsky-Giemsa stain.

Analysis of the visceral fat (omentum, pericardial fat) showed the strongest lymphocytic infiltration in subjects with NYHA class III-IV, both with cachexia and without cachexia. This variable was 53.4±7.8 % in the omentum and 49.7±8.4 % in the pericardium in patients with cachexia, and 42.1±6.7 % in the omentum and 42.6±8.8 % in the pericardium in patients without cachexia (compare to patients with NYHA I-II, who had the lymphocytic infiltration of 5.1±2.3 % in the omentum ($p1<0.001$, $p2<0.001$) and 4.9±2.6 % in the pericardium ($p1<0.001$, $p2<0.001$)).The amount of fibrous tissue in NYHA class III-IV patients without cachexia was higher than in the patients with NYHA class I-II: 15.2±4.9 % vs. 3.1±1.2 % in the omental adipose tissue ($p<0.001$), 14.8±5.4 % vs. 3.2±0.9 % in the adipose tissue of the pericardium ($p<0.001$), respectively.In NYHA III-IV patients with cachexia, the amount of fibrous tissue was significantly higher than in NYHA III-IV patients without cachexia: 24.8±3.7 % in the omentum ($p<0.001$) and 24.3±3.2 % in the pericardium ($p<0.001$).See figures 17-22.

Mean diameter of adipocytes was measured, with the following results:In CHF patients with NYHA class I-II, the diameter of adipocytes was 38.6±12.2 µm in the subcutaneous fat samples, 44.2±16.1 µm in the omentum, 42.3±11.4 µm in the pericardial fat. In CHF patients with NYHA class III-IV without cachexia, the diameter of adipocytes was 42.7±14.2 µm in the subcutaneous fat samples ($p=0.116$), 56.4±13.9 µm in the omentum ($p<0.001$), 52.2±11.3 µm in the pericardial fat ($p<0.001$). In NYHA class III-IV patients with cachexia, the diameter of adipocytes was 28.2±11.5 µm in the subcutaneous fat samples ($p=0.01$), 32.8±14.3 µm in the omentum ($p=0.028$), 30.3±12.4 µm in the pericardial fat ($p<0.001$).

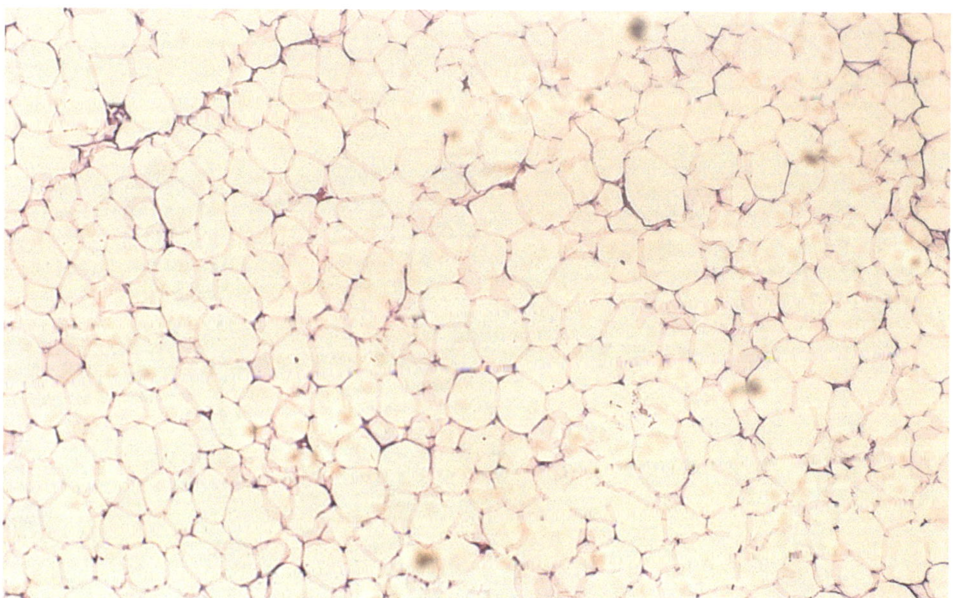

Fig. 17. Visceral adipose tissue (pericardial fat) in a CHF patient with NYHA class I. Romanowsky-Giemsa stain.

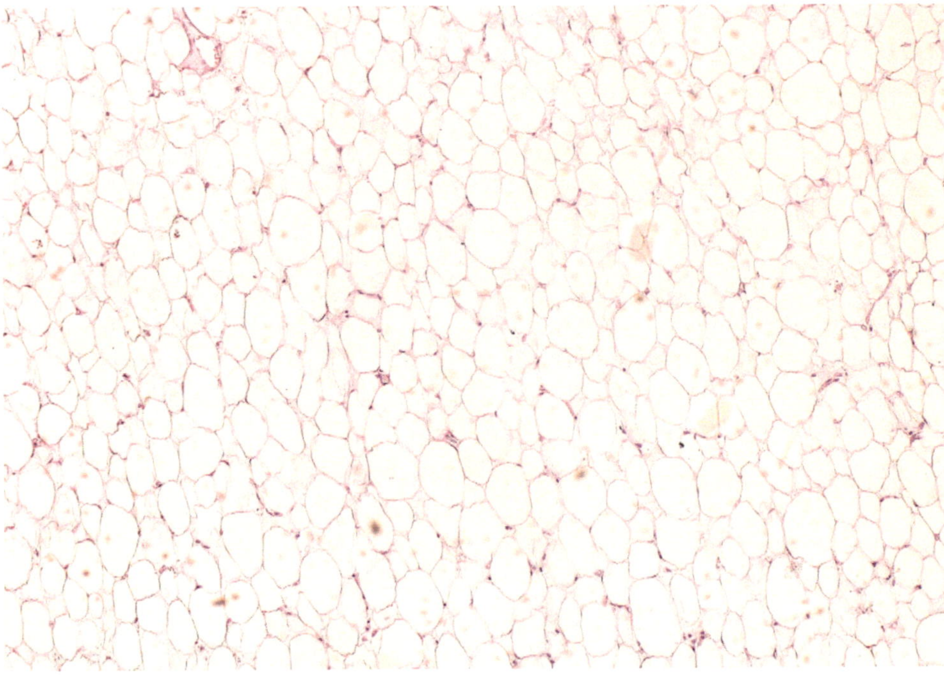

Fig. 18. Visceral adipose tissue (omentum) in a CHF patient with NYHA class I. Romanowsky-Giemsa stain.

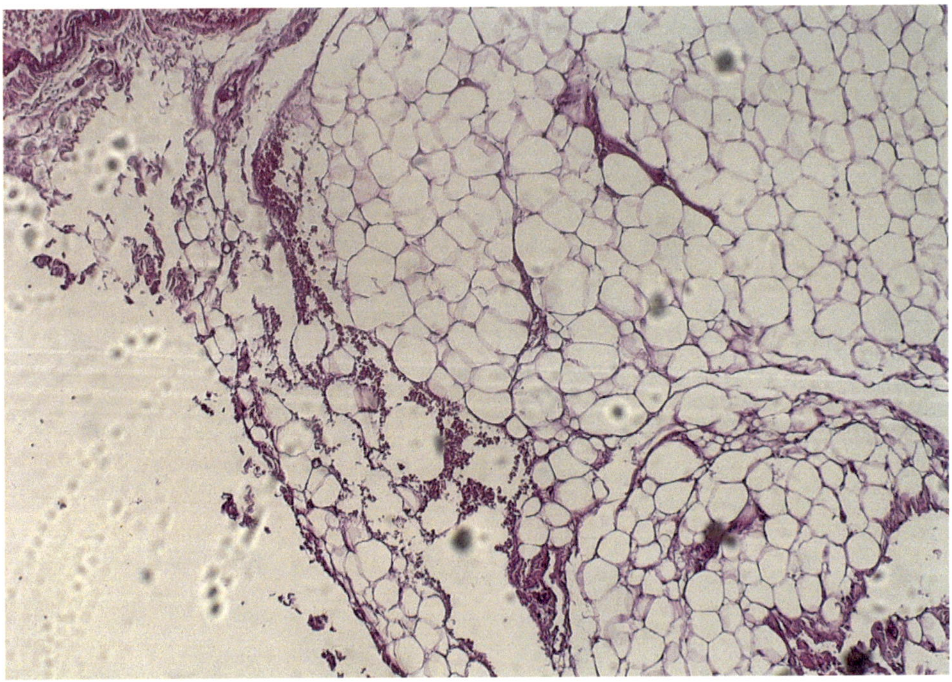

Fig. 19. Visceral adipose tissue (pericardial fat) in a CHF patient with NYHA class III.Romanowsky-Giemsa stain.

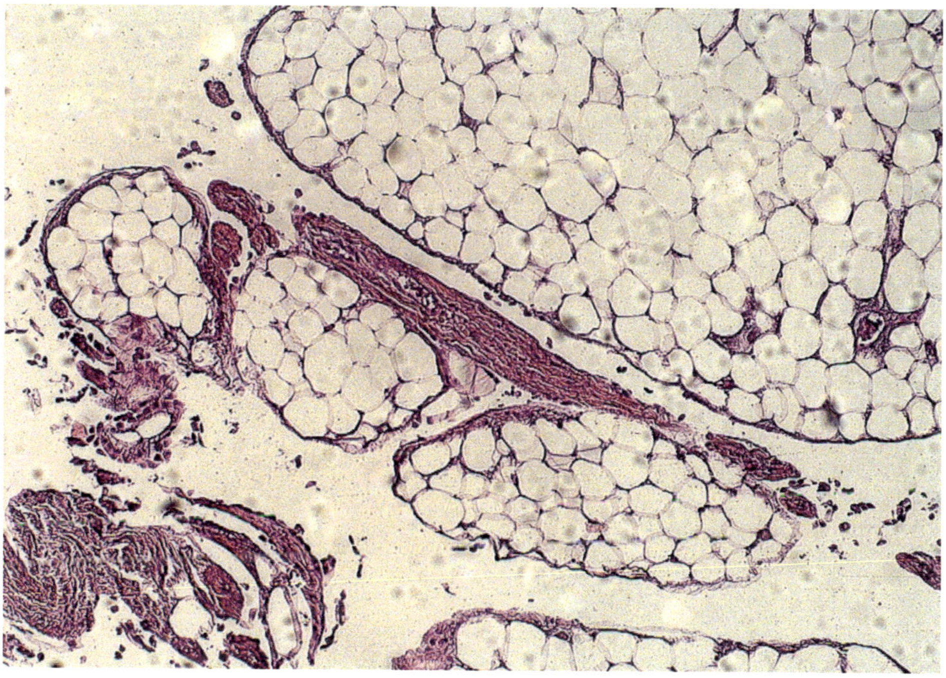

Fig. 20. Visceral adipose tissue (omentum) in a NYHA class III patient without cachexia. Van Gieson's stain.

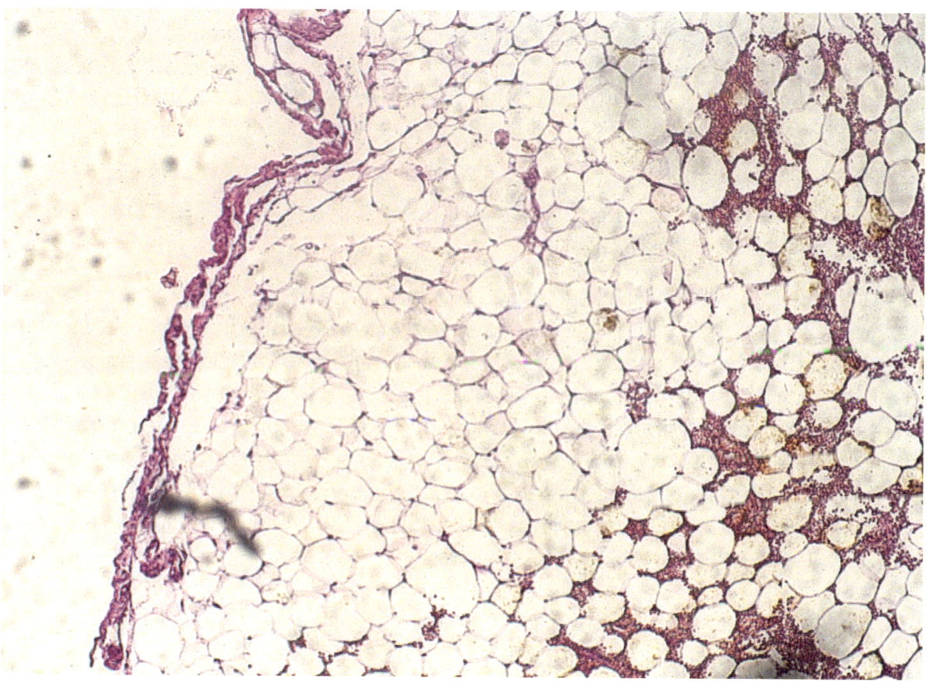

Fig. 21. Visceral adipose tissue (pericardial fat) in a CHF patient with NYHA class IV with cachexia.Romanowsky-Giemsa stain.

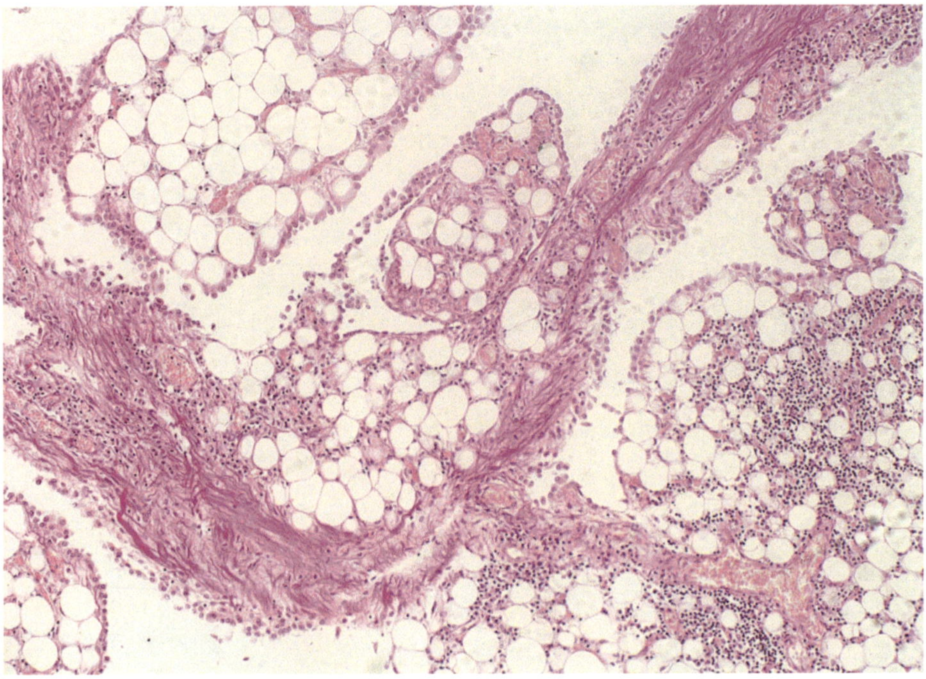

Fig. 22. Visceral adipose tissue (omentum) in a NYHA class IV patient with cachexia. Van Gieson's stain.

Therefore, the higher is NYHA class, the lower are the subcutaneous fat and the omentum weight. The higher is NYHA class, the more intensive is the chronic inflammation, manifested by the lymphocytic infiltration and the content of fibrous tissue, especially in the visceral fat.These changes are stronger in NYHA III-IV patients with cachexia.

In patients with NYHA III-IV and cachexia, a decrease in the content of adipose tissue was demonstrated to be the result of adipocyte shrinking, as well as substitution of the adipose tissue by fibrous tissue.

Currently, there is no solution for the problem of how to increase the body muscle mass and body fat mass in patients with cachexia, particularly with cardiac cachexia. Unfortunately, all attempts to use anabolic steroids in this patient population have been unsuccessful.We assumed that using nutritional support in this patient population would allow to change the nutritional status in addition to reducing the malabsorption syndrome. Moreover, nutritional mixes that have both local and systemic anti-inflammatory effect are currently available. Administration of these mixes might help fighting the inflammation observed in the large intestine of the CHF patients with higher classes of NYHA, as well as reducing their blood levels of pro-inflammatory cytokines.

3.6 Comparison of efficacy of Modulen vs. Peptamen added to standard-of-care therapy in CHF patients with NYHA III-IV

Screening was performed in a consecutive population of patients hospitalized to general internal medicine or cardiology departments (n=144).

Inclusion and exclusion criteria are shown in Table 5.

Inclusion criteria	Exclusion criteria
• CHF of ischemic origin • CHF history for more than 12 months • Age > 40 years old • Patient's consent to participation in the study	• Acute or chronic infectious diseases • Cancer within last 5 years • Severe impairment of liver or kidneys (AST, ALT > 3 x upper limit of normal, creatinine > 250 μmol/L) • Mental disorders • Primary or secondary immunodeficiency conditions • Alcohol or substance dependence • Any conditions that can cause cachexia (at investigator's discretion) • Lack of tolerance to enteral nutrition regimen • Unable to sign the informed consent • Unable to follow the study procedures

Table 5. Inclusion and exclusion criteria.

Chronic heart failure patients with NYHA class III-IV were randomized into three groups, 40 subjects in each:

- Patients in Group 1 received Modulen (balanced nutritional mix for enteral tube feeding or oral feeding) in addition to standard-of-care therapy.
- Patients in Group 2 received Peptamen (balanced nutritional mix for enteral tube feeding or oral feeding) in addition to standard-of-care therapy.
- Patients in Group 3 received the standard of care therapy only, as well as the necessary amount of nutrients in a standard diet designed for cardiology patients.

All patients received standard-of-care therapy, which included:

- ACE inhibitors/ angiotensin receptor antagonists (mean daily dose of 10 mg/160 mg);
- beta-blockers (prescribed from Day 5 after the start of the therapy, dose titration from the minimum therapeutic dose, mean daily dose was 12.5 mg of carvedilol per day);
- digoxin 0.00025 g per day (in case of atrial fibrillation with tachycardia or sinus rhythm with LVEF below 25 %);
- aspirin 125 mg/day (secondary prophylaxis method);
- loop diuretics (Lasix) with mean daily dose of 60 mg/day.

The following procedures were performed for every patient:medical history; physical examination, including measurement of weight, height, waist circumference, hip circumference, wrist circumference, arm circumference; casual BP; heart rate; fasting chemistry lab blood samples; 6-minute test; echocardiography for the measurement of the ejection fraction; caliper measurements; bioimpedance analysis of body composition to measure the lean body mass (LBM), body fat mass (BFM), total water content (TW); Clinical Status Assessment Score.

Group 1 patients received nutritional mix Modulen (100-130 g of dry mix), which accounted for 25 % of their daily energy demands, in addition to their basic diet.Group 2 patients received nutritional mix Peptamen (100-130 g of dry mix), which accounted for 25 % of their daily energy demands, in addition to their basic diet.Group 3 patients received their standard therapy only, as well as the necessary amount of nutrients within a standard diet, based on pre-calculated energy demands.All patients maintained their dietary diaries, which were used to adjust the diet on an individual basis.

The energy demands were calculated using Harris-Benedict formula with adjustment for body mass deficit, taking into account body temperature and activity of a patient.

Energy demands:

$$AEC = EOO*AF*TF*BMD \quad (1)$$

where:AEC – actual energy consumption (kcal/day);

EOO – basal metabolic rate, calculated using Harris-Benedict equations:

EOO (men) = 66 + (13.7*body mass, kg) + (5*height, cm) - (6.8*age)

EOO (women) = 655 + (9.6*body mass, kg) + (1.8*height, cm) - (4.7*age)

AF – activity factor (bed rest: 1.1, movement within room: 1.2, no limitations: 1.3), TF – temperature factor (36–37.0°C: 1.0, 37.1–38.0°C: 1.1, 38.1–39.0°C: 1.2), BMD – body mass deficit (10–20 %: 1.1, 20–30 %: 1.2, >30 %: 1.3).

This study enrolled 120 patients.Males: 18 subjects (45 %) in Group 1, 19 subjects (47.5 %) in Group 2, and 21 subjects (52.5 %) in Group 3.Females: 22 subjects (55 %) in Group 1, 21 subjects (52.5 %) in Group 2, and 19 subjects (47.5 %) in Group 3.

Total duration of CHF history was 15.3±4.3 months, 15.7±4.1 months, and 15.6±4.4 months for Group 1, Group 2, and Group 3, respectively.These characteristics were not significantly different between study groups.

Compensated type 2 diabetes mellitus was reported in 52.5 %, 55 %, and 42.5 % of subjects in Group 1, Group 2, and Group 3, respectively.

Charlson index was > 5 in all groups.

As demonstrated above, there were no statistically significant differences between groups in gender, age, and co-morbidity rates.

In all three groups, decreases of weight and LBM were demonstrated on Day 21 of the treatment period:in Group 1, Day 21 body weight was 56.4±2.6 kg (baseline 66.9±3.5 kg); in Group 2, Day 21 body weight was 56.4±2.1 kg (baseline 66.2±2.9 kg); in Group 3, Day 21 body weight was 55.4±1.7 kg (baseline 67.0±2.9 kg); in Group 1, Day 21 LBM was 40.9±1.7 kg (baseline LBM 47.2±1.9 kg); in Group 2, Day 21 LBM was 42.0±2.0 kg (baseline LBM 47.3±2.0 kg); in Group 3, Day 21 LBM was 41.2±1.9 kg (baseline LBM 46.9±1.8 kg).However, on Day 224, the body weight in Group 1 increased to 62.6±2.7 kg, but was significantly lower than in Group 2 (66.8±2.4 kg) and Group 3 (68.7±1.9 kg).The LBM also increased on Day 224, but it was lower than baseline LBM in Group 1 (44.4±1.6 kg), whereas it reached the baseline in Group 2 (47.4±2.2 kg) and significantly exceeded the baseline in Group 3 (48.1±1.9 kg).

In Group 2 and Group 3, a statistically significant decrease of total fluid content on Day 21 was demonstrated: 34.6±1.8 kg in Group 2 (baseline 47.3±2.1 kg) and 34.4±1.7 in Group 3 (baseline 47.1±1.7 kg).On Day 224, the total fluid content increased in both of these groups: 47.2±2.0 kg and 48.3±1.9, respectively.In Group 1, the total fluid content also decreased by Day 21 (34.3±1.9 kg) compared to baseline (46.8±2.0 kg), but there was no significant increase of the total fluid content on Day 224 (39.3±1.9 kg), unlike in other two groups.

On Day 224, the body fat mass increased significantly in Group 1 to 18.6±1.11 kg (baseline 16,8±1.13 kg), while no significant change in the body fat mass was reported for Group 2 and Group 3:16.8±1.13 kg (baseline 16.5±1.16 kg) in Group 2 and 16.6±1.33 kg (baseline 16.5±1.19 kg) in Group 3.

On Day 21, the BMI decreased from baseline in all groups:21.2±0.60 kg/m^2 in Group 1 (baseline 24.1±0.93 kg/m^2); 21.4±0.59 kg/m^2 in Group 2 (baseline 24.1±0.86 kg/m^2); and 21.5±0.64 kg/m^2 in Group 3 (baseline 24.3±1.01 kg/m^2).On Day 224, the BMI returned to baseline and was 23.7±0.62 kg/m^2 in Group 1, 23.7±0.58 kg/m^2 in Group 2, and 24.5±0.60 kg/m^2 in Group 3.

The body mass increased in all three study groups, but in patients on Modulen this was accountable to increase of muscle and fat mass, and not to increase of total fluid content.This suggests that administration of Modulen improves the nutritional status profile.

Assessment of NT-proBNP, adiponectin, leptin, CRP, IL-6, TNF-α during administration of Modulen and Peptamen added to standard-of-care therapy in CHF patients with NYHA class III-IV.

The level of NT-proBNP in all groups was over 3000 pg/mL.

Reduction of chronic inflammation intensity was demonstrated in patients receiving Modulen:on Day 224, there was a decrease in levels of CRP (4.7±0.4 mg/ml vs. baseline 8.9±0.7 mg/mL), IL-6 (5.2±0.4 U/L vs. baseline 11.8±0.8 U/L), TNF-α (3.4±0.2 U/L vs. baseline 6.8±0.4 U/L).Levels of adiponectin also declined in patients on Modulen: 15.8±1.5 µg/mL vs. baseline 24.4±1.5 µg/mL. No significant changes were demonstrated in Group 2 and Group 3.

There were no significant changes of leptin levels in any of the groups.

Assessment of hospitalization events showed the following results.In Group 1, during treatment with Modulen, 32 hospitalization events were reported per year: 22 hospitalizations were due to CHF decompensations, in 12 of these cases congestive pneumonia was also present; 2 events were due to myocardial infarctions, 5 events were for hypertensive crisis, with 2 of them progressing to CVA; 3 events were due to fibrillation paroxysms. Per-patient hospitalization rate was 0.55±0.01 event/person.There were 5 deaths over one year of observation in Group 1:2 deaths were caused by CHF decompensation, 2 deaths were caused by CVA, 1 death was caused by AMI.

In Group 1, during treatment with Peptamen, 38 hospitalization events were reported over one year of observation:of these, 27 hospitalization events were due to CHF decompensations, with 15 cases accompanied by congestive pneumonia; 3 events were due to acute myocardial infarctions; 7 events were due to hypertensive crisis, 1 of them progressed to CVA; 4 events were due to fibrillation paroxysms. Per-patient hospitalization rate was 0.95±0.02 event/person.There were 8 deaths over one year of observation in Group 2:5 deaths were caused by CHF decompensation, 2 deaths were caused by AMI, 1 death was caused by CVA.

In Group 3, 48 hospitalizations were reported over one year of observation: 41 events were due to CHF decompensations, in 22 of which congestive pneumonia was also present; 2 events were due to acute myocardial infarctions; 4 events were for hypertensive crisis, with 2 cases progressing to CVA; 1 event was due to a fibrillation paroxysm.Per-patient hospitalization rate was 1.2±0.03 event/person.There were 12 deaths over one year of observation in Group 3:8 deaths were caused by CHF decompensation, 2 deaths were caused by AMI, 2 deaths were caused by CVA.

4. Conclusion

Rates of hospitalization events and deaths over one year were lower in subjects receiving Modulen compared to Peptamen and standard-of-care therapy.

5. References

Anker S.D., Negassa A, Coats AJ et al. (2003). Prognostic importance of weight loss in chronic heart failure and the effect of treatment with angiotensin-converting-enzyme inhibitors: an observational study. *Lancet,*Vol.361, No.9363, (March 2003), pp.1077-1083, ISSN0140-6736

Dostalova I., Kavalkova P., Papezova H., Domluvilova D., Zikan V., Haluzik M. (2010).Association of macrophage inhibitory cytokine-1 with nutritional status, body composition and bone mineral density in patients with anorexia nervosa: the influence of partial realimentation.*Nutrition & Metabolism,*Vol.7, (April 2010), pp.34, ISSN 1743-7075

Francis G.S. (1998). Changing the remodeling process in heart failure: basic mechanism and laboratory results. *Current opinion in cardiology,* Vol.13, No.3, (May 1998), pp.156-161, ISSN 0268-4705

Harrington D., Anker S.D. (1997).Skeletal muscle function and its relation to exercise tolerance in CHF.*Journal of the American College of Cardiology,* Vol.30, No.7, (December 1997), pp.1758-1764, ISSN 0735-1097

Monteiro M.P., Ribeiro A.H., Nunes A.F. (2007).Increase in grelin levels after weight loss in obese zucker rats is prevented by gastric banding. *Obesity Surgery,*Vol.17, No.12, (November 2007), pp.1599-1607, ISSN 0960-8923

Moses A.W.G., Slater C., Preston T., Barber M.D., Fearon K.C.H. (2004). Reduced total energy expenditure and physical activity in cachectic patients with pancreatic cancer can be modulated by an energy and protein dense oral supplement enriched with n-3 fatty acids. *British Journal of Cancer,*Vol.90, No.5, (March 2004), pp.996-1002, ISSN 0007-0920

Nagaya N., Uematsu M., Kojima M. (2001). Elevated Circulating Level of Ghrelin in Cachexia Associated With Chronic Heart Failure. *Circulation,*Vol.104, No.17, (October 2001), pp. 2034-2038, ISSN 0009-7322

Springer J., Adams V., Anker S. D. (2010).Myostatin Regulator of Muscle Wasting in Heart Failure and Treatment Target for Cardiac Cachexia.*Circulation,*Vol.121, No.3, (January 2010), pp. 354-356, ISSN 0009-7322

20

Evaluation and Treatment of Hypotension in Premature Infants

Shoichi Ezaki and Masanori Tamura
Division of Neonatal Medicine, Center for Maternal, Fetal and Neonatal Medicine, Saitama Medical Center, Saitama Medical University, Japan

1. Introduction

Sixteen to 98% of extremely preterm infants are treated for hypotension within the first week of life. The enormous variation in this estimate is due to a lack of reliable evidence. While selecting a vasoactive agent, it is necessary to consider the goals of the therapy. To achieve those goals, the clinician must assess the mechanisms of action of the potential therapies. This chapter details the unique characteristics of the neonatal cardiovascular system and defines hypotension in preterm infants. It provides indications for treatment and appropriate therapies for individual cases.

2. Characteristic pathophysiology of hypotension in preterm infants

Blood pressure increases with advancing gestational and postnatal age, which is a developmentally regulated phenomenon (Noori and Seli, 2005). Since cardiac output (CO) and systemic vascular resistance (SVR) both contribute to blood pressure, elevation in blood pressure during development may be the result of increased CO, increased SVR, or both (Fig.1)

2.1 Hypovolemia

In preterm infants, absolute hypovolemia is the most frequent cause of hypotension. Peripheral vasodilation with or without myocardial failure is the most frequent primary etiological factor (Seli and Evans J, 2001). Absolute hypovolemia is defined as a loss of volume from the intravascular compartment; alternatively, relative hypovolemia is defined as vasodilatation with an inadequate volume to fill the expanded intravascular compartment. In both situations, the result is inadequate filling pressure (also known as preload) in the heart. If severe enough, hypovolemia can reduce CO, resulting in inadequate tissue perfusion and oxygenation (Fig 1).

In cases of absolute hypovolemia, the body releases corticosteroids, adrenaline, and noradrenaline, which cause vascular contraction in order to maintain blood pressure and filling pressure and cause increased heart rate and contractility to maintain systemic blood flow (SBF). However, in sick or immature infants, this response may be limited (Ng et al., 2001; Evans N, 2003). In addition, volume administration for the treatment of hypotension in sick infants has been reported to have a dopaminergic effect (Seli and Evans J, 2001).

In preterm infants with acute blood loss (e.g., intraventricular hemorrhage [IVH]) or excessive transepidermal water losses (e.g., gestational age ≤ 25 weeks), absolute hypovolemia should be considered the primary cause of hypotension.

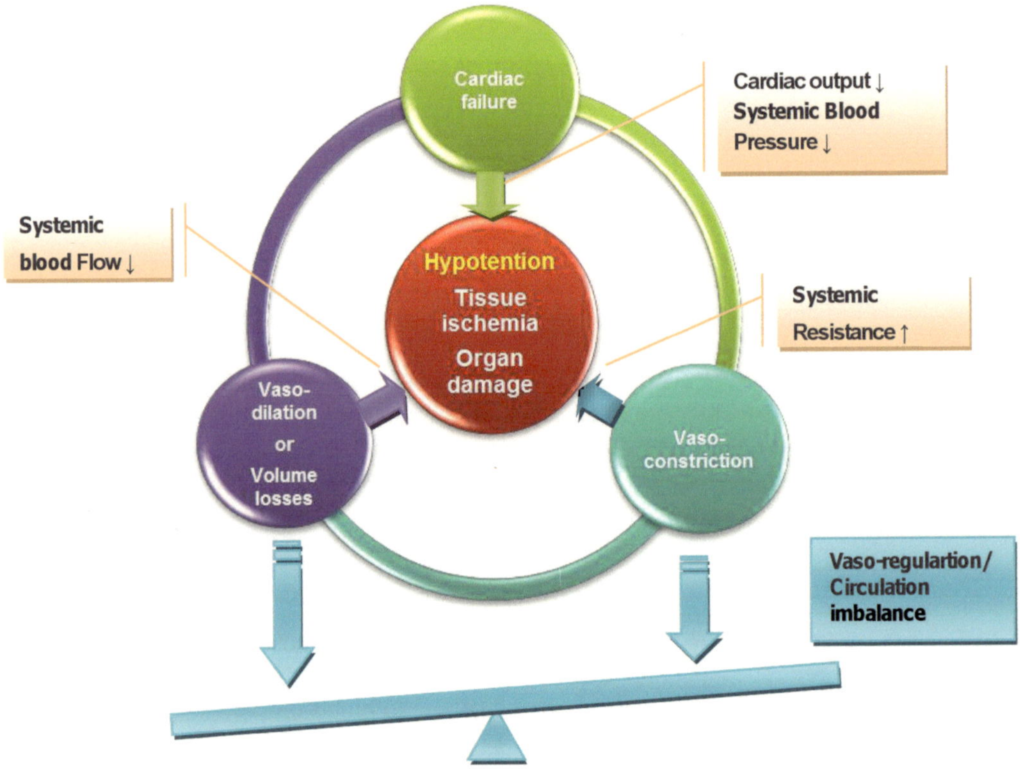

Fig. 1. Mechanism of preterm hypotension

2.2 Myocardial dysfunction

Myocardial contraction and relaxation depend on the regulation of cytosolic calcium concentration and the responsivity of myofilaments to changes in calcium content. Preterm infants, term infants, and adults all have the membrane systems that control cell calcium flux and the sarcomeres that make up the myofibrils. However, the components of each system undergo qualitative and quantitative changes during development. During in the prenatal and newborn periods, myocytes change in size and shape. There are also changes in the number of contractile elements and the nuclear-to-cellular volume ratio.

Cardiac contraction is an energy-dependent process that requires ATP, calcium, and an ATPase located at the myosin head. The processes of contraction and relaxation in immature myocardium as well as calcium homeostasis are different from those in mature myocardium. Specifically, immature myocytes do not rely as heavily on the release and re-uptake of calcium from the sarcoplasmic reticulum; instead, they depend more on extracellular calcium concentration. As such, the immature myocardium of the fetus and newborn depends on L-type calcium channels as a calcium source for contraction. Furthermore, immature myocytes have greater cell surface area-to-volume ratios, which may compensate for their underdeveloped T-tubule systems. The alterations in myocardial structure and function with maturation and the developmental changes in cardiovascular function provide the cellular and molecular bases for differences in myocardial contractility among preterm newborns, term newborns, and older infants (Rowland and Gutgesell, 1995; Noori and Seli, 2005).

Therefore, preterm infants with hypotension have a limited ability to increase CO in response to inotropes or changes in volume (Teitel and Sidi, 1985). Furthermore, they have an elevated sensitivity to increased afterload (Van Hare et al., 1990), which commonly leads to decreased CO (Belik and Light, 1989).

2.3 Abnormal peripheral vasoregulation

Immediately after birth, there is a sudden increase in SVR. This can have a deleterious effect on CO and potentially compromise organ blood flow. After the initial transition period, vasodilation predominates rather than vasoconstriction. Indeed, the complex regulation of vascular smooth muscle tone involves a delicate balance between vasodilators and vasoconstrictors (Fig. 1 and Fig. 2).

hANP: human atrial natriuretic peptide, NO: Nitric oxide, GTP: guanosine triphosphate, cGMP: cyclic guanosine monophosphate

The endogenous vasodilating factors include NO, eicosanoids, hAMP, and endothelin. The endogenous vasoconstrictive factors include catecholamines, vasopressin, and angiotensin II. The balance of these factors determines the blood vessel equilibrium and the tendency toward vasodilation or vasoconstriction (Fig.2). In Figure 2, the vasoconstriction pathway is shown in red, and the vasodilatation pathway is shown in blue. Phosphorylation of myosin is the critical step in vascular smooth muscle contraction. Vasoconstrictors, such as angiotensin II, vasopressin and norepinephrine, activate second messengers to increase cytosolic calcium concentration, which in turn activates myosin light chain kinase. Vasodilators, such as human atrial natriuretic peptide (hANP) and nitric oxide (NO), activate myosin phosphatase, which dephosphorylates myosin to cause vasorelaxation. The plasma membrane is shown at its resting potential (plus signs). cGMP denotes cyclic guanosine monophosphate (Landry and Oliver, 2001). In addition, potassium channels in the smooth muscle cell membrane have recently been implicated in the pathogenesis of vasodilatory shock (Liedel et al., 2002).

Under normal physiologic conditions, CO remains essentially unchanged throughout infancy. Therefore, the increased blood pressure with advancing gestational and postnatal age is primarily the result of increased SVR. Maturation of vascular smooth muscle, changes in the expression of vascular angiotensin II receptor subtypes, and maturation of the central autonomic and peripheral nervous systems play significant roles in increasing vascular tone and SVR. There are 2 major subtypes of angiotensin II receptors. AT1R, which is expressed in mature tissues and the umbilical artery, mediates smooth muscle contraction and regulates fluid and electrolyte balance. AT2R, which is expressed in fetal and newborn tissues, has an unknown function. The developmentally regulated transition from expression of AT2R to AT1R begins following the first 2 weeks of life and is complete by month 3 (Noori and Seli, 2005; Engle, 2001). The vasodilating factor NO increases under conditions of oxidative stress and sepsis. Because preterm infants are prone to these conditions (Ezaki et al., 2009a), their NO levels can easily increase. Together, these physiological characteristics of preterm infants make them susceptible to vasoregulatory dysfunction.

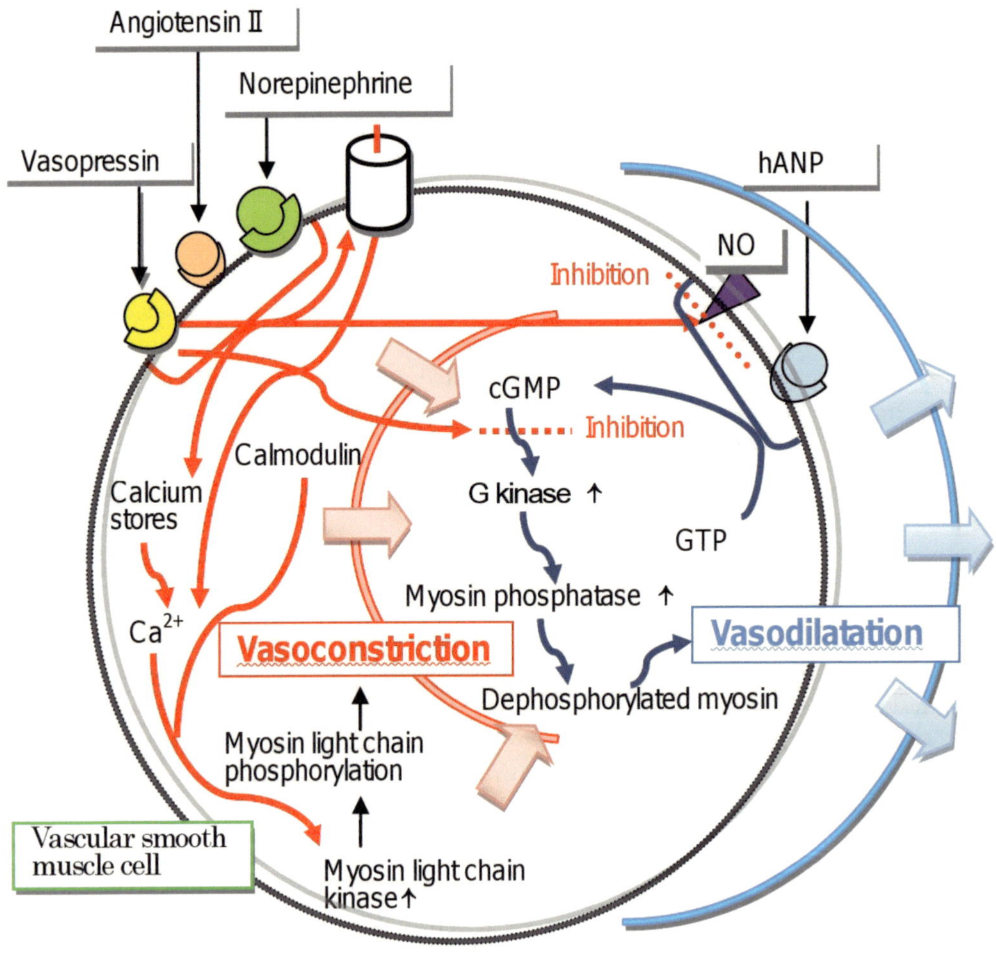

Fig. 2. Regulation of vascular smooth muscle tone

3. The significance of hypotension requiring treatment in preterm infants

3.1 Clinical outcomes

Hypotension is a common complication among preterm infants. Importantly, there is an association between systemic hypotension and neonatal morbidities, including IVH and neurodevelopmental disorders (Watkins et al., 1989; Goldstein et al., 1995). Unfortunately, common conditions among preterm infants, such as sepsis, renal failure, and neonatal asphyxia, can lead to the development of clinical hypotension and confer a poor prognosis.

3.2 Relationship between systemic blood flow and blood pressure

The most important goal in treating hypotension is to prevent cellular and tissue damage resulting from hypovolemia. Seli et al. and Greisen et al. have reported important considerations for the treatment of hypotension (Seli, 2006; Greisen, 2005). If effective treatment is not promptly initiated, the blood pressure may decrease further to the "ischemic threshold, which is said to be about 30 mmHg," resulting in tissue ischemia and permanent organ damage. For example, a loss of cerebral blood flow (CBF) triggers abnormal cerebral function and, finally, tissue ischemia (Fig. 3). Furthermore, high blood pressure is also deleterious. Although, exact value is not noted in existing reports, when blood pressure exceeds "intraventricular hemorrhage (IVH) threshold", risk of IVH increases (Fig. 3).

Loss of vascular autoregulation has not been formally proven as a cause of increased morbidity and mortality in preterm infants (McLean et al., 2008). However, it has consequences that negatively affect prognosis. For instance, loss of autoregulation often triggers IVH. In addition, the amount of blood shunted through the patent ductus arteriosus (PDA), present in preterm infants, can become unstable. Furthermore, the patient is likely to develop necrotizing enterocolitis (NEC) due to compromised blood flow to gastrointestinal tract. Finally, once the patient enters the ischemic stage, there is an increased incidence of periventricular leukomalacia (PVL) and severe renal failure. As such, although the exact reference blood pressure values that cause failure of autoregulation and CBF remain unclear, it is important that hypotension be treated properly.

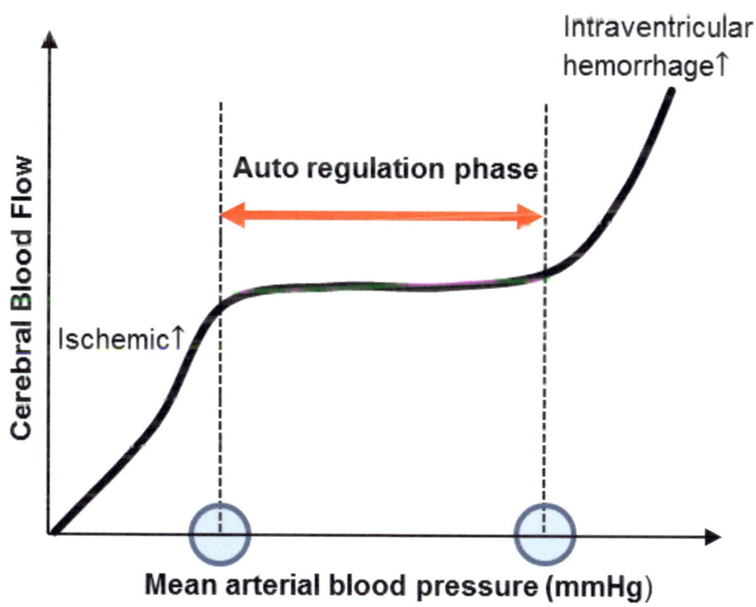

Fig. 3. Proposed relationship between blood flow and mean blood pressure in the cerebral circulation of the preterm infant

4. Definitions of normotension and hypotension in the preterm infant

Most preterm infants admitted to the neonatal intensive care unit (NICU) have medical conditions, such as respiratory disorders, electrolyte abnormalities, or neonatal asphyxia. In addition, because there is a wide range of ages and body weights, it is difficult to define hypotension as a single value in preterm infants. A neonate is considered to be hypotensive if the mean blood pressure is below the fifth or tenth percentile of the normative data according to gestational and postnatal age and weight (Cunningham et al., 1999). Another definition of hypotension is a mean blood pressure less than or equal to the patient's gestational age in weeks. Although this definition is a useful tool, it is only valid during the first 48 hours of life (Nuntnarumit et al., 1999). However, due to its simplicity, this value is a good indicator for neonatologists to suspect hypotension.

4.1.1 Definition of preterm hypotension and its relationship to low systemic perfusion

Figure 3 indicates blood pressure values that are thought result from a failure of autoregulation. Although they would be an ideal definition of hypotension, no consensus has yet been reached. Of preterm infants with a gestational age of 23–26 weeks, >90% have a mean blood pressure >30 mmHg (Nuntnarumit et al., 1999). Recent studies suggest that it may be as high as 28–30 mmHg, even among extremely low birth-weight infants (Munro et al., 2004).

4.1.2 Permissive hypotension

A recent study in very preterm neonates suggested that blood pressure below the clinically-accepted lower limit during the first postnatal days may not require intervention, as long as adequate tissue perfusion is maintained (Dempsey et al., 2009). This study suggested that although treatment must be initiated promptly, overzealous treatment may worsen the prognosis. Therefore, a diagnosis of hypotension must be based on clinical and laboratory findings.

4.2 Clinical signs

Many conditions may trigger hypotension in preterm infants (Table 1). The need for tests and treatments to prevent decreased tissue perfusion is examined.

Vasoregulation imbalance
Hemorrhage: Placental hemorrhage, abruption placenta prevail, feto-maternal hemorrhage, birth trauma-subaponeurotic bleed, massive pulmonary hemorrhage.
Other: Twin-to-twin transfusion, third-space losses, asphyxia, sepsis and septic shock, disseminated intravascular coagulopathy, NEC
Cardiogenic shock
Asphyxia, electrolyte abnormality, cardiac disease: arrhythmias, congenital heart disease, PDA, cardiomyopathy, myocarditis, air leak syndromes
Endocrine
Adrenal hemorrhage, adrenal insufficiency
Drug induced
Anesthetic drugs, sedative drugs

Table 1. Causes of hypotension in preterm infants

4.3 Hemodynamic monitoring in preterm infants

An ideal method for monitoring blood pressure would be simple, reliable, non-invasive, and painless and would provide continuous measurement. However, such an ideal method has not yet been developed. As such, the only reasonable approach to obtaining meaningful hemodynamic data in preterm infants is the use of complex, multi-channel, real-time monitoring towers combined with streamlined data-acquisition systems and observation of clinical symptoms.

4.3.1 Conventional assessment

Direct invasive measurements (via umbilical or peripheral artery catheterization) allow for constant monitoring of blood pressure in hypotensive preterm infants. Although this method is controversial, in our experience, blood pressure values obtained through intra-arterial catheterization are more accurate than non-intermittent blood pressure measurements taken during times of vasoconstriction. In addition, once intermittent blood pressure measurements become necessary, the patient's condition is often already severe, making the insertion of an arterial catheter impossible. It is important to note the risks of an indwelling catheter, including thrombus formation, hemorrhage, and infection.

In neonates admitted to the NICU, heart rate is continuously, accurately, and routinely monitored. However, factors such as anemia, drugs affecting the cardiovascular system, and infection can also affect heart rate. Therefore, heart rate monitoring has a limited role in the diagnosis of circulatory compromise.

Similarly, SpO2 measurements are performed routinely on neonates admitted to the NICU. This measures arterial oxygenation as an indicator of the arterial circulation. However, in contrast to adults, neonates have unique clinical complications. Clinical oximeters cannot detect carbon monoxide hemoglobin, methemoglobin, fetal hemoglobin, or other hemoglobin variations. Therefore, blood tests are needed for the accurate assessment a neonate's oxygenation status (Shiao and Ou, 2007). Nevertheless, SpO2 monitors are also useful for estimating the extent of the peripheral circulation on the basis of oxygenation waveforms.

Conventional monitoring of neonatal hemodynamics was restricted to intermittent evaluation of indirect clinical and laboratory indices of perfusion, such as peripheral-to-core temperature difference, skin color, urine output, capillary refill time, acid-base balance, and serum lactate levels. There are limited data available on capillary refill time in preterm infants. In the first 24 hours, the use of a capillary refill time of ≥ 3 seconds had a 55% sensitivity and 81% specificity for detecting low superior vena cava (SVC) flow (Osborn et al., 2004). In addition, abnormalities in skin color, urine output, base excess, and serum lactate often arise in other conditions of poor tissue oxygenation. For example, anemia can cause skin color abnormalities; kidney disease can cause abnormal urine output; dehydration and late metabolic acidosis can exacerbate BE and cause abnormal lactate levels. Hence, these measurements are not specific to hypotension and must be assessed in combination with other test findings.

4.3.2 Echocardiography

Echocardiographic examination may provide useful information regarding CO, contractility, pulmonary hemodynamics, and PDA shunting in hypotensive preterm infants. Recently, functional echocardiography has been increasingly used to assess CO, myocardial function, and organ blood flow in neonates requiring intensive care (Kluckow et al., 2007).

4.3.2.1 Systolic performance

Left ventricular systolic performance can be assessed by measuring the shortening factor (SF) and ejection fraction. Normal neonatal values for the SF are 28–40% (El-Khuffash and McNamara, 2011). A normal neonatal value for the ejection fraction is approximately 55% (Evans N and Kluckow, 1996).

4.3.2.2 Cardiac output

Normal left and right ventricular output ranges from 170 to 320 mL · kg-1 · min-1. Low left and right ventricular output is defined as < 150 mL · kg-1 · min-1 (normal values range from 170 to 320 mL · kg-1 · min-1) (Evans N and Kluckow, 1996). Superior Vena Cava Flow (SVC flow) in preterm infants is 50–110 mL · kg-1 · min-1. Low SVC flow is defined as below 30 mL · kg-1 · min-1 at the first 5 hours post-natally or below 46 mL · kg-1 · min-1 at the first 48 hours postnatally (Kluckow, 2005). Approximately 35% of preterm infants of < 30 weeks gestational age encounter a period of SVC flow below 40 mL · kg-1 · min-1 during the first 12 hours postnatally. After this point, SVC flow typically improves (Kluckow and Evans N, 2000).

4.3.2.3 Assessment of hypovolemia

The left ventricular end-diastolic diameter (LVEDD) is used to assess hypovolemia. LVEDD is measured at the point of maximal ventricular filling. Normally, the mean LVEDD increases from 11 mm at 23–25 weeks, 12 mm at 26–28 weeks, and 13 mm at 29–31 weeks to 14 mm at 32–33 weeks (Skelton et al., 1998). However, the utility of LVEDD as an indicator of hypovolemia in infants has not been systematically examined. In addition to LVEDD, other factors can affect left ventricular load in the transitional circulation (Evans N, 2003). However, once a preterm infant has been diagnosed with hypovolemia, LVEDD is a useful measurement for evaluation.

Thus, echocardiography is the most suitable test for evaluating cardiac activity and systemic perfusion in hypotensive preterm infants. Its drawback is that it does not allow for continuous observation. Additionally, there is no evidence that its use is associated with better outcomes. Alternatively, ultrasound Doppler, which continuously monitors CO, has also been used in neonates (Meyer et al., 2009).

4.3.3 Assessment of systemic and organ blood flow

Near-infrared spectroscopy (NIRS) measures hemoglobin flow and venous saturation in the forearm to calculate oxygen delivery and consumption and fractional oxygen extraction. In a previous study, Nagdyman et al. used NIRS to measure the cerebral tissue oxygenation index (TOI), regional cerebral oxygenation index (rSO2), venous oxygen saturation SjO2, and central SvO2 from the SVC. They found an association between cerebral TOI and SjO2, between cerebral TOI and SvO2, between cerebral rSO2 and SjO2, and between rSO2 and SvO2 (Nagdyman et al., 2008).

Peripheral and mucosal blood flow can be monitored using laser Doppler (Stark et al., 2009; Ishiguro et al., 2011), side-stream dark field imaging (Hiedl et al., 2010), and visible light T-

Sta (Van Bel et al., 2008) technologies. However, these devices have only been used in neonates for research purposes.

4.3.4 Further assessment of hypotension in preterm infants

As previously described, the diagnosis, treatment determination, and outcome evaluation of hypotension must be based on a combination of findings rather than a single marker. If possible, a time-course observation can improve the prognosis of hypotensive neonates.

Soleymani et al. designed a system for hemodynamic monitoring and data collection in neonates (Soleymani et al., 2010; Cavabvab et al., 2009). The system integrated conventional technologies (i.e., continuous monitoring of heart rate, blood pressure, SpO2, and transcutaneous CO2) with novel technologies, including impedance IEC for continuous assessment of CO and stroke volume and NIRS to monitor blood flow distribution to the brain, kidney, intestine, and/or muscle.

5. Treatment/ assessment of neonatal hemodynamics during postnatal transition

The first priority in treating hypotensive preterm infants is to maintain hemodynamics while the primary etiology is identified and its pathogenesis is addressed. Hemodynamic therapy consists of 3 broad categories: fluid resuscitation, vasopressor therapy, and inotropic therapy.

5.1 Fluid bolus

There is no evidence from randomized trials to support the routine use of early volume expansion in very preterm infants with hypotension. Fluid boli are useful in treating hypovolemia caused by twin-to-twin transfusion, third-space losses, or hemorrhage. However, circulating blood volumes are normal in most hypotensive infants, and there is little to no response to volume administration (Bauer et al., 1993). Moreover, preterm infants have immature cardiac contractile systems and vascular regulation; as such, volume management through fluid boli is not always effective.

Goldberg et al. observed an increased incidence of IVH among preterm infants receiving rapid volume expansion (Goldberg et al., 1980). Additionally, adverse neurological outcomes have been reported in preterm infants receiving colloid infusions (Greenough et al., 2002). The use of multiple fluid boli is also associated with an increased mortality in preterm infants (Ewer et al., 2003). Moreover, the administration of fluid boli has been reported be ineffective for cardiopulmonary resuscitation in cases other than at birth (Wyckoff et al., 2005).

There is insufficient evidence to determine the ideal type of volume expansion for preterm infants or for early red cell transfusions. Normal saline is equally effective as albumin in restoring blood pressure in hypotensive preterm infants. Normal saline is efficacious, safe, readily available, and inexpensive; therefore, it has become the fluid of choice for volume expansion (Oca et al., 2003). Furthermore, other crystalloids are costly and increase the risk of infection and neurodevelopmental deficits (Greenough et al., 2002).

5.2 Vasopressors and inotropes

5.2.1 Catecholamines

5.2.1.1 Mechanisms of action of catecholamines

The term "catecholamines" encompasses dopamine (DOA), NE (norepinephrine), and epinephrine (E). Catecholamines are produced by adrenal medullary cells and by neurons, specifically sympathetic postganglionic neurons. Indeed, adrenal medullary cells can be considered a subtype of postganglionic sympathetic neurons. Secretion of catecholamines by the adrenal medulla is regulated mainly by acetylcholine released from sympathetic nerve endings.

5.2.1.2 Biosynthesis of catecholamines (Fig.4)

First, tyrosine is hydroxylated to form dihydroxyphenylalanine (DOPA) in the rate-limiting step. DOPA is then converted into DOA through decarboxylation. DOA is packaged into secretory granules (chromaffin granules). Dopamine-β-hydroxylase inside the granules processes DOA to produce NE. In nerve cells, biosynthesis ends at this stage. In adrenal

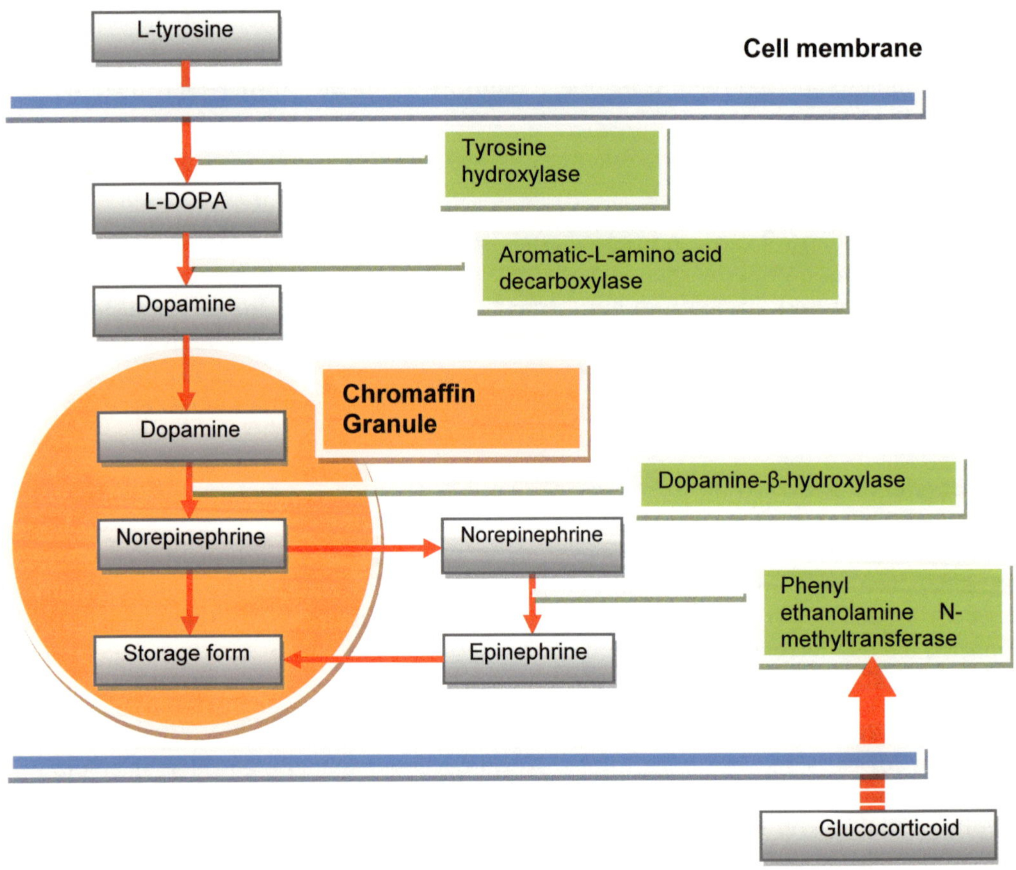

Fig. 4. Catecholamine biosynthesis

medullary cells, NE continues to be processed into E. Once NE is released from the secretory granules into the cytoplasm, it is processed by phenylethanolamine-N-methyltransferase (PNMT) to form E. E binds to a protein known as chromogranin and is recaptured into secretory granules, where it is stored (Goldstein et al., 2003).

The enzyme PNMT, which catalyzes the transformation of NE into E, is induced by glucocorticoids. The direction of blood flow in the adrenal gland travels from the cortex toward the medulla; as a result, medullary cells are in contact with the highest levels of cortisol. Therefore, E production may be regulated by adrenocortical cells.

Acetylcholine is secreted from preganglionic neurons upon stimulation of a sympathetic nerve. Acetylcholine acts at nicotinic receptors to depolarize chromaffin cells. This opens voltage-gated Ca2+ channels, increasing intracellular Ca2+ concentration.This is believed to result in the exocytosis of chromaffin granules.

5.2.1.3 Metabolism of catecholamines

E and NE secreted from the adrenal medulla are incorporated into various tissues and are metabolized by the kidneys. Their half-life in the blood is approximately 2 minutes. They are metabolized by 2 enzymes, catecholamine-O-methyltransferase (COMT) and monoamine oxidase (MAO), which convert them into metanephrine, normetanephrine, and vanillylmandelic acid. In addition to their actions on the heart and blood vessels, catecholamines act on the respiratory tract, gastrointestinal tract, urinary tract, sensory organs, skeletal muscles, adipose tissues, and pancreatic islets. With glucocorticoids, catecholamines also inhibit the proliferation of Th1 cells and promotes their differentiation into Th2 cells.

5.2.1.4 Adrenergic receptors

The physiological effects of catecholamines are elicited through receptors. The basic structure of adrenergic receptors is a seven-transmembrane protein that binds to GTP-binding proteins. There are 2 major types of adrenergic receptors, α and β, which are further classified into subtypes.

There are 2 major α-adrenergic receptor subtypes, α1 and α2, which are subdivided into several pharmacological subtypes. α1 receptors are present at postsynaptic membranes; their activation causes contraction of vascular smooth muscles. α2 receptors are present at presynaptic membranes and inhibit the release of NE caused by sympathetic stimulation. α2 receptors are also present in other various cells, such as blood platelets, pancreatic β-cells, and adipocytes. α1 receptors activate phospholipase C by conjugating with Gq protein. α2 receptors act by inhibiting the production of cAMP through inhibitory GTP-binding proteins (Gi).

β-adrenergic receptors are divided into 3 subtypes: β1, β2, and β3. β1 receptors are mainly distributed in the heart; β2 receptors are mainly distributed in blood vessels, bronchi, and glomerulus, and β3 receptors are mainly distributed in adipocytes. Therefore, β1 receptors promote cardiac stimulation; β2 receptors promote bronchodilation, vasodilation, and glycogenolysis in muscles, and β3 receptors promote lipolysis. β-adrenergic receptors increase the production of cAMP through stimulatory GTP-binding proteins, Gs. This activates cAMP-dependent protein kinase A.

5.2.1.5 Action of catecholamines

Catecholamines act through α and β receptors. The catecholamines differ in their action at α versus β receptors. For instance, while E acts on α and β receptors, NE acts mainly on α receptors (Fig. 5)

5.2.1.6 Cardiovascular effects of catecholamines

Through their actions at β1 receptors, catecholamines increase heart rate and cardiac contractile force. In coronary arteries, when the α-adrenergic effects of catecholamines trigger vasoconstriction, there is a compensatory β2-receptor-mediated vasodilation. In general, the vasodilatory effect predominates. Catecholamines also have vasoconstrictive α-adrenergic effects in arteries of the mucosa, kidney, spleen, and skeletal muscles and in venous vasculature. The β-adrenergic vasodilating effects of catecholamines include arterial vasodilation due to β2-adrenergic receptors in skeletal muscle. Because of their differential effects on adrenergic receptors, each catecholamine differently affects blood pressure and blood flow (Fig.6).

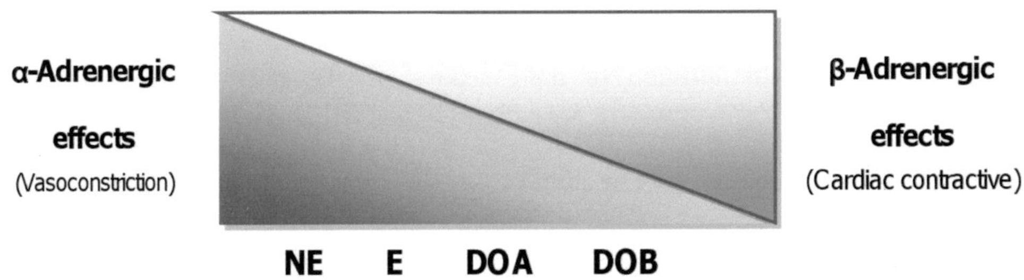

NE: Nor epinephrine, **E**: Epinephrine, **DOA** :Dopamine, **DOB**:Dobtamine

Fig. 5. α-and β-Adrenergic receptors effects of vasoactive inotropes

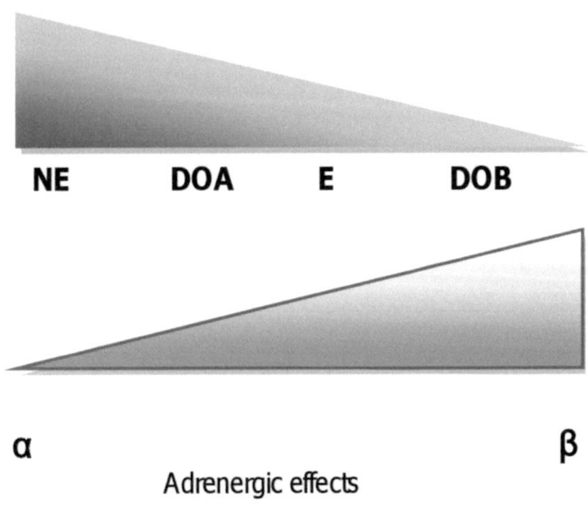

NE: Nor epinephrine, **E**: Epinephrine, **DOA** :Dopamine, **DOB**:Dobutamine

Fig. 6. Effects of catecholamines on blood pressure and blood flow (partly modified from Vincent, 2009)

5.2.1.7 Downregulation of adrenergic receptors

Recently, it has been proposed that exogenous catecholamine administration downregulates adrenergic receptors and their associated second-messenger systems (Hausdorff et al., 1999; Collins et al., 1991). During receptor downregulation, adrenergic receptors undergo lysosomal destruction; therefore, reversal of this process requires new protein synthesis.

5.2.1.8 Levels of catecholamines in hypotensive preterm infants

In extremely low birth-weight infants with hypotension, those in need of high doses of dopamine (DOA>10µg/kg/min) already had high levels of endogenous dopamine compared to those needing low doses of dopamine (DOA ≤10µg/kg/min) ($p<0.05$) (Ezaki et al., 2009b). The ratio of conversion from NE to E before the use of dopamine and 24 hours after administration were correlated in both infants who needed high doses of dopamine and in those who did not. This suggested that there was successful conversion of NE to E. In infants who did not need high doses of dopamine, there was a similar correlation between conversion of DOA to NE before and 24 hours after administration of dopamine. However, no correlation was found in infants who needed high doses of dopamine, suggesting that the conversion from DOA to NE was limited (Ezaki et al., 2009b) (Fig.7). Therefore, an understanding of the underlying pathological condition is important when administering catecholamines.

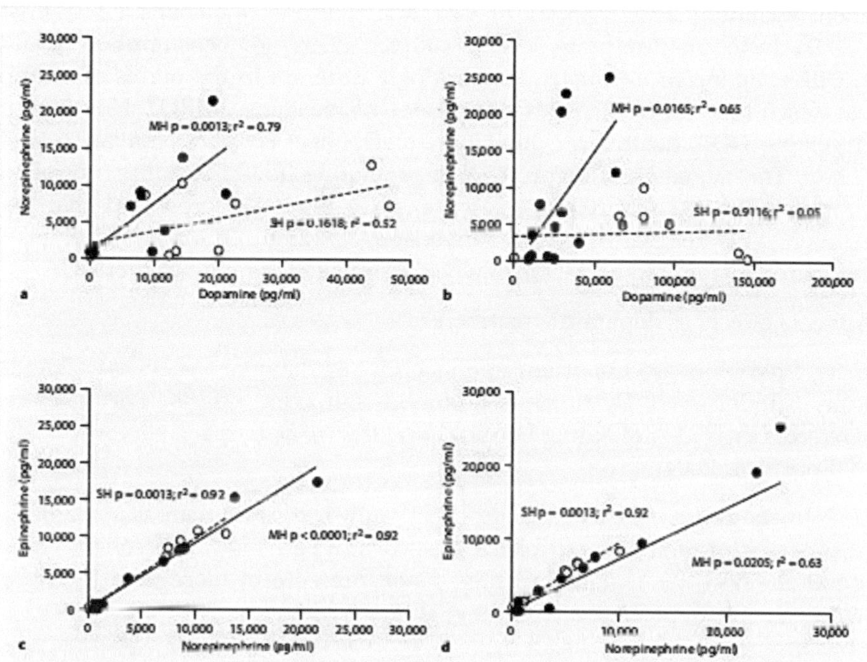

Fig. 7. Correlations between plasma levels of dopamine and norepinephrine at administration (a) and 24 h later (b) and between norepinephrine and epinephrine at administration (c) and 24 h later (d). The severe hypotension (SH, DOA>10µg/kg/min) group (n = 9) is represented by open circles with dotted regression lines, and the mild hypotension (MH, DOA≤10µg/kg/min) group (n = 13) is represented by closed circles with solid regression lines Correlation coefficients and p-values are shown in the respective graphs.

5.2.2 Dopamine

5.2.2.1 Treatment of dopamine in preterm hypotension

Dopamine is the most commonly used vasopressor/inotrope for the treatment of systemic hypotension in preterm infants (Seli,1996). DOA stimulates α-adrenergic receptors, β-adrenergic receptors, and dopaminergic receptors (See 5.2.1.4). DOA stimulates dopamine receptors at low doses (0.5 μg · kg-1 · min-1), mainly triggering effects in renal, mesenteric, and coronary blood vessels. At doses of 2–4 μg · kg-1 · min-1, DOA acts at α-adrenergic receptors, and at doses of 4–8 μg · kg-1 · min-1, DOA acts at β-adrenergic receptors (Seli, 2006).

With the exception of E administration, DOA administration is the most effective treatment for elevating blood pressure in preterm infants. The increase in CBF following DOA administration was found to be greater in hypotensive preterm infants compared to normotensive preterm infants, suggesting the presence of pressure-passive CBF in hypotensive neonates (Sassano et al., 2011). Therefore, we recommend the use of DOA as a first-line inotrope for the treatment of hypotension in preterm infants.

DOA is also an important neurotransmitter that affects both cerebral vasculature and neuronal activity. This is exemplified by pathological conditions caused by dopaminergic dysfunction, including abnormalities in CBF and neuronal metabolism (Edvinsson and Krause, 2002). In the mature brain, CBF is coupled to oxygen consumption (CMRO2). In contrast, CBF coupling to metabolism is strikingly different in the brains of very preterm infants, in which cerebral oxygen extraction, not CBF, sustains CMRO2. However, preterm infants receiving DOA treatment exhibit flow-metabolism coupling similar to that of the mature brain. This suggest a role for DOA in promoting flow-metabolism coupling in the preterm brain (Wong et al., 2009). In addition, we previously reported that high-dose administration of DOA can limit the conversion of NE to DOA (Ezaki et al., 2009b). Therefore, extreme caution must be taken when administering high doses of DOA.

5.2.2.2 Adverse effects of dopamine treatment

α2-adrenergic receptors are important in endocrine regulation; as such, even low doses of systemically administered DOA have profound endocrine effects. For instance, DOA infusion reduces thyroid stimulating hormone and thyroxine levels in very low birth-weight infants (Filippi et al., 2004).

Doses of DOA should rarely exceed 20 μg · kg-1 · min-1, because there is a risk of excessive α-adrenergic-receptor-mediated peripheral vasoconstriction and a subsequent reduction in CO (Rozé et al., 1993). DOA failed to raise blood pressure in more than 30% of preterm infants with systemic hypotension (Pellicer et al., 2005).

5.2.3 Norepinephrine

5.2.3.1 The use of norepinephrine in the treatment of preterm hypotension

NE is a potent vasopressor with α-and, to a lesser extent, β-1 receptor agonist activity (Hollenberg et al., 2004). In the adult, NE is primarily used as a vasopressor in states of hyperdynamic shock, in which SVR is decreased and mean arterial blood pressure is low (Corley, 2004). Experimental studies in fetal lambs have shown that NE may decrease basal pulmonary vascular tone (Houfflin-Debarge et al., 2001) and elevate pulmonary blood flow through activating α2-adrenergic receptors and NO release (Magnenant et al., 2003).

NE can reduce damage incurred by neuroinflammatory and neurodegenerative conditions. It induces the expression of the chemokine CCL2 in astrocytes, which is neuroprotective against excitotoxic damage (Madrigal et al., 2009). Indeed, early associative somatosensory conditioning requires NE (Landers and Sulliyan, 1999).

Thus, NE plays an important role not only in the cardiovascular system, but also in neonatal development. However, there are few studies on the use of NE in the treatment of hypotension in preterm infants. While no studies have compared NE to other drugs, its therapeutic effects in neonates have recently been reported (Paradisis and Osborn, 2004). The use of NE (0.5-0.75 μg · kg-1 · min-1) is effective in the treatment of term and near-term infants with septic shock that are resistant to DOA and dobutamine (Tourneux et al., 2008a). In neonates with persistent pulmonary hypertension-induced cardiac dysfunction, NE can reduce O2 requirements and normalize the systemic artery pressure (Tourneux et al., 2008b).

5.2.3.2 Adverse effects of norepinephrine treatment

In all previous reports describing the use of NE in neonates, NE was administered after other inotropes, making it impossible to describe the side effects solely attributable to NE. In addition, there are no reports on the long-term consequences of the use of NE in preterm infants. In general, excessive peripheral vasoconstriction causes a decrease in the contractile forces of the immature heart. This may result in tachycardia or decreased tissue perfusion. Therefore, capillary refill time, lactate levels, and peripheral and organ blood flow should be monitored.

5.2.4 Epinephrine

5.2.4.1 The use of epinephrine for the treatment of preterm hypotension

Low and moderate doses of E (0.125–0.5 μg · kg-1 · min-1) have found to be as effective as low and moderate doses of DOA (2.5–10 μg · kg-1 · min-1) for the treatment of hypotension in preterm infants (Valverde et al., 2006). In addition, the infusion of E increases mean arterial blood pressure and heart rate without decreasing urine output in very low birth-weight infants with hypotension that do not respond to dopamine infusion up to 15 μg · kg-1 · min-1 (Heckmann et al., 2002).

5.2.4.2 Adverse effects of epinephrine

Compared DOA, E use cases temporary dysfunction of carbohydrate and lactate metabolism (Valverde et al., 2006) and increased metabolic acidosis (Heckmann et al., 2002). E directly affects lactate metabolism by increasing lactate production and decreasing lactate metabolism, thus increasing serum lactate concentrations (Cheung et al., 1997). At very high doses, E induces vasoconstriction sufficient to counteract its inotropic benefits, and CO may fall (Barrington et al., 1995).

Pellicer et al. recently reported that the long-term prognosis of E use was the same as DOA use, and that both were safe (Pellicer et al., 2009). This important study provided an additional treatment option for preterm hypotension.

5.3 Non-catecholamine inotropic/pressor agents

5.3.1 Dobutamine

5.3.1.1 Physiology of dobutamine in preterm hypotension

Dobutamine is a racemic mixture of 2 isomers, the D-isomer with α1- and α2-adrenergic effects and the L-isomer with α1- and α1- adrenergic effects. Dobutamine is predominantly inotropic via stimulation of α1 receptors and has a variable effect on blood pressure (Hollenberg, 2011). Dobutamine administration results in a variable decrease in total SVR. Unlike DOA, dobutamine increases myocardial contractility exclusively through direct stimulation of myocardial adrenergic receptors (Noori et al., 2004).

5.3.1.2 The use of dobutamine for the treatment of preterm hypotension

At a dose of 2–15 µg · kg-1 · min-1, dobutamine increases CO mainly through augmenting stroke volume (Noori et al., 2004; Roze et al., 1993; Bhatt-Mehta and Nahata, 1989).

5.3.1.3 Adverse effects of dobutamine treatment

Adverse effects of dobutamine occur at high doses and include increased heart rate. At very high doses, dobutamine may increase blood pressure and SVR (Cheung et al., 1999), likely due to stimulation of á-receptors (Fig.5 and 6). One study suggested that dobutamine's potential benefit of increased oxygen delivery to the tissues was offset by increased tissue metabolic rate (Penny et al., 2001).

5.3.2 Vasopressin

5.3.2.1 Physiology of vasopressin in preterm infants

Vasopressin induces its physiological responses through 4 receptors, V1, V2, V3, and oxytocin receptors (OTR) (Holmes et al., 2001). When vasopressin binds to V1 receptors in vascular smooth muscle (Va1 receptors), it activates phospholipase C, triggering calcium release from intracellular calcium stores (Fig. 2). This results in vasoconstriction and a subsequent increase in blood pressure. Activation of V2 receptors in the stomach increases intracellular cyclic AMP levels through the mediation of adenylate cyclase and have an anti-diuretic effect. V3 receptors (also known as V1b receptors) are involved in vasopressin's adrenocorticotropic hormone (ACTH)-stimulating effects. Finally, OTR receptors mediate vasopressing's oxytocic effects on uterine contractility.

V2 receptors and OTR receptors also have vasodilating effects that are antagonistic to the effects of V1 receptors. In addition, V1 receptors and OTR receptors have diuretic effects, which are antagonistic to the anti-diuretic effects of V2 receptors. Vasopressin's effects are most adapted to disease-induced changes.

Previous reports have indicated that blood levels of endogenous vasopressin show a two-phased response in adults with shock (Holmes et al., 2001; Landry et al., 1997; Morales et al., 1999). During the initial phase of shock, endogenous vasopressin is released in large amounts and reaches high blood levels in order to maintain tissue perfusion. However, its concentration in the blood decreases over time. As such, vasopressin may be depleted due to its initial release in large amounts. The release of vasopressin from the pituitary gland may also be inhibited by NO produced by the vascular endothelium or due to autonomic nervous system disorders (Holmes et al., 2001; Landry et.al, 1997; Morales et al., 1999).

The effects of the small amounts of exogenous vasopressin may be a result of enhancing the effects of catecholamines, inhibiting inducible NO synthase (iNOS), inhibiting increased cGMP induced by NO and ANP, or inactivating KATP channels in vascular smooth muscles (Fig.2) (Landry et al., 2001; Hamu et al.,1999).

In preterm infants, the levels of vasopressin were high during the first 24 hours following birth (Ezaki et al., 2009b). The effects of these high levels of endogenous vasopressin on the cardiovascular system are not fully understood.

5.3.2.2 The use of vasopressin for the treatment of hypotension in preterm infants

Meyer et al. reported that vasopressin (0.035–0.36 U · kg-1 · hr-1) may be a promising rescue therapy for catecholamine-resistant shock in extremely-low-birth-weight infants with acute renal injury (Meyer et al., 2006). Similarly, Ikegami et al. found that administration of vasopressin (0.001–0.01 U · kg-1 · hr-1) was effective in extremely-low-birth-weight infants resistant to treatment with catecholamines and steroids (Ikegami et al., 2010).

5.3 Adverse effects of vasopressin treatment

The side effects of vasporessin include severe cutaneous ischemia, hepatic necrosis, neurological deficits, and dysmetria (Meyer et al., 2006; Rodríguez-Nunez et al., 2006; Zeballos et al., 2006). Unlike DOA, E, and dobutamine, there are few reports on the side effects of vasopressin. Moreover, it is unclear whether its side effects are dose-dependent and what the long-term prognoses are. However, vasopressin is a pharmacological agent that can be considered for use in patients in whom other drugs are ineffective.

5.4 Lusitropes

5.4.1 Physiology of phosphodiesterase-III inhibitors in preterm hypotension

Phosphodiesterase inhibitors increase intracellular cyclic AMP and thus have inotropic effects independent of α-adrenergic receptors. As such, they result in fewer chronotropic and arrhythmogenic effects than catecholamines. However, increased cyclic AMP in vascular smooth muscle cells can cause vasodilation, thus reducing SVR, which can exacerbate hypotension. In addition, this can reduce pulmonary artery pressure. (Chen et al.,1997,1998; Kato et al.,1998). Milrinone, a cyclic nucleotide phosphodiesterase-III inhibitor, improves contractility and reduces afterload in adults and newborns with cardiac dysfunction.

5.4.2 The use of phosphodiesterase-III inhibitors for the treatment of preterm hypotension

McNamara et al. reported that intravenous Milrinone (0.33–0.99 μg · kg-1 · min-1) administration produced early improvements in oxygenation without compromising systemic blood pressure in patients with severe persistent pulmonary hypertension (McNamara et al., 2006). One randomized clinical trial did not support the use of Milrinone (0.75 μg · kg-1 · min-1 for 3 hrs, then 0.2μ g · kg-1 · min-1 until 18 hours after birth) in the prevention of low SVC in the early transitional circulation of preterm infants (Paradisis et al., 2009).

5.4.3 Adverse effects of Milrinone treatment

Milrinone can cause hypotension and tachycardia (Chang et al., 1995). The long-term effects of Milrinone in preterm infants have not been reported.

5.5 Corticosteroids

5.5.1 Physiology of corticosteroids

The adrenal glands are involved in the growth and maturation of fetal organs during intrauterine life. In most mammals, a cortisol surge occurs as the full gestational term approaches; this triggers increased synthesis of pulmonary surfactant, reduced sensitivity of the arteries to prostaglandins, and increased conversion of pancreatic β-cells from T4 to T3 in the mature liver. These changes allow the fetus to survive in the extrauterine environment. There is also a surge in catecholamines produced by the adrenal medulla during delivery. This surge also allows adaptation to the extrauterine environment by influencing the cardiovascular system, including elevating the blood pressure and increasing the heart function, and by influencing glucose metabolism, fat metabolism, and water absorption in the lungs (Fisher, 2002).

The hypothalamic-pituitary-adrenal system in fetuses and neonates has been implicated in late-onset circulatory collapse (Masumoto et al., 2008) and in the fetal programming of the cardiovascular system. Preterm infants have low adrenal function due to their low levels of 3β-hydroxysteroid dehydrogenase (HSD) (Mesiano and Jaffe, 1997) and weak 11b-HSD2 activity (Donaldson et al.,1991).

Corticosteroids reverse neonatal hypotension by improving capillary-leak syndrome (Briegel et al., 1994), potentiating transmembrane calcium currents, increasing β-receptor sensitivity to catecholamines, reversing the downregulation of β-receptors, increasing the density of β-receptors, and inhibiting NO synthase expression (Prigent et al., 2004).

5.5.2 The use of corticosteroids in the treatment of preterm hypotension

Hydrocortisone administration is effective in the treatment of hypotension and vasopressor dependence in hypotensive preterm infants. Its clinical benefits include increasing blood pressure and decreasing the requirement for vasopressor administration (Higgins et al., 2010). Fernandez et al. have reviewed the use of hydrocortisone in the treatment of premature infants (Fernandez and Watterberg, 2009). Before initiating therapy with hydrocortisone in extremely preterm infants with refractory hypotension, a blood specimen should be analyzed for cortisol concentration. Pending that result, an initial dose of 1 mg/kg can be administered. If the blood pressure improves within 2 to 6 h, 0.5 mg/kg can be administered every 12 h (approximately 8–10 mg/m^2 per day). This long dosing interval is used, because hydrocortisone has a longer half-life in immature infants (Watterberg et al., 2005). This dosing strategy increases serum values by an average of 5 µg/100 ml; higher doses are associated with very high serum concentrations. If the initial cortisol concentration is high (>15–20 µg/100 ml), drug administration may be discontinued, especially in the absence of a clinical response.

5.5.3 Adverse effects of corticosteroid treatment

Although corticosteroid therapy improves blood pressure and circulation, there are many potential complications, including spontaneous gut perforation, hyperglycemia, and hypertension and long-term consequences, including cerebral palsy and intellectual impairment. These complications necessitate the judicious use of corticosteroids to support blood pressure in preterm infants (Yeh et al., 2004).

Hydrocortisone therapy administered simultaneously with indomethacin or ibuprofen has been associated with acute spontaneous gastrointestinal perforation in extremely preterm infants. Therefore, care should be taken to avoid concurrent therapy (Watterberg et al., 2004; Peltoniemi et al., 2005). Infants who develop spontaneous perforation often have high endogenous cortisol concentrations (Watterberg et al., 2004; Peltoniemi et al., 2005).

Watterberg et al. reported that early, low-dose hydrocortisone treatment was not associated with an increased risk of cerebral palsy. In fact, infants treated with hydrocortisone displayed improved developmental outcomes. Together with the short-term benefits, these data support the use of hydrocortisone for the treatment of adrenal insufficiency in extremely premature infants (Watterberg et al., 2007).

6. Conclusion

The major findings of the present chapter summarized in the following figure (Fig.8).

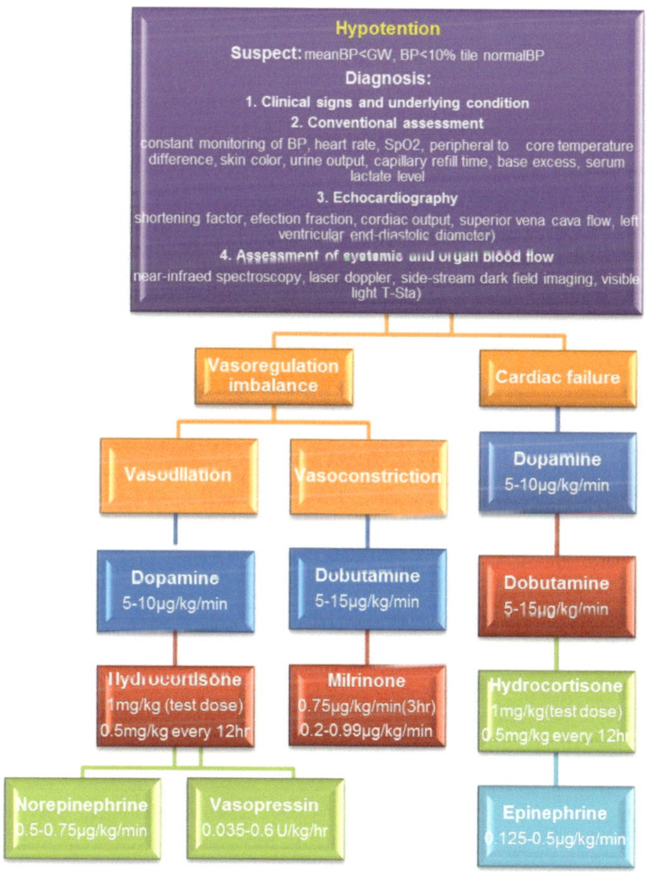

Fig. 8. Evaluation and treatment of hypotension in premature infants

7. Acknowledgment

We express gratitude to the efforts of the authors whose research is cited in this article. First author (FA)'s personal research on vasoactive factors in neonates was inspired by my wife, a physician who introduced me to the use of vasopressin for the management of shock. Therefore, FA offer my wife, Yuko Ezaki, my most sincere gratitude. Finally, FA dedicate this chapter to my famiiy: Munenori, Tomi, Yuko, Yoshiko, Yukiko, and Saeka Ezaki.

FA hope that this work will promote future advances in neonatal care.

8. References

Bauer, K. & Linderkamp, O. & Versmold, HT. (1993). Systolic blood pressure and blood volume in preterm infants. *Archives of disease in childhood,* Vol. 69, 5 Spec No, (Nov), pp. 521-522, ISSN 0003-9888

Barrington, KJ. & Finer, NN. & Chan, WK. (1995). A blind, randomized comparison of the circulatory effects of dopamine and epinephrine infusions in the newborn piglet during normoxia and hypoxia. *Critical Care Medicine,* Vol. 23, No. 4, (Apr). pp. 740-748, ISSN 0090-3493

Belik, J., Light, RB. (1989). Effect of increased afterload on right ventricular function in newborn pigs. *Journal* of *Applied Physiology,* Vol. 66, No. 2, (Feb), pp. 863-869, ISSN 8750-7587

Bhatt-Mehta, V. & Nahata, MC. (1989). Dopamine and dobutamine in pediatric therapy. *Pharmacotherapy,* Vol. 9, No. 5, (May), pp. 304-314, ISSN 0277-0008

Briegel, J. & Kellermann, W. & Forst, H et al. (1994). Low-dose hydrocortisone infusion attenuates the systemic inflammatory response syndrome. The Phospholipase A2 Study Group. *The Clinical investigator,* Vol. 72, No. 10, (Oct), pp. 782-787, ISSN 0941-0198

Cayabyab, R. & McLean, CW. & Seri, I. (2009). Definition of hypotension and assessment of hemodynamics in the preterm neonate. *Journal of Perinatology,* Vol. 29, Suppl. 2, (May), pp. S58-S62, ISSN 0743-8346

Chang, AC. & Atz, AM. & Wernovsky, G et al. (1995). Milrinone: systemic and pulmonary hemodynamic effects in neonates after cardiac surgery. *Critical care medicine,* Vol. 23, No. 11, (Nov), pp. 1907-1914, ISSN 0090-3493

Cheung, PY. & Barrington, KJ. & Pearson, RJ et al. (1997). Systemic, pulmonary and mesenteric perfusion and oxygenation effects of dopamine and epinephrine. *American Journal of Respiratory and Critical Care Medicine,* Vol. 155, No. 1, (Jan), pp. 32-37, ISSN 1073-449X

Cheung, PY. & Barrington, KJ. & Bigam, D. (1999). The hemodynamic effects of dobutamine infusion in the chronically instrumented newborn piglet. *Critical Care Medicine,* Vol. 27, No. 3, (Mar), pp. 558-564, ISSN 0090-3493

Chen, EP. & Bittner, HB. & Davis, RD Jr et al. (1997). Milrinone improves pulmonary hemodynamics and right ventricular function in chronic pulmonary hypertension. *The Annals of Thoracic* Surgery, Vol. 63, No. 3, (Mar), pp. 814-821, ISSN 0003-4975

Chen, EP. & Bittner, HB. & Davis, RD et al. (1998), Hemodynamic and inotropic effects of milrinone after heart transplantation in the setting of recipient pulmonary hypertension. *The Journal of Heart and Lung Transplantation*, Vol. 17, No. 7, (Jul), pp. 669-678, ISSN 1053-2498

Collins, S. & Caron, MG. & Lefkowitz, RJ. (1991). Regulation of adrenergic receptor responsiveness through modulation of receptor gene expression. *Annual Review of Physiology*, Vol. 53, pp. 497-508, ISSN 0066-4278

Corley, KT. (2004). Inotropes and vasopressors in adults and foals. *The Veterinary clinics of North America. Equine practice,* Vol. 20, No. 1, (Apr), pp. 77-106, ISSN 0749-0739

Cunningham, S. & Symon, AG. & Elton, RA et al. (1999). Intraarterial blood pressure reference ranges, death and morbidity in very low birth weight infants during the first seven days of life. *Early Human Development,* Vol. 56, No. 2-3, (Dec), pp. 151-165, ISSN 0378-378256.

Dempsey, EM. & Al Hazzani, F. & Barrington, KJ. (2009). Permissive hypotension in the extremely low birthweight infant with signs of good perfusion. *Archives of Disease in Childhood Fetal & Neonatal Edition,* Vol. 94, No. 4, (Jul), pp. F241-F244, ISSN 1359-2998

Donaldson, A. & Nicolini, U. & Symes, EK et al. (1991). Changes in concentrations of cortisol, dehydroepiandrosterone sulphate and progesterone in fetal and maternal serum during pregnancy. *Clinical endocrinology,* Vol. 35, No. 5,(Nov), pp. 447-451, ISSN 0300-0664

Edvinsson, L. & Krause, D. (2002). Catecholamines, In: *Cerebral blood flow and metabolism,* Edvinsson, L & Krause, D, (Eds.), 191-211, Lippincott Williams & Wilkins, ISBN 978-0781722599, Philadelphia

El-Khuffash, AF. & McNamara, PJ. (2011). Neonatologist-performed functional echocardiography in the neonatal intensive care unit. *Seminars in fetal & neonatal medicine,* Vol. 16, No. 1, (Feb), pp. 50-60, ISSN 1744-165X

Engle, WD. (2001). Blood pressure in the very low birth weight neonates. *Early Human Development,* Vol. 62, No. 2, (May), pp. 97-130, ISSN 0378-3782

Evans, N. (2003). Volume expansion during neonatal intensive care: do we know what we are doing? *Semin Neonatol,* Vol. 8, No. 4, (Aug), pp. 315-323, ISSN1744-165X52.

Evans, N. & Kluckow, M. (1996). Early determinants of right and left ventricular output in ventilated preterm infants. *Archives of disease in childhood. Fetal and neonatal edition,* Vol. 74, No. 2, (Mar), pp. F88-F94, ISSN 1359-2998

Ewer, AK. & Tyler, W. & Francis, A et al. (2003). Excessive volume expansion and neonatal death in preterm infants born at 27-28 weeks gestation. *Paediatric and Perinatal Epidemiology,* Vol. 17, No.2, (Apr), pp. 180-186, ISSN 0269-5022

Ezaki, S. & Suzuki, K. & Kurishima, C et al. (2009a). Resuscitation of preterm infants with reduced oxygen results in less oxidative stress than resuscitation with 100% oxygen. *Journal of clinical biochemistry and nutrition,* Vol. 44, No.1, (Jan), pp. 111-118, ISSN 0912-0009

Ezaki, S. & Suzuki, K. & Kurishima, C et al. (2009b). Levels of catecholamines, arginine vasopressin and atrial natriuretic peptide in hypotensive extremely low birth weight infants in the first 24 hours after birth. *Neonatology,* Vol. 95, No. 3, (Nov 4), pp. 248-255, ISSN 1661-7800

Fernandez, EF. & Watterberg, KL. (2009). Relative adrenal insufficiency in the preterm and term infant. *Journal of Perinatology,* Vol. 29, Suppl 2, (May), pp. S44-S49, ISSN 0743-8346

Fisher, D. (2002). Endocrinology of Fetal Development, In: *Williams Textbook of Endcrinology · 11th*, Kronenberg, HM. & Melmed, S, & Polonsky, KS. & Larsen, (Eds.), pp.756-776, WB Saunders, ISBN 978-1437703245, Phil ad elphia

Filippi, L. & Cecchi, A. & Tronchin, M et al. (2004). Dopamine infusion and hypothyroxinaemia in very low birth weight preterm infants. *Early Human Development*, Vol. 163, No. 1, (Jan), pp. 7-13, ISSN 0378-3782

Goldberg, RN. & Chung, D. & Goldman, SL et al. (1980). The association of rapid volume expansion and intraventricular hemorrhage in the preterm infant. *The Journal of Pediatrics*, Vol. 96, No. 6, (Jun), pp. 1060-1063, ISSN 0022-3476

Goldstein, DS. & Eisenhofer, G. & Kopin IJ. (2003). Sources and significance of plasma levels of catechols and their metabolites in humans. *Journal of Pharmacology and Experimental Therapeutics*, Vol. 305, No. 3, (Jun), PP. 800-811, ISSN 0022-3565

Goldstein, RF. & Thompson, RJ. & Oehler, JM et al. (1995). Influence of acidosis, hypoxemia, and hypotension on neurodevelopmental outcome in very low birth weight infants. *Pediatrics*, Vol. 95, No. 2, (Feb), pp. 238-243, ISSN 0031-4005

Greenough, A. & Cheesemen, P. & Kawadia, V et al. (2002). Colloid infusion in the perinatal period and abnormal neurodevelopmental outcome in very low birth weight infants. *European Journal of Pediatrics*, Vol. 161, No. 6, (Jun), pp. 319-323, ISSN 0340-6199

Greisen G. (2005). Autoregulation of cerebral blood flow in newborn babies. *Early Human Development*, Vol. 81, No. 5, (May), pp. 423-428, ISSN 0378-3782

Hausdorff, WP. & Hnatowich, M. & O'Dowd BF et al. (1990). A mutation of the beta 2-adrenergic receptor impairs agonist activation of adenylyl cyclase without affecting high affinity agonist binding. Distinct molecular determinants of the receptor are involved in physical coupling to and functional activation of Gs. *The Journal of Biological Chemistry*, Vol. 265, No. 3, (Jan), pp.1388-1393, ISSN 0021-9258

Hamu, Y. & Kanmura, Y. & Tsuneyoshi, I et al. (1999). The effects of vasopressin on endotoxin-induced attenuation of contractile responses in human gastroepiploic arteries in vitro. *Anesthesia & Analgesia*, Vol. 88, No. 3, (Mar), pp. 542-548, ISSN 0003-2999

Heckmann, M. & Trotter, A. & Pohlandt, F et al. (2002). Epinephrine treatment of hypotension in very low birthweight infants. *Acta Paediatrica*, Vol. 91. No. 5, (May), pp. 566-570, ISSN 0803-5253

Higgins, S. & Friedlich, P. & Seri, I. (2010). Hydrocortisone for hypotension and vasopressor dependence in preterm neonates: a meta-analysis. *Journal of Perinatology*, Vol. 30, No. 6, (Jun), pp. 373-378, ISSN 0743-8346

Hiedl, S. & Schwepcke, A. & Weber, F et al. (2010). Microcirculation in preterm infants: profound effects of patent ductus arteriosus. *The Journal of Pediatrics*, Vol. 156, No. 2, (Feb), pp. 191-196, ISSN 0022-3476

Hollenberg, SM. & Ahrens, TS. & Annane, D et al. (2004). Practice parameters for hemodynamic support of sepsis in adult patients: 2004 update. *Critical Care Medicine*, Vol. 32, No. 9, (Sep), pp, 1928-1948, ISSN 0090-3493

Hollenberg, SM. (2011). Vasoactive drugs in circulatory shock. *American Journal of Respiratory and Critical Care Medicine*, Vol. 183, No. 7, (Apr 1), pp. 847-855, ISSN 1073-449X

Holmes, CL. & Patel, BM. & Russell, JA et al. (2001). Physiology of vasopressin relevant to management of septic shock. *Chest*, Vol. 120, No. 3, (Sep), pp. 989-1002, ISSN 0012-3692

Ikegami, H. & Funato, M. & Tamai, H et al. (2010). Low-dose vasopressin infusion therapy for refractory hypotension in ELBW infants. *Pediatrics International*, Vol. 52, No. 3, (Jun), pp. 368-373, ISSN 1328-8067

Ishiguro, A. & Sekine, T. & Suzuki, K et al.(2011). Changes in skin and subcutaneous perfusion in very-low-birth-weight infants during the transitional period. *Neonatology*, Vol. 100, No. 2, (Mar), pp. 162-168, ISSN 1661-7800

Jaillard, S. & Houfflin-Debarge, V. & Riou Y et al. (2001). Effects of catecholamines on the pulmonary circulation in the ovine fetus. *American journal of physiology. Regulatory, integrative and comparative physiology*, Vol. 281, No. 2, (Aug), pp. R607-R614, ISSN 0363-6119

Kato, R. & Sato, J. & Nishino, T. (1998). Milrinone decreases both pulmonary arterial and venous resistances in the hypoxic dog. *British Journal of Anaesthesia* , Vol. 81, No. 6, (Dec), pp. 920-924, ISSN 0007-0912

Kluckow, M. & Evans, N. (2000). Superior vena cava flow in newborn infants: a novel marker of systemic blood flow. *Archives of Disease in Childhood Fetal & Neonatal Edition*, Vol. 82, No. 3, (May), pp. F182-F187, ISSN 1359-2998

Kluckow, M. & Seri, I. & Evans, N. (2007). Functional echocardiography: an emerging clinical tool for the neonatologist. *The Journal of Pediatrics*, Vol. 150, No. 2, (Feb), pp. 125-130, ISSN 0022-3476

Kluckow, M. (2005). Low systemic blood flow and pathophysiology of the preterm transitional circulation. *Early Human Development*, Vol. 81, No. 5, (May), pp. 429-437, ISSN: 0378-3782

Landry, DW. & Levin, HR. & Gallant, EM et al. (1997). Vasopressin deficiency contributes to the vasodilation of septic shock. *Circulation*, Vol. 95, No. 5, (Mar 4), pp. 1122-1125, ISSN 0009-7322

McNamara, PJ. & Laique, F. & Muang-In, S et al. (2006). Milrinone improves oxygenation in neonates with severe persistent pulmonary hypertension of the newborn. *Journal of Critical Care*, Vol. 21, No. 2, (Jun), pp. 217-222 ISSN 0883-9441

Landers, MS. & Sullivan, RM. (1999). Norepinephrine and associative conditioning in the neonatal rat somatosensory system. *Brain research. Developmental brain research*, Vol. 114, No.2, (May 14), pp. 261-264, ISSN 0165-3806

Landry, DW. & Oliver, JA. (2001). The pathogenesis of vasodilatory shock. *The New England Journal of Medicine*, Vol. 345, No. 8, (Aug 23), pp. 588-595, ISSN 0028-4793

Liedel, JL. & Meadow, W. & Nachman, J et al. (2002). Use of vasopressin in refractory hypotension in children with vasodilatory shock: five cases and a review of the literature. *Pediatric Critical Care Medicine*, Vol. 3, No. 1, (Jan), pp. 15-18, ISSN 1529-7535

Masumoto, K. & Kusuda, S. & Aoyagi, H et al. (2008). Comparison of serum cortisol concentrations in preterm infants with or without late-onset circulatory collapse due to adrenal insufficiency of prematurity. *Pediatric Research*, Vol. 63, No. 6, (Jun), pp. 686-690, ISSN 0031-3998

Magnenant, E. & Jaillard, S. & Deruelle, P et al. (2003). Role of the alpha2-adrenoceptors on the pulmonary circulation in the ovine fetus. *Pediatric Research*, Vol. 54, No. 1, (Jul), pp. 44-51, ISSN 0031-3998

Madrigal, JL. & Leza, JC. & Polak P et al. (2009). Astrocyte-derived MCP-1 mediates neuroprotective effects of noradrenaline. *Journal of Neuroscience*, Vol. 29, No. 1, (Jan 7), pp. 263-267, ISSN 0270-6474

McLean, CW. & Cayabyab, R. & Noori, S et al. (2008). Cerebral circulation and hypotension in the premature infant- diagnosis and treatment, In: *Neonatology Questions and Controversies: Neurology*, Perlman, JM. (Ed.), pp. 3–26, Saunders/Elsevier, ISBN, 978-1416031574, Philadelphia

Meyer, S. & Gottschling, S. & Baghai, A et al. (2006). Arginine-vasopressin in catecholamine-refractory septic versus non-septic shock in extremely low birth weight infants with acute renal injury. *Critical Care*, Vol. 10, No. 3, (May 5), R71, ISSN 1364-8535

Meyer, S. & Todd, D. & Shadboldt, B. (2009). Assessment of portable continuous wave Doppler ultrasound (ultrasonic cardiac output monitor) for cardiac output measurements in neonates. *Journal of Paediatrics and Child Health*, Vol. 45, No. 7-8, (Jul-Aug), pp. 464-468, ISSN 1034-4810

Mesiano, S. & Jaffe, RB. (1997). Developmental and functional biology of the primate fetal adrenal cortex. *Endocrine* Reviews, Vol. 18, No. 3, (Jun), pp. 378-403, ISSN 0163-769X

Morales, D. & Madigan, J. & Cullinane, S et al. (1999). Reversal by vasopressin of intractable hypotension in the late phase of hemorrhagic shock. *Circulation*, Vol. 100, No. 3, (Jul 20), pp. 226-229, ISSN 0009-7322

Munro, MJ. & Walker, AM. & Barfield, CP. (2004). Hypotensive extremely low birth weight infants have reduced cerebral blood flow. *Pediatrics*, Vol. 114, No. 6, (Dec), pp. 1591-1596, ISSN 0031-4005

Nagdyman, N & Ewert, P. & Peters, B et al. (2008). Comparison of different near-infrared spectroscopic cerebral oxygenation indices with central venous and jugular venous oxygenation saturation in children. *Pediatric Anesthesia*, Vol. 18, No. 2, (Feb), pp. 160-166, ISSN 1155-5645

Ng, PC. & Lam, CW. & Fok, TF et al. (2001) Refractory hypotension in preterm infants with adrenocortical insufficiency. *Archives of Disease in Childhood Fetal & Neonatal Edition*, Vol. 84, No. 2, (Mar), pp. F122-F124, ISSN 1359-2998

Noori, S. & Seri, I. (2005). Pathophysiology of newborn hypotension outside the transitional period. *Early Human Development*, Vol.81, No.5, (May), pp. 399-404, ISSN 0378-3782

Noori, S. & Friedlich, P. & Seri, I. (2004). Pharmacology Review: The Use of Dobutamine in the Treatment of Neonatal Cardiovascular Compromise. *NeoReviews. org*, Vol. 5, No. 1, (Jan 1), pp. e22-e26

Nuntnarumit, P. & Yang, W. & Bada-Ellzey, HS. (1999). Blood pressure measurements in the newborn. *Clinics in Perinatology*, Vol. 26, No. 4, (Dec), pp. 981-996, ISSN 0095-5108

Oca, MJ. & Nelson, M. & Donn, SM. (2003). Randomized trial of normal saline versus 5% albumin for the treatment of neonatal hypotension. *Journal of Perinatology*, Vol. 23, No. 6, (Sep), pp. 473-476, ISSN 0743-8346

Osborn, DA. & Evans, N. & Kluckow, M. (2004). Clinical detection of low upper body blood flow in very premature infants using blood pressure, capillary refill time, and central-peripheral temperature difference. *Archives of Disease in Childhood Fetal & Neonatal Edition*, Vol. 89, No. 2, (Mar), pp. F168-F173, ISSN 1359-2998

Paradisis, M. & Evans, N. & Kluckow, M et al. (2009). Randomized trial of milrinone versus placebo for prevention of low systemic blood flow in very preterm infants. *The Journal* of *Pediatrics*, Vol. 154, No. 2, (Feb), pp. 189-195, ISSN 0022-3476

Paradisis, M. & Osborn, DA. (2004). Adrenaline for prevention of morbidity and mortality in preterm infants with cardiovascular compromise. *Cochrane database of systematic reviews*, No.1, CD003958, ISSN 1469-493X

Pellicer, A. & Valverde, E. & Elorza, MD et al. (2005). Cardiovascular support for low birth weight infants and cerebral hemodynamics: a randomized, blinded, clinical trial. *Pediatrics*, Vol. 115, No. 6, (Jun), pp. 1501-1512, ISSN 0031-400568. Pellicer, A. & Bravo, MC. & Madero, R et al. (2009). Early systemic hypotension and vasopressor support in low birth weight infants: impact on neurodevelopment. *Pediatrics*, Vol. 123, No. 5, (May), pp. 1369-1376, ISSN 0031-4005

Penny, DJ. & Sano, T. & Smolich, JJ. (2001). Increased systemic oxygen consumption offsets improved oxygen delivery during dobutamine infusion in newborn lambs. *Intensive Care Medicine*, Vol. 27, No. 9, (Sep), pp. 1518-1525, ISSN 0342-4642

Peltoniemi, O. & Kari, MA. & Heinonen, K et al. (2005), Pretreatment cortisol values may predict responses to hydrocortisone administration for the prevention of bronchopulmonary dysplasia in high-risk infants. *The Journal of Pediatrics*, Vol. 146, No. 5, (May), pp. 632-637, ISSN 0022-3476

Prigent, H. & Maxime, V. & Annane, D. (2004). Clinical review: corticotherapy in sepsis. *Critical Care*, Vol. 8, No. 2, (Apr), pp.122-129, ISSN 1364-8535

Tourneux, P. & Rakza, T. & Abazine, A et al. (2008a). Noradrenaline for management of septic shock refractory to fluid loading and dopamine or dobutamine in full-term newborn infants. *Acta Paediatrica*, Vol. 97, No. 2, (Feb), pp. 177-180, ISSN 0803-5253

Tourneux, P. & Rakza, T. & Bouissou, A et al. (2008b). Pulmonary circulatory effects of norepinephrine in newborn infants with persistent pulmonary hypertension. *The Journal of Pediatrics*, Vol. 153, No. 3, (Sep), pp. 345-349, ISSN 0022-3476

Rodríguez-Núñez, A. & López-Herce, J. & Gil-Antón, J et al. (2006). Rescue treatment with terlipressin in children with refractory septic shock: a clinical study. *Critical Care*, Vol. 10, No. 1, (Jan 31), R20, ISSN 1364-8535

Rowland, DG. &, Gutgesell, HP. (1995). Noninvasive assessment of myocardial contractility, preload, and afterload in healthy newborn infants. *American Journal of Cardiology*,Vol. 75, No.12, (Apr 15), pp. 813-821, ISSN: 0002-9149

Rozé, JC. & Tohier, C. & Maingueneau C et.al. (1993). Response to dobutamine and dopamine in the hypotensive very preterm infant. *Archives of disease in childhood*, Vol. 69, 1 Spec No, (Jul), pp. 59-63, ISSN 0003-9888

Sassano-Higgins, S. & Friedlich, F. & Seri, I. (2011). A meta-analysis of dopamine use in hypotensive preterm infants: blood pressure and cerebral hemodynamics. *Journal of Perinatology*, Vol. 31, No. 10, (Oct 31), pp. 647-655, ISSN 0743-8346

Seri, I. (1995). Cardiovascular, renal, and endocrine actions of dopamine in neonates and children. *The Journal of Pediatrics*, Vol. 126, No. 3, (Mar), pp.333-344, ISSN 0022-3476

Seri, I. & Evans, J. (2001). Controversies in the diagnosis and management of hypotension in the newborn infant. *Current Opinion in Pediatrics*, Vol.13, No.2, (Apr), pp. 116-123, ISSN 1040-8703

Seri, I. (2006). Management of hypotension and low systemic blood flow in the very low birth weight neonate during the first postnatal week. *Journal of Perinatology*, Vol. 26, Suppl. 1, (May 26), pp. S8-S13, ISSN 0743-8346

Shiao, SY. & Ou, CN. (2007). Validation of oxygen saturation monitoring in neonates. *American Journal of Critical Care*, Vol. 16, No. 2, (Mar), pp. 168-178, ISSN 1062-3264

Skelton, R. & Gill, AB. & Parsons, JM. (1998). Reference ranges for cardiac dimensions and blood flow velocity in preterm infants. *Heart*, Vol. 80, No. 3, (Sep), pp. 281-285, ISSN 1468-201X 124, No. 1, (Jul), pp. 277-284, ISSN 0031-4005

Soleymani, S. & Cayabyab, R. & Borzage, TM et al. (2010). Comparison between charted and continuously recorded vital signs and hemodynamic data. *Annual PAS/SPR Meeting*, Vancouver, Abstract.

Stark, MJ. & Clifton, VL. & Wright, IM. (2009). Carbon monoxide is a significant mediator of cardiovascular status following preterm birth. *Pediatrics*, Vol.

Teitel, DF. & Sidi, D. (1985). Developmental changes in myocardial contractile reserve in the lamb. *Pediatric Research,* Vol. 19, No. 9, (Sep), pp. 948-955, ISSN 0031-3998

Valverde, E. & Pellicer, A. & Madero, R et al. (2006). Dopamine versus epinephrine for cardiovascular support in low birth weight infants: analysis of systemic effects and neonatal clinical outcomes. *Pediatrics*, Vol. 117, No. 6, (Jun), pp. e1213-e1222, 1098-4275

Van Hare, GF., & Hawkins, JA., & Schmidt, KG et al. (1990). The effects of increasing mean arterial pressure on left ventricular output in newborn lambs. *Circulation Research,* Vol. 67, No. 1, (Jul), pp. 78-83, ISSN 0009-7330

Van Bel, F. & Lemmers, P. & Naulaers, G. (2008). Monitoring neonatal regional cerebral oxygen saturation in clinical practice: value and pitfalls. *Neonatology*, Vol. 94, No. 4, (Sep 119), pp. 237-244, ISSN 1661-7800

Vincent, JL. (Ed.). (2009). *Critical care medicine: Churchill's ready reference,* Churchill Livingstone, pp. 12–13, ISBN 978-0080451367, Philadelphia

Watkins, AM. & West, CR. & Cooke, RW. (1989). Blood pressure and cerebral haemorrhage and ischaemia in very low birthweight infants. *Early Human Development,* Vol. 19, No. 2, (May), pp. 103-110, ISSN 0378-3782

Watterberg, KL. & Gerdes, JS. & Cole, CH et al. (2004). Prophylaxis of early adrenal insufficiency to prevent bronchopulmonary dysplasia: a multicenter trial. *Pediatrics,* Vol. 114, No.6, (Dec), pp. 1649-1657, ISSN 0031-4005

Watterberg, KL. & Shaffer, ML. & The PROPHET Study Group. (2005), Cortisol concentrations and apparent serum half-life during hydrocortisone therapy in extremely low birth weightinfants. *Pediatric academic societies annual meeting,* Vol 57, p. 1501

Watterberg, KL. & Shaffer, ML. & Mishefske, MJ et al. (2007). Growth and neurodevelopmental outcomes after early low-dose hydrocortisone treatment in extremelylow birth weight infants. *Pediatrics*, Vol. 120, No.1, (Jul), pp. 40-48, ISSN 0031-4005

Wong, FY. & Barfield, CP. & Horne, RS et al. (2009). Dopamine therapy promotes cerebral flow-metabolism coupling in preterm infants. *Intensive Care Medicine,* Vol. 35, No. 10, (Oct), pp. 1777-1782, ISSN 0342-4642

Wyckoff, MH. & Perlman, JM. & Laptook AR. (2005). Use of volume expansion during delivery room resuscitation in near-term and term infants. *Pediatrics,* Vol. 115, No. 4, (Apr), pp. 950-955, ISSN 0031-400

Yeh, TF. & Lin, YJ. & Lin, HC et al. (2004). Outcomes at school age after postnatal dexamethasone therapy for lung disease of prematurity. *The New England Journal* of *Medicine,* Vol. 350, No. 13, (Mar 25), pp. 1304-1313. ISSN 0028-4793.

Zeballos, G. & López-Herce, J. & Fernández, C et al. (2006). Rescue therapy with terlipressin by continuous infusion in a child with catecholamine-resistant septic shock. *Resuscitation*, Vol. 68, No. 1, (Jan), pp. 151-153 ISSN 0300-9572

21

Role of Echocardiography in Research into Neglected Cardiovascular Diseases in Sub-Saharan Africa

Ana Olga Mocumbi
National Health Institute & University Eduardo Mondlane, Mozambique

1. Introduction

Echocardiography is a non-invasive imaging technique that has been important in improving the quality and reliability of cardiovascular diagnosis, but access to it remains limited in most developing countries in Africa due to the costs of the technique and the lack of highly specialized personnel to perform it. Training in echocardiography is part of the postgraduate residency training requirements in cardiology in most African countries, despite the absence of an accreditation process such as that designed in Europe and United States of America (Ogah et al., 2006). While the use of transthoracic echocardiography has been spreading slowly around the continent, transesophageal echocardiography is still limited to few centers.

Barriers to obtaining ultrasound services in Sub-Saharan Africa include distance, time, cost of transfers and ultrasound charges (Shah et al., 2008). However, compared to other diagnostic imaging modalities echocardiography is safe, portable and inexpensive, uses simple power supply, and requires minimal maintenance. These characteristics make it the most suitable imaging technique for low-resource areas of Sub-Saharan Africa, where the introduction of smaller and battery-powered ultrasound machines is being used to reach out for people living in remote areas that traditionally did not have access to specialized cardiovascular diagnosis and care.

While witnessing an increasing awareness of the epidemic of cardiovascular disease, encompassing conditions such as hypertension, acute coronary syndrome, stroke and chronic heart failure, Sub-Saharan Africa still has a high burden of several infectious-related cardiovascular diseases and specific conditions such as cardiomyopathies. These neglected cardiovascular diseases include amongst others rheumatic heart disease (RHD) and endomyocardial fibrosis (EMF), both representing a considerable source of burden to the communities and playing a major role in determining premature mortality around the continent. Having recognized the potential of echocardiography as a research tool, African scientists have been using this technique to describe the epidemiology and profile of neglected cardiovascular conditions, as well as to bring new insights into the main causes of heart failure in both pediatric and adult populations (Mocumbi et al., 2008; Sani et al., 2007; Jaiyesimi & Antia, 1981a, b; Marijon et al., 2007; Adesanya 1979).

RHD and EMF have been the subject of community- and hospital-based research using echocardiography. This has resulted in an increase in the number of publications from Africa in indexed medical journals during the last decade. However, the increase is far from the desirable as the number of epidemiological and clinical studies using echocardiography augmented from 6 to 15 for RHD and from 2 to 4 for EMF (Figure 1).

In this chapter we review the recent use of transthoracic echocardiography worldwide for advancing knowledge about the pathogenesis and natural history of RHD and EMF, focusing on the modalities most readily available in low-resource settings, namely bidimensional, M-mode, pulsed and continuous Doppler. Finally, we discuss the specific role of echocardiography in fostering research into these two endemic diseases in Africa, and present the current challenges and opportunities of the use of this technique in Sub-Saharan Africa.

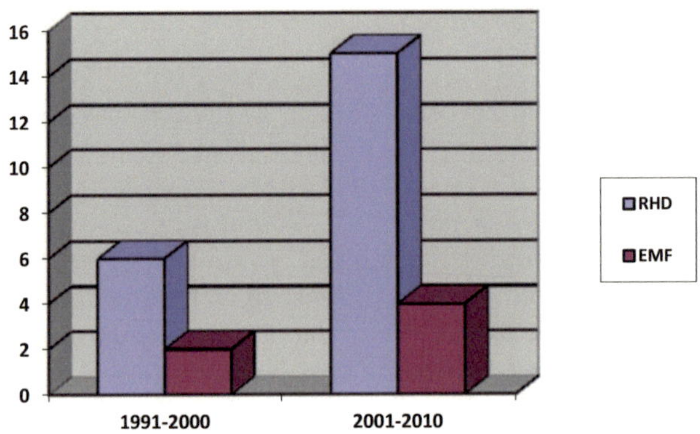

Fig. 1. Number of publications in indexed journals that reported hospital or community-based epidemiological and clinical studies using echocardiographic diagnosis for Rheumatic Heart Disease (RHD) and Endomyocardial Fibrosis (EMF) in the last two decades in Africa.

2. Endomyocardial fibrosis

EMF is a restrictive cardiomyopathy of unknown etiology characterised by progressive fibrous thickening of the ventricular endocardium, leading to restrictive physiology associated with atrioventricular valve dysfunction. Most of our knowledge of this condition comes from hospital-based studies in endemic areas of Uganda, Cote d'Ivoire, Nigeria, India and Brazil. Data on its exact epidemiology are scarce, but variations in geographical and ethnic distribution have been reported, stimulating the search for both environmental factors and genetic factors.

EMF is thought to be the commonest restrictive cardiomyopathy worldwide (Somers, 1990), affecting mainly children and adolescents of low-income communities from tropical regions of Africa, Asia and South America. Established and advanced disease can be easily diagnosed by clinical examination in endemic areas, but the finding of relatively asymptomatic individuals who present important echocardiographic abnormalities is not rare (Mocumbi et al., 2008; Salemi et al., 2005). The characterisation of early stages of the disease has not been systematically done, leading to major gaps in our knowledge of its pathogenesis and natural history.

The use of echocardiography for diagnosis of EMF, started almost half a century ago, has contributed to characterization of the disease and better understanding of its pathophysiology, resulting in improvements in management and prognosis. Several authors from different parts of the world have described the clinical and echocardiographic findings in EMF (Acquatella et al., 1979; Gonzalez-Lavin et al., 1982; Vijayaraghavan et al., 1983; Okereke et al., 1991; Rashwan et al.,1995), and more recently there have been attempts to use this technique for understanding its epidemiology (Mocumbi et al., 2008) as well define prognostic criteria prior to surgery (Mady et al., 2004).

2.1 Echocardiographic features

The hallmark of established EMF is the presence of thickened endocardium, ventricular obliteration and dilated atria. The typical image of restrictive cardiomyopathy is that of inversion of the size of heart cavities with small obliterated ventricles and dilated atria (Hassan et al., 2005; Berensztein et al., 2000). The wide spectrum of distribution and severity of the fibrotic lesions, as well as the changes in heart shape and distortion mandate a careful and comprehensive echocardiographic evaluation of each patient, using the usual and less conventional views.

The most characteristic echocardiographic features of EMF are large endocardial plaques, patchy endocardial thickening, obliteration of ventricular apices or valve recesses, ventricular and atrial thrombi, ventricular cavity volume reduction, enlarged atrium, restricted mobility of the atrioventricular valve leaflets, fusion of the papillary muscles to the wall and abnormalities of the ventricular regional wall motion (Okereke et al., 1991; Mady et al., 2005; Hassan et al., 2005; Berensztein et al., 2000). Less specific echocardiographic abnormalities include diffuse atrioventricular valve leaflet thickening, enhanced echodensity of the moderator band or trabeculae, abnormal movement of the interventricular septum and/or posterior LV wall, and presence of thickened left ventricular "false tendon" (Mocumbi et al., 2008). Moderate to massive pericardial effusion is a frequent finding in both left and right forms of EMF (George et al., 1982; Lowenthal & Teeger, 2000). Occasionally, endocardial calcification may be seen in the ventricles (Lowenthal & Teeger, 2000; Morrone et al., 1996; Trigo et al., 2010).

The pattern of distribution of the morphological and hemodynamic abnormalities allows the classification of EMF in different forms according to exclusive or predominant distribution of structural lesions in one or both sides of the heart. Hence the description of right, left and bilateral EMF.

2.1.1 Endocardial thickening

Thickening of the endocardium is the most characteristic feature of established EMF (Ojereke et al., 1991; Connor et al., 1967). It may consist of large plaques affecting one or both ventricles, as well as patchy endocardial thickening evenly distributed in the ventricular walls or affecting exclusively the interventricular septum. These abnormalities can be assessed by both bidimensional and M-mode. The most striking and constant features are increased amplitude echos at the right ventricular trabecular region, left ventricular apex and the region of the posterior mitral valve leaflet (Vijayaraghavan et al., 1983).

2.1.2 Ventricular thrombosis

Spontaneous contrast and ventricular thrombi are frequently seen in normally contracting ventricles in early stages of EMF, as part of the initial process that leads to endocardial fibrosis (Berensztein et al., 2000). The presence of ventricular thrombi, calcified or not, is a major determinant of management and prognosis.

2.1.3 Ventricular obliteration

This characteristic abnormality of EMF consists in partial or complete exclusion of a portion of the ventricle from the circulation (Figure 2). In right EMF the trabecular portion of the ventricle is separated from the remaining cavity by a large fibrotic endocardial plaque, underneath which there is myocardium of apparently normal texture (Trigo et al., 2010). Left ventricular obliteration affects both the apex and the recesses of the posterior mitral valve leaflet excluding these parts from the ventricular cavity (Berensztein et al., 2000). It is thought that obliteration by thrombi and subsequent scarring fibrosis are the mechanisms involved (Connor et al., 1967), both leading to reduction of the diastolic properties of the ventricles. Also, thrombi may involve the sub-valvar apparatus, leading to scarring and fusion of leaflets to the ventricular wall, therefore resulting in leaflet movement restriction and severe atrioventricular valve dysfunction.

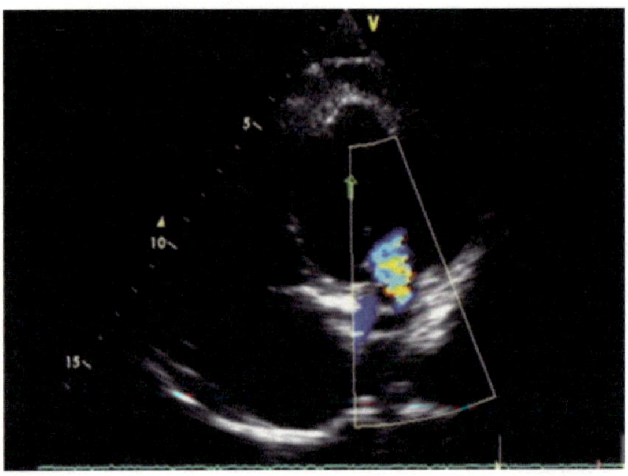

Fig. 2. Left-sided EMF with obliteration and endocardial thickening at the ventricular apex. The atypical mitral regurgitation jet is frequent in moderate disease.

With progression of the disease to more advanced stages cavity retraction occurs with further reduction of the effective ventricular cavity volume, seemingly due to progressive organization and fibrosis of the mural thrombi and adjacent endocardium. Particularly in the right ventricle, this process is associated with pulling of the wall by the retracted tricuspid valve apparatus, resulting in the distinctive finding of advanced right-sided EMF called "apical notch" (Figure 3). The apical notch gives the heart a shape that resembles the map of Africa, hence the designation "Heart of Africa" (Davies, 1960). On the left side the ventricular apex is never retracted; it becomes thicker leading to considerable reduction of the longitudinal diameter of the ventricle, resulting in a spherical ventricular shape.

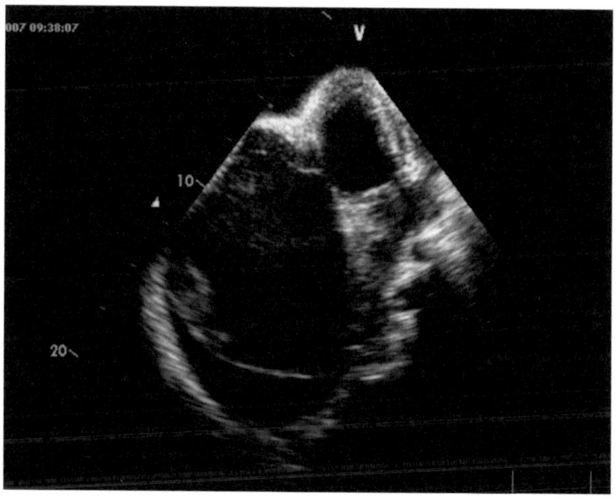

Fig. 3. Transthoracic image obtained during field research using a portable ultrasound machine showing retraction of the trabecular portion of the right ventricle with reduction of cavity size and aneurysmal right atrium in which a thrombus can be seen.

2.1.4 Diffuse leaflet thickening

Diffuse thickening of the atrioventricular valve leaflets occurs in some patients with EMF. This pattern helps differentiating left-sided EMF with predominant valvular lesion from chronic rheumatic disease of the mitral valve in endemic areas for both diseases. In chronic rheumatic mitral regurgitation leaflet thickening is usually restricted to or exaggerated at the tip of the valve, extends to the chordae, and is never associated to obliteration of the contralateral ventricle (Saraiva et al., 1999; Metras et al., 1983).

2.1.5 Septal motion abnormalities

The restricted movement of the fibrotic left ventricular apex and its obliteration are accompanied by compensatory contractile mechanism that results in exaggerated and distinctive motion of the basal portion of the left ventricle, the so-called Merlon sign (Vijayaraghavan et al., 1983; Berensztein et al., 2000). On M-mode the interventricular septum has a rapid anterior movement in early diastole (Acquatella et al., 1979) assuming an M-shaped movement. In some patients the septal motion may be reversed (paradoxical septal movement).

2.1.6 Restrictive filling pattern

A tall E wave with E/A ratio greater than 2, deceleration time less than 120ms and isovolumic relaxation time inferior to 160ms are the criteria used to define the presence of ventricular restrictive filling pattern. This evaluation is usually compromised by the presence of severe mitral regurgitation. The brisk early diastolic filling with poor filling in the remainder of diastole, the absence of respiratory changes, the presence of normal pericardium and the usual association to pericardial effusion, enable distinction from constrictive pericarditis.

2.1.7 Atrioventricular valve regurgitation

Mild mitral regurgitation is found in initial stages of left EMF. The jet is atypical and seems to start inside the ventricular cavity (figure 2). In severe left EMF thickening and scarring of the valve leaflets and the mitral valve apparatus lead to severe mitral regurgitation that is usually eccentric, due mainly to restricted movement of the posterior leaflet. The regurgitation has a high velocity jet directed to the posterior wall of the left atrium, reaching the pulmonary veins in most cases (Figure 4).

The tricuspid valve apparatus is distorted in EMF with restricted movement of the leaflets in early phases of the disease. In severe right EMF there is massive tricuspid annulus dilatation and non-turbulent low velocity regurgitant jet, witnessing the absence of pressure gradient between the two right cavities. In these cases the right filling pressures are very high, leading to severe dilatation of the cava system and reflux from the right atrium towards the supra-hepatic veins, a phenomenon easily accessed using pulsed and color Doppler.

2.1.8 Atrial dilatation

Both the restriction to ventricular filling and the atrioventricular valve regurgitation result in increase in atrial pressure, leading to progressive atrial dilatation. The consequence is further increase in atrioventricular valve annulus dilatation perpetuating the cycle and being responsible for the frequent finding of aneurysmal atria (Hassan et al., 2005; Berensztein et al., 2000). Annular dilatation, leaflet retraction and fibrosis of the sub-valvar apparatus lead to non-coaptation and free tricuspid valve regurgitation (Okereke et al., 1991), this later seen as a non-turbulent low velocity jet on color Doppler.

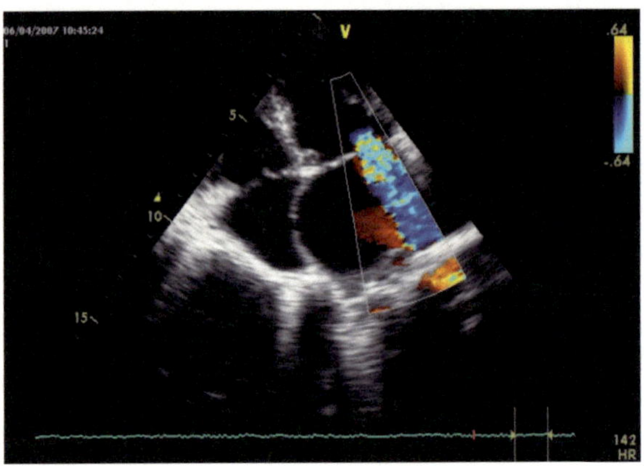

Fig. 4. Mitral regurgitation and left atrial dilatation on a patient with left EMF evaluated using portable ultrasound machine during a community-based study.

2.1.9 Semilunar valve abnormalities

The pulmonary valve is usually spared from structural abnormalities but there is often pulmonary regurgitation that allows estimation of the mean and diastolic pulmonary pressures. In severe cases due to the lack of pressure gradient between the atrium, the ventricle and the pulmonary artery, there is often diastolic opening of the pulmonary valve. The aortic valve is almost always normal, but in few cases there may be thickening of the cusps.

2.1.10 Abnormalities of the left side of the heart

Early left-sided EMF is characterized by thickening of the mitral leaflets, presence of apical thrombus, and/or obliteration of the apex or the recess between the posterior leaflet and the posterior wall. Thrombi may be found in the sub-valvar apparatus involving the free edges of both papillary muscles or in the apex. There is moderate left atrial dilatation but the valve remains non-regurgitant. The flow across the mitral valve reveals early diastolic filling followed by restriction pattern.

In the established left-sided EMF endocardial thickening is prominent in interventricular septum, the apex and posterior wall behind the recess of the posterior mitral leaflet, the ventricular cavity assumes a spherical shape and there is increased contractility at its basal portion. The left ventricular ejection fraction is usually not calculated due to the presence of mitral regurgitation and left ventricular distortion. The heart distortion and change in the position of the heart in the chest explains the fact that contractility is often graded using a visual scale. In patients without severe distortion of the left ventricular shape and no mitral regurgitation, the LV end-systolic and end-diastolic volumes and ejection fraction can be determined from the apical 4-chamber view according to the modified Simpson's rule or the Teicholz method (Feigenbaum, 1994).

Although in rare patients the mitral valve may be stenotic, most patients present an eccentric mitral regurgitation with signs of passive pulmonary hypertension. The left atrium maximal linear dimensions at the end of left ventricular systole are increased in all plans and, in severe cases the cavity may be aneurysmal. However, there is rarely left atrial thrombus.

Regarding the mitral valve there is leaflet thickening and shortage, leading to non-coaptation and severe mitral regurgitation. The posterior mitral valve leaflet appears to be tethered down to the left ventricular posterior wall, with reduced mobility during diastole. In severe cases the leaflet, its chordae and papillary muscle are completely adherent to the wall leading to massive regurgitation.

2.1.11 Abnormalities of the right side of the heart

The initial lesions on the right side consist of thickening of the moderator band. In the longitudinal view of the right ventricle and short axis of the left ventricle at the level of the aorta a stretched moderator band is seen, while in 4 chambers-view the ventricular cavity is separated into two cameras. There may be thickening of the tricuspid leaflets and the analysis of the tricuspid inflow by pulsed Doppler reveals abnormal compliance.

Right ventricular trabecular cavity obliteration is thought to start by separation of the trabecular chamber of the right ventricle from the rest of the cavity, as seen in 4-chambers view (Figure 5). It is usually accompanied by mild to moderate tricuspid regurgitation caused by restriction to the movement of the anterior and septal leaflets of the tricuspid valve. The leaflets may present attachments to the wall leading to an echocardiographic picture that may mimic "Ebstein Malformation" (Vaidyanathan et al., 2009), namely with dilatation of the tricuspid annulus, tricuspid regurgitation with jet originating from the level of non-cooptation of the leaflets, which is dislocated to the trabecular portion of the ventricle. The right ventricular systolic function, evaluated through a visual semi-quantitative scale using two-dimensional guided M-mode in several incidences (four-chambers, parasternal long axis, parasternal short axis and sub-costal views), is globally normal, but may be reduced when there are large endocardial plaques and cavity retraction.

Advanced right EMF is defined by retraction of the ventricular cavity due to elimination of the trabecular portion of the cavity, resulting in the pathognomonic finding of an "apical notch". The right ventricular outflow tract is dilated and hyperdynamic to compensate the loss of the trabecular portion, and the interventricular septal motion may be reversed.

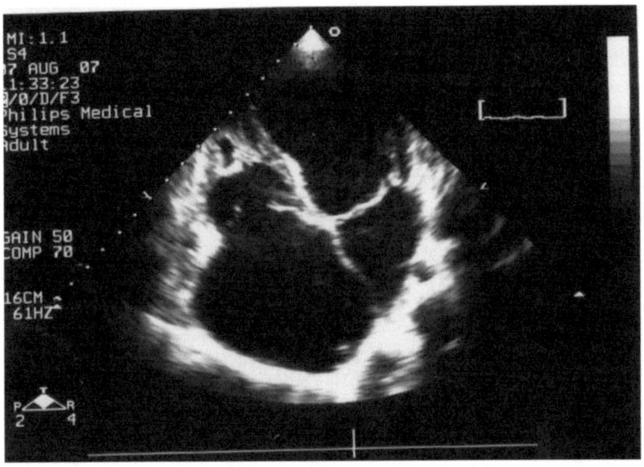

Fig. 5. Right EMF seen in 4-chambers view showing separation of the cavity in two portions, a feature that is characteristic prior to complete obliteration of the trabecular cavity.

Severe tricuspid regurgitation with no turbulence is characteristically associated to restriction of leaflet movements caused by involvement of the papillary muscles in the fibrotic process and to dilatation of the annulus that results from severe right atrial dilatation. At this stage most patients have spontaneous contrast inside the right atrium extending to the inflow tract of RV and also to the inferior vena cava and dilated supra-hepatic veins. Multiple thrombi may be found some moving freely and others attached to the atrial wall. The dilated inferior vena cava and supra-hepatic veins, usually with dynamic echos indicating stasis, do not show the normal respiratory changes, indicating increased systemic venous pressure. Pericardial, pleural and peritoneal effusions are also frequently present in patients in heart failure, best seen in subcostal view.

The colour Doppler is used for semi-quantitative estimation of tricuspid regurgitation severity, taking into account the width and depth of regurgitant jet inside the atrium seen from different views (four-chambers, short-axis and sub-costal). One criteria used to define severe tricuspid regurgitation is the lack of aliasing of the jet and its large width at origin, especially when there is non-coaptation of the tricuspid valve leaflets. The aneurismal right atrium results in heart distortion and compression of the left cavities making it difficult to evaluate the presence of mitral dysfunction. Abundant pericardial effusion and compression of left cavities compromise an adequate evaluation of the left ventricular function.

The lateral and supero-inferior dimensions of the right atrium are always increased and an aneurysmal atrium is usually found. The high pressure inside the atrial cavity pushes the interatrial septum towards the left side opening the *foramen ovale* in many occasions, and allowing a certain degree of right –to-left shunt that causes mild cyanosis. Compression of the left cavities by the severely dilated atrium and tense right ventricle at the level of the admission chamber may impede adequate ventricular filling as well as mask mitral regurgitation. On M-mode these findings are associated with interventricular paradoxical septal motion and small left ventricular cavity.

2.2 Pathological correlation

Surgery can be used to assess the accuracy of transthoracic echocardiography in determining the severity of EMF. This has been achieved by performing standardized transthoracic echocardiography on EMF patients prior to surgery, followed by detailed intra-operative examination of the abnormalities and histopathological evaluation of tissue obtained from excised biopsies (Mocumbi et al., 2010). In this series of patients from Mozambique the echocardiographic description coincided with the intraoperative findings in more than 80% of patients, the concordance being absolute for the most important pathological lesions of EMF, namely fusion of the posterior papillary muscle and leaflet to the wall, left ventricular apical fibrosis, thickening of the atrioventricular leaflets, right ventricular obliteration, right ventricular retraction and ventricular thrombi. This suggested that transthoracic echocardiography can be used in isolation for diagnosis and surgical management of chronic EMF in low-resource endemic areas.

2.3 Challenges and opportunities

Echocardiography can make a confident non-invasive diagnosis of EMF (Vijayaraghavan et al., 1983; Mocumbi et al., 2010), has been useful in determining patients who can benefit from surgery and allows evaluation of the response to treatment. Access to hand-carried echocardiography battery-operated systems has allowed for the first time the design and implementation of epidemiological research in a remote area in Mozambique. In this community, known to have a high attack rate of the disease from previous hospital-based data (Ferreira et al., 2002), 1063 individuals of all ages were randomly selected and submitted to transthoracic echocardiography using a standardized protocol (Mocumbi et al., 2008). A prevalence of 19.8% was found, with the majority of the individuals being asymptomatic and having mild or moderate disease.

For such disease with so many gaps in knowledge there is need to build regional or continental registries starting with phenotypic characterization of individuals in early stages of EMF through echocardiography, using standardized criteria that can be validated on follow-up studies in several endemic areas. This may contribute to uncover aspects related to its natural history, and constitute cohorts to test differences in genetic and to biological profile between healthy individuals and those affected by the disease in endemic areas. Follow-up of individuals with well-established echocardiographic phenotype may also be important to identify predictors of outcome using different disease management strategies.

3. Rheumatic heart disease

RHD is the most important form of acquired cardiovascular disease in children and adolescents in Africa. It is the only chronic sequelae of rheumatic fever (RF), a systemic disease that results from group A streptococcal infections.

Rheumatic Heart Disease (RHD) is still a major concern in Africa (World Health Organization, 2007) despite the dramatic declines in the incidence and prevalence of this condition that have occurred over the last 150 years in the developed world (Gordis, 1985). It is a disease traditionally associated with poverty and overcrowding, and this decline was achieved through improvement in living conditions and widespread use of penicillin for the treatment of streptococcal pharyngitis. The unacceptably high rates of RF/RHD in Sub-Saharan Africa lead to considerable use of health-care resources and a major impact on the patients, their families and the society as a whole.

Although RHD is still a neglected disease, there has been a new surge on research on this condition. This has been centered in developing countries and those populations within middle- and high-income countries where high burdens of disease still exist. Echocardiography is considered the adequate tool for identifying early stages of heart valve disease (Carapetis & Zuhlke, 2011).

3.1 Echocardiographic diagnosis

Echocardiography is an essential tool in diagnosis and management of RF and RHD. Several structural and hemodynamic abnormalities are important for classifying valve lesions, both in the acute and chronic phases of the disease. Even before the advent of colour Doppler flow imaging several studies had already highlighted the utility of echocardiography for the diagnosis of rheumatic carditis, and emphasized its value in defining the mechanisms of valve disease and heart failure associated with severe attacks of carditis (Vansan et al., 1996; Narula et al., 1999). Colour flow Doppler imaging was then considered a useful method of identifying subclinical mitral and aortic valvar disease at all stages of rheumatic fever when carditis cannot be otherwise detected (Folger et al., 1992). Regarding chronic rheumatic heart disease, echocardiography may be used to track the progression of valve abnormalities and to help determine the time for surgical intervention.

3.1.1 Acute carditis

In acute rheumatic disease Doppler-echocardiography identifies and quantifies valve abnormalities, ventricular dysfunction and pericardial effusion (Narula et al., 1999; Folger et al., 1992). The valve most commonly affected is the mitral, followed by the aortic valve (Folger et al., 1992). In the African context, severe pure rheumatic mitral regurgitation is as prevalent as pure stenosis but has an entirely different time course, surgical anatomy, and relation to disease activity, suggesting a separate pathophysiologic mechanism (Marcus et al., 1994).

The usual features of acute rheumatic valvulitis are annular dilatation, elongation of the chordae to the anterior leaflet, and postero-laterally directed mitral regurgitation jet (Vansan et al., 1996; Narula et al., 1999; Folger et al., 1992). Nodular thickening of valve leaflets also occurs (Vansan et al., 1996), and may represent echocardiographic equivalents of rheumatic verrucae seen universally at autopsy in patients who died of acute rheumatic fever (Baggenstoos & Titus., 1968) and noted macroscopically at surgery in a substantial proportion of patients subjected to valve surgery during the acute phase (Kinsley et al., 1981). When acute carditis courses with chordal thickening (Vijayalakshmi et al., 2008), it suggests acute rheumatic fever recurrence in patients with established rheumatic heart valve disease. Mild mitral regurgitation present during the acute phase usually resolves weeks to months after. In contrast, patients with moderate-to-severe carditis have persistent mitral and/or aortic regurgitation.

Valve insufficiency due to endocarditis, rather than myocardial dysfunction caused by myocarditis, is the dominant cause of heart failure in acute rheumatic fever, related to ventricular dilatation and/or restriction of leaflet mobility (Vansan et al., 1996). This has been supported by demonstration of the absence of cTnI elevations during rheumatic fever (Kamblock et al., 2003; Essop et al., 1993). The left ventricle is dilated with preserved or increased fractional shortening in most cases, but variable degree of ventricular dysfunction is not rare in the African setting probably due to the high prevalence of predisposing factors such as anemia.

3.1.2 Chronic rheumatic heart disease

Isolated mitral regurgitation or combined mitral and aortic regurgitation are the most common abnormalities found in chronic RHD (Vansan et al., 1996; Folger et al., 1992; Marcus et al., 1994). Several morphological abnormalities have been considered features of chronic mitral RHD namely (a) valve and/or chordal thickening; (b) restrictive leaflet motion due to chordal thickening, shortening or fusion, commissural fusion and leaflet calcification or thickening; and (c) chordal elongation, rupture or prolapse (Marijon et al., 2007; Paar et al., 2010; Namboodiri et al., 2009; Wilkins et al., 1988). In mitral regurgitation the posterior mitral leaflet is shortened and immobile because its submitral complex is also thickened, fused and shortened, resulting in a gap or non-coaptation of the two leaflets in many patients (Okubo et al., 1984). Mitral stenosis occurs when the leaflets of the affected valves become diffusely thickened, with fusion of the commissures and chordae tendineae, as well as increased echodensity of the mitral valve that may signify calcification. However, valvular calcification is rare in juvenile rheumatic heart disease, frequently seen in Africa (Yuko-Jowi et al., 2005). Left atrial thrombus is a common finding in mitral stenosis.

There are few studies of characterization of aortic valve abnormalities in rheumatic heart disease. Rheumatic aortic valve disease is usually diagnosed in combination with mitral disease, and after exclusion of congenital disease, mainly bicuspid aortic valve. Echocardiographic diagnosis has been based on morphological changes such as the presence of thickened leaflets, rolled leaflet edges, coaptation defect, deformed leaflets, commissural fusion, leaflet retraction, abnormal leaflet mobility, systolic doming of leaflet, hyperechogenicity of leaflet edges and prolapse are used (Marijon et al., 2007; Paar et al., 2010). For community studies a more accurate case-definition and assessment of severity is needed since follow up of patients with RHD shows that those with no or mild aortic valve disease at the time of mitral valve intervention rarely develop severe aortic valve disease, and seldom require aortic valve surgery over the long-term follow up, while the presence of mild aortic stenosis at baseline is predictive of relatively more rapid progression in the minority of cases (Namboodiri et al., 2009).

Two-dimensional echocardiographic criteria of organic rheumatic tricuspid valve disease include thickened leaflets with restriction in motion, diastolic doming, and encroachment of the leaflet tips on the wall of the ventricular inlet (Guyer et al., 1984; Meira et al., 2006). Since pulmonary hypertension is predominant in mitral valve disease, there is commonly annulus dilatation that results from right cavities dilatation and leads to tricuspid regurgitation. This must be differentiated from organic valve disease, which has usually morphological changes similar to that described above for the mitral valve.

3.1.3 Major valvular abnormalities

3.1.3.1 Restrictive or excessive leaflet motion

Restrictive leaflet motion is evident in most patients with established RHD requiring surgery MR (Chavaud et al., 2001), nearly one third of patients with acute RF (Vijayalakshmi et al., 2008; Marcus et al., 1989) and all those with rheumatic mitral stenosis (Wilkins et al., 1988; Naito et al., 1980; Prasad & Radhakrishnan, 1992; Van der Bel-Kahn & Becker, 1986). It is caused by chordal shortening, thickening and fusion, commissural fusion, and leaflet calcification and thickening (Chavaud et al., 2001; Van der Bel-Kahn & Becker, 1986; Carpentier, 1983). The terms used to characterize the abnormal and restricted mobility of the mitral leaflets include elbow, dog-leg and hockey-stick deformity (Paar et al., 2010; Webb et al., 2009; Steer et al., 2009; Reeves et al., 2011; Carapetis et al., 2008) (Figure 6).

Chordal elongation and rupture of the primary chords are the mechanisms responsible for mitral valve prolapse in RHD. These changes must be carefully looked for as they influence the surgical management (Chavaud et al., 2001; Marcus et al., 1989; Carpentier, 1983).

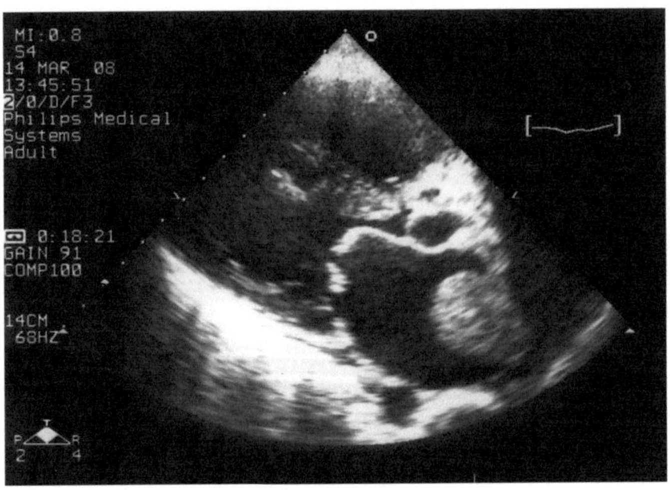

Fig. 6. Long axis parasternal view of a patient with mitral stenosis due to RHD showing thickening of the mitral and aortic valves, as well as restricted motion of the mitral leaflets. Notice a large left atrial thrombus.

3.1.3.2 Valve thickening

The rheumatic valve is fibrotic and firm, with thickening and fusion of leaflets and commissures (Van der Bel-Kahn & Becker, 1986), mostly seen in stenotic valves. Thickening of the mitral valve, especially the anterior mitral leaflet, appears to be a consistent feature of RHD (Figure 6), which can be adequately assessed in the parasternal long axial view where the anterior mitral valve because the ultrasound beam is perpendicular to the leaflet. Regarding the aortic valve both the parasternal and subcostal views allow adequate evaluation. Valve thickness of both mitral and aortic valves increases with age, based on an autopsy study (Sahsakul et al., 1988). However, in populations where RHD is prevalent there are very few additional conditions that are associated with increased thickness of the mitral valve in the age groups affected by RHVD, except for endemic areas for both RHD and EMF (Mocumbi et al., 2008).

3.2 Recent advances and research needs

The knowledge gap regarding epidemiology, pathogenesis and natural history of RF/RHD in Africa is related to several factors. First, group A streptococcal infections that precede RHD are subclinical, and most of the clinical cases are of a minor nature compared with other diseases afflicting children in this setting. Secondly, RF/RHD is not notifiable in most African countries and its impact is underestimated. Thirdly, many children are not brought to medical care when they complain of sore throat or a skin lesion. Finally, the diagnosis of rheumatic fever/carditis, requires clinical sophistication that exceeds the expertise available at many local hospitals that are manned by nurses or trained health care workers.

The echocardiographic diagnosis of RHD is not standardized and there are few studies looking systematically at criteria for diagnosing valve disease using modern echocardiographic tools. However, due to the persisting burden of the disease in some areas of the world echocardiography has been used in community studies in Mozambique and Cambodia (Marijon et al., 2007), Tonga (Carapetis et al., 2008), Nicaragua (Paar et al., 2010), Fiji (Steer et al., 2009; Reeves et al., 2011), Kenya (Anabwani et al., 1996), India (Thakur et al., 1996; Bhaya et al., 2010), Pakistan (Sadiq et al., 2009; Rizvi et al., 2004) and China (Zhimin 2006). These studies applied different inclusion and diagnostic criteria, raising the issue about the need for standardization of the definition of rheumatic heart valve disease by echocardiography.

Patients from African series present severe abnormalities at early ages (Sliwa et al., 2010; Marijon et al., 2008). Because rheumatic heart valve disease has an initial latent stage that can be detected by appropriate tests (among which echocardiography), has adequate affordable therapy, and may have its prognosis improved by interventions at an early stage, it should be the target of screening as a tool of preventive medicine.

3.2.1 Developing guidelines for echocardiographic screening

Early detection of "subclinical" rheumatic valve disease by echocardiography is vital, as it presents an opportunity for case detection at a time when prophylactic penicillin - to prevent recurrent episodes - can stop progression to important valve disease. This is very important in Africa, where most new patients admitted to hospitals have already advanced and complicated rheumatic valvular lesions (Sliwa et al., 2010), often resulting in heart failure and/or arrhythmia that cannot be adequately managed due to unavailability of open heart surgery. A current challenge for African scientists is therefore to make echocardiographic screening reliable, affordable and feasible in low-resource settings, using diagnostic criteria that are clear, simple, robust and reproducible. This would allow their incorporation in protocols for performing, reading and interpreting echocardiograms, in order to avoid over- and under-diagnosis.

Researchers from Africa have been involved in continental efforts to assess the epidemiology of RHD using echocardiography. This has started with the "**A**wareness, **S**urveillance, **A**dvocacy and **P**revention Strategy" lounged by the Pan African Society of Cardiology in 2005, which aims at reducing the burden of RF/RHD in the continent (Mayosi et al., 2006). More recently African researchers have been taking part in a global initiative aiming at standardization of echocardiographic screening that is led by the World Heart Federation (World Heart Federation, 2011).

3.2.2 Disseminating echocardiographic screening

The use of highly trained specialists for large scale echocardiographic screening of RHD in endemic areas of Africa is not practical (Figure 7) but the diffusion of ultrasound technology to nontraditional users has been rapid and far-reaching in the last years (Shah et al., 2008). Experiences for dissemination of echocardiography to non-traditional users in Rwanda and Tanzania have been designed aiming at the evaluation of pericardial effusion, rheumatic heart disease, congestive heart failure and estimation of global left ventricular function (Shah et al., 2008; Adler et al., 2008). The impact of this technology diffusion is being quantified, but early results show that ultrasound is a teachable skill, leads to accuracy of diagnosis, helps in management of common cardiovascular conditions, and improves professional satisfaction of local health providers (Shah et al., 2009). The role of task-shifting inside the health systems to allow non-cardiologists to perform echocardiographic screening for RHD must therefore be studied. However, there is need to carefully choose the health providers to be trained and implement measures of quality assessment and sustainability.

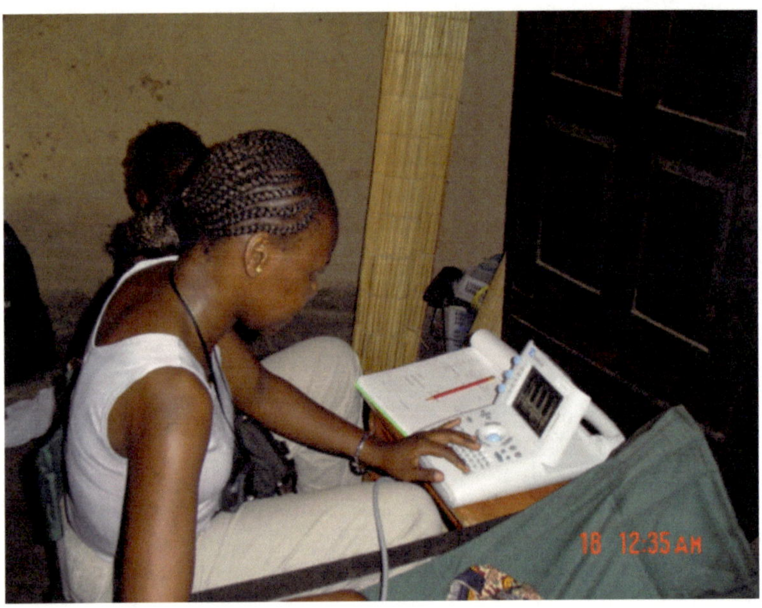

Fig. 7. Photograph of a researcher performing echocardiography in an Africa rural setting.

3.2.3 Definition of curricula and selection of ultrasound machines

Considering the unique pattern of cardiovascular disease in Africa, there is need for designing *curricula* and training materials tailored to the local needs, taking into consideration the differential diagnosis with conditions such as cardiomyopathy, which are also highly prevalent in the continent. In the particular conditions of health care provision in Africa the choice of the ultrasound machines is also of paramount importance. Machine specificities that are suitable for the African environment include durability, portability, battery-operated machines and high two-dimensional image quality. In portable machines a storage bag with room for gel, towels, probe covers and cleaning supplies is recommended (Shah et al., 2008).

4. Conclusions

There has been an increase in scientific publications from African researchers and institutions with the dissemination of echocardiography. Echocardiographic-driven research into neglected diseases such as endomyocardial fibrosis and rheumatic heart disease have contributed to uncover epidemiology and clinical profile of these conditions in the continent, confirming the role for this imaging technique in fostering research and improving quality of care in cardiovascular diseases in resource-deprived areas of Africa. Echocardiography may also help to quantify the health impact of certain neglected cardiovascular diseases in Africa, as well as assist in design and implementation of programs for surveillance, prevention and control of such conditions.

5. References

Anabwani GM, Bonhoeffer P. (1996). Prevalence of heart disease in school children in rural Kenya using colour-flow echocardiography. *East African Medical Journal*;73(4):215-217.

Acquatella H, Puigbo JJ, Suarez C, Mendoza J. (1979). Sudden early diastolic anterior movement of the septum in endomyocardial fibrosis. *Circulation*;59(4):847-848

Adesanya CO. (1979). M-mode echocardiography in the diagnosis of mitral stenosis. *Niger Med J*;9:533-537

Adler D, Mgalula K, Price D, Taylor O. (2008). Introduction of a portable ultrasound unit into the health services of the Lugufu refugee camp, Kigoma District, Tanzania. *Int J Emerg Med*;1:261-266

Baggenstoos AH, Titus JL. (1968). Rheumatic and collagen disorders of the heart. In: Gould SE, ed. Pathology of Heart and Blood Vessels. 3rd ed. Springield, III: Charles C Thomas Publisher;649-722

Berensztein CS, Pinero G, Marcotegui M, Brunoldi R, Blanco MV, Lerman J. (2000) Usefulness of echocardiography and Doppler echocardiographiy in endomyocardial fibrosis. *J Am Soc Echocardiog*; 13(3):226-30

Bhaya M, Panwar S, Beniwal R, Panwar RB. (2010) High prevalence of rheumatic heart disease detected by echocardiography in school children. *Echocardiography*; 27(4):448-453.

Carapetis J, Zuhlke L. (2011)Global research priorities in rheumatic fever and rheumatic heart disease. Annals of Pediatric *Cardiology*;4(1): 4-12.

Carapetis JR, Hardy M, Fakakovikaetau T, Taib R, Wilkinson L, Penny DJ, Steer AC. (2008) Evaluation of a screening protocol using auscultation and portable echocardiography to detect asymptomatic rheumatic heart disease in Tongan schoolchildren. *Nature Clinical Practice Cardiovascular Medicine*;5(7):411-417.

Carpentier A. (1983) Cardiac valve surgery - the "French correction". *J Thorac Cardiovasc Surg.*;86(3):323-337.

Chauvaud S, Fuzellier JF, Berrebi A, Deloche A, Fabiani JN, Carpentier A. (2001) Long-term (29 years) results of reconstructive surgery in rheumatic mitral valve insufficiency. *Circulation*;104(12 Suppl 1):I12-15;

Connor DH, Somers K, Hutt NSR, Manion WC, D'Arbela PGD. (1967) Endomyocardial fibrosis in Uganda (Davies'disease). Part I. *Am Heart J.*;74(5):687-709.

Davies, JNP. (1960) Some considerations regarding obscure diseases affecting the mural endocardium. *Am Heart J*;19(4):600-630

Essop MR, Wisenbaugh T, Sareli P. (1993) Evidence against a myocardial factor as the cause of left ventricular dilation in active rheumatic carditis. *J Am Coll Cardiol*;22:826-829

Feigenbaum, H. (1994) Echocardiographic evaluation of cardiac chambers, In: *Echocardiography*. 5th ed. Lippincott Williams & Wilkins. pp 134-180, ISBN 0-8121-1692-5 Philadelphia

Ferreira B, Matsika-Claquin MD, Hausse-Mocumbi AO, Sidi D, Paquet C. (2002) Origine geographique des cas de fibrose endomyocardique traitées a l'Hôpital Central de Maputo, entre 1987 et 1999 *Bull Soc Pathol Exot*, 95(4): 274-9.

Folger GM Jr, Hajar R, Robida A, Hajar HA. (1992) Occurrence of valvar heart disease in acute rheumatic fever without evident carditis: colour-flow Doppler identification. *Br Heart J*;67:434-439

George BO, Gaba FE, Talabi AI.(1982) M-mode echocardiographic features of endomyocardial fibrosis. *Br Heart J*.48(3):222-8.

Gonzalez-Lavin L, Friedman JP, Hecker SP, McFadden PM. Endomyocardial fibrosis: Diagnosis and treatment. Am Heart J 1982;105(4):699-705.

Gordis L. (1985) The virtual disappearance of rheumatic fever in the United States: lessons in the rise and fall of disease: T. Duckett Jones Memorial Lecture. *Circulation*;72:1155-62

Guyer De, Gillam LD, Foale RA, Clark MC, Dinsmore R, Palacios I, Block P, King ME, Weyman AE. (1984) Comparison of the echocardiographic and hemodynamic diagnosis of rheumatic tricuspid stenosis. *J Am Coll Cardiol* ;3(50):1135-44

Hassan W, Fawzy ME, Helaly SA, Hegazy H, Malik S. Pitfalls in Diagnosis and Clinical, Echocardiographic, and Hemodynamic Findings in Endomyocardial Fibrosis: a 25-year experience. Chest 2005;128:3985-92

Jaiyesimi F, Antia AU. (1981**a)** Congenital Heart Disease in Nigeria: a ten-year experience at UCH, Ibadan. *Ann Trop Paediatr*; 1;77-85

Jaiyesimi F, Antia AU. (1981**b)** Childhood rheumatic heart disease in Nigeria. *Trop Geogr Med*;33:8-13

Kamblock J, Payot L, Iung B, Costes P, Gillet T, Goanvic C, Lionet P, Pagis B, Pasche J, Roy C, Vahanian A, Papouin G. (2003) Does rheumatic myocarditis really exists?

Systematic study with echocardiography and cardiac troponin I blood levels. *Eur Heart J*;24:855-862

Kinsley RH, Girwood RW, Milner S.(1981) Surgical treatment during the acute phase of rheumatic carditis. In: Nyhus LM, ed *Surgery Annual*. East Norwalk, Conn: Appleton-Century-Crofts;13:299-323

Lowenthal MN, Teeger S. (2000) Endomyocardial fibrosis with pericardial effusion and endocardial calcification. *Isr Med Assoc J.*;2(3):249.

Mady C, Salemi VMC, Ianni BM, Arteaga E, Fernandes F, Ramires FJA. (2004) Quantitative Assessment of Left Ventricular Regional Wall Motion in Endomyocardial Fibrosis. *Arq Bras Cardiol*;84(3):241-244

Marcus RH, Sareli P, Pocock WA, Barlow JB. (1994) The spectrum of severe rheumatic mitral valve disease in a developing country: correlations among clinical presentation, survival pathological findings and hemodynamic sequelae. *Ann Intern Med*;120930;177-83

Marcus RH, Sareli P, Pocock WA, Meyer TE, Magalhaes MP, Grieve T, Antunes MJ, Barlow JB. (1989) Functional anatomy of severe mitral regurgitation in active rheumatic carditis. *Am J Cardiol*;63(9):577-584

Marijon E, Iung B, Mocumbi AO, Kamblock J, Thanh CV, Gamra H, Esteves C, Palacios IF, Vahanian A. (2008) What are the differences in presentation of candidates for mitral percutaneous commissurotomy across the world and do they influence the results of the procedure? *Arch Cardiovasc Dis*;101(10):611-7.

Marijon E, Ou P, Celermajer DS, Ferreira B, Mocumbi AO, Jani D, Paquet C, Jacob S, Sidi D, Jouven X. (2007) Prevalence of rheumatic heart disease detected by echocardiographic screening. *N Engl J Med*;357(5):470-476.

Mayosi B, Robertson K, Volmink J, Adebo W, Akinyore K, Amoah A, Bannerman C, Biesman-Simons S, Carapetis J, Cilliers A, Commerford P, Croasdale A, Damasceno A, Dean J, Dean M, de Souza R, Filipe A, Hugo-Hamman C, Jurgens-Clur SA, Kombila-Koumba P, Kotzenberg C, Lawrenson J, Manga P, Matenga J, Mathivha T, Mntla P, Mocumbi A, Mokone T, Ogola E, Omokhodion S, Palweni C, Pearce A, Salo A, Thomas B, Walker K, Wiysonge C, Zaher S. (2006) The Drakensberg declaration on the control of rheumatic fever and rheumatic heart disease in Africa. *S Afr Med J*; 96:246.

Meira Z, Goulart E, Mota C. (2006) Comparative Study of Clinical and Doppler Echocardiographic Evaluations of the Progression of Valve Diseases in Children and Adolescents with Rheumatic Fever. *Arq Bras Cardiol*;86 (1):32-8

Metras D, Ouezzin-Coulibaly A, Ouattara K, Bertrand E, Chauvet J. (1983) Endomyocardial fibrosis masquerading as rheumatic mitral incompetence. A report of six surgical cases. *J Thorac Cardiovasc Surg*;86(5):753-6.

Mocumbi AO, Carrilho C, Sarathchandra P, Ferreira MB, Yacoub MH, Burke M. (2010) Echocardiography accurately assesses the pathological abnormalities of chronic endomyocardial fibrosis. *Int J Cardiovasc Imaging*

Mocumbi AO, Ferreira MB, Sidi D, Yacoub MH. (2008) A population study of Endomyocardial Fibrosis in a rural area of Mozambique. *N Eng J Med*; 369:43-9.

Morrone LF, Moreira AE, Lopez M, Kajita LJ, Poterio DI, Arie S. (1996) Endomiocardiofibrose com Calcificação endocárdica maciça biventricular. *Arq Bras Cardiol*;67(2):103-5.

Naito M, Morganroth J, Mardelli TJ, Chen CC, Dreifus LS. (1980) Rheumatic mitral stenosis: cross-sectional echocardiographic analysis. *Am Heart J*;100(1): p. 34-40;

Namboodiri N, Remash K, Tharakan JA, Shajeem O, Nair K, Titus T, Ajitkumar VK, Sivasankaran S, Krishnamoorthy KM, Harikrishnan SP, Harikrishnan MS, Bijulal S. (2009) Natural history of aortic valve disease following intervention for rheumatic mitral valve disease. *J Heart Valve Dis*;18(1):61-7.

Narula J, Chandrasekar Y, Rahimtoola S. (1999) Diagnosis of active carditis: the echos of change. *Circulation*;100:1576-1581

Ogah OS, Adebanjo AT, Otukoya AS, Jagusa TJ. (2006) Echocardiography in Nigeria: use, problems, reproducibility and potentials. *Cardiovascular Ultrasound*; 4: 13 doi:10.1186/1476-7120-4-13

Okereke OUJ, Chikwendu VC, Ihenacho HNC, Ikeh VO. (1991) Non-invasive diagnosis of endomyocardial fibrosis in Nigeria using two-dimensional echocardiography. *Tropical Cardiology*;17(67):97-103

Okubo S, Nagata S, Masuda Y, Kawazoe K, Atobe M, Manabe H. (1984) Clinical features of rheumatic heart disease in Bangladesh. *Jpn Circ J*;48(12):1345-9

Paar JA, Berrios NM, Rose JD, Caceres M, Pena R, Perez W, Chen-Mok M, Jolles E, Dale JB. (2010) Prevalence of rheumatic heart disease in children and young adults in Nicaragua. *Am J Cardiol.*;2010: 105(12):1809-1814.

Prasad k, Radhakrishnan S. (1992) Echocardiographic variables affecting surgical outcome in patients undergoing closed mitral commissurotomy. *Int J Cardiol*;37(2): p. 237-42;

Rashwan MA, Ayman M, Ashour S, Hassanin MM, Zeina AA. (1995) Endomyocardial fibrosis in Egypt: an illustrated review. *Br Heart J*;73:284-9.

Reeves BM, Kado J, Brook M. (2011) High prevalence of rheumatic heart disease in Fiji detected by echocardiography screening. *Journal of Paediatrics and Child Health*: 47(7):473-8

Rizvi SF, Khan MA, Kundi A, Marsh DR, Samad A, Pasha O. (2004) Status of rheumatic heart disease in rural Pakistan. *Heart*;90:394-399

Sadiq M, Islam K, Abid R, Latif F, Rehman AU, Waheed A, Azhar M, Khan JS. (2009) Prevalence of rheumatic heart disease in school children of urban Lahore. *Heart*;95(5):353-357.

Shah S, Noble VE, Umulisa I, Dushimiyimana JMV, Bukhman G, Mukherjee J, Rich M, Epino H. (2008) Development of an ultrasound training curriculum in a limited resource international setting: successes and challenges of ultrasound training in rural Rwanda. *Int J Emerg Med*; 1:193-196

Shah SP, Epino H, Bukhman G, Umulisa I, Dushimiyimana JMV, Reichman A, Noble VE. (2009) Impact of the introduction of ultrasound services in a limited resource setting: rural Rwanda 2008. *BMC International Health and Human Rights*, 9:4

Sahsakul Y, Edwards WD, Naessens JM, Tajik AJ. (1988)Age-related changes in aortic and mitral valve thickness: implications for two-dimensional echocardiography based on an autopsy study of 200 normal human hearts. *Am J Cardiol*;62: 424-430

Salemi VMC, Rochitte CE, Barbosa MM, Mady C. (2005) Clinical and echocardiographic dissociation in a patient with right ventricular endomyocardial fibrosis. *Heart*;91(11):1399

Sani M, Mukhtar-Yola M, Karaye K, Karaye KM. Spectrum of congenital heart disease in a tropical environment: an echocardiographic study. Journal of the National Medical Association 2007;99(6):665-9

Saraiva LR, Carneiro RW, Arruda MB, Brindeiro Filho D, Lira V. (1999) Mitral valve disease with rheumatic appearance in the presence of left ventricular endomyocardial fibrosis. *Arq Bras Cardiol.*;72(3):327-32.

Sliwa K, Carrington M, Mayosi BM, Zigiriadis E, Mvungi R, Stewart S. (2010) Incidence and characteristics of newly diagnosed rheumatic heart disease in urban African adults: insights from the heart of Soweto study. *Eur Heart J*;31(6):719-27.

Somers K. (1990) Restrictive Cardiomyopathies. In Pediatric Cardiology. International Congress Series 906. Pongpanich B, Sueblinvong V, Vongprateep C (eds). Excerpta Medica, Amsterdam.

Steer AC, Kado J, Wilson N, Tuiketei T, Batzloff M, Waqatakirewa L, Mulholland EK, Carapetis JR. (2009) High prevalence of rheumatic heart disease by clinical and echocardiographic screening among children in Fiji. *Journal of Heart Valve Disease*;18(3):327-335; discussion 336.

Thakur JS, Negi PC, Ahluwalia SK, Vaidya NK. (1996) Epidemiological survey of rheumatic heart disease among school children in the Shimla Hills of northern India: prevalence and risk factors. *Journal of Epidemiology & Community Health*;50(1):62-67.

Trigo J, Camacho A, Gago P, Candeias R, Santos W, Marques N, Matos P, Brandão V, Gomes V. (2010) Fibrose endomiocárdica com calcificação maçica do ventrículo esquerdo. *Rev Port Cardiol*;29(0):445-449

Vaidyanathan K, Agarwal R, Sahayaraj A, Sankar M, Cherian KM. (2009) Endomyocardial fibrosis mimicking Ebstein's anomaly. *Tex Heart Inst J*;36(3):250-1

Van der Bel-Kahn J, Becker AE.(198) The surgical pathology of rheumatic and floppy mitral valves. Distinctive morphologic features upon gross examination. *Am J Surg Path*;10(4):282-292

Vansan R, Shrisvastava S, Vijayakumar M, Narang R, Lister B, Narula J. (1996) Echocardiographic evaluation of patients with acute rheumatic fever and rheumatic carditis. *Circulation*;94:73-82

Vijayalakshmi IB, Vishnuprabhu RO, Chitra N, Rajasri R, Anuradha TV. (2008) The efficacy of echocardiographic criterions for the diagnosis of carditis in acute rheumatic fever. *Cardiol Young*;18(6):586-92.

Vijayaraghavan G, Davies J, Sadanandan S, Spry CJF, Gibson DG, Goodwin JF. (1983) Echocardiographic features of tropical endomyocardial disease in South India. *Br Heart J*;50:450-9

WHO Report of the Regional Committee of Africa 2005. (2005) Available at: http://www.afro.who.int/rc55/documents/afr_rc55_12_cardiovascular.pdf.

Wilkins G, Weyman A Abascal V, Block P, Palacios I. (1988) Percutaneous ballon dilatation of the mitral valve: an analysis of echocardiographic variables related to outcome and the mechanisms of dilatation. *Br Heart J*;60:299-308.

www.world-heart-federation.org

Yuko-Jowi C, Bakari M. (2005) Echocardiographic patterns of juvenile rheumatic heart disease at Kenyatta National Hospital, Nairobi. *East Afr Med J*;82(10):514-9

Zhimin W, Yubao Z, Lei S, Xianliang Z, Wei Z, Li S, Hao W, Jianjun L, Detrano R, Rutai H. (2006) Prevalence of chronic rheumatic heart disease in Chinese adults. *Int J Cardiol*;107(3):356-359.

22

Psychophysiological Cardiovascular Functioning in Hostile Defensive Women

Francisco Palmero and Cristina Guerrero
Universitat Jaume I
Spain

1. Introduction

Cardiovascular diseases are the leading causes of death and disability in the world, in both developed and developing countries, and also in both sexes. In fact one third of annual deaths worldwide are due to cardiovascular problems, according to the WHO (World Health Organization) estimated 17.3 million people died from CVDs in 2008, over 80% of CVD deaths take place in low- and middle-income countries, and by 2030, almost 23.6 million people will die from CVDs (in http://www.who.int/cardiovascular_diseases). Therefore, is a serious problem, and not only in industrialized countries, indeed, is an epidemic that not only continues but it is precisely in the developing countries, where it currently is increasing dramatically. On the other hand, prevalence and mortality from these diseases among *women* has increased in an exaggerated way. This for several reasons: first, as mentioned, in women the death rate from CVDs has increased significantly, equaling or exceeding that of the male population, so we think it is of great importance to focus on studies considering this sector only a few risk factors have also increased; second, the sample with which we had consisted mostly of women, given the characteristics of it (psychology undergraduates), which were removed the few men who participated in the study. Thus, from these data and indications, and since most studies have focused on people of both sexes or only male, we considered appropriate to carry out research with a sample of only women.

Moreover the etiology of CVD is multidimensional, that is, factors involving genetic, physiological, chemical, nutritional, environmental and psychosocial, and moreover, is not fully known. It is known that a number of cardiovascular risk factors that may contribute to the development, progression or maintenance of CVD, called "classic risk factors". Among the most important are: age, sex, cholesterol, hypertension, smoking, physical inactivity and obesity. However, surprisingly, these factors fail to explain more than 50% of the variance in predicting cardiovascular risk, whether considered independently or when considered together (Chesney, 1996; Gump & Matthews, 1999). Nevertheless a large proportion of CVDs are preventable, but they continue to increase mainly because preventive measures are inadequate.

Therefore, research about this topic has been long and extensive, especially directed to seek and discover other factors, beyond the "classics", are also contributing to the development

CVD (Brydon et al., 2010; Chida & Steptoe, 2009; Everson-Rose & Lewis, 2005; Jorgensen & Kolodziej, 2007; Vella & Friedman, 2009). We refer to *psychosocial factors*. Thus, the relationship between different psychosocial variables and the risk of CVD has been studied extensively since the mid past century, mainly for these two reasons.

2. Psychosocial risk factors and cardiovascular disease

In the search and exploration for other risk factors that may explain the etiology of CVD, psychosocial factors have gained importance to such an extent that research has been able to explain the mechanisms of action of these variables on CVD. The results obtained in various research studies have confirmed the relationship between psychosocial factors and the atheromatous plaque, which constitutes the basic injury occurring in CVD (Kaplan, et al, 1983; Kaplan, et al, 1987; Manuck, et al, 1983; Manuck, Kaplan & Matthews, 1986; Manuck, et al, 1989; Jennings, et al, 2004; Vale, 2005). The mechanisms involved in its formation, which are mechanical and chemical factors are seriously affected by psychosocial processes, and especially by the stress response. In these processes, emotions cause a faster heart rate and higher blood pressure, leading to increased blood flow and turbulence. In addition, there is a mobilization of lipids which exceeds the body's metabolic requirements, and which facilitates aggregation to artery walls and heart tissue. This relationship between psychosocial factors and CVD has received the generic name of "Hypothesis of the cardiovascular reactivity", and has been supported by various prospective studies (Keys & Taylor, 1971; Schiffer, et al, 1976; Manuck, et al, 1992; Steptoe, et al, 2000).

To date, research has shown that individuals who tend to display strong responses and reactivity are at increased risk of CVD (Manuck et al., 1992; Palmero et al., 2006; Treiber, et al, 2003; Matthews, et al, 2006). The argument that defends this refers to the stereotype response: if the cardiovascular reactivity is a characteristic of an individual and is physiological stable and consistent, then the same response patterns will be seen every time the individual is faced with a situation of stress. Evidently with certain limitations, laboratory situations can be regarded as a procedure that provides information on an individual's physiological functioning in real life (Allen, et al, 1987; Allen & Matthews, 1997; Palmero, et al, 2002; Moseley & Linden, 2006; Palmero, et al, 2007). Thus individuals, whose pattern of cardiovascular functioning is characterized by the expression of exaggerated responses, are those who, with time, are likely to experience some cardiovascular dysfunction (Everson, et al, 1996; Markovitz, et al, 1998; Strike, et al, 2003). Given this relationship between excessive cardiovascular response and CVD, research efforts have focused on finding any variable causing an increase in such responses as this will mean an increase in the likelihood of suffering from one of these diseases.

From the study on the classic Type A behavior pattern through the anger-hostility complex and hostility were conducted, in recent years, research has focused on the *defensive hostility* (high hostility and high defensiveness) as a risk factor in CVD (Guerrero & Palmero, 2010; Helmers & Krantz, 1996; Jamner, et al, 1991; Larson & Langer, 1997; Shapiro, et al, 1995; Palmero, et al, 2007; Vella & Friedman, 2007). The trait of defensive hostility reflects an approach–avoid conflict between the desire for social approval and distrust of those who can provide such support, and currently can be considered as one of the psychosocial factors with more weight and empirical support in its relationship with CVD.

Several studies of CVD patients demonstrate that subjects with high scores in defensive hostility show higher rates of ischemia during a mental stress situation, greater damage by infusion and a longer duration of ischemia during daily activities (Helmers, et al, 1995). As well, a field study conducted with paramedics showed a higher cardiac response by people with a high hostility defensive when they deal with stress situations (Jamner, et al, 1991). These results, usually obtained from real situations, appear to be supported by laboratory studies (Jorgensen, et al, 1995; Shapiro, et al, 1995; Helmers & Krantz, 1996; Larson & Langer, 1997; Palmero et al., 2002; Palmero et al., 2007), which indicates the existence of a subgroup of people who are characterized by high "Defensive Hostility" (DH), as well as a greater cardiovascular response. In general, DH individuals show greater cardiovascular response during the task phase that other groups can be formed when combining hostility and defensiveness variables (Larson & Langer, 1997). And, unlike this group, find another subgroup which is characterized by low hostility and low defensiveness and show a lower cardiovascular response -low risk group-.

However as these studies show, various inconsistencies were also found, which originated, at least in part, from the different tasks used to measure the cardiovascular variables. These results suggest the relevance of broadening the research spectrum whose aim it is to strengthen the association between psychological variables and cardiovascular response from the understanding that the exaggerated response would be the link between these and CVD. In other words, it seems appropriate to establish whether defensive hostility can be seen as the toxic component in relation to CVD.

Therefore, the *general objective* pursued with this study refers to the delimitation of the effects of defensive hostility on cardiovascular response in women, in a real stress situation. Specifically, exploring the relationship between defensive hostility, which is a better predictor than hostility alone, and cardiovascular responses (HR, SBP and DBP) in this tonic dimension. That is, considering all three phases of the experiment (adaptation: A, task: T and recovery: R) to establish the significance of the functional psychophysiological profiles in the four experimental groups (DH: high hostility-high defensiveness, HH: high hostility-low defensiveness, Def: low hostility-high defensiveness, LH: low hostility-low defensiveness).

From these premises and the proposed main objective has been carried out this research with the ultimate aim to contribute both to the development of the theoretical basis on psychosocial variables that can be considered as cardiovascular risk factors and its subsequent application in clinical practice as well as contribute to methodological development in the field of psychophysiological research.

The *general hypothesis* suggests that individuals with high scores in defensive hostility display the highest values with the psychophysiological variables. Specifically, we expect that these individuals show the greatest average values recorded in the variables (HR, SBP and DBP), and in all the phases of the experiment (A, T and R), compared to those shown by the individuals of the other three groups. In addition, DH group will be characterized by less adaptive psychophysiological profile.

3. Empirical study

3.1 Study design

In this section we show data from a recent study published by the authors (Guerrero and Palmero, 2010). One hundred and thirty female students from a *Universitat Jaume I* participated in this research. The mean age of the participants was 20.34 years (*SD*=2.06). The criteria to form the groups were the scores obtained with both the Ho Inventory (Cook & Medley, 1954) and the Social Desirability Questionnaire (Crowne & Marlowe, 1960). We used the median as the cut-off point to classify participants as "high" or "low" in each variable, thus the sample was composed as follows: 30 Defensive Hostility (DH), 40 High Hostility (HH), 42 Defensive (Def), and 18 Low Hostility (LH).

3.2 Instrumentation

Cardiovascular responses were measured with the registration system Biopac MP150 with NIBP module 100A, both were connected to a personal computer to monitor and store all the responses. Specifically, this registration system was used to measure the physiological responses: heart rate, systolic blood pressure and diastolic blood pressure. Also, this system recorded these cardiovascular parameters continuously and noninvasively.

Hostility was measured with the Hostility Inventory of Cook and Medley (1954), specifically the Composite Hostility Score (Chost) consisting in three subscales: cynicism, hostile feelings and aggressive responses. In previous studies, this information led to a scale being provided with a greater ability to predict the response and cardiovascular reactivity in comparison with the Ho scale provided as a whole (Barefoot et al., 1989; Christensen & Smith, 1993; Guerrero, 2008).

Defensiveness was measured with the Spanish version (Ávila & Tomé, 1989) of the Social Desirability Questionnaire of Crowne and Marlowe (1960). It consists of 33 items of choice alternatives (true or false) that reflect socially desirable behaviors and cognitions.

Also, reports and self-reports were also used to collect some data on behavioral habits related to health issues, and various personal and socio-demographic data.

3.3 Study procedure

A real academic exam was used as a situation of stress. More specifically, we used an exam of the degree of Psychology; this situation represents a real mental stress task for students.

Data were collected individually in one session. Following informed consent, each subject completed a questionnaire of demographics, previous medical history and noted any medication. Then, they went into the experimental cabin where they were asked to sit comfortably in an armchair and a sensor was connected to their non dominant wrist. From this time onward, both instructions and exam questions were submitted through the projector.

Following this registration session, it was necessary to remove the sensors and to go to another room to complete the corresponding scales. Finally, they were thanked for their collaboration and left.

The recording session consisted in three phases: adaptation (A), task (T) and recovery (R), with duration of 10, 20 and 10 minutes, respectively.

a. *Adaptation phase* (10 min): there was no stimulus. The purpose of this period was for participants to become familiar with the environment. The psychophysiological variables were recorded in their tonic dimension to establish baseline levels with the aim of obtaining the participants' usual levels under rest conditions.
b. *Task phase* (20 min): the 20 stimuli that formed the experimental task were presented: an objective test of 20 questions with four alternative answers. The stimuli were separated by a one-minute period, and the duration of this phase was therefore 20 minutes. This phase was considered an overall stressful period, and its variables were recorded in their phasic dimension.
c. *Recovery phase* (10 min): no stimulus was presented. The variables were considered in their tonic dimension to see how these variables recovered their usual levels after the stress situation. These data allow us to ascertain how long the organism needs to achieve its usual values following a situation of stress. This is extremely relevant when considering the consequences caused by the stress situation from a neuroendocrinological viewpoint because the greater the time needed by the organism to recover its baseline levels, the greater the exposure to the effects of substances released by the organism because of this situation of stress (catecolamnines and cortisol).

3.4 Statistical analysis

The first approaches were the descriptive analysis and correlations, and an analysis of variance (ANOVA) was carried out for a more detailed analysis of the results. Then, according to the main objective, that of analyzing the relationship between defensive hostility and the cardiovascular responses to study the functional significance of each group's profiles during all three phases, namely in their tonic dimension, an ANOVA was carried out whose design was 4 groups (DH, HH, LH and Def) x 3 phases (adaptation, task and recovery) with repeated measures for the phase variable. Subsequently, a univariate analysis of variance has been conducted for each phase to obtain a more accurate description of the potential differences encountered should such differences be given from the post hoc Tukey test with which the groups involved in them will be determined.

3.5 Study results

Data will be presented in the following figures, which reflect the psychophysiological profiles obtained from analysis of data for each physiological variable separately.

Although, before that, we like to refer to the profiles described by Kelsey (1993) on which we relied. There are different ways to respond physiologically to stressful events, which depends on external factors (situational) and internal factors (personality variables). In this regard, and from the classic proposal Kelsey, we noted three response patterns, which reflect corresponding profiles associated with different forms of reaction to stressful events: *habituation, sensitization* and support or *constant*.

- Habituation.

When you perceive a situation as potentially threatening or novel, occurs an increase in cardiovascular reactivity. After an exposure time in such a situation, and after that initial increase, there is a phenomenon of habituation, during which we see a progressive decrease of the initial values. This phenomenon is considered essential in the process of adaptation and regulation of humans and lower animals, demonstrating the ability to self-regulatory organism, that is, it can be activate to deal with a potentially dangerous or threatening situation and, in turn, is able to return to baseline (BL) once the situation has gone or is under control.

- Sensitization.

In this case, the individual responds to an agent or stressor stimulus with a high cardiovascular reactivity (the phenomenon of sensitization), similar to the previous pattern but without habituation occur. Instead, it produces a progressive increase in reactivity over the situation. It shows a organism's inability to return to baseline, which is highly detrimental to the heart muscle and overall health.

- Constant.

In this third pattern occurs an initial increase, similar to that of the other two patterns, but no habituation or sensitization occurs. This increase remains constant throughout the stress. Thus, this pattern is also maladaptive; since there is no preparation behavior is essential in the adaptation to the environment (Cannon, 1932) or has the ability to return to baseline levels.

From these profiles is observed that only the first is adaptive, decreasing when the individual cardiovascular reactivity to stressful events faced long periods of time. On the one hand, the initial increase in activation allows for better coping with the situation and the subsequent decline after a period of time, it is necessary to avoid damaging the body and maintain homeostasis (Palmero, Breva, et al., 1994; Palmero, Espinosa et al., 1995).

Concerning *heart rate* in Figure 1 shows the obtained profiles by different groups.

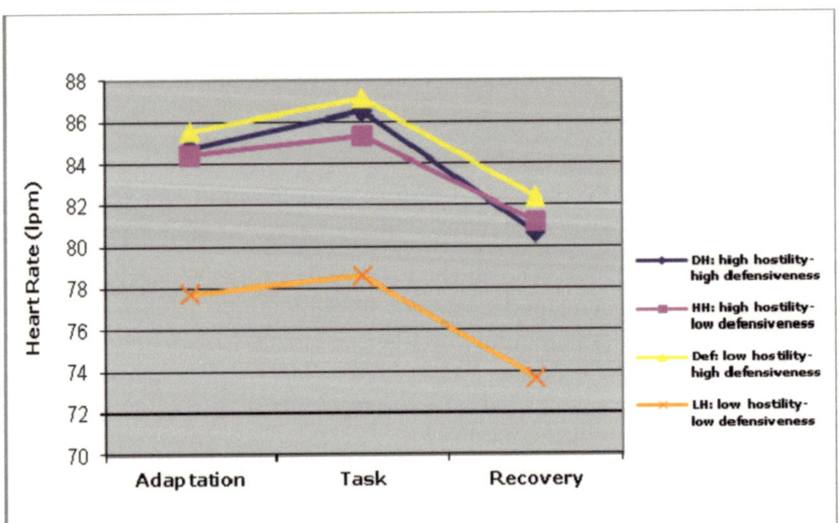

Fig. 1. Heart rate and defensive hostility during three phases.

As for the functional significance of the various profiles, as seen in Figure 1, all groups show the habituation trend, so profiles are adaptive. Although, LH group shows the more adaptive pattern, as it presents a greater and faster recovery to their baseline levels.

Concerning to *systolic blood pressure* as seen in Figure 2, all groups show the habituation trend. Again, LH group presents a more adaptive pattern, with lower values in the recovery phase.

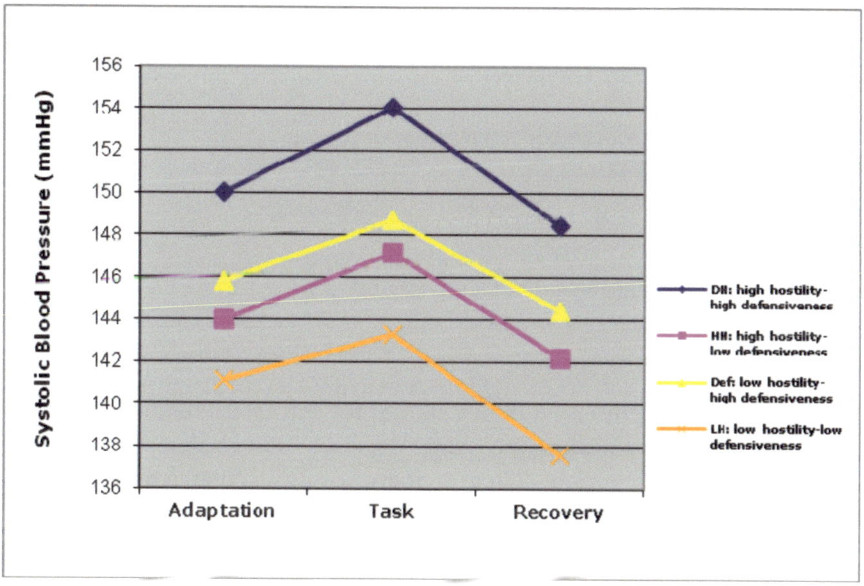

Fig. 2. Systolic blood pressure and defensive hostility during three phases.

Here we also find that DH is the group that obtained the greatest values in systolic pressure in all three phases.

An additional interesting fact is the effect of variable defensiveness, although the difference was not statistically significant, we see that the two groups with high defensiveness, DH and Def, presented the higher SBP values in all three phases (A, T and R)

Concerning *diastolic blood* pressure as seen in Figure 3, all groups show the habituation trend, and again LH group presents a more adaptive pattern.

Again, we see that DH is the group that shows the highest values in all three phases. In this case also notes the effect of variable defensiveness, although neither are statistically significant differences. Two groups with high defensiveness, DH and Def, presented the higher DBP values, but only in adaptation and task phases.

Figure 2 and 3 demonstrate clear differences between SBP and DBP between the psychophysiological patters of extreme groups: DH presents higher values than LH group. And the other two groups are in an intermediate position, with values very similar among them and throughout the three phases.

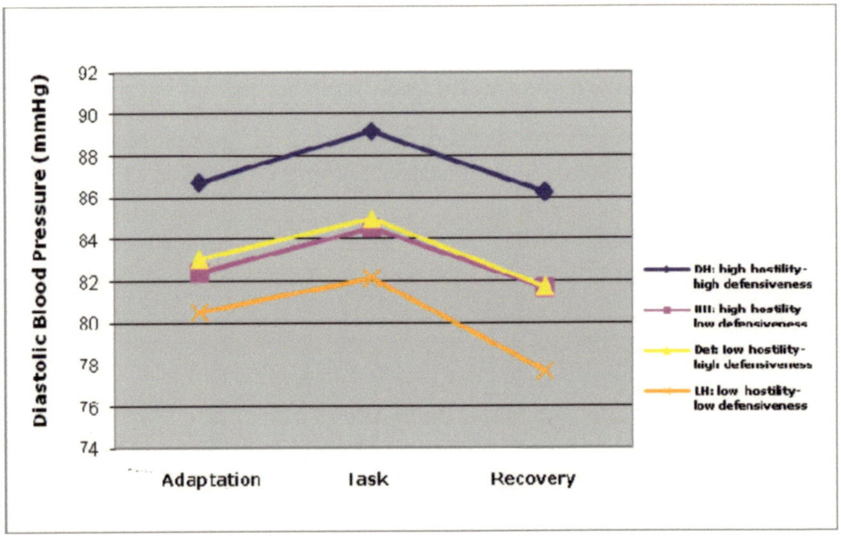

Fig. 3. Diastolic blood pressure and defensive hostility during three phases.

4. Conclusion

In general, the DH group presented higher values for the cardiovascular variables during the three phases, as well as a slow recovery. Thus, we believe that *defensive hostility* has proved to be a more appropriate criterion than hostility alone when determining the possible risk of cardiovascular dysfunction.

So, consistent with our main objective, and in relation to establishing the functional significance of the general profiles in the four groups through considering the three experiment phases, our results are in the expected direction. Specifically, the DH group obtains the highest values in the three phases and variables, particularly in the blood pressure index. Additionally, extending the findings available to therefore include the recovery phase, we have found that this group of individuals takes longer to recover after a stress situation, that is, they score the highest values encountered during the recovery phase.

About the *cardiovascular parameters*, the three most commonly used in these studies were HR, SBP and DBP (Swain & Suls, 1996), to combine the criteria and to enhance the comparison between different results from various research studies. All the parameters have been captured, recorded, stored and analyzed in a highly reliable, non invasive and continuous manner, which is especially relevant in the case of blood pressure. They are easily accessible and provide us with highly reliable information on cardiac and vascular functioning over different time periods, that is, to reflect the changing psychophysiology profile of individuals at all times.

Among these parameters, we note blood pressure reflects the greatest differences between the two extreme groups (DH and LH): introducing a greater response, activation and recovery for the DH group. On the other hand, HR reveals a clear difference in the lowest values submitted by the low-risk group (LH) compared to a more homogeneous response from the other three groups in all the phases. So, we suggest that the cardiovascular functioning of hostile defensive individuals in such situations is best reflected through blood pressure, specifically through diastolic pressure, an index which seems to appear truer for the recovery phase, as reflected by the significant differences found between the two extreme groups.

More specifically, showing each cardiovascular physiological variable separately, the following was observed.

Regarding the *HR*, although there is no effect of interaction between hostility and defensiveness, since the group HD presents values very similar to those groups HH and Def, HR shows how the low-risk group, LH , presents the lowest values along the three phases compared to the other groups.

We must also emphasize for the three groups with higher levels in HR, which is the group Def -although differences are not statistically significant- which presents the highest levels in all three phases, reflecting a major effect of the variable defensiveness, specifically in the adaptation and task phases where groups with high defensiveness (DH and Def) show the highest levels.

Our data also specifies that it is in the recovery phase where there are statistically significant differences between the Def group and the LH group.

Regarding the *SBP*, beside show the effect of interaction between hostility and defensiveness, a fact that reflects the important values of the DH group, the main effect of the defensiveness variable also exist in three phases, which means that subjects with high scores in defensiveness obtain higher values than subjects with low scores in defensiveness.

In addition, our data indicate that statistically significant differences that exist between DH and LH groups are specifically at the task and the recovery phases, in turn, indicates that there are no differences between groups with respect to their baseline levels.

The fact that the DH group presents higher scores for these values, leads us to suggest that defensive hostility rather than hostility alone better predicts the cardiovascular function in situations of stress.

Regarding the *DBP*, it seems that the real meaning of this variable can be seen only with the consideration of defensive hostility, such as denoting the effects of interaction in all three phases. Like the previous case, our data indicate that statistically significant differences also exist between DH and Def groups, but in this case appear in the recovery phase. There was also a main effect of the defensiveness variable, but is almost imperceptible.

Regarding the *functionality of the profiles* all four groups in three variables were adaptive. But in blood pressure case, it seems interesting to note that while the four groups that tend to indicate profiles of habituation, the fact that the individuals' defensive hostile obtains these statistically significant values during the recovery phase means that this group of individuals takes significantly longer to return to the baseline values of situations without stress. Thus, the profile of hostile defensive subjects would be less adaptive, because in this group the recovery is more slow and gradual. The profiles of the three remaining groups are adaptive, with a faster recovery.

Specifically, in our view, while DBP continues the pattern of other variables during the task, and displays an interaction effect between hostility and defensiveness, it is the most important variable to detect the cardiovascular functioning of hostile defensive individuals in the recovery phase. Once again, these arguments lead us to suggest that it is desirable to consider this variable, along with the inclusion of the recovery phase.

In short, along with the results corresponding to the tonic dimension of the cardiovascular variables being studied, it appears that *defensive hostility* is more appropriate than hostility alone to understand cardiovascular functioning in stressful situations. So, defensive hostility identifies a dimension of personality that, ultimately, would be a better predictor of the cardiovascular response in particular and of cardiovascular disease in general. It would be more fitting than hostility alone to explain and understand cardiovascular functioning in stressful situations.

The DH group, which shows that those individuals with high scores in hostility and high scores in defensiveness, are those who reflect the highest values in activation and cardiovascular response, but only when faced with the demands of a challenging task. For this reason, and as we have pointed out, it seems appropriate to use a real situation of stress as an experimental task because this specific environment is the best scenario to see the psychophysiological response style that characterizes the individuals being studied. In addition, if the situation of stress is sufficiently long, there is also the possibility of locating the adjustment mechanism of individuals to the sustained demands of this stressful activity. Those hostile individuals seeking to perform an action that is not disagreeable to others display the greatest difficulty in controlling their hostile experiences. The result of this inability to properly monitor hostility experiences produces a sustained increase in the activation of the sympathetic system which, in turn, gives rise to significant increases in the cardiovascular variables studied: HR, SBP and DBP. One particular sensitivity of the SBP is to capture this sympathetic activation which suggests its suitability differential in such studies.

Thus, these findings show the relationship between defensive hostility and cardiovascular functioning in situations of stress by the various cardiovascular register indexes (HR, SBP and DBP) and by considering the various parameters analyzed, namely response, activation and cardiovascular recovery, have been demonstrated. As mentioned above, we believe that defensive hostility has proved to be a more appropriate criterion than hostility alone when determining the possible risk of cardiovascular dysfunction.

Regarding the three *experimental phases*, we can state the following. About the *recovery phase*, we think that its inclusion in the experimental research laboratory is especially important since it provides vital information on restoring physiological parameters. This phase is a basic and essential element in the detection of the possible risks of future dysfunctions (Guerrero & Palmero, 2006). As seen, the recovery phase profile in the DH group has shown a slower recovery, especially in terms of blood pressure, and more specifically in DBP. Thus, the inclusion of the recovery phase in this type of experimental laboratory, it constitutes a basic and essential element in the detection of possible risks of future dysfunctions. From a neuroendocrinological viewpoint, it is important to consider the consequences caused by the situation since the more time the organism needs to recover the baseline levels, the greater the exposure to the effects of the substances released (catecholamines and cortisol).

About the *task phase*, by considering the *duration* parameter, which is scarcely taken into account in such research, we believe it appropriate to propose an experimental task that is long enough to establish a genuine cardiovascular functioning, that is more likely to be correct, by appreciating how the adjustment to a stressful situation is produced, or not. The fact that short or moderately long tasks have been systematically used may have masked the dysfunctional connotations of the response profiles in the different groups.

Regarding the *tasks* used as a stressful situation in the laboratory, the importance of creating and using a type of task that involves a real stress situation must be highlighted, that is, one as close as possible to everyday situations. Thus, one can understand some of the inconsistencies found which, in turn, provide the ecological laboratory experiments in this field with more validity. In this respect, we believe that the task used in this research, a real exam, is a task with connotations of personal and social threats, which also requires investing considerable effort to be able to deal with it actively and successfully, and this has been reflected by the significant differences obtained in the three experiment phases.

Concluding, in our modest opinion, with this and other research we have conducted we provide more empirical support about the great relevance within the theoretical framework on DH as a possible psychosocial cardiovascular risk factor also in women. However, as a future research direction, probable variability among females as compared to males necessitates concentrated research in this area, and we recognize the need for separate data analysis for males. Also, the study should be replicate with other samples to see if there are similar results and generalize these obtained data.

5. References

Allen, M.T. & Matthews, K.A. (1997). Hemodynamic responses to laboratory stressors in children and adolescents: The influences of age, race, and gender. *Psychophysiology, 34*, 329-339.

Allen, M.T., Sherwood, A., Obrist, P.A., Crowell, M.D., & Grange, L.A. (1987). Stability of cardiovascular reactivity to laboratory stressors: A 2 ½ year follow-up. *Journal of Psychosomatic Research, 31*, 639-645.

Brydon L., Strike P.C., Bhattacharyya M.R., Whitehead D.L., McEwan J., Zachary I., and Steptoe A. (2010). Hostility and physiological responses to laboratory stress in acute coronary syndrome patients. *J Psychosom Res*, 68 (2), 109-116.

Cannon, W.B. (1932). *The wisdom of the body*. New York: Norton.

Chida Y. and Steptoe A. (2009). The Association of Anger and Hostility with Future Coronary Heart Disease. A Meta Analytic Review of Prospective Evidence. *J Am Coll Cardiol*, 53 (11), 936-946.

Cook, W.W. & Medley, D.M. (1954). Proposed hostility and pharisaic-virtue scales for the MMPI. *Journal of Applied Psychology, 38*, 414-418.

Crowne, D. P. & Marlowe, D. (1960). A new scale of social desirability independent of psychopathology. *Journal of Consulting Psychology, 24* (4), 349-354.

Chesney, M.A. (1996). New behavioral risk factors for coronary heart disease: Implications for intervention. In K. Orth-Gomer y N. Schneiderman (eds.): *Behavioral Medicine Approaches to Cardiovascular Disease Prevention* (pp. 169-182). Mahwah, NJ: Erlbaum.

Everson, S.A., Kaplan, G.A., Goldberg, D.E., & Salonen, J.T. (1996). Anticipatory blood pressure response to exercise predicts future high blood pressure in middle-aged men. *Hypertension, 27,* 1059-1064.

Everson-Rose, S.A.; Lewis, T.T. (2005). Psychosocial factors and cardiovascular diseases. *Annual Review of Public Health, 26,* 469-500.

Guerrero, C., and Palmero, F. (2006). Percepción de control y respuestas cardiovasculares. *International Journal of Cliniccal and Health Psychology, 6* (1), 145-168.

Guerrero, C. (2008). Metodología en psicofisiología cardiovascular: procedimiento alternativo para la medición de la reactividad y su relación con la hostilidad defensiva. Tesis doctoral publicada. Universitat Jaume I, Castellón. En http://www.tesisenxarxa.net/TDX- 0206108-131614/index.html.

Guerrero, C., and Palmero, F. (2010). Impact of defensive hostility in cardiovascular disease. *Behavioral Medicine, 36* (3), 77-84.

Gump, B.B. &Matthews, K.A. (1999). Do background stressors influence reactivity to and recovery from acute stressors? *Journal of Applied Social Psychology, 29,* 469-494.

Helmers, K. F., Krantz, D. S., Merz, C. N. B., Klein, J., Kop, W. J., Gottdiener, J.S., & Rozanzki, A. (1995). Defensive hostility: Relationship to multiple markers of cardiac ischemia in patients with coronary disease. *Health Psychology, 14,* 202-209.

Helmers, K.F. & Krantz, D.S. (1996). Defensive hostility, gender and cardiovascular levels and responses to stress. *Annals of Behavioral Medicine, 18,* 246-254.

Jamner, L.D., Shapiro, D. Goldstein, I.B., & Hug, R. (1991). Ambulatory blood pressure and heart rate in paramedics: Effects of cynical hostility and defensiveness. *Psychosomatic Medicine, 51,* 285-289.

Jennings, J.R., Kamarck, T.W., Everson-Rose, S.A., Kaplan, G.A., Manuck, S.B., & Salonen, J.T. (2004). Exaggerated blood pressure responses during mental stress are prospectively related to enhanced carotid atherosclerosis in middle-aged Finnish men. *Circulation, 110*: 2198–2203.

Jorgensen, R.S.; Abdul-Karim, K.; Kahan, T.A., & Frankowsi, J.J. (1995). Defensiveness, cynical hostility and cardiovascular reactivity: A moderator analysis. *Psychotherapy and Psychosomatics, 64(3-4),* 156-161.

Jorgensen, R.S., and Kolodziej, M.E. (2007). Suppressed anger, evaluative threat, and cardiovascular reactivity: a tripartite profile approach. *International Journal of Psychophysiology,* 66(2), 102-8.

Kaplan, J.R., Manuck, S.B., Adams, M.R., Weingand, K.W., & Clarkson, T. B. (1987). Inhibition of coronary atherosclerosis by propanolol in behaviorally predisposed monkeys fed an atherogenic diet. *Circulation, 76,* 1364-1372.

Kaplan, J.R., Manuck, S.B., Clarkson, T.B., Lusso, F.M., Taub, D.M., & Miller, E.W. (1983). Social stress and atherosclerosis in normocholesterolemic monkeys. *Science, 220,* 733-735.

Keys, A. & Taylor, H.L. (1971). Mortality and coronary heart disease among men studied for 23 years. *Archives of Internal Medicine, 128,* 201-214.

Larson, MR. & Langer, AW. (1997). Defensive hostility and anger expression: relationship to additional heart rate reactivity during active coping. *Psychophysiology, 34,* 177-184.

Manuck, S.B., Kaplan, J.R., & Clarkson, T.B. (1983). Behaviorally induced heart rate reactivity and atherosclerosis in cynomolgus monkeys. *Psychosomatic Medicine, 45,* 95-108.

Manuck, S.B., Kaplan, J.R., & Matthews, K.A. (1986). Behavioral antecedents of coronary heart disease and atherosclerosis. *Arteriosclerosis, 7,* 485-491.

Manuck, S.B., Kaplan, J.R., Adams, M.R., & Clarkson, T.B. (1989). Behavioral elicited heart rate reactivity and atherosclerosis in female cynomolgus monkeys. *Psychosomatic Medicine, 51,* 306-318.

Manuck, S.B., Olsson, G., Hjemdahl, P., & Rehnqvist, N. (1992). Does cardiovascular reactivity to mental stress have prognostic value in postinfarction patients? A pilot study. *Psychosomatic Medicine, 54,* 102-108.

Markovitz, J.H., Raczynski, J.M., Wallace, D., Chettur, V., & Chesney, M.A. (1998). Cardiovascular reactivity to video game predicts subsequent blood pressure increases in young men: The CARDIA study. *Psychosomatic Medicine, 60,* 186-191.

Matthews, K.A., Zhu, S., Tucker, D.C, & Whooley, M.A. (2006). Blood pressure reactivity to psychological stress and coronary calcification in the coronary artery risk development in young adults study. *Hypertension, 47*(3): 391-395.

Mente, A. & Helmers, K.F. (1999). Defensive hostility and cardiovascular response to stress in young men. *Personality and Individual Differences, 27(4),* 683-694.

Moseley, J.V. & Linden, W. (2006). Predicting blood pressure and heart rate change with cardiovascular reactivity and recovery: results from 3-year and 10-year follow up. *Psychosomatic Medicine, 68*: 833-843.

Palmero, F., Guerrero, C., Gómez, C. y Carpi, A. (2006). Certezas y controversias en el estudio de la emoción. *Revista Electrónica de Motivación y Emoción, 9,* 23-24. *Psychosomatic Medicine, 68*: 833-843.

Palmero, F., Breva, A. & Landeta, O. (2002). Hostilidad defensiva y reactividad cardiovascular en una situación de estrés real. *Ansiedad y Estrés, 8*(2-3), 115-142.

Palmero, F., Iñiguez, C., Guerrero, C., Carpi, A., Díez, J.L. & Diago, J.L. (2007). Hostilidad, psicofisiología y salud cardiovascular. *Avances de Psicología Latinoamérica. Colombia, 25* (1), 22-43.

Schiffer, F., Hartley, L.H., Schulman, C.L., & Abelmann, W.H. (1976). The quiz electrocardiogram: A new diagnostic and research technique for evaluating the relation between emotional stress and ischemic heart disease. *American Journal of Cardiology, 37,* 41-47.

Shapiro, D., Goldstein, I.B., & Jamner, L.D. (1995). Effects of anger/hostility, defensiveness, gender, and family history of hypertension on cardiovascular reactivity. *Psychophysiology, 32,* 425-435.

Steptoe, A., Cropley, M., & Jockes, K. (2000). Task demands and the pressures of everyday life: Associations between cardiovascular reactivity and work blood pressure and heart rate. *Health Psychology, 19,* 46-54.

Strike, P.C., Magid, K., Brydon L., Edwards, S., McEwan, J.R., & Steptoe, A. (2003). Exaggerated platelet and hemodynamic reactivity to mental stress in men with coronary artery disease. *Psychosomatic Medicine, 66*: 492–500.

Swain, A., & Suls, J. (1996). Reproducibility of blood pressure and heart rate reactivity: A meta-analysis. *Psychophysiology, 33,* 162-174.

Treiber, F.A., Kamarck, T., Schneiderman, N., Sheffield, D., Kapuku, G, & Taylor, T. (2003). Cardiovascular Reactivity and Development of Preclinical and Clinical Disease States. *Psychosomatic Medicine, 65,* 46-62.

Vale, S. (2005). Psychosocial stress and cardiovascular diseases. *Postgraduate Medical Journal, 81,* 429-435.

Vella, E.J. (2003). *Autonomic Characteristics of Defensive Hostility: Reactivity and Recovery to Active and Passive Stressors.* Published thesis. Blacksburg, Virginia.

Vella, E.J. y Friedman, B.H. (2007). Autonomic characteristics of defensive hostility: Reactivity and recovery to active and passive stressors. *International Journal of Psychophysiology, 66,* 95-101.

Vella, E.J., and Friedman, B.H. (2009). Hostility and anger-in: Cardiovascular reactivity and recovery to mental arithmetic stress. *Int J Psychophysiol,* 72, 253-259.